First Principles of Gastroenterology

THE BASIS OF DISEASE AND AN APPROACH TO MANAGEMENT

THIRD EDITION

First Principles of Gastroenterology

THE BASIS OF DISEASE AND AN APPROACH TO MANAGEMENT

THIRD EDITION

A. B. R. THOMSON
and E. A. SHAFFER, editors

ASSOCIATION
CANADIENNE DE
GASTROENTEROLOGIE

CANADIAN
ASSOCIATION OF
GASTROENTEROLOGY

Sponsored by
the Canadian Association of Gastroenterology
and Astra Pharma Inc.

The publication of this book was sponsored by the Canadian Association of Gastroenterology and supported by an education grant from Astra Pharma Inc.

Publishers:

Canadian Association of Gastroenterology
c/o Dr. A.B.R. Thomson
University of Alberta
519 Newton Research Building
11315-87 Ave.
Edmonton, Alberta T6G 2C2

Astra Pharma Inc.
1004 Middlegate Road
Mississauga, Ontario
L4Y 1M4

Canadian Cataloguing in Publication Data

Main entry under title:

First principles of gastroenterology : the basis of disease and an approach to management
3rd ed.
Co-published by Astra Pharma Inc.
Issued also in French under title: Principes fondamentaux de gastro-entérologie
Includes bibliographical references and index.
ISBN 0-920163-16-5 (bound) ISBN 0-920163-14-9 (pbk.)

1. Gastrointestinal system – Diseases.
2. Gastrointestinal system – Diseases – Treatment.
3. Digestive organs – Diseases. 4. Digestive organs – Diseases – Treatment.
I. Shaffer, E.A. (Eldon A.), 1941– . II. Thomson, A.B.R. (Alan Bryan Robert), 1943– . III. Astra Pharma Inc. IV. Canadian Association of Gastroenterology.

RC801.F57 1997   616.3'3   C97-931220-5

Project Management: MacLean Communications, Milton, Ontario
                        Tel: (905) 878-9752   Fax: (905) 878-1948
Copy Editor: Cy Strom, Toronto, Ontario (416) 214-0183

Printed on recycled paper and bound in Canada.

Dedication

Without the caring support from our families for our academic work, the meaning of our accomplishments would diminish. We acknowledge and express our sincere thanks for the encouragement and loving support of Jeannette, James, Matthew, Jessica and Benjamin Thomson, and of Beryl, Andrea, Emily and Alexandra Shaffer.

This work is also dedicated to Audrey and Bryan Thomson on the occasion of their 78th and 80th birthdays.

We also wish to express our appreciation for the assistance of Ms. Kathy Dixon and Mr. Cy Strom for their production and editing expertise. The comments of Dr. Tom Lay were very helpful and much appreciated.

A.B.R. Thomson
E.A. Shaffer

Preface

Growth in the field of gastroenterology and hepatology is exponential and inexorable. Not only has it provided the scientific basis for how we manage our patients, but it also has brought with it a problem: an ever-expanding wealth of information that needs clarification. There are several important large tomes dedicated to diseases of the gastrointestinal and hepatobiliary system. Information in these is encyclopedic and not readily synthesized into the practice of medicine or as a learning experience for trainees. To answer this need, a multi-authored text, *First Principles of Gastroenterology*, was first brought out five years ago and then revised three years ago. It provided valuable information for students, residents and practicing physicians, be they internists, hepatologists or gastroenterologists. It was also unique, having both English-speaking and French-speaking contributors and being published in both languages. A first!

The text has been an overwhelming success, with extremely positive feedback from physicians and academic centers. Because of this and the opportunity to "do better," a third edition was born. The second edition introduced an important section on pediatric gastroenterology and nutrition, greatly extended topics on HIV disease and inflammatory bowel disease, a multi-authored approach to liver disease and, most important, an update. This third edition has continued the extensive revisions and updates, and includes an important new section on bowel ischemia. Many talented authorities from across Canada have contributed to this edition. New section leaders were used in some sections, and other new authors have been brought in. The learning objectives lists have been further revised and standardized. More figures have been added to illustrate and clarify the text. We have aimed at making this work attractive and worthwhile to a broad spectrum of readers from a variety of disciplines and with different levels of experience.

Work on this text has truly reached from sea to sea, and is both Canadian and *canadien*. Medicine unites and this book is also meant to unite our hearts and minds as we care for the patients to whom many of us dedicate our lives in service.

The editors wish to acknowledge the generous sponsorship by Astra Pharma Inc., particularly Mr. Peter Dixon for his unstinting efforts. We also recognize the valued contributions by graduate medical students, fellows training in gastroenterology and members of the Canadian Association of Gastroenterology.

The renewal process is perpetual. The fourth edition is already in the gestational phase.

A.B.R. Thomson
E.A. Shaffer

First Principles
of Gastroenterology

THE BASIS OF DISEASE AND
AN APPROACH TO MANAGEMENT

THIRD EDITION

1

Common Symptoms and Signs in Gastroenterology

R.R. Gillies, W.G. Thompson, M.C. Champion,
S. Grégoire, S. Meban, D.G. Patel, L.J. Scully,
A.S.C. Sekar, R.F. Bursey, J.M. Fardy and
D.G. MacIntosh

1. INTRODUCTION / W.G. Thompson

The key to accurate diagnosis and effective management of gastrointestinal problems is flawless history-taking. Since up to 50% of gastrointestinal disorders are associated with no anatomical change, no physical findings and no positive test result, diagnosis and therapy must often be based on the medical interview. The gastrointestinal history must include an accurate description of the symptom itself, a past history of gastrointestinal disorders or surgery, a meticulous search for symptoms that might suggest organic disease (such as gastrointestinal hemorrhage, anemia or weight loss) and finally, a careful assessment of the patient's psychosocial state, with particular attention directed toward traumatic events or concerns associated with the onset of the patient's complaints.

The physician should determine the time of onset of the symptom, its occurrence in the past, its periodicity, its location and radiation if appropriate, its aggravating and relieving factors, and its relationship to other symptoms. A review of past history should include not only any previous gastrointestinal surgery or diseases, but also systemic illnesses (such as diabetes or severe cardiovascular disease) that might affect the gut. One should pay particular attention to such symptoms as gastrointestinal hemorrhage, profound weight loss, voluminous diarrhea or episodes of extreme abdominal pain, which might indicate organic disease. Similarly, such phenomena as anemia, fever or incapacity to work may indicate a more serious gastrointestinal disorder demanding treatment and follow-up. A family history of inflammatory bowel disease or bowel cancer may indicate a more careful investigation as well.

When considering a gastrointestinal complaint, the astute physician cannot ignore the patient's psyche. Many studies establish that those who bring gastrointestinal complaints to a physician, even if they are organic in nature, frequently have psychosocial disabilities. Failure to identify and manage the patient's reaction to his or her psychosocial environment (whether it be hostility toward a spouse, an abnormal fear of cancer or a profound loss) may lead to an unsatisfactory therapeutic outcome.

The following is a synopsis of the common gastrointestinal symptoms. These notes include a description of the symptom itself, a word about how the symptom is generated, the important historical features and associated physical findings, and a brief approach to diagnosis and management. These serve as introductory comments; greater detail can be found throughout the text in discussions of specific diseases. The final section of this chapter presents a sequential approach to the examination of the abdomen.

2. GLOBUS / W.G. Thompson

2.1 Synonyms
Globus hystericus; lump in the throat.

2.2 Description
Globus is a lump in the throat or a perceived inability to swallow unassociated with meals. Nearly one out of every two persons experiences this symptom, often at the time of an intense emotional experience.

2.3 Mechanism
Globus is a "functional" disorder since no pathologic or pathophysiologic abnormality has been clearly identified. Many believe that globus is due to a dysmotility of the upper esophageal sphincter.

2.4 Important Historical Features
Generally speaking, patients with globus can swallow meals normally but feel an inability to swallow their saliva between meals. The tendency of globus to occur when the patient is experiencing intense emotion has led in the past to the use of the epithet "globus hystericus." Since one-half of the population experiences this symptom, the term *hystericus* hardly seems justified. Patients may have psychogenic features such as anxiety, but are not overt in displaying other conversion features. There are no physical findings.

2.5 Differential Diagnosis
Globus is easily distinguished from true dysphagia by its occurrence between meals and by the lack of difficulty in swallowing such items as bread and meat. The sensation is continuous.

2.6 Management

There is no treatment beyond reassurance. No diagnostic tests are indicated. Deep-seated emotional features may warrant a psychiatric opinion.

3. HEARTBURN / W.G. Thompson

3.1 Synonyms

Pyrosis.

3.2 Description

Heartburn is a burning sensation experienced behind the sternum. It characteristically occurs or is worsened when the subject is bending over, straining or lying down, especially after a meal. It is aggravated by certain foods (acidic drinks, chocolate, coffee), obesity or anxiety. Unlike angina, it is not usually worsened by exercise or exertion.

3.3 Related Symptoms

Heartburn may be associated with a sensation of reflux into the gullet, or even actual regurgitation into the mouth (with the risk of aspiration). It should be distinguished from *rumination*, in which the subject regurgitates meals routinely and then swallows them again, usually with no consequence beyond disgust in the observer.

3.4 Mechanism

Heartburn is associated with reflux of gastric contents (usually acidic) into the esophagus. The mechanism is complex. Decreased tone or inappropriate relaxation of the lower esophageal sphincter favors reflux. Anatomic disturbances such as obesity or hiatus hernia may also be important. In diseases in which peristalsis of the esophagus is disturbed (e.g., scleroderma) any acid that does reflux into the esophagus will not be adequately cleared.

Contrary to popular opinion, the presence of a hiatus hernia has a minor role in the genesis of heartburn (Figure 1). Both hiatus hernia and heartburn occur in approximately one-third of subjects (not necessarily the same third). Thus, individual cases may have heartburn without hiatus hernia and vice versa.

The mechanism of the pain is obscure. There appear to be no nerve endings for pain in the esophageal mucosa. Severe esophagitis may exist in the absence of heartburn or indeed of any symptoms. Conversely, individuals with heartburn may have an apparently normal esophagus. This gives rise to the suspicion that gastroesophageal reflux may be associated with a disturbance in esophageal motility that is responsible for the sensation of heartburn.

GASTROESOPHAGEAL REFLUX

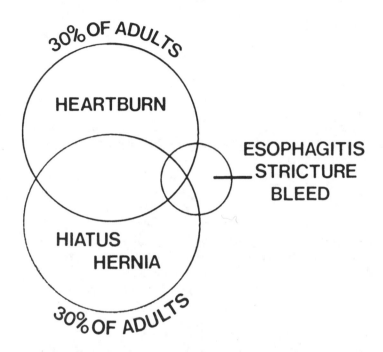

FIGURE 1.   Heartburn and hiatus hernia each occurs in about 30% of adults, so some overlap is inevitable; a causal relationship has not been established. Complicated GERD may occur with heartburn, hiatus hernia, both or neither.

3.5 **History and Physical**
When heartburn is suspected, one should determine the effect of position, food, stress and exercise on the discomfort. The interviewer should carefully exclude such symptoms as dysphagia, odynophagia, weight loss, bleeding and anemia, which indicate complications of reflux or more serious esophageal disease.

There are no physical findings that can be associated with heartburn. The presence of substernal or costochondral tenderness suggests a musculoskeletal origin for the symptom.

3.6 **Differential Diagnosis**
The presence of heartburn implies that the individual has gastroesophageal

reflux disease (GERD). If the burning retrosternal sensation is aggravated by bending and relieved by antacids, then no further investigation is necessary. Some, however, have a retrosternal sensation that cannot be distinguished from that of angina pectoris, particularly if it is in some way related to effort, relieved by nitroglycerin and associated with other features of heart disease. As discussed in the chapter on the esophagus, esophageal spasm may be responsible for chest pain. However, it is often difficult to prove this relationship even with sophisticated motility equipment. Musculoskeletal disturbances such as costochondritis may be responsible for chest pain; they are characterized by local tenderness.

3.7 Approach to Investigation and Management
One-third of adults have experienced heartburn and one in ten suffer heartburn at least once per week. If the heartburn is not incapacitating and is unaccompanied by dysphagia or anemia, then a trial of therapy is a reasonable first approach. Foods that delay gastric emptying (e.g., fat) or that weaken the lower esophageal sphincter (e.g., chocolate, onions) should be avoided. Antacids or alginate compounds such as Gaviscon® are usually successful in relieving the symptoms or even preventing them. Having small meals, fasting before bedtime, elevating the head of the bed and avoiding bending or exertion on a full stomach may be beneficial as well.

In the event that such simple management fails to relieve heartburn, or that dysphagia, anemia or bleeding occurs, then some investigation is necessary. An endoscopy provides the most information, since it allows the degree of inflammation of the esophagus to be assessed. This permits the physician to plan treatment on the basis of its security. Generally speaking, mild esophagitis may be successfully managed with an H_2 blocker, while severe (grade 3 or 4) esophagitis will require a proton-pump inhibitor. In either case, long-term treatment is usually required. If a stricture is present, it should be biopsied. If the stricture proves to be nonmalignant, dilation may be carried out. A more detailed discussion of pharmacologic therapy for gastroesophageal reflux disease is found in Chapter 5, "The Esophagus."

4. WATERBRASH / W.G. Thompson

4.1 Description
Waterbrash is the spontaneous flooding of the mouth with a clear, slightly salty fluid, which may be of sufficient quantity to require expectoration.

4.2 Mechanism
The source of the fluid appears to be the salivary glands. It is believed to result

from a vagal cholinergic reflex, with afferents originating in the upper gastrointestinal tract and efferents destined for the salivary glands.

4.3 Important Historical Points
The fluid, with a neutral or somewhat salty taste, is quite distinct from the acidic or bitter contents that are refluxed from the stomach. The symptom commonly accompanies upper gastrointestinal distress such as heartburn, peptic ulcer disease and even acute gastroenteritis. By itself, it has no pathologic significance.

4.4 Differential Diagnosis
Waterbrash must be distinguished from gastroesophageal reflux disease and rumination. Diagnosis and management depend upon the underlying upper gastrointestinal disorder.

5. DYSPHAGIA / A.S.C. Sekar

5.1 Description
Dysphagia means difficulty in swallowing. Some patients describe food sticking in the throat or retrosternally.

5.2 Important Historical Points and Differential Diagnosis
A careful history is important. Mechanical narrowing is a common cause; an inflammatory stricture must be distinguished from a carcinoma. If the dysphagia is relatively short in duration (e.g., only a few months) and is worsening, this suggests a progressive mechanical narrowing of the lumen such as may occur with an esophageal carcinoma. With benign disease, symptoms are often present for a longer period of time than with carcinoma. A previous history of heartburn or acid regurgitation in a patient with progressive dysphagia might point to an esophageal stricture secondary to gastroesophageal reflux disease. Not all patients with a benign esophageal stricture have a clear history of preceding heartburn or acid regurgitation. This is particularly true in the elderly patient. A history of ingestion of caustic agents such as lye suggests an esophageal stricture secondary to severe chemical esophagitis.

Infections of the esophagus can also cause difficult swallowing. Infections, usually due to Candida albicans or herpes virus, are often accompanied by significant pain on swallowing, termed *odynophagia*. Often the odynophagia is so severe that the patient even has difficulty swallowing his or her saliva. Although herpes esophagitis can occur in relatively healthy patients, Candida esophagitis is associated with diabetes, an underlying malignancy or immunosuppression.

The patient may point to the site of obstruction, but this is not always reliable. A stricture of the lower esophagus may be experienced at the xiphoid area or as high as the throat. Upper esophageal obstruction is experienced high in the throat region, not low in the chest.

Dysphagia can also occur with motor disorders of the esophagus. These conditions include esophageal spasm and achalasia. With motor disorders of the esophagus, the dysphagia may be for both solids and liquids. The dysphagia is intermittent and may have a long history. Sometimes with esophageal spasm the dysphagia may be accompanied by pain (odynophagia), especially with extremely cold or hot liquids. These patients are usually able to wash down impacted particles of food, whereas patients with a mechanical cause (such as a stricture) may need to regurgitate impacted particles of food to obtain relief.

A common cause of intermittent dysphagia is a mucosal ring at the gastroesophageal junction (lower esophageal or Schatzki's ring). On occasion when a relatively large bolus of food is swallowed the ring can cause mechanical obstruction, producing a dramatic onset of acute dysphagia (sometimes associated with pain). Often such patients will have to leave the table and regurgitate. Patients with a Schatzki's ring usually have symptoms for many years before they seek medical attention.

A rare cause of upper esophageal dysphagia is the Paterson-Kelly syndrome or Plummer-Vinson syndrome. Here, a chronic iron deficiency anemia is associated with narrowing of the upper esophagus due to a web.

Cricopharyngeal dysphagia may be due to a cricopharyngeal or Zenker's diverticulum, which develops from an abnormality of the cricopharyngeal sphincter. Patients with a diverticulum often complain of regurgitating food that they swallowed a day or so earlier.

There are non-esophageal causes of dysphagia. Underlying neuromuscular disease may cause cricopharyngeal dysphagia, where patients have difficulty initiating a swallow. A large goiter or mediastinal tumor can cause extrinsic compression of the upper esophagus.

5.3 Approach to Diagnosis and Management

A barium swallow is the most important initial investigation in the diagnosis of dysphagia. It might reveal a Zenker's diverticulum, an esophageal stricture (benign or malignant) or a Schatzki's ring. If inflammation of the esophagus is suspected, endoscopy with biopsies is indicated. If a stricture is identified on a barium swallow, endoscopy with biopsies is necessary to determine whether this stricture is benign or malignant. Also, benign strictures can be dilated following the endoscopic diagnosis. A barium swallow may help diagnose motility disturbances such as esophageal spasm and achalasia.

Esophageal manometry is often required to confirm such motility disturbances.

Once a cause of dysphagia has been established, management will depend on the cause. For example, reflux esophagitis will be managed with the usual antireflux measures, with or without prokinetic drugs such as domperidone, H_2-receptor antagonists such as ranitidine or a proton pump antagonist such as omeprazole. Esophageal strictures can be dilated following endoscopy. Esophageal carcinoma requires either surgery, radiation or palliative insertion of prosthesis. Esophageal motility disturbances can sometimes be managed medically with nitroglycerin or calcium channel blocking agents. Achalasia and esophageal spasm sometimes require surgical myotomy or pneumatic dilation.

6. DYSPEPSIA / W.G. Thompson

6.1 Synonyms
Indigestion.

6.2 Description
Dyspepsia is an imprecise term. It is best described as a chronic (over three months), recurrent, often meal-related epigastric discomfort, pain or fullness. The location of the pain and the relationship to meals resemble the classic description of peptic ulcer disease, so the physician must consider the possibility that a dyspeptic patient has a peptic ulcer. Dyspepsia is usually a daily experience, yet is seldom disabling.

6.3 Mechanism
The mechanism of dyspepsia is uncertain. Even in those dyspeptic patients who have a peptic ulcer, the cause of the pain is uncertain. It is disputed whether the discomfort is related to (1) impaired gastric emptying, (2) a disorder of the basic electrical rhythm of the stomach or (3) pyloroduodenal dysmotility. None are proven.

Although many patients believe that specific foods are responsible for dyspepsia, only fat appears to be a consistent offender. Fat may induce dyspepsia by slowing gastric emptying or by releasing cholecystokinin, which is known to affect the smooth muscle of the upper gastrointestinal tract.

Other upper gastrointestinal symptoms relate to dyspepsia. These include nausea, vomiting (rarely), belching and a feeling of gaseous distention. Terms such as gallbladder dyspepsia, pancreatic dyspepsia, appendiceal dyspepsia and gaseous dyspepsia are misleading and serve no useful purpose. There should be no confusion between the episodic nature and severity of pain due to biliary colic or pancreatic disease and the more predictable and regular occurrence of dyspepsia. Indeed, dyspeptic symptoms are equally common in those who have and in those who do not have gallstones.

It is important as well to distinguish dyspepsia from the recumbency-aggravated retrosternal burning that we call "heartburn." Heartburn results from gastroesophageal reflux and has different diagnostic and therapeutic approaches than dyspepsia.

6.4 Important Historical Points
In an individual case it is almost impossible to distinguish ulcer from non-ulcer dyspepsia. Large studies have shown that, statistically, epigastric pain occurring at night and relieved with antacids is more likely to be associated with peptic ulcer disease. The pain of dyspepsia is not incapacitating. Of course, evidence of complications such as bleeding, weight loss or vomiting would not be expected in nonulcer dyspepsia. The pain or discomfort of the irritable bowel syndrome may occur in the epigastrium. This is generally distinguished from discomfort originating in the upper gastrointestinal tract by its association with defecation and a coexistent alteration in bowel habit.

On physical examination epigastric tenderness will not distinguish between ulcer and nonulcer dyspepsia. In the latter there should be no complications suggestive of peptic ulcer disease, such as peritoneal signs, a succussion splash or the presence of an epigastric mass.

6.5 Approach to Diagnosis and Management
Dyspepsia occurs in about 10% of the population, many of whom do not seek medical help. Of those who do, approximately one-third will not have a peptic ulcer. There is little evidence that those who have nonulcer dyspepsia will eventually develop an ulcer. Yet the symptoms usually persist for long periods in the patient's life.

Thus, investigation and management will depend upon the establishment of a clear diagnosis at the outset, the cost of investigation and the cost of treatment. Since anti-ulcer medication is very effective and seemingly safe, one attitude would be to treat all such individuals without investigation. In the United States, where x-ray and endoscopy are very expensive and the cost must be borne by the individual, indiscriminate therapy has achieved some currency. In such countries as Canada, where drug costs are similar but procedural costs are much less and are not borne by the individual, it seems more efficacious to establish the diagnosis at the outset before committing the patient to drug therapy. Now that we know that most non–NSAID-induced ulcers are due to the presence of Helicobacter pylori and are cured once these gastric bacteria are killed, other approaches are proposed. The current recommendation is that those who have both an ulcer and H. pylori should be given appropriate antibiotics. Those without an ulcer will not benefit from eradication of the organism. New strategies suggest testing dyspeptics for H. pylori and endoscoping only those who test positive. Others would treat indiscriminately. Cost and outcome analysis has not established which is the best approach. More details on this fast-evolving issue are found in Chapter 6, "The Stomach and Duodenum."

Although a carefully conducted upper gastrointestinal series will discover most ulcers, endoscopy is more accurate and will detect mucosal lesions as well. The advantage of early diagnosis is that if no ulcer is found then the futile use of expensive, systemic drugs can be avoided in those with nonulcer dyspepsia. Further, the uncertainty factor in failing to establish a diagnosis compounds inappropriate therapy and aggravates patient unease.

7. NAUSEA AND VOMITING / M.C. Champion

7.1 Synonyms
Barf, upchuck, bring up.

7.2 Description
Nausea is a psychic as well as physical experience and defies precise definition. Vomiting is evacuation of the stomach contents through the mouth. Nausea normally precedes vomiting. There can be associated tachycardia, hypersalivation, waterbrash and excessive perspiration.

7.3 Mechanism (Figure 2)
A variety of stimuli may produce nausea (labyrinthine stimulation, pain, unpleasant memories). The neural pathways mediating nausea are not known, but evidence suggests that they are the same pathways that mediate vomiting. During nausea, gastric tone and peristalsis are reduced. The tone of the duodenum and proximal jejunum tends to be increased, with frequent reflux of duodenal contents into the stomach.

Vomiting occurs as the gastric contents are forcefully brought up to and out of the mouth. This occurs by forceful sustained contraction of the abdominal muscles at a time when the cardia of the stomach is raised and open and the pylorus is contracted. Elevation of the cardia eliminates the intra-abdominal portion of the esophagus and relaxes the lower esophageal sphincter. This allows the stomach contents to enter the esophagus. The act of vomiting is completed with rapid upward displacement of the diaphragm and reversal of thoracic pressure from negative to positive. The glottis closes, the soft palate rises, the mouth opens and the stomach contents are expelled. The control of

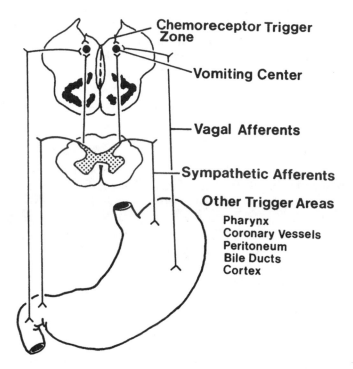

Chemoreceptor Trigger Zone

Vomiting Center

Vagal Afferents

Sympathetic Afferents

Other Trigger Areas
Pharynx
Coronary Vessels
Peritoneum
Bile Ducts
Cortex

FIGURE 2.   The vomiting center and chemoreceptor trigger zone control vomiting. Peripheral trigger areas send visceral afferent impulses, which excite the vomiting center into action.

vomiting consists of two anatomically and functionally separate units, a vomiting center and a chemoreceptor trigger zone. The vomiting center is in the reticular formation of the medulla and is excited directly by visceral afferent impulses (sympathetic and vagal) arising from the gastrointestinal tract and other peripheral trigger areas. These trigger areas are found in the pharynx, cardiac vessels, peritoneum, bile ducts, cortex and stomach. The chemoreceptor trigger zone is on the floor of the fourth ventricle, on the blood side of the blood–brain barrier. The chemoreceptor trigger zone is unable to cause vomiting without an intact vomiting center.

7.4 History and Physical
Patients may complain of nausea and hypersalivation. With gastrointestinal causes of the nausea (and vomiting) there may be associated symptoms of heartburn or epigastric pain. Prior to vomiting, patients may retch (spasmodic, abortive respiratory movements with the glottis closed).

History-taking should probe for precipitating factors, other symptoms that suggest the underlying cause, drug use and dietary habits. The history should also explore psychological trauma or disturbances of body image suggestive of anorexia nervosa.

Physical examination is often normal. An abdominal mass may point to an underlying cause (e.g., gastric carcinoma). Prolonged vomiting may cause dehydration.

7.5 Differential Diagnosis
Prolonged nausea, by itself, rarely has an organic origin. There are many causes of nausea and vomiting, including intracerebral problems (e.g., hydrocephalus, brain tumor), stimulation of the peripheral trigger areas (e.g., severe chest pain, pain from kidney stones), systemic disease (malignancy), medications and pregnancy. Upper gastrointestinal diseases (esophagitis, peptic ulcer disease, gastric carcinoma) are common. Early morning nausea and vomiting suggest pregnancy, gastroesophageal reflux disease, alcohol withdrawal, a metabolic cause (e.g., uremia) or a psychogenic origin.

7.6 Approach to Diagnosis and Management
In approaching a patient with nausea and vomiting, one should look for and correct any underlying causes. Prolonged vomiting may cause dehydration and the patient may need to be rehydrated intravenously. Medications should be discontinued.

There are many drugs that have anti-emetic actions. Antihistamines act on the vestibular apparatus as well as on the chemoreceptor trigger zone. Phenothiazines also exert their action on the chemoreceptor trigger zone. Metoclopramide and domperidone are both anti-emetics and gastric prokinetics (which stimulate the stomach to empty). Domperidone exerts its action on the chemoreceptor trigger zone, whereas metoclopramide also crosses the blood–brain barrier and affects the vomiting center. Cisapride, a newer gastric prokinetic, has no effect on the chemoreceptor trigger zone or vomiting center. Like the other prokinetic agents, it may improve nausea and vomiting if they are due to gastric stasis or gastroparesis.

8. ANOREXIA / M.C. Champion

8.1 Description
Anorexia is the lack (or loss) of appetite. Anorexia is a common and important, but nonspecific, symptom. It can be a presenting feature in patients with organic or psychological disease. Anorexia and weight loss may be the early signs of malignancy.

8.2 Mechanism
The hypothalamus plays a major role in regulating the intake of food. At one time it was generally held that a "satiety center" and a "feeding center" in the hypothalamus exerted the fundamental control over food intake. Stimulation of the satiety center was believed to inhibit the feeding center and gastric hunger contractions. The feeding center was considered to be an integrative station that coordinates complex reflexes associated with food intake. However, it is now believed that control of appetite is best considered as multiple neuropharmacologic interactions in the hypothalamus rather than the effect of a distinct satiety center and feeding center.

8.3 History and Physical
The history should detect other symptoms that may suggest underlying organic or psychological disease. A calorie count is also helpful to assess the actual intake of food. The amount and duration of weight loss should also be documented.

Physical examination may be normal except for evidence of weight loss. It may point to the underlying organic problem, such as cardiac failure or malignancy.

8.4 Differential Diagnosis
Many (and perhaps most) illnesses feature a loss of appetite. These range from gastrointestinal disease to malignancy, chronic renal failure, congestive heart failure and many psychiatric diseases, such as depression and anorexia nervosa.

8.5 Approach to Investigation and Management
Investigation should exclude organic disease. The approach depends upon the patient's symptoms and signs. If no physical ailment is discovered, careful screening may be necessary to exclude psychiatric disease.

9. GAS AND BLOATING / W.G. Thompson

9.1 Synonyms and Related Terms
Burbulence, flatulence, burp, belch, borborygmi, gaseous distention, wind, flatus, fart.

Gas and bloating embrace three unrelated phenomena. *Farting* is a physiologic phenomenon due to the production of gas by colon bacteria. Excessive belching or burping is associated with *aerophagia* (air swallowing). This is also partly physiological, but it may become exaggerated through habit. The mechanism of *bloating* is obscure. These phenomena are unrelated, yet they often occur together.

9.2 Gas, Wind, Flatus

9.2.1 *MECHANISM*

Farting is a physiologic excretory process. Normally, the gut contains 100 to 200 mL of gas. An average person on a normal diet emits about 1 L per day. We pass 50 to 500 mL a mean of 13.6 times per day, although there is great variation from person to person and from time to time. Those prone to produce greater amounts of gas or who are unduly sensitive may suffer socially. Most emitted gas originates in the colon. Some carbohydrates such as cellulose, glycoproteins and other ingested materials, not assimilated in the small intestine, arrive intact in the colon where resident bacteria digest them to produce hydrogen, carbon dioxide, methane and trace gases.

Intestinal floras differ from person to person. Some bacteria produce hydrogen, while others consume it. In one person out of three, an organism called Methanobrevibacter smithii converts hydrogen to methane. The presence of this organism and the methane-producing trait are a result of early environment. Spouses do not share the trait with one another. Another product of fermentation, carbon dioxide, is also released when hydrochloric acid reacts with bicarbonate in the intestines. However, this gas is quickly absorbed. Hydrogen, carbon dioxide, methane and swallowed nitrogen comprise 99% of colon gas. The remaining 1% consists of trace gases that compensate for their small quantities by their strong odors. Smelly gases include hydrogen sulfide ammonia, skatole, indole and volatile fatty acids.

Borborygmi is the name given to the noises generated as air and fluid gurgle through the gut. Farting and borborygmi do not account for bloating.

9.3 Aerophagia

9.3.1 *MECHANISM*

During inspiration, the normally negative intraesophageal pressure draws in ambient air. Forced inspiration against a closed glottis (intentionally closed windpipe) draws in even more air. The air may be forced out again as intraesophageal pressure increases with expiration. Adolescents love to shock their elders with voluntary belching. As a practical application, those who have lost their larynx because of cancer put this learnable skill to use in generating esophageal speech. More commonly, aerophagia is an unwanted habit in those who repeatedly belch in response to other gut symptoms.

Some air is ingested with each swallow, perhaps more with food. Nervous patients undergoing abdominal x-rays accumulate more intestinal gas than those who are relaxed. Other mechanisms of aerophagia include thumb sucking, gum chewing, drinking carbonated drinks, rapid eating and wearing poor dentures. Stomach gas has the same composition as the atmosphere.

In achalasia, where the lower esophageal sphincter cannot relax, the stomach is gasless. In bowel obstruction or a gastrocolic fistula colon gases reach the stomach. Sometimes gastric stasis permits bacteria to grow and produce hydrogen in the stomach. Normally, gastric gas is swallowed air.

9.3.2 CLINICAL MANIFESTATIONS OF AEROPHAGIA

Belching is to bring forth wind noisily from the stomach. The word *burp* means to "cause to belch," as one would burp a baby, but colloquially, the terms are used interchangeably. A belch after a large meal is a physiologic venting of air from the stomach. A meal stretching the muscle of the stomach, which can stretch to accommodate food, causes distress with little increase in intragastric pressure. A satisfying belch eases the discomfort. Some individuals seem unduly sensitive to intragastric pressure. People with gastroenteritis, heartburn or ulcers swallow more frequently. If release of gas transiently relieves the distended feeling, a cycle of air swallowing and belching may be established. The swallow-belch cycle may continue long after the original discomfort is forgotten.

Of course, venting gas is important, as those unable to do so will attest. When the lower esophageal sphincter is reinforced by antireflux surgery, belching may be impossible. Bedridden patients such as those recovering from surgery may trap air in the stomach. In the supine position gastric contents seal the gastroesophageal junction so that air cannot escape until the subject assumes the prone position.

While a patient may insist that his or her stomach is producing prodigious amounts of gas, in reality air is drawn into the esophagus and released. A little may even reach the stomach. Some can belch on command, and the inspiration against a closed glottis is demonstrable. Most sufferers are relieved to have their habit pointed out, but some are incredulous. Quitting the habit is often difficult. Repeated and intractable belching is termed *eructio nervosa*.

9.4 Functional Abdominal Bloating

9.4.1 MECHANISM

Those complaining of bloating and distention are often convinced that it is due to excess intestinal gas. Although the sensation may induce aerophagia, it seldom results from it. Farting may temporarily relieve bloating, but intestinal gas production does not cause it. Research has demonstrated that gas volume in bloaters is not abnormal. Despite visible distention, x-rays and computerized tomography (CT) show no large collections of intestinal gas. The distention disappears with sleep and general anesthesia.

Gut hypersensitivity may explain the sensation of abdominal bloating. The hypersensitive gut feels full at lower than normal filling, and abdominal muscles relax to accommodate the perceived distention. The stomach is and feels distended with normal amounts of air.

Abdominal girth of female irritable bowel syndrome (IBS) patients complaining of distention may increase 3 to 4 cm over an eight-hour day. CT has demonstrated the change in profile despite unchanged gas content or distribution. There were no corresponding changes in control subjects. Lumbar lordosis (arching of the spine) is sometimes increased. When women deliberately protrude their abdomens, the configuration is different from when they are bloated, so a conscious mechanism poorly explains increased abdominal girth. Perhaps abdominal muscles are weakened. The reality of the phenomenon is indisputable; the mechanism remains a mystery.

9.4.2 CLINICAL FEATURES

Bloating occurs in 30% of adults and is frequent in 10%. Amongst those with the irritable bowel syndrome and dyspepsia the figures are much higher. It is often the most troublesome feature of these conditions. Typically, the abdomen is flat upon awakening, but distends progressively during the day, only for the distention to disappear with sleep. Women complain of the need to let out their clothing and sometimes volunteer "It's as if I'm six months pregnant." Many report that bloating occurs quickly, in some cases within a minute. It is often aggravated by eating and relieved by lying down. Menstrual periods and stress affect a few cases. Usually, it is most obvious in the lower abdomen, but many report it near the umbilicus or all over the belly.

9.4.3 DIFFERENTIAL DIAGNOSIS

Observable bloating has been called *hysterical nongaseous bloating*, *pseudotumor* or *pseudocyesis* (false pregnancy). If distention is present at the time of the examination (more likely late in the day), the phenomenon is likely functional. There is no abdominal tympany to suggest gaseous intestines, and sometimes the distended abdomen can be mistaken for ascites or a tumor.

Bloating is often associated with dyspepsia or IBS. On its own, it is not a symptom of organic disease and should prompt no investigation. In intestinal obstruction or postoperative ileus (paralyzed intestines), gas accumulates and distends the gut to cause discomfort and pain. In such a case, there are other symptoms and signs with which to make a diagnosis.

10. CONSTIPATION / W.G. Thompson

10.1 Synonyms
Costiveness, obstipation.

TABLE 1.   Causes of chronic constipation

Functional
Irritable bowel syndrome

Motility disorders of unknown mechanism
Atonic colon
Failure of defecation
   Obstruction by hyperactive anal sphincter
   Impaired rectoanal reflex

Pharmacologic
Opiates, antidepressants, calcium
Laxative abuse

Organic
Hypothyroidism
Depression
Hirschsprung's disease
Pseudo-obstruction
   Hollow viscera myopathy
   Hollow viscera neuropathy
Obstructing lesions (e.g., carcinoma, diverticulitis)

10.2 **Description**
Constipation defies accurate definition. What is "normal" frequency? Ninety-five percent or more of the population have between three movements per day and three movements per week. Some people consider that fewer than three movements a week without discomfort or dissatisfaction is normal. The effort needed to pass the stool and the consistency of the stool are probably of greater importance. Most would agree that hard bowel movements that are difficult to pass constitute constipation even if they occur as often as daily. One definition of constipation is the need to strain at stool on more than 25% of occasions. Thus constipation may be defined as persistent symptoms of difficult, infrequent or seemingly incomplete evacuation.

10.3 **Mechanism**
The causes of constipation are summarized in Table 1; organic causes are discussed elsewhere in this text. The commonest kind of constipation is that associated with the spastic colon type of irritable bowel. In this instance, the stool is hard, difficult to pass, and often scybalous (i.e., like rabbit stools or sheep stools). Frequently, passage of such stools is accompanied by abdominal pain.

Some other functional causes of constipation are difficult to define. In simple atonic constipation, stool in the rectum fails to stimulate the defecation reflex. That is, a full rectum fails to initiate the evacuating response of the internal sphincter. In others, there is no gastrocolonic response to a meal. Still others are part of a generalized motility disorder called chronic idiopathic intestinal pseudo-obstruction. This disorder may be confined to the colon, but often affects other parts of the gastrointestinal tract. In this group must be included problems associated with long-standing use or abuse of laxatives. It is not certain whether the laxative use causes or results from the motility disorder.

10.4 Important Historical Points and Physical Examination Features
The physician's questions should elicit details about the nature of the stool. The presence of hard, pellet-like, difficult-to-pass stools, sometimes with a little bit of blood coating the edge, in an otherwise healthy young person strongly suggests the irritable bowel syndrome. On rectal examination or sigmoidoscopy the rectum is often empty or contains only scybala. This type of constipation is often interspersed with periods of normalcy or diarrhea.

The atonic type of constipation, on the other hand, is associated with a full colon and/or rectum. Often, examination of the abdomen reveals distention, and one may palpate large amounts of stool in the more proximal colon.

Various sensory or anorectal dysfunctions may also cause constipation.

Constipation and blood mixed with the stool raise the possibility of an obstructing lesion, such as a carcinoma. Hirschsprung's disease may present in adults, although usually there is a history of childhood disability. Other possibilities include a spinal lesion, hypothyroidism, hypercalcemia or drug use (e.g., opiates).

10.5 Approach to Diagnosis
Sigmoidoscopic examination using either the rigid or flexible instrument is necessary to rule out local diseases such as fissures, fistulas or distal proctitis. Many cancers are within the range of the sigmoidoscope. One might also detect melanosis coli, a pigment in the rectal mucosa that indicates chronic laxative use.

If the constipated patient is over 40, has blood or pus in the stool, or has had significant weight loss, a barium enema is indicated to rule out polyps, cancer or Crohn's disease of the colon.

A gut transit study may be revealing. Twenty radiopaque markers are ingested and daily plain abdominal x-rays are taken. If 80% of the markers have disappeared in five days, the transit time is said to be normal. In cases of longer transit, the position of the markers may help distinguish colonic inertia from anorectal disorder. More sophisticated studies are then required.

10.6 **Approach to Management**

Obviously, the best management of constipation is to treat any underlying disease. For the spastic type of irritable colon, a good response can be expected if sufficient bulk is added to the diet. It is best to avoid the chronic use of stimulant laxatives because of their potential to damage the myenteric plexus in the colon. If overused, laxatives may cause excessive loss of fluids and electrolytes. Colonic inertia or anorectal dysfunction causing severe constipation or obstipation requires specialist care.

11. **DIARRHEA** / W.G. Thompson

11.1 **Synonyms**

Lax bowels, the flux.

11.2 **Description**

Diarrhea is best described as too frequent passage of too loose (unformed) stools. Diarrhea is frequently accompanied by urgency, and occasionally incontinence. When considering a patient with diarrhea the following must be considered: frequency (>3 movements/day), consistency (loose/watery), urgency, volume (>200 g/day) and whether the condition is continuous. Persistent, frequent, loose, urgent, large-volume stools are most likely to have a pathology. Lesser and intermittent symptoms are more likely to be functional.

11.3 **Mechanism**

Diarrhea is due to one or more of four mechanisms: osmotic attraction of water into the lumen of the gut, secretion of excess fluid into the gut (or decreased absorption), exudation of fluid from the inflamed surface of the gut, and rapid gastrointestinal transit.

Osmotic diarrhea results if the osmotic pressure of intestinal contents is higher than that of the serum. This may result from malabsorption of fat (e.g., in celiac disease) or of lactose (e.g., in intestinal lactase deficiency). Certain laxatives, such as lactulose and magnesium hydroxide, exert their cathartic effect largely through osmosis. Certain artificial sweeteners, such as sorbitol and mannitol, have a similar effect. Characteristically, osmotic diarrhea ceases when the patient fasts.

Secretory diarrhea occurs when there is a net secretion of water into the lumen. This may occur with bacterial toxins, such as those produced by E. coli or Vibrio cholerae, or with hormones, such as vasoactive intestinal polypeptide (VIP), which is produced by rare islet cell tumors (pancreatic cholera). These provoke adenylate cyclase activity in the enterocyte (intestinal epithelial cell), increase cyclic AMP and turn on intestinal secretion. A similar effect may occur as a result of excess bile salts in the colon (choleretic enteropathy) and from the cathartic affect of hydroxylated fatty acids resulting from the bacterial action on malabsorbed fat. Such a diarrhea does not diminish with fasting. Osmotic and secretory diarrhea result from abnormalities in the small intestine such that the flow of water through the ileocecal area overcomes the absorptive capacity of the colon.

Exudative diarrhea results from direct damage to the small or large intestinal mucosa. This interferes with the absorption of sodium salts and water and is complicated by exudation of serum proteins, blood and pus. Infectious or inflammatory disorders of the gut cause this kind of diarrhea.

Acceleration of intestinal transit may result in diarrhea (e.g., as a result of hyperthyroidism). The rapid flow-through impairs the ability of the gut to absorb water, resulting in diarrhea.

In most instances of diarrhea two or more of these four mechanisms are at work, so these pathogenetic concepts are seldom of great help in diagnosis.

11.4 **Important Historical Points and Physical Examination Features**

It is important to establish the frequency of defecation, the duration of the diarrhea, the nature of the stool and its volume. If diarrhea has been present for less than two weeks, it is most likely a result of an infection or toxin. A history of many previous attacks, on the other hand, may indicate a recurrence of inflammatory bowel disease. The frequency of the stool gives some idea of severity; one should establish whether incontinence is also present. To elicit the latter history may require direct or leading questions. Stool from malabsorption is often foul-smelling and contains oil droplets. A history of nutrient deficiency, anemia or weight loss also suggests malabsorption. Watery diarrhea, particularly when large in volume, supports a diagnosis of small bowel disease. However, a large villous adenoma of the distal colon may produce a watery diarrhea. The presence of blood or pus in the stool suggests an exudative diarrhea, a type of diarrhea that is often relatively small in volume and indicative of colitis. Loose bowel movements interspersed with normal or even constipated ones are evidence of the irritable bowel syndrome.

There are many causes of diarrhea, some of which are summarized in Table 2. The presence of profound weight loss and malnutrition in a young person points to a malabsorption syndrome due to small bowel or pancreatic disease or to inflammatory bowel disease. Metabolic conditions such as hyperthyroidism or the overuse of (magnesium-containing) antacids or laxatives might also be responsible for chronic diarrhea.

Travel to tropical countries can be marred by an attack of so-called traveler's diarrhea. The most common cause is toxigenic E. coli (it is known as toxigenic because a toxin is produced). However, a large variety of intestinal

TABLE 2. Anatomic approach to the causes of chronic diarrhea

Gastric
Dumping syndrome

Small intestine
Celiac disease
Lymphoma
Whipple's disease
Parasitic infection (Giardia lamblia)
Abnormal intestinal tract motility with bacterial overgrowth (scleroderma, amyloidosis, diabetes, hyperthyroidism)

Large bowel
Villous adenoma (adenocarcinoma)
Inflammatory bowel disease (ulcerative colitis, Crohn's disease)
Irritable bowel (diarrhea phase)
Functional diarrhea
AIDS-related infections

Pancreatic
Chronic pancreatitis
Islet cell tumors
    Gastrin secretions
    VIP secretions

Drugs
Antacids
Antibiotics
Alcohol
Antimetabolites
Laxatives
Digitalis
Colchicine
Sorbitol, fructose
Many others

Metabolic
Hyperthyroidism
Hypoparathyroidism
Addison's disease
Diabetes
Carcinoid syndrome

infestations can occur with travel. Pseudomembranous colitis may occur with-in weeks of the use of antibiotics. Campylobacter or cryptococcosis may be acquired from pets. Contaminated water may result in giardiasis, amebiasis or cryptococcosis. Chronic use of alcohol may damage the small intestinal mucosa. Diabetics frequently have diarrhea because of autonomic neuropathy, perhaps with bacterial overgrowth.

Finally, it is essential to establish if the patient is homosexual. Almost any of the usual gastrointestinal pathogens can be spread by homosexual activity, including lymphogranuloma venereum and gonococcus. In addition to the "gay bowel syndrome," homosexuals are liable to the gastrointestinal compli-cations of AIDS.

11.5 Differential Diagnosis and Management
The differential diagnosis is very complex. A careful history is often the most important diagnostic tool. Patients examined for the first time deserve at least a sigmoidoscopy to rule out local colon disease. If a small intestinal diarrhea is suspected, a three-day collection of stool to determine daily weight and fat content is necessary. If there is steatorrhea, or if stool weight exceeds 500 g per day, there is likely to be small intestinal or pancreatic disease. Smaller vol-umes, particularly if accompanied by blood, point to inflammation of the colon.

The recent onset of acute diarrhea requires careful examination of the stool for pus cells and culture for bacterial pathogens, or a study for ova and para-sites in the case of suspected protozoa. Viral studies are important in infants, and special studies are required in AIDS.

12. MALNUTRITION / D.G. Patel

12.1 Description
Nutrition may be defined as the process by which an organism utilizes food. This complex process involves ingestion, digestion, absorption, transport, uti-lization and excretion. Any alteration in one or many of these factors can pro-duce malnutrition. Globally, primary malnutrition due to lack of food is the most common cause of malnutrition. Malnutrition in the Western world is mainly due to inadequate intake of nutrients, malabsorption and/or the hyper-catabolism accompanying a critical illness. Protein-energy undernutrition is increasingly recognized in eating disorders such as anorexia nervosa.

12.2 Mechanism
The malnutrition associated with gastrointestinal disorders is usually multifactorial and varies with the nature and activity of the disease.

1. Lack of food intake due to anorexia or food-related symptoms such as dysphagia, pain or vomiting.
2. Maldigestion due to pancreatic disease. Deficiency of bile salts due to cholestatic hepatobiliary disease or to ileal disease leads to maldigestion of triglyceride and lipid-soluble vitamins. Steatorrhea (fat malabsorption) produces negative caloric balance and deficiency of fat-soluble vitamins.
3. Malabsorption due to mucosal disease of the small intestine or loss of surface area due to intestinal bypass, fistula or resection.
4. Excessive loss of nutrients, as in protein-losing enteropathy and loss of zinc in diarrheal illness.
5. Therapeutic agents that may selectively affect nutrient utilization – e.g., cholestyramine use for bile acid–induced diarrhea can worsen steatorrhea.
6. Alcoholism – an extremely common cause of malnutrition in the Western world. Social and economic status, behavior problems, isolation and depression cause reduced intake of nutrients. Alcoholics rarely consume a well-balanced diet and depend very heavily on "empty" calories from alcohol. Protein and vitamin deficiencies, particularly of the B-complex group, are extremely common. Alcohol is a toxic agent that even in the presence of adequate nutritional intake can produce damage to the pancreas, liver and small bowel mucosa, aggravating malnutrition.

12.3 Signs of Malnutrition

1. Weight loss in the absence of edema is a good indicator of energy deficiency.
2. Muscle wasting, particularly in the temporal area and dorsum of the hand between thumb and index finger, suggests protein-calorie deficiency.
3. Dry, scaly skin with pigmentation results from vitamin and trace metal deficiency.
4. Angular mouth fissure (cheilosis) is due to riboflavin deficiency.
5. Glossitis and depapillation of the tongue are due to B_{12}, folate or iron deficiency.
6. Hepatomegaly may be due to fatty liver, a common finding in protein malnutrition or alcoholism.
7. Peripheral neuropathy (decreased position sense), decreased vibration sense or ataxia may result from B_{12} deficiency.
8. Weakness and paresthesia of the legs are signs of nutritional polyneuropathy, especially in alcoholics (due to thiamine or pyridoxine deficiency).
9. Anemia due to iron, folate or B_{12} deficiency or chronic disorders.
10. Peripheral edema.
11. Hypoalbuminemia.

13. **ACUTE ABDOMEN** / S. Meban

13.1 **Description**
The term *acute abdomen* describes an urgent situation in which abdominal symptoms onset suddenly and are sufficiently severe to suggest a potentially lethal condition. Pain is usually the predominant feature. Since many "acute abdomens" require prompt treatment, it is important to make a diagnosis as soon as possible.

13.2 **Mechanism**
Acute abdominal pain may be referred to the abdominal wall from the intra-abdominal organs or may involve direct stimulation of the somatic nerves in the abdominal wall. Less commonly, pain may be referred to the abdomen from extra-abdominal sites. On occasion, acute abdominal pain is a feature of systemic disease.

Visceral pain. This type of pain is carried by the sympathetic autonomic nerves and enters the spinal cord from T6 to L2. The parasympathetic system also carries pain sensation from the pelvic organs via S2, 3 and 4. The nerve supply to viscera arising from the primitive gut is bilateral, and pain is usually experienced in the midline. Foregut pain is epigastric in location. Midgut pain is umbilical, and hindgut pain is felt in the hypogastrium. Organs that are bilateral give rise to pain that is confined to one or the other side of the body.

Somatic pain. Somatic afferents supplying the abdominal wall enter the spinal cord between T5 and L2. Additionally, the undersurface of the diaphragm has innervation from the phrenic nerve (C3, 4 and 5). Thus, irritation of the diaphragm may refer pain to the shoulder.

The stimulus to pain may be chemical irritation from a perforated peptic ulcer or bacterial contamination from perforation of the colon. Other stimuli include ischemia and distention (or stretching) of the gut or parietal peritoneum. Direct pressure on a nerve by a prolapsed intervertebral disc or tumor may result in abdominal pain.

Pain perception may be altered by aberrant function of the pain-conducting pathways. There is also marked variation in the pain "threshold" of individuals.

13.3 **History**
Severe pain of sudden onset suggests a catastrophic event – e.g., perforation of an ulcer, mesenteric embolism or rupture of aortic aneurysm. The level of referral gives a clue to the organ in which the pain originates. Visceral pain is less precise in location than somatic pain.

Steady, severe pain is usually more ominous than colicky pain. Biliary colic is a misnomer, in that the pain is often steady (unlike the true colic of bowel obstruction or a ureteric stone). The latter corresponds to peristaltic waves and eases or disappears between waves.

Radiation patterns are important clues. Irritation of the diaphragm from blood in the peritoneal cavity may cause shoulder tip pain. Biliary pain may radiate to the right scapular region.

13.4 Associated Symptoms

Anorexia, nausea and vomiting are nonspecific but more common in disease of the GI tract. Abdominal distention and change in bowel habit suggest obstruction. Blood in the stool may come from ulceration, tumor or infarction. In women an accurate menstrual history aids the diagnosis of ovarian disease, ectopic pregnancy and pelvic inflammatory disease.

13.5 Physical Examination

Examination is carried out with the patient in the supine position. Preferably, analgesia should be delayed until a diagnosis is made to avoid masking physical signs.

Inspection should note any abdominal distention or local masses. The patient with peritonitis lies immobile, as any movement increases peritoneal irritation. With colic the patient may be restless, seeking a more comfortable position.

Gentle palpation may detect masses. It also detects tenderness and muscle guarding or rigidity, which might suggest peritoneal irritation.

Percussion is useful to assess the nature of abdominal distention or to outline masses. Percussion is also helpful as a "mini rebound" test that more accurately localizes the point of maximum tenderness. It is also much less distressing to the patient with peritonitis.

Auscultation may reveal a range of bowel sounds, from the silent abdomen of peritonitis to the hyperactive sounds of bowel obstruction. Bruits suggest vascular disease, but an epigastric bruit may also be found normally.

Rectal examination should be carried out and recorded by at least one examiner. Tenderness above the peritoneal reflection indicates pelvic peritonitis (e.g., appendicitis or diverticulitis).

Pelvic examination may be necessary to help exclude a gynecological cause of abdominal pain.

13.6 Differential Diagnosis

Apart from abdominal and extra-abdominal causes of abdominal pain, one should also consider nonsurgical causes such as diabetic ketoacidosis.

13.7 **Approach to Diagnosis**

In most cases a good history and a thorough physical examination provide the clinical diagnosis. Complete blood count (CBC) and urinalysis are standard, in addition to serum amylase and electrolytes when indicated. A serum lactate level should be done if bowel ischemia is suspected. Chest x-ray and views of the abdomen help narrow the differential diagnosis.

More sophisticated tests may be necessary. Ultrasound is very useful in the diagnosis of biliary tract disease. Plain films of the abdomen will show large bowel obstruction, but a barium enema may be required to show the level of obstruction and to exclude pseudo-obstruction. Intravenous pyelography can demonstrate kidney nonfunction or hydroureter in suspected renal pain. An opaque calculus may be seen on plain abdominal x-rays. In suspected bowel ischemia, mesenteric angiography is essential. In diverticulitis a Gastrografin® enema can be helpful. Increasingly the abdominal CT scan is being used for diagnosis of the acute abdomen. The most appropriate investigation should be discussed with a radiologist.

13.8 **Approach to Management**

This will depend on diagnosis. In the early stages it may be impossible to distinguish the colic of acute enteritis from appendicitis. Only careful observation and repeated examination allow differentiation. Many abdominal pains settle without a confirmed diagnosis. Occasionally peritonitis requires laparotomy without a clear-cut preoperative diagnosis.

14. **CHRONIC ABDOMEN /** W.G. Thompson

14.1 **Synonyms**

Recurrent abdominal pain; recurrent abdominal pain in children.

14.2 **Description**

Ten percent of children suffer recurrent abdominal pain and approximately 20% of adults have abdominal pain at least six times per year unrelated to menstruation. The pain is chronic when it has been present for six months or more. It may be related to gastrointestinal functions such as eating and defecation. It is often a feature of dyspepsia or the irritable bowel syndrome. Occasionally, the pain has no relationship to bodily functions, and no gastrointestinal, hepatobiliary, genital or renal cause for the pain can be found.

14.3 **Causes and Mechanism**

The mechanisms of abdominal pain are discussed above, in Section 13 ("Acute Abdomen"). Of course, chronic abdominal pain may be caused by many organic diseases. *Peptic ulcer* generally produces pain after meals or on an empty stomach and is relieved by food or antacid. Abdominal pain awakening the patient at night is a particularly discriminating feature.

Biliary colic may be due to cystic or common bile duct obstruction by a stone. Characteristically this pain is significant enough to awaken the patient at night or require a visit to the emergency room for analgesia. It lasts from 1 hour to 12 hours; beyond that time consider acute cholecystitis or pancreatitis. Attacks are sporadic and at intervals, not continuous. Biliary pain is located in the epigastrium, the right upper quadrant and/or the right scapula. It leaves the patient shaken but well. Should the gallbladder become inflamed, cholecystitis results. Obstruction of the common bile duct with a stone results in pain, jaundice and sometimes fever (cholangitis).

Pancreatitis is a devastating illness, with steady epigastric pain radiating to the back and sometimes accompanied by shock. It almost always requires admission to hospital.

Ischemic bowel disease, subacute bowel obstruction caused by Crohn's disease, *neoplasm* or *volvulus* may present with recurrent bouts of abdominal pain, often related to eating. These conditions are usually progressive and accompanied by physical signs.

In a patient with *diverticular disease*, a peridiverticular abscess may develop, causing recurrent bouts of severe left lower quadrant abdominal pain and fever. Usually, diverticula are asymptomatic and symptoms that do occur are those of coincident irritable bowel syndrome.

Renal colic due to a stone in the ureter is rarely chronic but may be recurrent. It consists of severe flank pain radiating to the groin and testicle, and may be accompanied by hematuria. Typically, a patient smitten with renal colic is unable to lie still.

Gynecologic conditions ranging from mittelschmerz (ruptured ovarian cyst) to pelvic inflammatory disease may account for recurrent abdominal pain. Menstruation-related pain in a young woman suggests endometriosis. Chronic pelvic pain often relates to the irritable bowel syndrome.

Chronic appendicitis probably does not exist.

The chronic abdomen is seldom explained by the above mechanisms. *Functional abdominal pain* may originate in any part of the gastrointestinal tract or biliary tree. It is unrelated to bodily function and may be continuous. It is uncertain whether the pain is due to a normal perception of abnormal gut motility or an abnormal perception of normal motility, or indeed if it is due to the gut at all; there are frequently accompanying psychosocial difficulties.

14.4 Important Historical Points and Physical Examination Features
Pain, when related to a bodily function – defecation, eating, micturition or

menstruation – focuses the investigation upon the involved system. Certain physical findings (such as an abdominal mass, or blood or mass upon rectal examination) point to specific organic diseases. Fever, weight loss, rectal bleeding and/or anemia indicate further tests. These features are absent in chronic functional abdominal pain.

14.5 Differential Diagnosis, Diagnosis and Management

Management of the organic causes of the chronic abdomen can be directed at the underlying disease process. In many instances, however, there is no organic basis. Here, the physician's responsibility is to reassure the patient that no serious disease exists, and help the patient coexist with the symptoms in the light of the patient's social background. One might improve digestion through regular and better eating habits, and treat bowel dysfunction, particularly constipation, with increased dietary bulk.

14.6 Pain and Emotion

There are patients who have severe recurrent abdominal pain unrelated to bodily function or organic disease. Such patients see many doctors without satisfaction; the genesis of the symptom is thought to be psychogenic. This pain is often given such descriptors as "illness behavior" and "pain proneness." Some have hypochondriasis and do not improve when organic disease has been disproved. An extreme example is the Münchausen syndrome, where the patient deliberately relates a tall tale of medical duress in order to precipitate treatment, perhaps even surgery.

Functional pain is frequent in those who have recent conflicts, have experienced a death in the family, or have become overly concerned with fatal illness. Depression and anxiety are frequent. Here, it is important not to carry out extensive investigation in a fruitless search for an elusive cause. This only reinforces the patient's belief that something is wrong and undermines the patient's confidence in the benign diagnosis.

Such pain may be an emotional expression, in which case regular visits are necessary to allow the patient to vent his or her problems. Drugs, especially narcotics, should be used with restraint, and the physician should strive to develop a strong doctor–patient relationship while dealing with the patient's depression, anxiety, frustration and often hostility. These patients test our skill in the art rather than the science of medicine.

15. JAUNDICE / L.J. Scully

15.1 Definition

A state characterized by increased serum bilirubin levels and a yellow appearance due to deposition of bile pigment in the skin and mucus membranes.

15.2 Mechanism

Bilirubin is a waste product of hemoglobin metabolism. Interruption of the breakdown pathway at any of a number of steps, or a marked increase in load due to red cell destruction, results in an increase in serum bilirubin and (if high enough) clinical jaundice.

Under normal circumstances senescent red blood cells are taken up and destroyed in the reticuloendothelial system. Through a number of steps the heme molecule of hemoglobin is converted to bilirubin and, tightly bound to albumin, is transported in the plasma to the liver cells. Hepatocytes take up bilirubin, conjugate it to glucuronide and excrete the bilirubin diglucuronide in bile into the duodenum. In the bowel, bacteria break down bilirubin to urobilinogen, 80% of which is excreted in the feces, contributing to the normal stool color. The remaining 20% is reabsorbed and excreted in bile and urine (enterohepatic circulation of urobilinogen).

Functional or anatomic obstruction at almost any level in this pathway (from hemoglobin breakdown to uptake by the hepatocellular membrane to excretion into the biliary system) will result in jaundice, with an increase in serum bilirubin. A large increase in the breakdown products of hemoglobin alone (e.g., hemolytic anemia) will cause an increase in serum unconjugated bilirubin. If the problem lies after the uptake and conjugation step, the increase is in serum conjugated bilirubin. Causes of jaundice are usually classified as (1) hemolysis, (2) genetic defects in bilirubin handling, (3) hepatocellular disease and (4) obstruction.

15.3 Clinical Presentation

Clinical jaundice is detected when the serum bilirubin level reaches 2–4 mg/dL (40–80 µmol/L). It is usually preceded by a few days of pale stools (as excretion of bilirubin into the intestine is decreased) and dark urine (due to increased glomerular filtration of conjugated bilirubin). Jaundice is usually first detected in the sclera, although the bilirubin is actually deposited in the overlying conjunctival membranes. Yellow skin without scleral icterus should suggest carotenemia or the ingestion of such drugs as quinacrine.

Most patients with jaundice, excluding those in whom it is secondary to hemolysis, have nausea, anorexia and discomfort over the liver. There may be hepatomegaly, masses in the epigastrium or pancreas or a dilated gallbladder. Signs of chronic liver disease such as spider nevi or palmar erythema are important. Pruritus may result, presumably from the deposition of bile salts (or a retained pruritogen normally excreted in bile) in the skin.

FIGURE 3.   Causes of hyperbilirubinemia.

Several genetic defects in the conjugation or excretion of bilirubin may cause long-standing unconjugated or conjugated hyperbilirubinemia.

15.4 Approach to Diagnosis

Initially the most important information is whether the jaundice is due to conjugated or unconjugated hyperbilirubinemia (Figure 3). Serum bilirubin can be fractionated from "total" into conjugated and unconjugated, but the presence of bile in the urine determined by a test strip at the bedside confirms that the bilirubin rise is predominantly in the conjugated form. If the bilirubin is unconjugated, hemolysis or genetic defects are implicated. If the bilirubin is conjugated, "liver biochemical tests" (AST, ALT, GGT and alkaline phosphatase) will help determine if the jaundice is primarily due to obstruction/ cholestasis (high GGT and alkaline phosphatase) or hepatocellular damage (high AST and ALT). Cholestatic jaundice requires ultrasound as the best, first test to detect biliary tract disease. If the jaundice is cholestatic, then an ultrasound of the abdomen is required to determine if there is obstruction of the ducts or intrahepatic bile duct dilatation.

15.5 Management

The management of obstructive jaundice is directed toward the cause where possible (e.g., removal of obstructing gallstone). Jaundice secondary to hepatocellular disease, such as viral hepatitis, does not require any specific treatment. Jaundice due to alcohol, toxin or drug requires withdrawal of the offending agent.

16. ASCITES IN CHRONIC LIVER DISEASE / L.J. Scully

16.1 Definition
Ascites is the accumulation of nonsanguinous fluid in the peritoneal cavity.

16.2 Mechanisms
With significant liver disease, albumin synthesis is reduced. Low serum albumin results in a decrease in intravascular osmotic pressure. This causes renal blood flow changes, resulting in sodium and water retention. Increased aldosterone levels, possibly due to decreased catabolism of this hormone by the liver, also contribute. There is a generalized salt and water retention, but the fluid accumulation may be confined to the peritoneal cavity or may be associated with peripheral edema. Ascites develops because of increased portal pressure and the transudation of fluid from the capillaries in the portal system to the peritoneal cavity. Hepatic lymph production also increases and extravasates directly into the peritoneal cavity.

16.3 Signs and Symptoms
Ascites most commonly presents with increasing abdominal girth, often associated with an uncomfortable feeling of distention, and sometimes nausea and anorexia. Shortness of breath may develop, resulting from either elevation of the diaphragm or pleural effusion. Ankle edema may accompany ascites.

Clinical examination reveals flank fullness on inspection. "Shifting dullness" or a "fluid thrill" may be elicited. Smaller amounts of fluid may be detected on ultrasound when clinical signs are absent. One should look for other signs of portal hypertension, such as dilated abdominal wall veins or an enlarged spleen.

16.4 Differential Diagnosis
Newly developed ascites must have a diagnostic aspiration to determine the albumin level, cell count and cytology. The fluid should be clear and straw-colored. Occasionally, lymph can accumulate in the peritoneal cavity, causing "chylous ascites," which requires different management. Ascitic fluid may become infected, in which case the white blood cell count will be elevated in the fluid. If the fluid is sanguinous, other causes – such as infection or malignancy – must be sought. The serum ascites albumin gradient is the best way of confirming if the ascitic fluid is secondary to portal hypertension. In this situation the gradient is high – i.e., >11 g/L – whereas it is low if the ascites is due to peritoneal carcinomatosis. This is far more accurate than our previous assessment of transudative versus exudative ascites.

TABLE 3.   The important causes of upper GI bleeding

Duodenal ulcer
Gastric ulcer
Gastric erosions
Ulcerative esophagitis
Esophagogastric varices
Mallory-Weiss tear
Carcinoma, lymphoma
Angiodysplasia

16.5 Approach to Management

Management initially includes bed rest and salt restriction. Most cases also require adding a diuretic such as spironolactone. Careful aspiration of large quantities (up to 8 L) of ascitic fluid may be necessary in some resistant cases; this can be safely performed, and if the serum albumin level is very low an intravenous infusion of albumin is given before the paracentesis.

17. GASTROINTESTINAL BLEEDING / R.R. Gillies

17.1 Description

Blood issuing from the GI tract is a cause for alarm, and justifiably so! The visible evidence is described as hematemesis, hematochezia and/or melena.

Hematemesis – vomited blood, either red (fresh) or dark brown (altered by reaction with HCl) – comes from a source proximal to the duodenojejunal junction.

Hematochezia – blood in the stool – comes from the left colon, or even above if the volume of blood is large and the transit rapid.

Melena – black, tarry, smelly stool, looser and larger with larger hemorrhages – comes from the upper GI tract, in which case bacterial action has longer to break down the blood. It may even come from the lower tract when transit is delayed. The important causes of upper gastrointestinal bleeding are shown in Table 3, and of lower gastrointestinal bleeding in Table 4.

17.2 Important Historical Points and Physical Examination Features

Vomiting blood usually signifies a major hemorrhage. In a briskly bleeding duodenal ulcer, rapid transit may result in passage of red blood and clots per rectum without vomiting. Even before being passed per rectum, a large hemorrhage into the upper tract will announce itself by hyperactive bowel sounds. It is obvious that such a large-volume blood loss will have major cardiovas-

TABLE 4.   The important causes of lower GI bleeding

Hemorrhoids, anal fissure
Carcinoma, adenomatous polyps
Angiodysplasia
Ulcerative colitis
Crohn's disease
Diverticular disease
Ischemic colitis
Certain bacterial infections
Amebic colitis
Meckel's diverticulum

---

cular effects compared to a rectal lesion causing passage of red blood and clots.

The symptoms associated with blood loss may occur before any blood appears externally (e.g., the features of an acute anemia – weakness, faintness, sweating, pallor, thirst and collapse). While the first clues as to the site of bleeding are gathered, we need to know more about how the patient is tolerating the blood loss. A rapid, thready pulse; hypotension; cold, sweaty skin; and pallor tell us that emergency restoration of blood volume is needed to keep the patient alive. Vital signs may be normal while the patient is recumbent, but a blood pressure fall of 15 mm Hg when the patient sits up indicates a significant blood loss. Cardiovascular compensation may be perfect – for the moment! A large-diameter IV line (at least 18 gauge) must be inserted. The patient should be given first saline or plasma and then, as soon as it is available, blood as indicated by any features of hypovolemia.

Once resuscitation is under way, one can assess the site and etiology of the bleeding. First, take a detailed history, particularly noting upper and lower GI symptoms, previous episodes of bleeding, previous GI surgery, ASA or NSAID intake, ethanol abuse, and diseases or treatments that could cause clotting defects. Ulcer pain often stops as bleeding starts; ulcer pain does not precede ulcer bleeding in 20–25% of cases.

Next, do a thorough physical examination, with attention to vascular lesions of the skin and mucosa, ecchymoses, the liver, peripheral signs of cirrhosis, splenomegaly and prominent superficial abdominal veins. Inspection of the nares and oropharynx avoids the embarrassment of missing epistaxis as a source of swallowed blood. Rectal examination allows stool examination.

17.3 **Approach to Diagnosis** (Figure 4)
When the passage of blood from either end of the GI tract has been reported

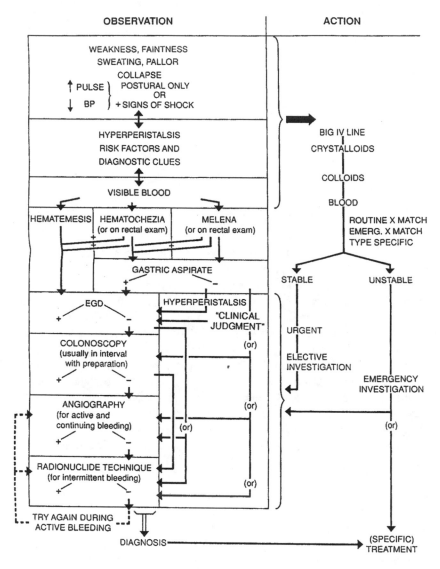

FIGURE 4.   GI bleeding decision tree.

but not observed, or when hematochezia or melena without hematemesis has been observed, the passage of a nasogastric tube for a single aspiration will help determine if bleeding is proximal or distal to the pylorus. Providing the patient's response to IV volume replacement is satisfactory, one can make a decision as to the timing and type of investigation needed to identify the cause of bleeding. Upper GI endoscopy is the most reliable technique to detect lesions proximal to the duodenojejunal junction. Sometimes perendoscopic injection, heater probe application or snare-cautery polypectomy may be employed to stop bleeding from identified lesions. Whether endoscopy is emergent, urgent or elective depends on the status of the patient. Remember that the status may rapidly deteriorate. One must be prepared to change the plan just as rapidly.

Bleeding lower GI tract lesions may be identified and treated endoscopically. Usually this is feasible only later, after proper bowel preparation removes the accumulated blood. When active bleeding continues from the small or large bowel, mesenteric angiography is the best choice to discover the bleeding site. If the bleeding is less brisk and is intermittent, radionuclide imaging may point to the site. Bleeding must occur during either test to make it useful.

When all else fails, total enteroscopy – endoscopy of the entire small bowel – should be done. Usually this is more efficient at laparotomy where the surgeon can assist by manipulating the loops of bowel over the advancing scope.

17.4 Approach to Management
Remember that the objective is a live patient. Continued, careful assessment of the patient's cardiovascular response to blood loss and replacement will guide interventions, including surgical. Specific treatment depends upon the underlying disease and will be dealt with in subsequent sections.

18. ABDOMINAL MASS / S. Grégoire

18.1 Description
When an abdominal mass is discovered on physical examination, one must define its nature. Using a systematic approach often permits the identification of the mass before the use of sophisticated tests.

18.2 Important Points in History and Physical Examination
Important clues in the history and general physical examination may help to identify the enlarged viscus. For example, in a young patient presenting with diarrhea, weight loss and abdominal pain, finding a right lower quadrant mass would suggest inflammatory bowel disease. However, an abdominal mass may be discovered during physical examination of an asymptomatic individual. Certain observations made during the abdominal examination may be helpful. (See also Section 20.)

18.2.1 *INSPECTION*

Where is the mass located? A practical approach is to divide the abdomen into four quadrants (see Section 20.1). Starting from the principle that an abdominal mass originates from an organ, surface anatomy may suggest which one is enlarged. A mass seen in the left lower quadrant, for example, could be of colonic or ovarian origin but, unless there is situs inversus, one would not consider an appendiceal abscess!

Does the mass move with respiration? In the upper abdomen a mobile intra-abdominal mass will move downward with inspiration, while a more fixed organ (e.g., aorta, pancreas) or an abdominal wall mass (e.g., hematoma of rectus muscle) will not.

Is there visible peristalsis?

18.2.2 *AUSCULTATION*

Careful auscultation for bowel sounds, bruit or rub over an abdominal mass is part of the systematic approach.

18.2.3 *DEFINING THE CONTOUR AND SURFACE OF THE MASS*

This is achieved by inspection, percussion and palpation. Is the organ air-filled (e.g., stomach) or fluid-filled? Is it a well-defined mass (e.g., liver, spleen) or are its borders difficult to define (matted loops of small bowel)? Is the surface regular? An enlarged liver due to fatty infiltration may have a smooth surface, while a cirrhotic organ is usually irregular and nodular. What is the consistency of the mass? Firm? Hard or soft? Is it pulsatile? In the absence of ascites, ballottement of an organ situated in either upper quadrant more likely identifies an enlarged kidney (more posterior structure) than hepatomegaly or splenomegaly.

18.3 **Differential Diagnosis**

The following suggests an approach to the differential diagnosis of an abdominal mass located in each quadrant:

18.3.1 *RIGHT UPPER QUADRANT*

This location suggests liver, right kidney, gallbladder and, less commonly, a colon or gastroduodenal mass. A pancreatic mass is rarely palpable.

18.3.1.1 *Liver*

As a subdiaphragmatic organ, the liver moves downward with inspiration. This anterior organ has an easily palpable lower border, which permits assessment of its consistency. A bruit or venous hum can be heard in certain conditions. An enlarged left lobe can usually be felt in the epigastric area.

18.3.1.2 *Right kidney*
The kidney may protrude anteriorly when enlarged and be difficult to differentiate from a Riedel's lobe of the liver. It may be balloted.

18.3.1.3 *Gallbladder*
This oval-shaped organ moves downward with inspiration and is usually smooth and regular.

18.3.1.4 *Colon*
Colon masses are deep and ill-defined, and do not move with respiration. High-pitched bowel sounds suggest obstruction.

18.3.2 *LEFT UPPER QUADRANT*
Location in the left upper quadrant suggests spleen or left kidney. Less commonly, a colonic (splenic flexure) or gastric mass can be felt. A pancreatic mass is rarely palpable.

18.3.2.1 *Spleen*
This anterior organ moves downward with inspiration. Since it has an oblique longitudinal axis, it extends toward the right lower quadrant when enlarged. It has a medial notch and the edge is sharp.

18.3.2.2 *Left kidney*
Its more posterior position and the presence of ballottement helps distinguish the left kidney from the spleen.

18.3.2.3 *Colon, pancreas, stomach*
It is practically impossible to differentiate masses in these by physical examination. The history helps but often one must resort to radiology or endoscopy.

18.3.3 *RIGHT LOWER QUADRANT*
A mass in this area has its origin either in the lower GI tract (colon, distal small bowel, appendix) or in a pelvic structure (ovary, uterus, fallopian tube).

18.3.3.1 *Lower GI tract*
These deeper organs are usually ill-defined. Clinical context is important. Inflammatory bowel disease usually would be associated with pain on palpation but carcinoma of the cecum would be painless.

18.3.3.2 *Pelvic organs*
Bimanual palpation is the preferred method.

18.3.4 *LEFT LOWER QUADRANT*
As with a right lower quadrant mass, the differential diagnosis here is between lower GI (in this quadrant the sigmoid colon) and pelvic origin. The shape of the organ and pelvic examination should help differentiate the two.

18.4 Approach to Diagnosis
To complete the assessment of an abdominal mass, one may choose among several different investigational tools. The use of specific tests depends on availability and on the organ studied.

Generally, ultrasound is useful. This noninvasive, safe, cheap and widely available method identifies the mass and provides information on its origin and nature. Ultrasound may also be used to direct a biopsy. Other noninvasive modalities are nuclear imaging and CT scan. Hollow organs may be demonstrated radiographically through the use of contrast media (e.g., barium enema, GI series, ultrasound, intravenous pyelogram, endoscopic retrograde cholangiopancreatography, etc.). Sometimes, laparotomy or laparoscopy will be necessary to make the diagnosis.

19. PROCTALGIA FUGAX / W.G. Thompson

19.1 Description
Proctalgia fugax is a sudden severe pain in the anus lasting several seconds or minutes and then disappearing completely.

19.2 Mechanism
The pathophysiology of proctalgia fugax is uncertain. Although some observations (under obviously fortuitous circumstances) suggest a rectal motility disorder, the symptom appears more likely to result from spasm of the skeletal muscle of the pelvic floor (specifically, the puborectalis).

19.3 History and Physical Examination
Proctalgia fugax occurs in about 14% of adults and is somewhat more common in females than males. The pain may be excruciating, but since it is so short-lived patients seldom report it to their physician. In 90% of instances it lasts less than five minutes and in many cases less than a minute. About one-third of patients suffer attacks following defecation. A small minority report attacks following sexual activity. There are no physical signs.

19.4 Differential Diagnosis
Perianal disease may cause pain but it usually accompanies, rather than follows, defecation. One should be particularly careful to exclude the presence

of an anal fissure, which may be difficult to see on anal inspection. Pain originating from the coccyx may be accompanied by coccygeal tenderness both externally and from within the rectum. An acute attack of anal pain lasting several hours may indicate a thrombosed hemorrhoid. However, constant pain for many months or years is unlikely to have an organic explanation.

19.5 Management
Beyond reassurance there is no treatment.

20. EXAMINATION OF THE ABDOMEN / R.F. Bursey, J.M. Fardy and D.G. MacIntosh

Examination of the abdomen is an important component of the clinical assessment of anyone presenting with suspected disease of the gastrointestinal tract. As in all other parts of the examination, care must be taken to show respect and concern for the patient while ensuring an appropriate and thorough examination.

While performing the examination it is useful to keep in mind the concepts of sensitivity and specificity. How confident can we be that a suspected physical finding is in fact present and has clinical significance? For example, how sensitive and specific is our bedside examination for hepatomegaly? What is the clinical significance of an epigastric bruit heard in a thin 20-year-old female versus a 55-year-old hypertensive, obese male?

In the following sections we will describe an appropriate sequential examination of the abdomen and highlight some of the potential pitfalls of this process.

20.1 Inspection
Ensure that the abdomen is exposed from the costal margin to symphysis pubis. When describing the location of an abnormality it is useful to divide the abdomen into four quadrants with a perpendicular line through the umbilicus from the xiphoid process to the symphysis pubis. A horizontal line through the umbilicus then allows the abdomen to be divided into 4 areas: the left upper, right upper, left lower and right lower quadrants (Figure 5). On occasion it may be helpful to divide the abdomen into 9 regions with the spaces marked by vertical lines through the left and right mid-clavicular lines and horizontal lines passing through the subcostal margins and anterior iliac crests (Figure 6).

The overall appearance such as scaphoid, protruberant, or obese should be described, and the location of any surgical scars noted. One should look for any abnormal surface markings, including cutaneous lesions as well as vascular markings. A comment should also be made about the apparent ease of

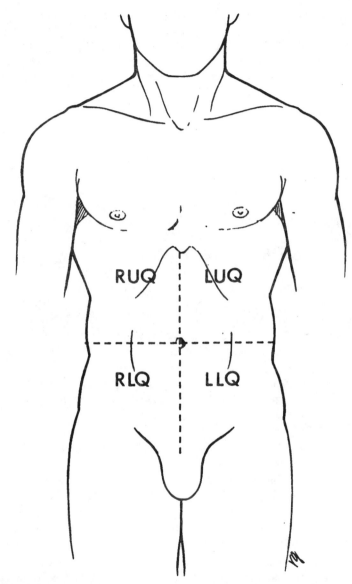

FIGURE 5. Division of the abdomen into four quadrants: the left upper quadrant, right upper quadrant, left lower quadrant and right lower quadrant.

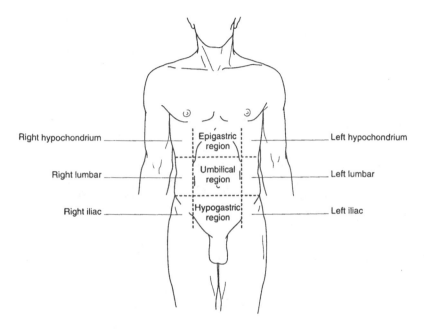

Right hypochondrium — Epigastric region — Left hypochondrium

Right lumbar — Umbilical region — Left lumbar

Right iliac — Hypogastric region — Left iliac

FIGURE 6.   Division of the abdomen into nine regions.

movement of the abdominal wall with respiration and change in body position. Occasionally organomegaly or a mass will be visible. It is helpful to look at the abdomen from the foot of the bed as well.

20.2 Auscultation

It is useful to auscultate the abdomen prior to palpation or percussion, as bowel sounds induced by further examination may mask vascular bruits or pleural rubs. When listening for vascular bruits it is useful to keep in mind the surface markings. The aorta enters the abdomen at or just to the left of the xiphoid process and bifurcates to the left and right common iliac arteries at the level of the umbilicus. The renal arteries are found approximately one-half the distance between the xiphoid process and the umbilicus, and auscultation is best performed within 2 cm of the midline. Bruits are often best heard at the bifurcation of major vessels; therefore it is also appropriate to listen at the bifurcation of the common iliacs into the internal and external iliacs, approximately halfway between the umbilicus and the inguinal ligament. One should listen over the inguinal ligament for femoral bruits as well.

A venous hum is best heard overlying the portal vein, which is found in an area approximated by an elliptical shape between the umbilicus and the mid-clavicular line where it crosses the right subcostal margin. Arterial bruits are usually heard only during systole and best heard with the diaphragm of the stethoscope, as they are high pitched. A venous hum is more likely to be continuous and best heard with the bell of the stethoscope, as this is a low-pitched sound. There are, however, no studies to suggest these findings are helpful or reliable in routine examination. Venous hum can occur in portal venous hypertension of any cause. Undifferentiated liver patients in one study had a prevalence of bruits reported as less than 3%. The ability of clinicians to distinguish hepatic arterial bruits from other arterial bruits such as a renal artery bruit has not been studied.

Friction rubs may occur overlying the liver or spleen and are always abnormal, though rare. Even with careful auscultation of patients with known liver tumors, fewer than 10% are found to have a rub.

20.2.1 BOWEL SOUNDS
Auscultation for bowel sounds is a rather controversial subject. Bowel sounds should be listened for prior to palpation or percussion, but the yield of this examination is low. The diaphragm of the stethoscope should be placed on the abdomen, as least initially in the right lower quadrant near the ileocecal valve. The particular characteristics of the bowel sounds or even absence of them is not diagnostic of a particular condition, perhaps except for the very high pitched noises of acute small bowel obstruction. In fact, it is probably more helpful in this regard to observe how the bowel sounds change over a period of several hours.

20.3 Palpation
Palpation of the abdomen should be done in an orderly sequence with the patient in the supine position. Light palpation should be done first in all four quadrants assessing for areas of potential tenderness. Light palpation is a one-handed technique. If no areas of obvious tenderness are elicited, then deep palpation is performed, again in all four quadrants using a two-handed technique. Pressure is applied with one hand over the other hand, which is placed on the abdominal wall, as it is thought that deep palpation with one hand may lead to the inadvertent nonrecognition of suble fullness or mass if the hand applying deep pressure is also responsible for detecting the abnormality. The accuracy of this is untested. It is stated that if a patient has difficulty relaxing the abdominal wall musculature, then placing the soles of the patient's feet on the bed with hips and knees flexed will aid relaxation; in all likelihood, however, a calm, organized approach with verbal reassurance by the examiner will be just as effective.

The techniques of palpation of liver and spleen are discussed in Sections 20.5 and 20.6.

20.4 Percussion

Percussion of the abdomen will detect the presence of bowel gas. The technique as it relates to defining organomegaly and the presence of fluid is discussed in later sections.

20.5 Examination of the Liver

Examination of the liver consists mainly of palpation for the lower edge of the liver and percussion to determine the span. This examination is performed after inspection for right upper quadrant swelling and extrahepatic signs of liver disease. To palpate the lower edge of the liver the examiner starts with gentle pressure in the right lower quadrant of the abdomen. The patient is asked to breathe gently and slowly, in order to bring the liver edge down to the examining fingertips of the right hand. The examiner moves the right hand in a cephalad direction about 2 cm with each breath. If the edge is not felt, no further examination is required. If liver disease is suspected the lower liver edge can be located by percussion.

If the edge is located, mark the lower border in the mid-clavicular line. Percuss for the upper border starting in the third intercostal space with a finger that is held flat and lies within the space. Move down one interspace at a time until the percussion note changes from resonant to dull. To confirm the change of percussion note strike the third and fourth fingers laid in adjacent interspaces. The note on the top finger should be resonant and on the lower dull. Measure the distance between the upper and lower percussion edges in the mid-clavicular line. Determination of the liver span can be done with firm or gentle percussion to locate the lower border. Gentle percussion is the recommended technique, as this method appears to better estimate liver span as judged by ultrasound. Remember that the upper edge of the liver is dome shaped and not straight across.

The scratch test has been used to find the lower liver margin. The diaphragm of the stethoscope is placed at the right costal margin in the mid-clavicular line. A finger moves up the abdomen in the mid-clavicular line, scratching gently and with consistent pressure. When the liver edge is reached, there is a sudden increase in the scratching sound heard through the stethoscope. In one comparative study the scratch test was not felt to offer any advantage over the techniques of palpation and percussion.

When the liver edge is palpable, trace the edge working laterally to medially. Try to determine the characteristics of its surface – for example, soft, firm or nodular. These characteristics may help in the assessment of patients with liver disease; however, agreement about the characteristics is poor, even among experts. Auscultation is rarely helpful. An attempt should be made to assess the left lobe in the epigastrium using these techniques.

What is the significance of a palpable liver edge? A recent review suggested that a palpable liver is not necessarily enlarged or diseased. When clinical examination is compared to nuclear medicine scanning, about one-half of palpable livers are not enlarged. The inability to feel a liver edge does not rule out hepatomegaly, but does reduce its likelihood.

What is the normal percussion span? Only one study has been done to establish the normal span. Castell examined 116 healthy subjects using firm percussion. The mean span in the mid-clavicular line was 7 cm in women and 10.5 cm in men. The following nomograms were developed to predict estimated liver dullness in a normal population using firm percussion technique: Male liver dullness equals (0.032 × weight in pounds) + (0.183 × height in inches) − 7.86. The female liver dullness equals (0.027 × weight in pounds) + (0.22 × height in inches) − 10.75. The 95% confidence intervals were ±2.64 cm. Therefore a 5 ft. 10 inch, 175 lb. male would have an estimated liver span of 10.2 cm (range 7.6–12.8) and a 5 ft. 5 inch, 130 lb. female would have an estimated liver span of 7.1 cm (4.5–9.7 cm) by this formula.

20.6 Examination of the Spleen

The normal spleen is a curved, wedge-shaped organ located beneath the rib cage in the upper left quadrant. The spleen lies beneath the left tenth rib and normally weighs about 150 g, measuring approximately 12 cm in length, 7 cm in width and 3 cm in thickness. The normal spleen usually cannot be palpated, but as it enlarges it descends below the rib cage, across the abdomen toward the right lower quadrant. An enlarged spleen may have a palpable notch along its medial edge.

Examination of the spleen should begin with observation of the left upper quadrant for an obvious mass, though such a mass is quite uncommon. The examiner should then proceed with percussion over the area of the spleen to look for evidence of dullness, implying splenetic enlargement. The two most useful methods are percussion over Traube's space and Castell's sign.

The surface markings for Traube's space are the left sixth rib, the left mid-axillary line and the left costal margin. An enlarged spleen may cause dullness over Traube's space. Percussion should be carried out at one or more levels of Traube's space from medial to lateral. This maneuver has a sensitivity and specificity between 60 and 70% for splenetic enlargement; however, the sensitivity and specificity increases to approximately 80% in non-obese patients who are fasting.

Castell's method involves percussion in the lowest intercostal space in the left anterior axillary line. In normal individuals this area is resonant on percussion and remains resonant on inspiration. In patients with mild splenic enlargement this area will be resonant on percussion and become dull on maximal inspiration. This method has a sensitivity and specificity of approximately 80% for detection of splenic enlargement and would seem particularly suited for detection of a minimally enlarged spleen that may not be palpable.

Palpation of the spleen should begin in the right lower quadrant and proceed toward the left upper quadrant in order to follow the path of splenic enlargement. Palpation should initially be carried out in the supine position with a bimanual technique using the left hand to gently lift the lowermost portion of the left rib cage anteriorly. The fingertips of the right hand are used to palpate gently for the spleen tip on inspiration. The hand is moved from the right lower quadrant, advancing toward the left upper quadrant. If the spleen is not palpated in the supine position the patient should be moved into the right lateral decubitus position and again with bimanual technique the spleen tip should be sought using the fingertips of the right hand on inspiration. This technique has a sensitivity of about 70% and specificity of 90% for splenic enlargement.

20.7 Examination for Suspected Ascites

The presence of ascites – free fluid within the abdominal cavity – is always due to an underlying pathological process. Most often the underlying etiology is cirrhosis of any type. Other potential causes include severe right-sided heart failure, lymphatic obstruction, primary intra-abdominal malignancy and peritoneal metastases. It is easy to identify large-volume ascites clinically, but the sensitivity of the examination techniques falls with lower volumes of fluid. Ultrasound, which can detect as little as 100 mL of free fluid, is the gold standard against which the clinical diagnostic maneuvers are compared.

An approach involves inspection for bulging flanks, followed by palpation for the presence or absence of fluid waves combined with percussion to demonstrate flank dullness as well as shifting dullness. One has to be aware that adipose tissue in the flanks may be occasionally mistaken for free fluid. To demonstrate a fluid wave it is necessary to enlist the aid of the patient or another individual. With the patient in the supine position, place one hand on the patient's flank. With the other hand briskly tap the other flank. A third hand is placed in the mid-abdomen with sufficient pressure applied to dampen any wave that may pass through adipose tissue in the anterior abdominal wall. If fluid is present a shock wave will be felt with the palpating hand. The sensitivity of this technique is approximately 50% but it has a specificity of greater than 80%.

When percussing for free fluid one should place the finger parallel to the expected edge and percuss from resonance in the mid-abdomen to dullness in the flanks. This area is then marked and the patient rolled to the opposite side. For example, if flank dullness is demonstrated on the left then the patient should be rolled onto the right side. One should allow approximately 30 seconds for the fluid to move between the mesentery and loops of bowel into the inferior portion of the abdomen. The previous area of dullness in the left flank should now be resonant. It does not matter which side one chooses to start with. In three separate studies shifting dullness had a sensitivity that ranged from 60–88% and a specificity that ranged from 56–90%.

In one study involving six gastroenterologists and 50 hospitalized alcoholic patients, the overall agreement was 75% for the presence or absence of ascites and reached 95% among senior physicians.

Interestingly, symptoms are often as useful as physical examination techniques for the clinical diagnosis of ascites. The most useful findings to make a diagnosis of ascites are a positive fluid wave, shifting dullness or peripheral edema. The absence of these findings is useful in ruling out ascites, as is a negative history of ankle swelling or increasing abdominal girth.

SUGGESTED READING LIST

Section 20 Examination of the Abdomen
Castell DO, O'Brien KD, Muench H, Chalmers TC. Estimation of liver size by percussion in normal individuals. Ann Intern Med 1969; 70(6):1183–1189.

Grover SA, Barkun AN, Sackett DL. Does this patient have splenomegaly? JAMA 1993; 270:2218–2221.

Naylor CD. Physical examination of the liver. JAMA 1994; 271:1859–1865.

Sapira JD. The art and science of bedside teaching. In: Urban & Schwarzenberg 1990.

Williams JW, Jr, Simel DL. Does this patient have ascites? How to divine fluid in the abdomen. JAMA 1992; 267:2645–2648.

2

Nutrition in Gastrointestinal Disease

J.S. Whittaker, U.P. Steinbrecher, M. Lemoyne and
H.J. Freeman

1. INTRODUCTION

Food assimilation is the major function of the gastrointestinal tract, and
important manifestations of many gastrointestinal diseases are their nutritional effects. Digestion and absorption of nutrients are discussed elsewhere. This
chapter reviews physiologic considerations that are essential for planning
proper nutritional management. The focus will be on the role of the liver in
regulating the supply of carbohydrate and lipid fuels as well as ensuring the
availability of essential substrates to peripheral tissues. The clinical features
of malnutrition and specific effects of malnutrition on the gastrointestinal tract
and liver will be discussed along with diet therapy in gastrointestinal disease.
Finally, an approach to clinical nutrition will be presented, including nutritional assessment and the rational use of enteral and parenteral nutritional support.

2. ESSENTIAL PHYSIOLOGIC CONCEPTS IN NUTRITION

To maintain a continuous supply of nutrients in the bloodstream in the face of
intermittent dietary intake, a complex set of regulatory mechanisms have
evolved. These allow the storage of nutrients during feeding, and their release
from storage pools during the interdigestive period so as to maintain nutrient
levels in the bloodstream within remarkably narrow limits. Short-term regulation between the fed state and the interdigestive state is mediated principally by (1) the concentration of several key substrates and (2) a set of regulatory hormones, which include insulin, glucagon, catecholamines and corticosteroids (Table 1).

TABLE 1. Hormonal regulation of nutrient metabolism

Hormone	Principal metabolic actions
Insulin	Increases glucose uptake in peripheral tissues
	Stimulates protein synthesis
	Inhibits lipolysis and glycolysis
Glucagon	Increases cyclic AMP levels in the liver and adipose tissue, with stimulation of fatty acid mobilization, glycogenolysis, glycolysis and gluconeogenesis
Catecholamines	Increase cyclic AMP levels in the liver, skeletal muscle and adipose tissue, with release of glucose, free fatty acids and lactate
Corticosteroids	Increase gluconeogenesis
	Increase amino acid mobilization from the periphery (chiefly skeletal muscle)
	Increase fatty acid release from extremities
	Decrease glucose utilization by peripheral tissues

The fate of glucose in the fed and the fasting states is detailed in Figure 1. Glucose is rapidly absorbed following ingestion as starch, disaccharides or monosaccharides. The glucose is transported via the portal system to the liver, which extracts a considerable fraction of portal venous glucose. The remainder enters the systemic circulation and causes pancreatic secretion of insulin. The high portal vein insulin and glucose concentrations lead to hepatic glucose uptake with conversion to glycogen and fatty acids. The peripheral rise in insulin, which occurs in association with the rise in plasma glucose concentration, causes a large peripheral uptake of glucose, first by muscle cells, and second by adipocytes. Glucose is the essential substrate for brain, renal medulla and red cell metabolism; other organs mainly use fatty acids for energy. The rise in plasma insulin also leads to amino acid uptake by muscle and has an antiproteolytic effect. These effects on muscle protein have led to the designation of insulin as an "anabolic hormone." In the postabsorptive or interdigestive state, plasma glucose is low, with low plasma insulin levels. The low plasma insulin influences the metabolism of all three macronutrients (i.e., carbohydrates, fat and protein). Glycogenolysis occurs in the liver to maintain plasma glucose levels. The low plasma insulin also allows lipolysis to take place, such that fatty acids can be utilized as the major energy substrate. Finally, the low plasma insulin leads to proteolysis, particularly of muscle protein, which leads to release of alanine and glutamine, which can be used for gluconeogenesis in the liver. This gluconeogenesis occurs in concert with glycogenolysis to assure an ongoing supply of glucose for the body.

A. Fed state

B. Interdigestive state

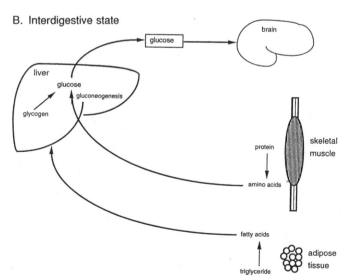

FIGURE 1.   Carbohydrate and protein metabolism.

Other hormones, such as glucagon, catecholamines and growth hormone, play less important roles in macronutrient metabolism, but in general have been termed the "stress hormones," since they are released during times of stress and have anti-insulin effects. In particular, if for any reason there is a low blood sugar, all these hormones are released and will promote an elevation in plasma glucose.

The flux of lipid nutrients in the fed and the interdigestive states is contrasted in Figure 2. In the fed state, fat enters the circulation from the intestine as chylomicrons, which are large droplets of triglyceride emulsified by a surface monolayer of phospholipid and apolipoproteins. Additional apolipoproteins are transferred onto the chylomicrons from HDL. The artificial fat emulsions used for parenteral nutrition are very similar to chylomicrons in that they contain a core of triglyceride with a surface monolayer of phospholipid. They initially contain no apolipoproteins, but acquire these from HDL very rapidly once they have entered the circulation. One of the apolipoproteins, apolipoprotein C-II, is particularly important in that it is an essential cofactor for the action of lipoprotein lipase. This enzyme is attached to the capillary endothelium in tissues, such as the heart and adipose tissue, that are active in utilizing fatty acids. Chylomicrons bind to the enzyme and the core triglyceride is rapidly hydrolyzed. The released fatty acids are then taken up and utilized in the peripheral tissues. As the chylomicron particle shrinks in size, the excess surface material is transferred back to HDL, and ultimately the remnant particles are cleared via a specific receptor in the liver. The process of lipolysis is extremely efficient, and the half-life of chylomicron triglyceride in the circulation is normally less than 15 minutes. The lower panel of Figure 2 depicts the postabsorptive or interdigestive state. Chylomicrons are absent, but triglyceride fuels are available in the circulation in the form of VLDL, which are secreted by the liver. The substrates for triglyceride assembly include free fatty acids released from adipose tissue through the action of a hormone-sensitive lipase, and fatty acids synthesized in the liver from acetyl-CoA. The newly secreted VLDL acquire apolipoproteins and cholesterol ester from HDL. Lipolysis of VLDL in peripheral tissues is mediated by lipoprotein lipase. As the particle decreases in size, free cholesterol transfers to HDL, where it is esterified through the action of lecithin-cholesterol acyltransferase (LCAT), and the resultant cholesterol ester is then transferred back to the lipolyzed particle, where it forms part of the core. When lipolysis is completed, what is left behind is termed an LDL particle. This is smaller and more dense than VLDL, has lost all apolipoproteins except apolipoprotein B, and has a core of cholesterol ester rather than triglyceride. LDL is cleared relatively slowly, with a half-life of several days. The uptake of LDL is medi-

A. Fed state

B. Postabsorptive state

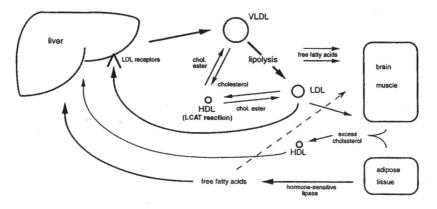

FIGURE 2.   Lipoprotein metabolism.

ated by a specific membrane receptor, termed the LDL receptor, whose activity in turn is regulated by intracellular cholesterol levels. The most active tissues (on a weight basis) for LDL clearance are steroidogenic tissues, such as the adrenals, gonads and the liver; because of its size, the liver accounts for over half of total LDL catabolism. As peripheral tissues cannot degrade cholesterol, excess cholesterol is returned to the liver via HDL, where it is used for bile acid synthesis or excreted in the bile.

In addition to the short-term regulation mediated by substrates and hormones outlined above, additional adaptive responses occur in response to particular dietary circumstances. For example, a diet rich in carbohydrate at the expense of fat will lead to the induction of enzymes involved in glycolysis, the pentose phosphate pathway and fatty acid synthesis (e.g., glucokinase, glucose-6-phosphate dehydrogenase, 6-phosphogluconate dehydrogenase, acetyl-CoA carboxylase). A diet containing predominantly fat at the expense of carbohydrate will lead to induction of fatty acid oxidation, with increased acyl-CoA-carnitine acyltransferase, and induction of enzymes involved in gluconeogenesis, including glucose-6-phosphatase, fructose diphosphatase and transaminases. A diet rich in protein but low in carbohydrate will also lead to induction of gluconeogenic enzymes and transaminases, as well as other enzymes involved in amino acid interconversion and degradation, and induction of urea cycle enzymes to deal with the enhanced production of ammonia.

Starvation leads to a number of adaptive responses. There is a depletion of liver glycogen within 24 to 48 hours, with stimulation of gluconeogenic enzymes to allow the production of glucose from amino acids released through protein breakdown in skeletal muscle. Lipolysis in adipose tissue leads to increased fatty acid levels and activation of enzymes responsible for β-oxidation of fatty acid in the liver (acyl-CoA-carnitine acyltransferase). In addition to acetyl-CoA, fatty acid oxidation generates ketone bodies. One important adaptive response to starvation is the induction of 3-hydroxybutyrate dehydrogenase in the brain, which allows this organ to utilize ketone bodies as a fuel. Decreased dependence on glucose reduces the need for excess gluconeogenesis and spares muscle protein. In a relatively lean 70 kg man with 12% body fat, survival without food can be expected to be about 60 days or longer.

3. CLINICAL AND LABORATORY FEATURES OF PROTEIN-ENERGY MALNUTRITION

Protein-energy malnutrition may result from a number of causes. These are shown in Table 2. Intake or assimilation may be impaired or, alternatively,

TABLE 2.   Causes of protein-energy malnutrition

Impaired intake
Insufficient quantity or quality
Impaired intake due to systemic disease (e.g., cerebrovascular accident, chronic infections)
Impaired intake due to localized gastrointestinal disease (e.g., benign or malignant esophageal
   stricture)

Impaired digestion and/or absorption
Selective enzyme defect (e.g., enterokinase deficiency, trypsinogen deficiency)
Generalized enzyme defect (e.g., pancreatic exocrine insufficiency)
Impaired small intestinal assimilation (e.g., celiac disease)

Excessive enteric protein loss
Gastric or intestinal mucosal disease (e.g., Ménétrier's disease, intestinal lymphangiectasia)
Extraintestinal disease with lymphatic blockage (e.g., pericarditis, lymphoma)

Disorders with multiple causes
Advanced malignancy
Chronic renal failure with uremia
Other chronic debilitating diseases

---

losses may be increased, as occurs with excessive enteric protein loss in protein-losing enteropathies. In some disorders, multiple causes may be present. Moreover, requirements may be significantly increased in some patients as a result of growth, pregnancy, tissue injury or a superimposed disease process. In some patients with chronic debilitating diseases, multiple factors may be responsible.

Attempts have been made to classify malnutrition into a predominantly protein-depleted (i.e., kwashiorkor) or calorie- (energy-) starved (i.e., marasmus) state. In kwashiorkor, the subject ingests a moderate number of calories, usually as complex carbohydrate (e.g., rice), but very little protein. The carbohydrate is absorbed as glucose, causing rises in plasma glucose and insulin, and leading to decreased lipolysis and proteolysis. The liver is therefore supplied with inadequate amino acids, with little oral intake and little peripheral mobilization from skeletal muscle stores. Transport of triglyceride made from ingested glucose is impaired since there is inadequate production of apoprotein, which is needed for the formation of VLDL. The liver becomes fatty and enlarged. Furthermore, other proteins, including albumin, are inadequately produced by the liver in kwashiorkor, and serum albumin falls, with resulting peripheral edema. With marasmus the subject takes inadequate amounts of protein and calories. The low caloric intake means that only small amounts of carbohydrate are taken; plasma glucose and insulin are low. Hence, lipolysis and proteolysis occur, with adequate delivery of amino acids from muscle to the liver for protein production. Fatty liver does not occur, and serum albumin levels tend to be normal, with no peripheral edema. Often patients fall between these two extremes of nutritional states, but there are examples of kwashiorkor and marasmus in Western clinical practice. Anorexia nervosa is a classic example of marasmus. Marked muscle wasting and loss of subcutaneous tissue (adipose tissue) occur with normal-sized nonfatty livers and no peripheral edema. In contrast, the intensive care unit patient who has received intravenous dextrose (glucose) without amino acids for a prolonged period will often show a fatty liver and marked hypoalbuminemia and edema.

Clinical features of protein-energy malnutrition vary depending on the severity and duration of nutrient deficiency, age at onset and the presence or absence of other contributing or conditioning factors. With minimal deficiency, abnormalities may be subtle – particularly in adults, in whom there are no growth requirements. In these patients muscle wasting and loss of subcutaneous fat may be present. Weakness and minimal changes in psychomotor function may develop. Nontender parotid enlargement may occur, sometimes bilaterally. Patchy brown pigmentation, particularly over the malar eminences of the face, may occur. A lackluster appearance with thinning and increased shedding of hair from the sides of the head, particularly on combing or brushing, may develop. Bradycardia may occur. Variable degrees of hepatomegaly may result, sometimes with steatosis. In patients with protein-energy malnutrition following jejunoileal bypass a wide spectrum of histopathologic change has been observed, similar to findings frequently associated with alcoholic liver disease. Other changes in the liver that may occur in nutritional disorders are listed in Table 3.

In adults with severe protein-energy malnutrition and in growing children, clinical features may be even more significant. Muscle wasting, subcutaneous fat loss, dependent edema and weight loss may be marked. Severe mental apathy and reduced physical activity may occur. Abnormalities in the hair, particularly of children, may be striking. Severe dyspigmentation may develop, especially distally; rarely, alternating strands of light and dark hair are observed. Hair may be removed without pain. Nails may become brittle, with horizontal grooves. An asymmetrical confluent pattern of skin hyperpigmentation may be seen, particularly over perineal and exposed areas, such as the face. Extensive desquamation may occur, leaving depigmented areas of superficial ulcers, particularly on the buttocks and backs of the thighs. Gastrointestinal symptoms are common but variable. These include marked consti-

TABLE 3. Effects of specific nutritional disorders on the liver

Nutritional disorders	Effects on the liver
Common conditions	
Alcoholism	Steatosis, alcoholic hepatitis and cirrhosis
Obesity	Steatosis, steatohepatitis and cholelithiasis
Uncontrolled diabetes	Glycogenosis, steatosis and steatohepatitis
Protein deficiency	Pigment stones
Kwashiorkor	Steatosis and decreased protein synthesis
Fasting	Mild unconjugated hyperbilirubinemia, especially in Gilbert's syndrome
Uncommon conditions	
Jejunoileal bypass	Steatosis and steatohepatitis
Gross dietary iron excess	Bantu siderosis/hemochromatosis
Senecio alkaloids	Veno-occlusive disease
Dietary aflatoxins	Hepatocellular carcinoma (?)
Chronic arsenic ingestion	Noncirrhotic portal hypertension, angiosarcoma and hepatocellular carcinoma
Hypervitaminosis A	Hepatic fibrosis and cirrhosis

pation, diarrhea, anorexia or hyperphagia, nausea, vomiting and dehydration. Laboratory features are also variable. Serum proteins may be substantially reduced, including serum albumin and some higher-molecular-weight transfer proteins, such as transferrin, ceruloplasmin, lipoproteins, thyroxin and cortisol binding proteins. Serum amino acid analysis may show a decrease in essential amino acids (i.e., leucine, isoleucine, valine, methionine), and either normal or depressed levels of nonessentials (i.e., glycine, serine, glutamine). The urinary excretion of urea, creatinine and hydroxyproline may decrease. Severe electrolyte abnormalities develop, although serum levels may be normal.

Clinical vitamin deficiencies are listed in Table 4. Except for cheilosis and glossitis, which are seen with multiple vitamin B deficiencies, physical findings of single or isolated vitamin deficiencies are seldom observed in protein-calorie malnourished patients in developed countries. Trace elements are elements that are required in small quantities (mg amounts or less) for normal growth and/or function. Essential trace elements for humans include iron, iodine, zinc, chromium, copper, selenium and cobalt, and possibly molybdenum, manganese and vanadium. Except for iron deficiency due to blood loss and/or poor intake, deficiency states of trace elements are rare in subjects with some oral intake, since only minute amounts are required.

TABLE 4. Vitamin deficiency syndromes

Vitamin	Name of deficiency state	Clinical occurrence	Common clinical features
1. Water-soluble			
B$_1$ (thiamine)	Beriberi: Dry (neurologic) Wet (cardiac)	Refeeding after starvation	Neurologic: Peripheral neuropathy, Wernicke-Korsakoff Cardiac: Heart failure
	Wernicke-Korsakoff syndrome		
B$_2$ (riboflavin)	—	Rare	B-complex deficiency*
B$_6$ (pyridoxine)	—	Only with pyridoxine-antagonist drugs (isoniazid, cycloserine, penicillamine)	Neurologic: Convulsions B-complex deficiency* Anemia
B$_{12}$ (cyanocobalamin)	Pernicious anemia (when secondary to idiopathic gastric atrophy)	Achlorhydria Terminal ileal disease or resection Bacterial overgrowth Diphyllobothrium latum Pancreatic insufficiency	Hematologic: Pancytopenia Neurologic: Subacute combined degeneration Peripheral neuropathy Glossitis
Folic acid	—	Pregnancy Poor intake Malabsorption	Hematologic: Pancytopenia Glossitis
Niacin	Pellagra	Poor diet	Characteristic dermatitis Dementia Diarrhea
Pantothenic acid	—	Rare	—
Biotin	—	Excess egg white ingestion ? TPN	Dermatitis Glossitis Anorexia
C (ascorbic acid)	Scurvy	Infants, the elderly and alcoholics with very poor intake	Purpura Gum disease (when teeth present)

TABLE 4. Vitamin deficiency syndromes (cont'd)

Vitamin	Name of deficiency state	Clinical occurrence	Common clinical features
2. Fat-soluble			
A	—	Third World children Severe low intake	Night blindness, corneal changes, xerophthalmia, xeroderma and hyperkeratosis
D	—	Inadequate sun exposure Inadequate intake Renal disease	Osteomalacia (rickets in children) Hypocalcemia
E	—	Cholestatic liver disease (especially children)	Neurologic: Posterior column degeneration, areflexia
K	—	Warfarin anticoagulant Long-term antibiotics (especially with TPN) Newborn infants	Hemorrhage with prolonged prothrombin time

*B-complex deficiency: cheilosis, angular stomatitis, glossitis.

4. EFFECTS OF MALNUTRITION ON THE GASTROINTESTINAL TRACT AND PANCREAS

Protein-energy malnutrition may produce major structural and functional changes in the gastrointestinal tract and pancreas, which, in turn, may aggravate the underlying poor nutritional condition. In severe protein-energy malnutrition, for example, acinar cell atrophy occurs and exocrine cells have decreased numbers of zymogen granules. Pancreatic secretion may be reduced following stimulation with cholecystokinin and/or secretin. With malnutrition, the activities of enzymes contained in pancreatic juice (i.e., trypsin, chymotrypsin, lipase, amylase) are reduced. With reversal of malnutrition these can return to normal levels, but this may require several weeks.

In addition to pancreatic exocrine changes, the entire wall and mucosal lining of the stomach and intestine may be reduced in thickness. This change appears to be reversible, as a more normal macroscopic appearance can follow nutritional repletion. Microscopically, marked changes may develop, including severe "flattening" of the small intestinal mucosa, similar to celiac disease. In contrast to celiac disease, however, reduced numbers of crypt mitoses are seen; the mucosa is hypoplastic rather than hyperplastic. In this setting, correction of the nutritional state per se can produce a complete reversion to normal. Nonspecific ultrastructural changes also occur, including epithelial cell lipid droplets. Changes may be present throughout the small intestine in an irregular patchy distribution, although the jejunum appears to be most severely affected. Qualitative and quantitative changes in the intestinal microflora, particularly anaerobes, also occur in protein-energy malnutrition. However, their role in altering mucosal structure and function requires definition. Some brush-border enzymes (i.e., disaccharidases) may be reduced; as a result, malabsorption of a variety of substances (e.g., lactose) may be observed. Altered uptake of glucose and D-xylose has also been reported, and steatorrhea may be present with impaired absorption of fat and some fat-soluble vitamins. In addition, there may be increased protein loss from the gut, leading to increased fecal nitrogen loss. Finally, specific nutrients may be deficient and cause alterations in certain tissues. For example, folic acid and vitamin B_{12} deficiencies have well-recognized effects on rapidly dividing hematopoietic precursor cells in the bone marrow; for similar reasons, as shown in Table 5, analogous changes may be anticipated in the small intestinal epithelium.

There is increasing evidence that the colonic mucosa uses short-chain fatty acids (especially butyrate) as an energy source. In patients who undergo a colostomy, the bowel that is left distally does not have a fecal stream. The mucosa of this bowel may develop inflammation, called "diversion colitis."

TABLE 5. Effects of depletion of specific nutrients on the intestine

Nutrient	Effects
Protein-energy malnutrition (e.g., especially, kwashiorkor)	Total or subtotal villous "atrophy" and crypt hypoplasia
Folic acid deficiency	Total or subtotal villous "atrophy" and crypt hypoplasia; macrocytic and/or "megaloblastic" enterocytes
Vitamin B_{12} deficiency	Total or subtotal villous "atrophy" and crypt hypoplasia; macrocytic and/or "megaloblastic" enterocytes
Vitamin E deficiency	(?) Small intestinal ceroidosis (i.e., "brown bowel syndrome")
Vitamin A deficiency	Reduced numbers of intestinal goblet cells

This condition can be corrected by administering short-chain fatty acid enemas. A major source of the short-chain fatty acids in the colon is fermented dietary fiber, and thus fiber may be considered a "nutrient."

5. DIETARY THERAPY IN GASTROINTESTINAL DISEASE

5.1 General Principles
A number of specific diets are useful in different gastrointestinal disorders. These may involve diet restriction or supplementation, or alternatively, a change in the consistency or content of specific nutrients. In patients with steatorrhea, for example, luminal fatty acids are present and involved in the pathogenesis of diarrhea. In these patients, reduction in diarrhea can be accomplished, in part, by a reduction in the oral intake of triglycerides; a low-fat diet may be beneficial. In some patients with steatorrhea, supplementation with medium-chain triglycerides may be useful because these are hydrolyzed more rapidly by pancreatic enzymes, do not require bile acid micelles for absorption, and are primarily directed to the portal rather than the lymphatic circulation. Because medium-chain triglycerides undergo ω-oxidation to metabolically nonutilizable dicarboxylic acids, the effective caloric content of medium-chain triglycerides is less than expected. Medium-chain triglycerides in a daily dose of 60 mL will provide approximately 460 calories. Low-fat dietary supplements may be provided in the form of a number of commercially available products prepared as complete nutritional supplements. Fat-soluble vitamins can be replaced using oral water-miscible formulations, if

steatorrhea is present. For vitamin K, a water-soluble form is available. Fat-soluble vitamins require bile acid micelles for absorption; thus, if steatorrhea is due to bile acid depletion (as might occur in the short bowel syndrome following surgical resection for extensive Crohn's disease), increased amounts of vitamins may be required.

Bloating and cramping pain may follow ingestion of lactose-containing foods. This may be due to lactase deficiency (e.g., small bowel disease, "ethnic" lactase deficiency). Dietary lactose restriction may be indicated in patients if there is a history of lactose intolerance or a positive lactose tolerance test (i.e., rise in blood sugar less than 20 mg/dL after 50 g of lactose) accompanied by characteristic symptoms. An alternative test involves measurement of breath hydrogen; a rise of more than 20 ppm is consistent with lactose intolerance. Lactose may be found in milk, including buttermilk, even if it has been naturally fermented. Commercial yogurt should also be avoided, since this often has milk or cream added after fermentation to avoid the sour taste produced by fermenting lactose. Ice cream and sherbets have high lactose concentrations and should be avoided. Cheese or desserts made from milk or milk chocolate as well as sauces or stuffings made from milk, cream or cheese should also be avoided. Calcium supplements may be necessary with dairy product restriction, particularly in postmenopausal women. Liquid dairy products may be used to a limited extent by patients who have lactose intolerance; in these patients, a yeast enzyme preparation (i.e., lactase from Kluyveromyces lactis) added to milk at 4°C (15 drops/L) can hydrolyze up to 99% of the lactose in 24 hours. Nonliquid dairy products cannot be treated with enzyme preparations, although lactase tablets may be chewed prior to eating solid food.

5.2 Celiac Disease

Celiac disease, also known as gluten-sensitive enteropathy or celiac sprue, is a malabsorption disorder resulting from ingestion of proteins derived from certain cereal grains of the grass family, Gramineae: wheat, rye, barley and possibly oats. It is believed that the alcohol-soluble gliadin fraction of wheat gluten or similar alcohol-soluble proteins from the other grains (termed *prolamins*) cause the intestinal damage. Consequently, absolute restriction is required for life. Table 6 provides some dietary guidelines for celiac disease patients. Gluten, however, is a particularly ubiquitous substance and can be found in coffee, catsup, dip, frozen TV dinners, ice cream and even in the capsules of medications! Although wheat, rye, barley and possibly oats are important, corn and rice do not appear to activate celiac disease. Data on other grains are not as clear. Buckwheat is not derived from the grass family and is usually permitted. Millet and sorghum are often allowed, but have not been

TABLE 6. Dietary guidelines for celiac disease patients

Foods to avoid
Wheat, rye, barley, oat products
Triticale (wheat–rye hybrid)
Millet and sorghum
Malt and hydrolyzed vegetable protein

Acceptable foods
Corn, rice, buckwheat products
Wine and distilled alcoholic beverages
Fruits and vegetables
Meat
Nuts
Dairy products (unless lactose-intolerant)

---

thoroughly evaluated. Triticale, a hybrid of wheat and rye, should be avoided. Rye whiskey, Scotch whiskey and other cereal-derived alcohols can be consumed, since gluten is not present in distilled spirits. Similarly, brandy and wine made from fruit pose no difficulties. Beer and ale are produced from barley; it is not entirely clear if they can activate disease and would best be avoided. Malt made from barley should be avoided, as well as hydrolyzed vegetable proteins used as flavor enhancers in processed foods, since they may be made from soy, wheat and other cereal proteins.

For both symptomatic and asymptomatic patients with celiac disease, a lifelong gluten-free diet is recommended. Multivitamin supplements are frequently required and specific vitamin, mineral and trace element deficiencies should be corrected. Iron and folate supplementation may be needed and poor absorption of oral iron may sometimes necessitate parenteral administration. Supplements of calcium and vitamin D may be required to prevent mobilization of skeletal calcium, and in some patients magnesium may be needed.

5.3 Inflammatory Bowel Disease

Malnutrition in patients with inflammatory bowel disease, especially Crohn's disease, is a frequent problem. Weight loss may be seen in over 65% of patients and growth retardation may be observed in up to 40% of children. As shown in Table 7, there are multiple causes for malnutrition, especially in patients with Crohn's disease with small bowel involvement. The goal of nutritional management is to ensure adequate nutrient intake with modifications that reduce symptoms. Although only limited studies are available, evidence suggests that energy expenditure is no greater than one would predict for a healthy individual unless the disease is complicated by fever or sepsis.

TABLE 7.   Malnutrition in inflammatory bowel disease

Reduced oral intake
Disease-induced (e.g., postprandial abdominal pain and diarrhea, sitophobia, anorexia, nausea
   and vomiting)
Iatrogenic (e.g., restrictive diets, "fad" diets)

Malabsorption
Reduced absorptive surface (e.g., shortened small intestine due to prior resection, diseased
   segments)
Bacterial overgrowth (e.g., associated with strictures and bypassed loops, stasis)
Bile salt deficiency after ileal resection (e.g., impaired micelle formation and steatorrhea)
Lactase deficiency (e.g., associated with small bowel disease)
Drug-induced malabsorption

Increased nutrient loss
Protein-losing enteropathy
Diarrhea losses of electrolytes, minerals and trace elements (e.g., potassium, zinc)
Gastrointestinal blood loss (e.g., iron loss)

Drug-induced malabsorption
Cholestyramine (e.g., bile acids; fat; fat-soluble vitamins, including vitamins D and K)
Sulfasalazine (e.g., folic deficiency associated with reduced absorption and increased
   requirement related to hemolysis)
Steroids (e.g., calcium absorption and mobilization)

Increased requirements
Chronic inflammatory disease, fever, superimposed infection

There may be increased caloric as well as nutrient requirements, however, particularly if gastrointestinal losses are substantial and malabsorption is significant. Attention should also be placed on micronutrient deficiencies in these patients, particularly if concomitant malabsorption is present. For example, patients with significant ileal disease or resection require regularly administered parenteral vitamin B_{12}.

Frequently, the diet consistency or form will require modification to permit intake of adequate amounts of various nutrients. Thus, a low-fiber or low-residue diet may be recommended if symptoms are associated with stenotic bowel segments. In some, symptoms may be improved by a diet with increased fiber. Increased amounts of pectin or guar, for example, may be helpful in patients with increased stool water content, as these fibers tend to have a significant water-retaining capacity.

Lactose intolerance may be common in patients with inflammatory bowel disease, particularly with small intestinal involvement, as well as in ethnic groups with a high frequency of primary lactase deficiency. Recent reports suggest that lactose intolerance in Crohn's disease is not as common as previously thought. In patients with a limited ileal resection, diarrhea may result from impaired ileal bile salt reabsorption. With more extensive ileal resection, particularly if over 100 cm, bile salt depletion may occur. As a result, micelle formation may be suboptimal, and fat malabsorption results. In addition, fecal fat and/or fatty acids may bind to calcium, magnesium, zinc and copper; increased fecal losses of these divalent cations may result. Increased fat-soluble vitamin loss may occur. Finally, patients with Crohn's disease and an ileal resection with steatorrhea are more prone to develop calcium oxalate kidney stones. This is due to increased urinary oxalate concentrations associated with enhanced absorption of dietary oxalate, largely in the colon. Steatorrhea causes enteric hyperoxaluria because calcium binds to unabsorbed fatty acids. As a result, more oxalate is available for passive colonic diffusion. In addition, fatty acids appear to increase colonic permeability to oxalate. By reducing dietary fat, oxalate absorption is also reduced.

Specific drugs may also alter nutrient absorption. For example, sulfasalazine is a competitive inhibitor of intestinal folate absorption. In addition, patients on sulfasalazine may have hemolysis secondary to red cell oxidant injury from sulfapyridine. Thus, folate requirements are increased.

6. DIETARY THERAPY IN LIVER DISEASE

Two important manifestations of chronic liver disease, ascites and portal-systemic encephalopathy, can be effectively treated with dietary modifications. The prime dietary objective in the treatment of ascites is sodium restriction. Some authorities have recommended restriction of dietary sodium intake to as little as 10–20 mmol/day for patients with symptomatic, large-volume ascites. However, it is almost impossible to design a palatable diet or provide sufficient protein to maintain nitrogen balance with such stringent restrictions, and therefore these will not be satisfactory for long-term use. Well-motivated patients can often be maintained on a 40 mmol sodium diet (equivalent to about 1 g of sodium or 2.5 g of sodium chloride).

The treatment of portal-systemic encephalopathy includes dietary protein restriction. Management will obviously need to be individualized for patients with fulminant hepatic failure or stage IV coma, but patients with chronic liver disease and mild to moderate encephalopathy should usually have dietary protein intake restricted to 0.5–0.8 g/kg body weight. Even more rigorous restriction may be necessary to control encephalopathy in the short term, but is difficult to maintain for prolonged periods because of limited patient compliance and negative nitrogen balance. It is believed that vegetable protein may be less ammoniagenic than meat, but part of this may relate to decreased efficiency of absorption of vegetable protein. Disproportionately high levels of aromatic amino acids are found in plasma of patients with decompensated cirrhosis. Hence, nutritional supplements rich in branched-chain amino acids have been advocated; however, unequivocal evidence for their efficacy is lacking.

Patients with advanced cirrhosis often have hepatic glycogen depletion. During fasting, glucagon and catecholamines will be released to maintain blood glucose levels. In the absence of hepatic glycogen stores, this requires gluconeogenesis, and the substrate is provided to a significant extent from muscle catabolism. Utilization of the amino acids for gluconeogenesis will lead to ammonia production. It is not known whether dietary manipulations designed to provide a continuous supply of glucose, and therefore to reduce gluconeogenesis, would improve the hyperammonemia in these individuals. Cholestatic liver diseases, including primary biliary cirrhosis (PBC), secondary biliary cirrhosis, sclerosing cholangitis and biliary atresia, may be accompanied by malabsorption of fat-soluble vitamins. Vitamin K deficiency can be easily confirmed with the demonstration of a prolonged prothrombin time that corrects with administration of parenteral vitamin K. Assays for vitamins D, A and E are generally available only in specialized laboratories. If confirmatory tests are not available and if there are strong clinical grounds for suspecting a deficiency state, appropriate replacement therapy should be initiated. Table 8 lists a number of hereditary liver diseases for which appropriate therapy includes specific dietary interventions.

7. NUTRITION INTERVENTION

7.1 Nitrogen Requirements
In a well-nourished adult in steady state, total nitrogen intake will equal nitrogen output in urine, stool and skin. This is termed (zero) "nitrogen balance." Nitrogen is assimilated almost exclusively as protein, and, on average, 6.25 g protein is equivalent to 1 g nitrogen. The nitrogen is excreted predominantly as urea in the urine, but stool and skin losses account for about 2–3 g daily. If a 70 kg man consumes 1 g protein/kg (= 70 g protein or 11.2 g N), then about 8–9 g of nitrogen can be expected in the urine, assuming nitrogen balance. In the steady state, ingestion of more nitrogen will merely result in excretion of more nitrogen in the urine. In growing children or in malnourished adults, the nutritional goal is a positive nitrogen balance, meaning that body tissue is being formed in excess of what is being broken down (i.e., there is net growth).

Nitrogen balance studies have shown that well-nourished adults can maintain nitrogen balance when given as little as 0.5 g/kg protein intake, if energy

TABLE 8.   Diet therapy for hereditary liver diseases

Disorder	Dietary intervention
Tyrosinemia	Low-phenylalanine diet
Hereditary fructose intolerance	Low-fructose, low-sucrose diet
Galactosemia	Galactose-free diet
Glycogen storage disease	Continuous glucose feeding
Cerebrotendinous xanthomatosis	Deoxycholic acid supplementation
Wilson's disease	Low-copper diet, zinc supplementation (together with chelating agent)
Hemochromatosis	Avoidance of excess dietary iron, selection of foods containing phytates or tannins to reduce iron absorption (together with appropriate phlebotomy treatment)
Cystic fibrosis	Low-fat diet, pancreatic enzyme supplements, fat-soluble vitamin supplements

requirements are met or exceeded. It is important that the protein supplied be of high quality; it should include all essential amino acids and a balanced mix of nonessential amino acids. Malnourished, septic, injured or burned patients will require more protein, in the order of 1.5–2.0 g/kg daily. Pregnant patients should also be given 1.5 g/kg protein daily. It is less clear that patients with conditions associated with protein loss, such as nephrotic syndrome and protein-losing enteropathy, benefit from extra protein intake.

7.2 Energy Requirements
Basal energy requirements in healthy subjects are accurately predicted by the Harris-Benedict equation:

MALES: Energy (kcal/d) = 66 + (13.75 × W) + (5.00 × H) − (6.78 × A)

FEMALES: Energy (kcal/d) = 655 + (9.56 × W) + (1.85 × H) − (4.68 × A) where W = weight in kg, H = height in cm and A = age in years.

Basal energy requirements, as predicted by these equations, increase in the presence of fever (13% per °C), sepsis or injury (up to 20–30%), and burns (up to 100%). Modest physical activity usually requires about 30% above basal requirements.

7.3 Types of Nutritional Intervention

The options for refeeding include oral refeeding, tube feeding and total parenteral nutrition. An assessment by a dietitian regarding current food intake and food preferences is essential. It may well be possible by determining food preferences to provide a well-balanced, nutritionally complete diet. In addition, supplements of high-calorie, high-protein foods such as milkshakes or commercially prepared liquid formula diets may allow for adequate intake. If the patient will not or cannot eat, however, nutritional intervention may be indicated. Examples of patients who will not eat include those with anorexia due to tumor or chemotherapy, and those with anorexia nervosa. Such patients generally have a normal or near-normal nonobstructed bowel, and can be fed enterally. Patients who cannot eat because of severe gastrointestinal illness include those with bowel obstruction or ileus. If nutritional intervention is required in these patients, parenteral (intravenous) nutrition will be necessary.

7.3.1 *ENTERAL NUTRITION*

Enteral nutrition generally refers to nutrition provided through a tube that has been inserted into the gastrointestinal tract. Usually the tube is a fine-bore (10 French [3.3 mm] or less) Silastic® or polyurethane tube placed via the nose into the stomach, duodenum or jejunum. When long-term feeding is required, it is often preferable for cosmetic and comfort reasons to perform a gastrostomy, which can now be done endoscopically or radiologically with only local anesthetic and mild sedation. If pulmonary aspiration is a potential problem, the tube should be placed into the jejunum.

A multitude of commercial enteral formulas are available for infusion. The formulas have been traditionally divided into polymeric, oligomeric and modular. Polymeric formulas (also called defined formula diets) provide nitrogen as whole protein, often casein, egg white solids or soy protein. Carbohydrate is provided as corn syrup, maltodextrins or glucose oligosaccharides, with sucrose added for sweetness in oral formulas. Fat is usually provided as soy oil, although corn oil and safflower oil may be used. Medium-chain triglycerides (MCT oil) are rarely used. Protein may be provided as milk (usually dry or skim), with lactose as a major carbohydrate. These formulas are contraindicated in patients with lactose intolerance.

Oligomeric formulas (also called elemental diets) provide nitrogen as oligopeptides from partially hydrolyzed whole protein or as crystalline amino acids. Carbohydrate tends to be provided as glucose oligosaccharides or glucose. Fat is usually present in small quantities, enough to meet the requirement for linoleic acid (an essential fatty acid), which is about 2–4% of total calories. MCT oil is added to some formulas. The oligomeric diets were formulated to require minimal digestion by the gastrointestinal tract, with little necessity for bile and pancreatic secretions, and minimal "work" by the enterocyte in terms of brush-border enzyme activity or re-esterification. Hence, these diets have been commercially promoted as ideal for patients with decreased bile output (cholestasis), pancreatic insufficiency and short bowel. However, there is little evidence that these diets are superior to polymeric diets, except with pancreatic insufficiency. Crohn's disease is another condition in which elemental diets may be superior to polymeric diets, although this too remains controversial. Furthermore, since the diet is "predigested," osmolality is high. Finally, the high cost of these diets (often 5 to 10 times that of polymeric diets) rarely justifies their use except in patients with severe pancreatic disease or possibly Crohn's disease.

Most of these formulas provide enough protein, calories, water, electrolytes, minerals, vitamins and trace elements in 2 L/day for most "nonstressed" patients. In other words, these diets are "complete." Excess requirements may exist in patients with multiple injuries, major infections or burns.

Modular formulas are those that contain or predominantly contain one kind of nutrient. There are commercially available modules for protein, fat, carbohydrates, vitamins, electrolytes and trace elements. These modules are not required for the majority of patients, and are rarely used. However, they may be used if different nitrogen-to-calorie ratios are indicated for a patient. Examples of this might include burns or protein-losing enteropathy, if more protein is to be given, or liver disease, if less protein is to be given. Modular feeding is time-consuming, since solutions must be mixed by the hospital, and are more expensive than "complete" formulas.

Finally, specialized amino acid solutions have been made for use in special circumstances – for example, liver disease, renal disease and "stress," such as trauma and sepsis. For liver disease, these solutions are composed mostly or exclusively of branched-chain amino acids, whereas for renal disease the solutions are predominantly essential amino acids. In general, these solutions are expensive and their efficacy is controversial.

Complications of enteral feeding may be divided into aspiration, mechanical, gastrointestinal and metabolic. In general, enteral feeding is well tolerated, and provided the complications are known, preventive and/or corrective measures may be undertaken to minimize patient risk.

Aspiration of the infused formula, with development of pneumonia, is a potentially lethal complication of tube feeding. Proper positioning of the tube requires radiographic verification. Risk factors for aspiration include patients on a ventilator and those with gastroesophageal reflux, poor or absent gag reflex, and impaired mentation. To minimize aspiration, it is suggested that patients, when possible, be fed with the head of the bed elevated 20–30°. Gastric contents should initially be checked by aspirating the tube every four to six hours, and if residue is present more than two hours following infusion, it should be temporarily stopped. Unfortunately, the small nasoenteric tubes in current use often collapse when aspirated, so small returns do not guarantee that the stomach is not becoming distended with fluid. Hence, examination for epigastric distention and succussion splash should be done. If there is any concern, an upright (if possible) plain film to assess gastric size may be useful. It has also been suggested that the feeding tube be placed into the small bowel well beyond the pylorus to minimize aspiration in those at risk.

Mechanical problems in patients with nasoenteric tubes include problems in the upper respiratory tract, esophagitis with development of esophageal ulceration and stenosis, tracheoesophageal fistula, and gastric outlet and small bowel obstruction. Upper respiratory problems include pharyngeal irritation, nasal erosions and necrosis, sinusitis and otitis media. These mechanical problems can be largely avoided by the use of soft, small-bore nasoenteric tubes.

Gastrointestinal problems related to nasoenteric feeding are common, occurring in 20–30% of patients. The most frequent complaints are nausea, vomiting, abdominal distention and altered bowel habit. Symptoms may be minimized by feeding at a slow rate with dilute solutions, but these symptoms may be just as common as with full-rate, full-strength solutions. Alternatively, a different enteral solution may be tried. If a lactose-containing solution is being used (generally not recommended for tube feeding), changing to a lactose-free solution is indicated. For constipation, fiber-containing solutions may be tried, although they are often unhelpful. Fiber, however, is a potential energy source for the colon, as previously discussed, and may therefore be important for maintenance of the colonic mucosa. At the present time, fiber-containing solutions are not routinely used.

Metabolic complications include overhydration, dehydration, hyperglycemia (including hyperosmolar nonketotic coma) and electrolyte disturbances. Electrolyte problems include hyponatremia, hyper- and hypokalemia, hyper- and hypophosphatemia and hypomagnesemia. In healthy, reasonably nourished individuals with normal cardiac, liver and renal function, these problems are not common. It is recommended that appropriate blood tests be done at intervals over the first few weeks to check for these potential problems.

7.3.2 *TOTAL PARENTERAL NUTRITION*

Total parenteral nutrition (TPN) involves intravenous administration of all known essential nutrients. This form of therapy is as effective as oral or enteral intake in terms of growth and maintaining body nitrogen. Indications include inability to eat for a minimum of 7 to 10 days with a nonfunctional gut. Total parenteral nutrition is also used for "bowel rest," especially in Crohn's disease, intestinal fistulas and pancreatitis, even if adequate absorption is possible. Several studies suggest, however, that bowel rest is not helpful in Crohn's disease. Furthermore, other studies have shown that elemental diets can be used instead of TPN, except when bowel obstruction is present. In general, if the gut is functional, enteral feeding is preferred since it is safer, cheaper and more physiologic.

7.3.2.1 *Solutions*

7.3.2.1.1 *Amino acids* "Protein" is supplied as synthetic crystalline, L-amino acid solutions; these are commercially available in 7–10% concentrations. Most available amino acid mixtures are devised for patients without special requirements. Solutions with added branched-chain amino acids are available for hepatic failure, and solutions with essential amino acids are available for renal failure.

7.3.2.1.2 *Fat* There is a human requirement for linoleic acid, which is a precursor of arachidonic acid, which is in turn a precursor of prostaglandins. Linoleic acid, an essential fatty acid, cannot be produced by humans. It has been recommended that this be supplied as 4% or more of total caloric intake. Commercial fat solutions consist of soybean or safflower oil, emulsified with egg phospholipid, and made isotonic at 300 mOsmol/L with added glycerol. Commercially available fat emulsions are available at concentrations of 10% or 20%.

7.3.2.1.3 *Carbohydrate* Glucose is the preferred carbohydrate for intravenous use. Glucose is widely available in concentrations from 5–70%. The osmolality of these solutions may be markedly hyperosmolar up to about 2,500 mOsmol/L.

7.3.2.1.4 *Nonprotein energy source* Once the initial 100 g of glucose is provided for use in the brain, renal medulla and red blood cells, glucose and fat are equally effective in preserving body nitrogen after an equilibration period of four to five days. Glucose is very inexpensive as an energy source, but requires insulin for uptake into cells, and hyperglycemia can be a problem when large amounts of glucose are utilized. The high osmolality of glucose solutions means that only dilute solutions can be used in peripheral veins, and if glucose is used as a major energy source, a large central vein is necessary to prevent thrombosis. Furthermore, glucose has a respiratory quotient (R.Q. = CO_2 produced/O_2 consumed) of 1.0, meaning that large amounts of carbon dioxide may be produced. Finally, glucose infusion leads to catecholamine release and increased metabolic rate, further increasing CO_2 production. These changes may be deleterious for patients being weaned from ventilators, or with borderline respiratory function.

Lipid solutions offer the benefit of being iso-osmolar, containing linoleic acid and having a lower respiratory quotient of 0.7, with less carbon dioxide production. Drawbacks include somewhat higher cost compared to glucose, and poor tolerance in patients with hyperlipidemia.

7.3.2.2 *Routes of delivery*

7.3.2.2.1 *Central* The most flexible way to deliver total parenteral nutrition is through a large central vein, usually the superior vena cava, via either the internal jugular or subclavian approach. With the large flow through the superior vena cava, solution osmolality is not of great concern, and thrombosis of this vessel is rare.

7.3.2.2.2 *Peripheral* Ten percent amino acid solutions approach 1,000 mOsmol/L, and 50% dextrose solutions are over 2,500 mOsmol/L, while intravenous fat solutions are, as mentioned, iso-osmolar at about 300 mOsmol/L. Therefore, fat must become the major caloric source in a system that infuses total parenteral nutrition into a peripheral vein. There is a minimum requirement of a 1:1 ratio of amino acid/dextrose solution to the lipid solution. The typical peripheral total parenteral nutrition regimen will consist of 1 L of 5% amino acid/10% dextrose solution, Y-connected to 1.5 L of 10% lipid. This provides 50 g "protein," 350 kcal as glucose and 1,650 kcal as lipid, with the final osmolality over 600 mOsmol/L. Because of this hypertonicity, it is still necessary to rotate the catheter site every 48 hours to prevent phlebitis.

7.3.2.3 *Complications*
Complications of total parenteral nutrition may be divided into local and systemic. Local problems relate to the catheter site, and in the case of central lines involve all the complications of central catheters, including inadvertent arterial catheterization with bleeding, pneumothorax, hemothorax and inadvertent infusion of solutions into the pleural cavity. The complication of pneumothorax is much more common with subclavian insertion than with internal

jugular insertion, meaning that internal jugular insertion is a safer technique, overall. Air embolism may occur at the time of insertion or any time thereafter with a central line. Catheter embolization may occur, and as mentioned, thrombosis has been reported, particularly with the use of stiff catheters. For long-term use, Silastic® catheters are preferred. It is essential that catheter placement be done by persons with considerable experience to minimize these complications.

Systemic complications include sepsis, metabolic problems and bone disease. Bacteremia or fungemia occurs in 3–7% of patients given total parenteral nutrition, and this appears to arise predominantly from the hub where the catheter joins the intravenous tubing. Catheters are always inserted in a strictly aseptic manner, with personnel fully gowned and gloved. Metabolic problems include hyperglycemia, which can be treated by reducing the amount of glucose given in the solutions, hypertriglyceridemia when excess calories and/or excess lipid is given, and alterations in electrolytes. In particular, total parenteral nutrition causes anabolism with increased intracellular water, so that potassium and phosphate are driven into cells, leading to possible hypokalemia and hypophosphatemia. These complications are very uncommon if adequate amounts of these electrolytes are provided and careful monitoring is performed. Liver disease remains a frustrating complication of total parenteral nutrition and occurs in up to 90% of cases, but in most cases the changes are restricted to enzyme elevations. In general, mild elevations in AST and alkaline phosphatase occur in the second week, with occasional elevations in bilirubin occurring later. Liver biopsy may show mild cholestasis. Overfeeding, particularly with glucose calories, may result in steatosis; this can be treated by reducing total calories and glucose. Rarely, long-term TPN (extending over years) may result in cirrhosis without a well-defined cause.

3

Gastroenterology and Medical Ethics

J.J. Sidorov

Basic moral principles and rules of medical ethics are as old as the medical profession itself. They were succinctly formulated in such codes as the Hippocratic Oath and Maimonides' Prayer, and have served for centuries as an unchanged moral base for medical practice. Major social and moral changes, particularly those of the second half of the 20th century, have challenged many of these classical values and modified others: witness the introduction of new attitudes toward sexuality and developments in transplantation of human tissues and organs, and opposing views on abortion. Promotion of the patient's autonomy and of human rights has led to the firm establishment of the right of the individual patient to be fully informed and consulted on all medical considerations and decisions related to his or her well-being, health and even death. The influence of such professionals as philosophers, ethicists, sociologists, anthropologists and lawyers has altered concepts of the patient–doctor relationship.

The change from a classical paternalistic to a modern participatory patient–doctor relationship has significantly altered the pattern of medical practice. When a patient consults a physician, a contractual arrangement takes place. The patient provides the physician with the personal, intimate information necessary for proper evaluation and rational management. Complete patient care must take into consideration the patient as a total person, including his or her personal moral values.

The rapid expansion of medical knowledge and technology has also introduced a range of expensive, complex, and often aggressive diagnostic and therapeutic procedures. The rising costs of many new, highly skilled, labor-intensive techniques have led to the rationing of our progressively diminishing health-care resources and raised difficult questions of fairness and priori-

TABLE 1.   Ethical principles and professional obligations

Ethical principles	Professional obligations
Beneficence	Confidentiality
Nonmaleficence	Fidelity (promise-keeping)
Respect for autonomy	Interest
Justice, fairness	Veracity (truth-telling)

ties: who gets what and why, at whose expense, and under what circumstances?

Application of current biomedical ethical principles to the changing clinical and social situation has thus become an essential part of the practice of modern medicine (Table 1).

Gastroenterologists share common ethical principles with and encounter problems similar to those faced by their colleagues in other medical disciplines. Like other specialists, gastroenterologists must often apply general medical ethical principles to specific areas of their activities. One such area is diagnostic and therapeutic endoscopy. Others include the treatment of patients with new, potent drugs, the active participation of gastroenterologists in drug trial studies, and their relationship with industry.

Transplantation of the liver, intestine and pancreas also raises ethical issues, particularly related to economy of resources. The demands that organ transplantation places on society lead to political rather than purely medical decisions concerning the allocation of resources and assignment of priorities. These decisions are not only based on the principle of individual beneficence, but they also are greatly influenced by social perceptions of justice and fairness. Gastroenterologists are being exposed to escalating pressure to control costs, ration resources and act as gatekeepers for organ transplantation. In addition to purely medical decisions, assessing patient suitability involves ethical issues. Should, for example, an individual with self-induced liver disease from abusing alcohol or other drugs, or from following a particular lifestyle, be accepted for transplantation?

Commerce involving organs or parts of organs is another area of ethical concern. Organ sale elsewhere in the world has been justified in that it is the only way to meet current needs. The issue is clouded by a lack of absolute ethical standards that could be uniformly applied in all parts of the world. Although medicine is generally transcultural, ethics is often culture-specific, as it depends on historical, religious, social and cultural factors. Ethical principles applicable to contemporary Western societies do not apply to parts of the world with completely different cultural and social traditions.

The availability of cadaveric organs is the main limiting factor in adult liver transplantation in Canada. According to a recent study, at least 37 patients died in Canada in 1991 while waiting for a new liver.

The Council on Ethics and Judicial Affairs of the American Medical Association has recommended a system of mandated choice, in which "everyone would be asked whether they consent to organ donation."

The Council of Europe has adopted a policy in 13 countries of "presumed consent" in which the onus is placed on the individual to opt out of cadaveric organ donation.

No such system exists in Canada. Canadian physicians therefore find themselves morally responsible for ensuring that no potentially available organ is wasted. Accordingly, a failure to secure such an organ, either by discouraging a donation as a result of personal bias, or failing through a passive attitude to consider the possibility and appropriateness of timely retrieval of a patient's organs, amounts to withholding a potentially lifesaving treatment from a waiting recipient.

The advent of fiberoptic endoscopy has had a major impact on research and clinical practice in gastroenterology. Ethical issues peculiar to gastrointestinal endoscopy are often not obvious. Gross violations of a code of ethics are easily detected and identified. The difficulty arises, however, when assessing skill, competence and quality control. It is often difficult to draw a clear line between professional competence and the safety of a procedure on one hand, and ethical behavior on the other.

Ethical considerations arising from invasive diagnostic and therapeutic gastroenterological procedures have been recently addressed in Canada by the Canadian Association of Gastroenterology in its consensus report "Consensus in Endoscopy." The patient's informed consent, based on a full understanding of risks and benefits, must be obtained prior to the procedure and sedation. While society's resources should be economically utilized, economic constraints should not adversely influence the quality of the care.

In addition to mandatory training requirements, the physician's technical and cognitive skills must be maintained through strict adherence to specified standards and must be further improved through constant learning.

Performance of endoscopic procedures in excess of diagnostic and therapeutic requirements and beyond the needs of approved research is unethical.

An innovative procedure or a significant modification of a standard procedure cannot be undertaken without prior approval by the institutional review board or the hospital ethics committee, and without the fully informed consent of the patient.

Life-support measures that provide nutrition through a variety of oral, enteral and parenteral routes have become the principal form of treatment of not only critically ill patients, but often also patients who are terminally ill.

Nonetheless, the belief that nutritional support is beneficial to terminally ill patients has been recently questioned.

Recent reports provide increasing evidence that withholding artificial nutrition and hydration is actually devoid of suffering, providing that oral food and liquids are given as requested by the patient and that proper care is taken of mouth and lips. While insufficient to maintain the patient's weight and life, this limited nutrition and hydration keeps the patient comfortable.

Since food and water have a strong emotional connotation as the essence of life, any attempt at withholding these is strongly resisted by care-givers. Furthermore, some physicians may not only try to persuade but may also resort to coercion and force a patient to accept a given form of artificial feeding. Strong ethical arguments are nevertheless being put forward that prolonging the life of a terminally ill patient through artificial nutrition and hydration prolongs suffering and delays the natural process of death. It therefore violates the ethical principle of beneficence and nonmaleficence. When carried out against the patient's expressed wish or through coercion it also violates the principle of autonomy.

Close cooperation between the pharmaceutical industry and the medical profession has greatly contributed to recent progress in research and to educational opportunities. The development of new drugs requires clinical trials. Development of a new drug from the initial invention of a chemical structure until its final approval for general use takes an average of 10 to 15 years and may cost up to $100 million before realizing any financial return. The industry is quite aware that commercial objectives must not override ethical considerations and has developed the guidelines governing the conduct of such studies. By subscribing to such codes, the industry has accepted responsibility for proper monitoring and supervision of sound clinical trials. For their part, those physicians involved in a clinical study must possess adequate knowledge and devote the necessary time to ensure that no breach of ethical principles occurs.

It is unethical to enter a patient into a trial unless the investigator truly believes that the new drug or procedure will provide benefits beyond those already available. The investigator must be free to publish the results regardless of the outcome, unencumbered by the private interests of the sponsor. The principal investigator shares with the sponsor the responsibility for the scientific validity, ethical content and correctness of the clinical evaluation of the product undergoing trial. The investigator may be remunerated for clinical work (such as physical examination, endoscopies and other technical procedures) if charged for at standard rates. It is unethical, however, to derive personal financial benefit as a reward for participating in or conducting the study.

Medical research using human subjects requires careful scrutiny. A recent study by an international group of reviewers found that a significant proportion of studies involving humans, and published in some of the leading gastroenterology journals, failed to meet ethical standards as defined by the reviewers. Approximately 40% would have been rejected by reviewers had they been members of the review boards at the institutions where the work was done. Some 12% of these "rejections" involved perceived danger to participating patients; the remainder involved poor study design or problems of statistical analysis. Between 10 and 15% of medications used were subsequently discovered to be potentially toxic.

There seem to be several places where a potential deficiency may originate. Concern about personal career development and academic pressure to demonstrate research productivity might induce an investigator to disregard what might at first appear to be a trivial issue. Casual supervision and inadequate quality control by senior, experienced and established investigators could be another factor. Poorly conducted research leading to faulty conclusions based on avoidable deficiencies and errors is unethical. Just because a project has received the approval of an institutional review board, there is no guarantee that it will remain ethical throughout. Finally, the system of peer review, the traditional method of ensuring the quality of scientific investigation, is not infallible. Close supervision based on clearly defined institutional publication policies and periodic careful review of the study's progress may eliminate many of these ethical pitfalls. The ethical component must be part of the scientific review.

The complexity of current scientific, technical, philosophical and social developments and other conditions in the second half of 20th century present a plethora of ethical issues that we need to consider in our daily work – clinical practice, research or teaching. We should always consider the patient not only as a collection of symptoms, signs and pathological processes but also as an individual with emotions, problems and moral standards. Biomedical ethics is an integral part of such care. Familiarity with basic bioethical principles (Table 1) is as essential for the practice of medicine as the knowledge of pathophysiology is for the understanding of the disease process.

SUGGESTED READING LIST

Bailey RJ, Barkun A, Brow J, et al. Consensus in endoscopy. Can J Gastroenterol 1996; 10:237–242.

Bricker BM. Industrial marketing and medical ethics. N Engl J Med 1989; 320:1690–1692.

Canada. Health Protection Branch, Health and Welfare Canada. Code of good monitoring practice for clinical investigators. 1983.

CMA guidelines for drug–company supported CME. CMAJ 1986; 135:384A.

Davies IB, Grind IM, Pottage A, Turner P. Development of new drugs in man: a review. J Roy Soc Med 1986; 79:96–99.

DeDombal PT, Holt PR, Sidorov JJ. Ethics in gastroenterology: proceedings of a workshop meeting of the World Organisation of Gastroenterology held at St. George's House, Windsor Castle, Berkshire, England, 29 April – 2 May 1986. Leeds: University of Leeds Printing Service, 1986:21–24.

Duggan JM. Resource allocation and bioethics. Lancet 1989; 1:772–773.

Engler RL, Covell JW, Friedman PJ, Kitcher PS, Peters RM. Misrepresentation and responsibility in medical research. N Engl J Med 1987; 317:1383–1389.

Gibinski K. Ethics and training in digestive endoscopy. Endoscopy 1989; 21:232–233.

Grad MR. Human experimentation and informed consent. CMAJ 1984; 131:932–935.

Leaf A. The doctor's dilemma — and society's too. N Engl J Med 1984; 310:718–720.

MCann RM, Hall WJ, Groth-Juncker A. Comfort care for terminally ill patients. JAMA 1994; 272:1263–1266.

McGregor M. Pharmaceutical "generosity" and the medical profession. Ann RCPSC 1988; 21:289.

Mullen MA, Kohut N, Sam M, Blendis L, Singer PA. Access to adult liver transplantation in Canada: a survey and ethical analysis. CMAJ 1996; 154:337–342.

Omery A, Caswell D. A nursing perspective on the ethical issues surrounding liver transplantation. Heart and Lung 1988; 17:626–630.

Rawlins MD. Doctors and the drug makers. Lancet 1984; 2:276–278.

Reagan MD. Health care rationing: what does it mean? N Engl J Med 1988; 319:1149–1151.

Reagan MD. Physicians as gatekeepers: a complex challenge. N Engl J Med 1987; 317:1731–1733.

The Royal College of Physicians of London. The relationship between physicians and the pharmaceutical industry: a report of the Royal College of Physicians. J Roy Col Phy of London 1986; 20:235–241.

Sabesin SM, Williams JW, Evans LS. Ethical and economic issues. In: Maddrey WC (ed.), Transplantation of the liver. New York: Elsevier, 1988:331–343.

Sidorov JJ. Ethical dilemmas in gastroenterology. Med North Am 1995; 472–476.

Sidorov JJ. Ethics in gastrointestinal research. Scand J Gastroenterol 1988; 23(Suppl. 144):100–113.

Singer PA, Siegler M, Whitington RF, et al. Ethics of liver transplantation with living donors. N Engl J Med 1989; 321:620–621.

Sircus W. Ethics of diagnostic and therapeutic endoscopic procedures. Scand J Gastroenterol 1988; 23(Suppl. 144):105–106.

Thompson WG. The ethics of physician–pharmaceutical company relationships. CMAJ 1988; 129:835–836.

Williams JR. Human organ sales. Ann RCPSC 1985; 18:401–404.

Younger SJ, Allen M, Bartlet ET, et al. Psychosocial and ethical implications of organ retrieval. N Engl J Med 1985; 313:321–323.

4

Pharmaceutical Research and Clinical Trials: The Basis for New Knowledge

A. Archambault and B.G. Feagan

1. INTRODUCTION

The scientific study of new drugs is an important research activity that requires close cooperation between investigators in industry and in academia. Despite the relatively small size of the Canadian pharmaceutical market (3% of global drug expenditures), Canadian investigators have played a leading role in the development of new drug treatments for both peptic ulcer disease and inflammatory bowel disease. Since the development of a new drug may require 10 to 15 years of investment in research before a product reaches the market, and only one out of 8,000 substances initially tested in animal models can be expected to result in the development of a useful treatment in humans, this activity is both time-consuming and expensive. The goal of this chapter is to familiarize the reader with the activities necessary for the development of new drug treatments.

2. CLINICAL RESEARCH REGULATIONS AND SUPERVISION

Investigators, sponsors and institutional authorities share equal responsibility for producing high-quality data and following ethical recommendations for the conduct of biomedical research involving human subjects. The Declaration of Helsinki – first proposed in Finland in 1964 and later revised by the World Medical Assembly in Hong Kong in 1989 – is a universally accepted ethical code.

In 1987 the Medical Research Council of Canada (MRC) approved guidelines for research involving human subjects. The latest guidelines for good clinical research practices are stipulated in a document entitled "Conduct of

Clinical Investigations"; they were officially adopted by the Health Protection Branch (HPB) of the Canadian government in 1989.

In the United States, federal regulations concerning the development of new drugs and their subsequent admissibility for clinical investigation were in place as early as 1938. Following the tragic events surrounding the use of thalidomide in the 1950s, important amendments were adopted: review of preclinical data, the informed consent of patients and the reporting of preclinical findings became mandatory in 1962. In an attempt to standardize compliance with regulatory requirements, good clinical practice (GCP) rules for sponsors (1977) and for investigators (1978) were developed by industry. The investigational new drug (IND) regulation was established in 1987.

The most recent and comprehensive set of guidelines for drug trials emerged in October 1990 as a result of a meeting where the tenets of good practice were compared by scientists from the European Community and North America. Uniform standards were subsequently defined.

Although some differences exist among countries in the government regulations governing clinical research in humans, these guidelines are becoming more uniform.

3. CLINICAL RESEARCH DEVELOPMENT

The research process includes both preclinical studies and clinical trials.

3.1 Preclinical Studies

The pharmaceutical industry must identify chemical structures for synthesis and subsequently assess the biological effects of these compounds in laboratory and animal models. Compounds that show promising biological effects are selected for further study.

Preclinical studies are usually conducted in the research laboratory of pharmaceutical companies or in university centers. Once a potential compound has been identified, a pharmacological expert analyzes the main biological effects of the drug, its duration of action and the adverse effects of the compound in various animal species. Pharmacokinetic studies performed in animals define the absorption, volume of distribution, metabolism and excretion of the candidate compound. Toxicological studies are performed to identify any possible mutagenic or teratogenic effects of the drug. Compounds that meet the requirements of these early studies are further assessed to determine the optimal dosage and route of administration. From these studies a drug may be selected for further development. These goals usually can be achieved within two to four years. At this time a submission to the regulatory authorities for authorization to administer the potential new drug (IND: investigational new drug) to humans is applied for. The latter process involves a well-defined procedure that may require an additional few months for approval. During this process the preclinical data are reviewed by an appropriate national regulatory body, such as the U.S. Food and Drug Administration (FDA) or the HPB in Canada. These agencies follow similar procedures, and for this reason multicenter studies are often performed using similar protocols in the two countries.

3.2 Clinical Trials

Four phases of clinical drug development are recognized.

3.2.1 PHASE I

These studies are carried out in small numbers of *normal, healthy volunteers*. The primary objective is to test the compound for safety and tolerability. These studies are done initially with a single dose, then with multiple doses. Pharmacokinetic and pharmacodynamic studies in humans must be performed with close medical surveillance and continuous monitoring of patients for adverse effects. During the time that Phase I studies are underway, animal studies for toxicity and potential carcinogenicity are continued.

3.2.2 PHASE II

At this phase, pilot studies to evaluate the efficacy and safety of a new drug are performed in *patients with the specific disease of interest*. The studies are usually short-term and may either be placebo-controlled or employ a comparison with a standard therapy. The emphasis in Phase II is on the definition of the most appropriate dose, dosing interval and route of administration. These studies often provide information that is vital for the design of Phase III trials. The latter provide definitive data regarding the efficacy and safety of a new drug.

Animal studies for toxicity and carcinogenicity continue during this phase.

3.2.3 PHASE III

These studies, which are usually conducted in a large number of patients, are designed to demonstrate either short- or long-term efficacy and provide further safety data. A Phase III trial usually compares a fixed dose of the new drug to conventional therapy under conditions that approximate those of usual clinical care. The therapeutic profile of the drug is defined by the results of these studies, which determine the final indications, dosage, route of administration, contraindications, adverse effects and possible drug interactions.

The duration of Phases II and III is often in the range of three to five years.

Following accumulation of appropriate Phase II and III data, a submission to regulatory authorities is filed (NDS: New Drug Submission). These data are then scrutinized by the appropriate government experts. In Canada it may require an additional two years before approval to market the product is received.

3.2.4 PHASE IV
Following approval for general use, the evaluative process continues. Clinical studies are performed with approved or marketed drugs to gather more information on possible adverse events, to compare them with alternative treatments, and to detect interactions with other drugs. Due to the low prevalence of most serious adverse events, Phase IV observational studies (postmarket surveillance) are often the only means of adequately defining the safety profile of new compounds. During this period, new indications, new formulations or effective combinations of the new drug with existing therapies may be explored. The knowledge of a new pharmaceutical grows gradually through the various phases of clinical research, and it is never 100% complete. All relevant findings must be documented and reported, regardless of the time that has passed since the initial approval of the drug for general use.

4. METHODOLOGY IN CLINICAL RESEARCH

The randomized, controlled trial is the benchmark for the evaluation of new drug therapies. Random allocation is a powerful means of controlling for the potential effects of confounders and serves to minimize bias (systematic deviation from the truth) on the part of physicians and patients. Concealing the treatment allocation from the patient and investigator (blinding), which reduces the potential for bias, is also a fundamental component of a rigorously designed clinical trial. Considerable controversy has arisen regarding the use of placebo controls in evaluating new drugs. Some authors have argued against their use on the basis that patients are denied treatment of proven efficacy and thus may experience some degree of morbidity by participation in a placebo-controlled study. However, a placebo comparison allows an evaluation of the new therapy against the alternative of no treatment, and thus is scientifically valid and ethical when the standard therapy has only modest efficacy or causes important adverse effects. In Phase III trials it is vital that investigators choose as a primary measure of response an outcome that is clinically meaningful. In the past there has been an over-reliance on surrogate markers of efficacy such as improvements in laboratory tests. In some instances these have been shown not to correlate with clinically meaningful events. Investigators should consider utilization of quality of life measures as measures of response in addition to the more conventional outcomes of death, occurrence of disease-related complications and clinical activity indices. Once an appropriate outcome has been identified, the planning of a clinical trial requires input from a biostatistician. Careful consideration is given to the number of patients required, which is dependent upon the alpha (false positive) and beta (false negative) error rates selected by the investigator, the size of treatment effect that is considered to be clinically meaningful and the estimated rate of occurrence of the outcome of interest in the placebo (or standard therapy) group. If interim analyses are planned, these must be defined prior to initiation of the study, and appropriate statistical techniques employed to account for the increase in the alpha error rate that results from the use of multiple statistical testing procedures.

5. PLANNING OF CLINICAL TRIALS

5.1 Protocol Design and Implementation

The study protocol should explicitly state the rationale for studying the drug in the disease of interest. The source and chemical nature of the compound, its pharmacology and toxicology, and the data obtained in previous clinical investigations must be present in appropriate detail. All study protocols must be approved by the appropriate regulatory authorities. The objectives of the study must be clearly stated and appropriate methodology employed to ensure that these are met. The study treatment schedule should define the drug administration (dosage, strength, route of administration, the blinding process, packaging and labeling) in sufficient detail.

The inclusion and exclusion criteria, baseline, pre- and post-treatment measurement and evaluation visits and procedures for reporting adverse events and treatment overdoses must be clearly specified.

A study discontinuation procedure is defined in the event of lack of efficacy, intolerable side effects, poor patient compliance or the occurrence of a treatment endpoint.

Detailed definitions of the statistical analysis, data management procedures, administrative structure of the study and insurance and liability requirements are also necessary.

The protocol should contain a description of the background information that is provided to the patient and the informed consent document. For the patient's protection, lay language must be used. Diary forms and informed consent papers must be translated into the patient's primary language.

Once a protocol has been developed, an appropriate study administrative structure should be organized. An executive (steering) committee is constituted, which is responsible for the strategic aspects of conducting the trial. Usually other committees are organized to oversee the operational aspects of the trial, to monitor the safety of participants, and to adjudicate key outcomes.

5.2 Selection of Investigators and Centers

The selection of the investigators for clinical research will depend on the nature of the drug and the phase of the investigation. Experts in clinical pharmacology are selected for Phase I and II studies; experts in medical practice or medical specialties will usually be selected for Phase III and IV studies. The principal investigator in each center is responsible for the study in accordance with the protocol and for the accurate and complete reporting of the results: he or she must sign a formal statement of agreement for the study and its commitments and provide copies for the sponsor and government authorities. Investigators are selected on the basis of several criteria, including their past record in peer-reviewed medical research, their current interest in the proposed study and available time to participate. Appropriate on-site hospital or private clinic facilities with adequate space, equipment, safe drug storage, assistance from a research nurse and access to a certified laboratory are essential prerequisites for participation in clinical trials. The laboratory must be able to conduct the study according to the guidelines of good laboratory practices (GLP) adopted by the FDA in 1978. In addition, the investigators should be able to make an estimate of the number of study subjects available at their centers so a recruitment projection can be derived. The investigators must agree to have their facility and data audited at any time by the sponsor's representatives or by the regulatory authorities (FDA or HPB).

6. INFORMED CONSENT FORM AND ETHICAL ISSUES

The informed consent form is a written description of the nature and purpose of the trial. This document includes an explanation of the nature of randomization and includes a description of the benefits, foreseeable risks, discomforts and potential side effects of participating in the study. The consent form should inform the patient that he or she has the right to withdraw from the study at any time without prejudice, and that alternative treatments are available, should he or she decide not to participate in the study. The consent form is presented to the patient, preferably in the presence of an impartial witness, by the investigator or a qualified delegate; sufficient time must be allowed for the patient to consider the information and to ask questions.

This form is an acknowledgment that specific information has been given; it is never proof that the subject has been fully informed. It does not indicate the degree of comprehension or autonomy of the patient. Even if the informed consent is for the protection of the investigator and the patient, it has no legal power in North America.

7. CLINICAL MONITORING

An essential aspect of the conduct of clinical research is monitoring. All aspects of these investigations must be open and verifiable upon independent audit.

Accountability of the drug dispensed to the patients includes surveillance of the expiry date, lot numbers, stability and storage conditions. Compliance with the study medication requirements should be assessed by direct questioning and/or pill counts. All unused medication should be returned to the investigator.

The patient's condition before, during and after the treatment period, laboratory data, concomitant therapy, and adverse events should be accurately recorded using standardized procedures at specified times. Information that is recorded in the case report form should be consistent with information documented in the patient's medical record. Principles of good clinical practice (GCP) should be followed. The number and extent of audits will vary from study to study, depending upon specific requirements.

At the completion of the study, the final evaluation of data for both efficacy and safety is undertaken by an adjudication committee. This committee ensures the accuracy, completeness and legibility of the data. Finally, the results and conclusion of the study are summarized in a final report which must be reviewed and signed by the investigators. Publication of the data in a peer-reviewed medical journal follows.

8. INSTITUTIONAL REVIEW COMMITTEE (IRC)

No patient can be enrolled in a clinical trial before an institutional review committee has accepted the protocol and the informed consent form.

During this process, the scientific aspects of a trial are evaluated by experienced clinical researchers in each institution where the study is performed. Modifications to the protocol suggested by the IRC should be carefully considered by the investigators.

The committee should comprise at least five sufficiently qualified members: both sexes must be represented and members should be sensitive to local racial and cultural issues. There should be at least one nonscientific member and one member who is not affiliated with the institution. There should be no conflicting interests for any of the committee members.

The elements of the informed consent to be considered by the members of the committee are numerous. These are specifically outlined in the Declaration of Helsinki.

Confirmation of acceptance of a study by the IRC must be transmitted with the signed agreement form to the government authorities.

9. CONCLUSION

The efficacy and safety of a drug must be well established by appropriate therapeutic trials before it can be accepted for clinical use. Internationally accepted regulatory standards, scientific principles of clinical trial design and good clinical practice rules have evolved to meet these requirements. This chapter should provide the medical student with some basic information concerning drug development and with a better understanding of this important area of clinical research.

BIBLIOGRAPHY

Canada. Health Protection Branch, Health and Welfare Canada. Drugs Directorate guidelines.
a. Preparation of human new drug submissions (1991).
b. Conduct of clinical investigations. No. H42-2/14 (July 1989).

Canada. Medical Research Council of Canada. Guidelines on research involving human subjects. Minister of Supply and Services Canada, 1987. No. MR 21-5/1987E.

The clinical trial in Canada, USA, in Nordic and EEC countries. 2nd Symposium on drug development sponsored by the Faculty of Pharmacy of the Université de Montréal and the Health Protection Branch, Canada, May 6–7, 1990, Montréal, Québec. Montréal: Université de Montréal, 1990 (binder).

Declaration of Helsinki: Recommendations Guiding Physicians in Biomedical Research Involving Human Subjects.

France. Ministère des affaires sociales et de l'emploi. Ministre chargé de la santé et de la famille. Bulletin officiel. Direction des journaux officiels, 26, rue Desaix, 75105 Paris, France.

Good Clinical Research Practices Limited. Clinical study monitoring (binder).
Three-day course presented in Mississauga, Ontario, March 1991.
Bolaychuk WP, Ph.D.
Ball GT, C.D., Ph.D.
Kimpton DJ.
European office: Round Windows, Grayshott Road, Headly Down, Hampshire, U.K. GU 358JL.

Guidelines for research and ethical rules from FDA (U.S.A.)

Review articles. Drug Information Journal (January/June 1982):7–96.

5
The Esophagus
W.G. Paterson and S. Mayrand

1. INTRODUCTION

The esophagus is a hollow muscular organ whose primary function is to propel into the stomach the food or fluid bolus that it receives from the pharynx. Symptoms of esophageal disease are among the most commonly encountered in gastroenterology. Fortunately, most symptoms are due to benign disease that can be easily remedied. The physician must be on the lookout, however, for the more serious disorders, which can present with a similar spectrum of symptoms. This chapter will focus on the pathophysiology, diagnosis and management of the more common esophageal disorders. Rare diseases involving the esophagus will be dealt with only briefly.

2. ANATOMY

2.1 Muscular Anatomy

The esophagus is a hollow muscular tube closed proximally by the upper esophageal sphincter (UES) and distally by the lower esophageal sphincter (LES). The UES consists predominantly of the cricopharyngeus and the caudal fibers of the inferior pharyngeal constrictor muscles. The UES forms a transverse slit at the C5–C6 vertebral level due to surrounding bony structures and cartilage. In the proximal one-quarter to one-third of the esophagus, the muscle is striated. There is then a transition zone of variable length where there is a mixture of both smooth and striated muscle. The distal one-half to one-third of the esophageal body and LES are composed of smooth muscle. The LES is located at the junction between the esophagus and stomach, usually localized at or just below the diaphragmatic hiatus. Despite its distinct physiological function, it is not easily distinguished anatomically.

2.2 Innervation

The motor innervation of the esophagus is via the vagus nerves. The cell bodies of the vagal efferent fibers innervating the UES and the proximal striated- muscle esophagus arise in the nucleus ambiguus, whereas fibers destined for the distal smooth-muscle segment and the LES originate in the dorsal motor nucleus. The esophagus and LES also receive sympathetic nerve supply (both motor and sensory) arising from spinal segments T1–T10. Sensory innervation is also carried via the vagus and consists of bipolar nerves that have their cell bodies in the nodose ganglion and project from there to the brainstem.

2.3 Blood Supply

Arterial blood supply to the UES and cervical esophagus is via branches of the inferior thyroid artery. Most of the thoracic esophagus is supplied by paired aortic esophageal arteries or terminal branches of bronchial arteries. The LES and the most distal segment of the esophagus are supplied by the left gastric artery and by a branch of the left phrenic artery. Venous drainage is via an extensive submucosal plexus that drains into the superior vena cava from the proximal esophagus and into the azygous system from the mid-esophagus. In the distal esophagus, collaterals from the left gastric vein (a branch of the portal vein) and the azygos interconnect in the submucosa. This connection between the portal and systemic venous systems is clinically important; when there is hypertension, variceal dilation can occur in this area. These submucosal esophageal varices can be the source of major gastrointestinal hemorrhage.

2.4 Lymphatic Drainage

In the proximal third of the esophagus, lymphatics drain into the deep cervical lymph nodes, whereas in the middle third, drainage is into the superior and posterior mediastinal nodes. The distal-third lymphatics follow the left gastric artery to the gastric and celiac lymph nodes. There is considerable interconnection among these three drainage regions.

2.5 Histology

The wall of the esophagus consists of mucosa, submucosa and muscularis propria. Unlike other areas of the gut, it does not have a distinct serosal covering, but is covered by a thin layer of loose connective tissue. The mucosa consists of stratified squamous epithelium in all regions of the esophagus except the LES, where both squamous and columnar epithelium may coexist. Beneath the epithelium are the lamina propria and the longitudinally oriented muscularis mucosa. The submucosa contains connective tissue as well as lymphocytes, plasma cells and nerve cells (Meissner's plexus). The muscularis propria consists of an inner circular and an outer longitudinal muscle layer. The circular muscle layer provides the sequential peristaltic contraction that propels the food bolus toward the stomach. Between the circular and longitudinal muscle layers lies another nerve plexus called the myenteric or Auerbach's plexus, which mediates much of the intrinsic nervous control of esophageal motor function.

3. PHYSIOLOGY

The major function of the esophagus is to propel swallowed food or fluid into the stomach. This is carried out by sequential or "peristaltic" contraction of the esophageal body in concert with appropriately timed relaxation of the upper and lower esophageal sphincters. The esophagus also clears any refluxed gastric contents back into the stomach and takes part in such reflex activities as vomiting and belching.

3.1 Deglutition: Primary Peristalsis
The act of deglutition is a complex reflex activity. The initial phase is under voluntary control. Food is chewed, mixed with saliva and formed into an appropriately sized bolus before being thrust to the posterior pharynx by the tongue. Once the bolus reaches the posterior pharynx, receptors are activated that initiate the involuntary phase of deglutition. This involves the carefully sequenced contraction of myriad head and neck muscles. The food bolus is rapidly engulfed and pushed toward the esophagus by the pharyngeal constrictor muscles. Simultaneously there is activation of muscles that lift the palate and close off and elevate the larynx in order to prevent misdirection of the bolus. Almost immediately upon activation of this reflex, the UES opens just long enough to allow the food bolus to pass through; it then rapidly shuts to prevent retrograde passage of the bolus. The oropharyngeal phase is thus completed and the esophageal phase takes over. This involves two major phenomena: (1) the sequential contraction of the circular muscle of the esophageal body, which results in a contractile wave that migrates toward the stomach; and (2) the relaxation and opening of the LES, which allows the bolus to pass. The peristaltic sequence and associated UES and LES relaxation induced by swallowing are termed *primary peristalsis*. These can be assessed manometrically using an intraluminal tube to measure pressures. The typical sequence seen during primary peristalsis is depicted in Figure 1. *Secondary peristalsis* refers to a peristaltic sequence that occurs in response to distention of the esophagus. This is a localized peristaltic wave that usually begins just above the area of distention. It is associated with LES relaxation, but not with UES relaxation or deglutition.

FIGURE 1. Schematic representation of primary peristalsis as recorded by intraluminal manometry. Swallowing is marked by a rapid pharyngeal contraction coincident with abrupt relaxation of the UES. This is followed by postrelaxation contraction of the UES and sequential contraction of the esophageal body, which produces a pressure wave that migrates toward the stomach. A swallowed food bolus is pushed in front of this migrating contraction wave. The LES relaxes within 1 to 2 seconds of the onset of swallowing and remains relaxed until the esophageal pressure wave has reached the distal esophagus. LES pressure then recovers and is followed by a postrelaxation contraction, which occurs in continuity with the distal esophageal contraction.

SOURCE: Goyal RK, Paterson WG. Esophageal motility. In: Wood JD (ed.), Handbook of physiology: motility and circulation, vol. 4. Washington DC: American Physiological Society, 1989. Used with permission.

3.2 Upper Esophageal Sphincter Function

The UES serves as a pressure barrier to prevent retrograde flow of esophageal contents and the entry of air into the esophagus during inspiration. This high-pressure zone is created by tonic contraction of the UES muscles, which is produced by tonic neuronal discharge of vagal lower motor neurons. With deglutition this neuronal discharge ceases temporarily and permits relaxation of the UES. UES opening will not occur with relaxation of the muscles alone; it requires elevation and anterior displacement of the larynx, which is mediated by contraction of the suprahyoid muscles. Relaxation lasts for only one second and is followed by a postrelaxation contraction (Figure 1).

3.3 Esophageal Body Peristalsis

There is a fundamental difference in the control mechanisms of peristalsis between the upper (striated-muscle) esophagus and the lower (smooth-muscle) esophagus. In the striated-muscle segment, peristalsis is produced by sequential firing of vagal lower motor neurons so that upper segments contract first and more aboral segments subsequently. In the smooth-muscle segment, the vagal preganglionic efferent fibers have some role in the aboral sequencing of contraction, but intrinsic neurons are also capable of evoking peristalsis independently of the extrinsic nervous system. Transection of vagal motor fibers to the esophagus in experimental animals will abolish primary peristalsis throughout the esophagus; however, in this setting, distention-induced or secondary peristalsis will be maintained in the smooth-muscle but not in the striated-muscle segment. Furthermore, if vagal efferent fibers are stimulated electrically (Figure 2), a simultaneous contraction will be produced in the striated-muscle esophagus that begins with the onset of the electrical stimulus, lasts throughout the stimulus, and ends abruptly when the stimulus is terminated. In the smooth-muscle esophagus, however, the response to vagal efferent nerve stimulation is quite different, in that the onset of contractions is delayed relative to the onset of the stimulus. The latency to onset of the contraction increases in the more distal segments of the esophagus (i.e., the evoked contractions are peristaltic).

This experimental observation indicates that intrinsic neuromuscular mechanisms exist and can mediate peristalsis on their own. Further evidence for this mechanism is found in studies where strips of esophageal circular smooth muscle are stimulated electrically in vitro. The latency to contraction after stimulation is shortest in the strips taken from the proximal smooth-muscle segment and increases progressively in the more distal strips.

This latency gradient of contraction is clearly important in the production of esophageal peristalsis. Although the exact mechanisms are unclear, initial or deglutitive inhibition is important. With primary or secondary peristalsis, a

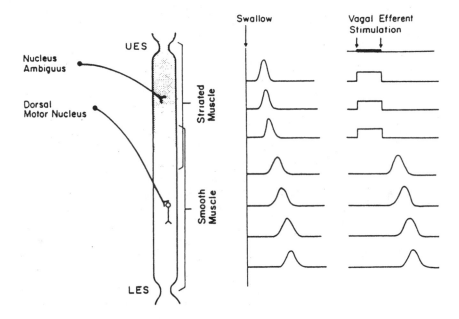

FIGURE 2. Schematic representation of esophageal peristaltic contractions as evoked by swallowing and vagal efferent nerve stimulation. Swallowing evokes sequential esophageal contractions that pass smoothly from the striated- to the smooth-muscle segment. Electrical stimulation of the distal cut end of a vagus nerve, which simultaneously activates all vagal efferent fibers, evokes peristaltic contractions only in the smooth-muscle segment of the esophagus. In the striated-muscle esophagus, vagal stimulation causes simultaneous contractions that occur only during the period of stimulation. This demonstrates that the striated-muscle esophagus is dependent on central neuronal sequencing for its peristaltic contraction, whereas intrinsic neuronal mechanisms are capable of producing a persistaltic sequence in the smooth-muscle segment.
SOURCE: Goyal RK, Paterson WG. Esophageal motility. In: Wood JD (ed.), Handbook of physiology: motility and circulation, vol. 4. Washington DC: American Physiological Society, 1989. Used with permission.

wave of neurally mediated inhibition initially spreads rapidly down the esophagus. This is caused by the release of a nonadrenergic, noncholinergic inhibitory neurotransmitter (most likely nitric oxide) that produces hyperpolarization (inhibition) of the circular smooth muscle. It is only after recovery from the initial hyperpolarization that esophageal muscle contraction (which is mediated primarily by cholinergic neurons) can occur. Thus, the duration of this initial inhibition is important with respect to the differential timing of the subsequent contraction. Derangements of the mechanisms behind this latency gradient lead to nonperistaltic contractions and dysphagia. Such derangements could result from problems with either the intrinsic neural mechanisms (enteric nervous system) or the central neuronal sequencing.

3.4 Lower Esophageal Sphincter Function

The LES is an intraluminal high-pressure zone caused by tonic contraction of a region of physiologically distinct circular smooth muscle at the junction of the esophagus and stomach. This results in a pressure barrier that separates the esophagus from the stomach and serves to prevent reflux of gastric contents up into the esophagus. In normal individuals, resting LES pressure averages between 10 and 30 mm Hg above intragastric pressure. Patients with very feeble resting LES pressure are prone to develop gastroesophageal reflux disease (GERD). Unlike that of the UES, the resting tone of the LES is primarily due to myogenic factors that result in tonic contraction of the sphincter. Extrinsic innervation as well as circulating hormones can modify the resting tone; however, the muscle fibers themselves have inherent properties that result in their being tonically contracted.

At the time of deglutition or when the esophagus is distended, the LES promptly relaxes. Swallow-induced LES relaxation is mediated by vagal efferent fibers that synapse on nonadrenergic, noncholinergic inhibitory neurons of the myenteric plexus. The inhibitory neurotransmitter released from these intrinsic neurons is probably nitric oxide. LES relaxation usually lasts about five to seven seconds, and is sufficient to abolish the gastroesophageal pressure barrier. This permits the food bolus to pass unimpeded from the esophagus to the stomach. The LES also relaxes to permit belching or vomiting. Inadequate LES relaxation is seen in achalasia and results in dysphagia.

4. SYMPTOMS AND SIGNS OF ESOPHAGEAL DISEASES

4.1 Symptoms

4.1.1 *DYSPHAGIA*

This sensation of food sticking during swallowing is a manifestation of impaired transit of food through the mouth, pharynx or esophagus. It is important to differentiate oropharyngeal ("transfer") dysphagia from esophageal dysphagia. If the patient has problems getting the bolus out of the mouth, then one can be certain of an oropharyngeal cause; if the food sticks retrosternally, an esophageal cause is indicated. Some patients, however, will sense food sticking at the level of the suprasternal notch when the actual obstruction is the distal esophagus. Thus, it can be difficult to determine the site of the problem when patients refer their dysphagia to the suprasternal notch or throat area. With these patients it is important to elicit any ancillary symptoms of oropharyngeal-type dysphagia, such as choking or nasal regurgitation. It may also be helpful to observe the patient swallowing in an attempt to determine the timing of the symptom; with esophageal dysphagia referred to the suprasternal notch, the sensation of dysphagia onsets several seconds after swallowing begins.

The history can also be used to help differentiate structural from functional (i.e., motility disorders) causes of dysphagia. Dysphagia that is episodic and occurs with both liquids and solids from the outset suggests a motor disorder, whereas when the dysphagia is initially for solids such as meat and bread, and then progresses with time to semisolids and liquids, one should suspect a structural cause (e.g., stricture). If such a progression is rapid and associated with significant weight loss, a malignant stricture is suspected.

Associated symptoms help determine the etiology of dysphagia. For instance, a reflux-induced stricture should be suspected if the dysphagia is associated with heartburn or regurgitation, esophageal cancer if there is associated mid-back pain and weight loss, a motor disorder such as diffuse esophageal spasm if there is angina-like chest pain, and a "scleroderma esophagus" if there is arthralgia, skin changes or Raynaud's phenomenon.

4.1.2 ODYNOPHAGIA

This refers to the sensation of pain on swallowing. Local inflammation or neoplasia in the mouth and pharynx can produce such pain. When the pain is retrosternal, one should suspect nonreflux-induced forms of esophagitis, such as infection, radiation or pill-induced (chemical) injury. Less commonly it occurs with esophageal cancer, a deep esophageal ulcer (e.g., Barrett's ulcer) or esophageal motor disorders.

4.1.3 HEARTBURN OR PYROSIS

The sensation here is one of retrosternal burning. Typically it begins in the low retrosternal area and radiates up to the throat. It may be precipitated by bending over or lying down, and usually begins shortly after consuming certain foods or beverages. It is often associated with regurgitation of acidic material into the back of the throat. "Heartburn" with these features indicates gastroesophageal reflux. This very common symptom has been experienced at one time or another by over one-third of the population and therefore does not necessarily indicate serious disease. Many patients will complain of "heartburn," but this should not be taken at face value: this term is used by some patients to describe unrelated symptomatology. It is therefore important to have patients describe exactly what they mean by the term *heartburn*.

4.1.4 REGURGITATION

This refers to the spontaneous appearance of food or fluid in the back of the throat or in the mouth. Some patients describe this symptom as "vomiting"; therefore it is important to determine whether there is associated nausea, retching, etc., when patients present with "vomiting." The taste and consistency of the regurgitated material is an important historical detail. Regurgitation of acidic or bile-stained fluid indicates gastroesophageal reflux. Regurgitation of undigested food or stagnant fluid devoid of an acidic taste indicates an esophageal transport problem (e.g., achalasia). (With achlorhydria, gastric contents also lack acid.) In motor disorders and mechanical obstruction of the esophagus, food may become stuck and then rather quickly will be regurgitated if it does not pass through into the stomach. Some patients regurgitate food back into their mouths after a meal only to chew and swallow it all over again. This is called *rumination* and, although a rarity in humans, it is a normal physiological event in certain animals.

4.1.5 NONHEARTBURN CHEST PAIN

This can also indicate esophageal disease. Chest pain, and in particular middorsal pain, is seen in advanced esophageal cancer. The most common type of nonheartburn esophageal chest pain, however, is a pain that is qualitatively similar to the pain of ischemic heart disease. This pain can be squeezing or crushing and can radiate into the jaw or arms. Unlike ischemic heart pain, angina-like chest pain of esophageal origin is not predictably elicited by exertion and often occurs spontaneously, in relationship to meals or in the middle of the night. It is associated with other esophageal symptoms. Clearly, patients with this type of pain need to have ischemic heart disease excluded. Once this is done, many will be found to have some form of esophageal motor disorder. In addition, this angina-like pain can be precipitated by gastroesophageal reflux.

4.1.6 WATERBRASH

This sudden appearance of copious amounts of saliva in the mouth must be differentiated from regurgitation of fluid. With waterbrash, acid reflux into the esophagus stimulates hypersalivation via a (cholinergic) neural reflex.

4.1.7 BLEEDING

This may be a symptom of certain esophageal diseases. Mucosal laceration in the region of the gastroesophageal junction (*Mallory-Weiss tear*), as a consequence of retching or vomiting, is a common cause of upper gastrointestinal tract bleeding. Esophageal varices can cause massive hematemesis and melena. Deep esophageal ulcers may also bleed massively, but this is uncommon.

Usually the bleeding from ulcerative lesions of the esophagus or esophageal cancer is occult. When the patient does present with hematemesis or melena from esophagitis, the rate of bleeding is usually slow; therefore, significant hemodynamic compromise is uncommon.

4.1.8 *RESPIRATORY/LARYNGEAL SYMPTOMS*

These may be a manifestation of esophageal disease or oropharyngeal swallowing disorders. Aspiration at the time of swallowing will cause coughing, choking and eventual hoarseness. In addition, patients with motor disorders or gastroesophageal reflux disease (GERD) may regurgitate esophageal or gastric contents up into the larynx and subsequently aspirate. These patients may present with pneumonia, chronic cough, wheezing, hoarseness or laryngitis. Gastroesophageal reflux may also trigger coughing and wheezing via a vasovagal reflex.

4.2 **Signs**

It is uncommon for esophageal disease to be associated with specific physical findings. Signs of weight loss and malnutrition can be found if the esophageal problem is so severe that adequate caloric intake is not maintained. There may be signs of metastatic disease (e.g., hepatomegaly, supraclavicular lymphadenopathy) in esophageal cancer. Patients with GERD rarely have respiratory tract signs such as wheezing, hoarseness or lung consolidation. It is important to look for signs of connective tissue disease (especially scleroderma) in patients with reflux symptoms or dysphagia.

The physical examination is more often helpful in patients with oropharyngeal dysphagia. Careful examination of the head and neck for structural and neurologic abnormalities is mandatory. It is also important to look for more generalized neurologic or connective tissue abnormalities. Observing the patient swallow is also useful when oropharyngeal dysphagia is present.

5. INVESTIGATIONS USED IN THE DIAGNOSIS OF ESOPHAGEAL DISEASE

5.1 **Barium X-ray**

This most commonly used method of investigating the esophagus evaluates both structural lesions and motor disorders. It is the single most important test in evaluating patients with dysphagia. Proper communication between physician and radiologist is vital. Videotaping the barium swallow allows for playback and slow-motion review. This is very helpful in assessing the rapid events of the oropharyngeal phase of swallowing. Use of marshmallows, barium-coated cookies and different consistencies of barium further assesses swallowing disorders, as delays in transport may not be apparent with simple liquid barium. The disadvantage of barium x-rays is that they are relatively insensitive in detecting mucosal disease, even if air contrast technique is added.

5.2 Endoscopy with Mucosal Biopsy and Brush Cytology

Fiberoptic endoscopy directly visualizes the esophageal mucosa as well as other areas of the upper gastrointestinal tract. Its direct view is superior to barium x-rays for assessing mucosal disease of the esophagus, and the esophagoscope permits assessment of structural lesions that are identified. Furthermore, pinch biopsies and/or brush cytology of specific lesions are easily obtained through the endoscope. Microscopic evidence of esophagitis may be found even when the mucosa looks grossly normal. Endoscopy is the single most useful test in the evaluation of patients with reflux symptoms, as it permits one to establish the presence or absence of esophagitis or Barrett's esophagus (Section 7.3). Endoscopy gives little reliable information regarding esophageal function.

5.3 Bernstein (Acid Perfusion) Test

This tests the sensitivity of the patient's esophagus to acid perfusion. A tube is placed into the distal esophagus and saline, acid and then antacid are infused sequentially, with the patient kept unaware as to what is being administered. The patient is questioned periodically about the presence or absence of symptoms and their quality. This test is useful in determining whether a patient's atypical chest or epigastric pain is secondary to acid reflux. The test is positive if the patient's presenting pain is reproduced during acid perfusion and relieved by antacid perfusion.

5.4 Esophageal Manometry

This involves recording intraluminal pressures at multiple sites along the esophagus (Figure 1). The most commonly used method involves a perfused multilumen catheter bundle with side holes at 5 cm intervals. Each catheter is connected to a pressure transducer, which in turn is attached to a physiograph. LES pressure and swallow-induced LES relaxation are measured, as are pressure responses to swallowing at several esophageal sites. Pharyngeal peristalsis and UES function can also be measured. Esophageal manometry is the "gold standard" in the assessment of esophageal motor disorders. Motor dysfunction, however, may be intermittent and therefore not detected at the time of the study. Manometry is now commonly combined with provocative tests (acid perfusion, balloon distention and/or pharmacological stimulation of the esophagus with bethanechol or edrophonium) in an attempt to evoke abnormal contractions and reproduce the patient's chest pain (Section 11).

5.5 pH Reflux Studies

These are performed using a pH electrode passed via the nose or mouth into the distal esophagus. The traditional short-duration study measures acid reflux events (pH drop to < 4) after various postural maneuvers. This has now been largely replaced by a miniature system that with computer assistance allows 24-hour ambulatory studies. The results of this test are compared to a healthy control population to determine whether an abnormal degree of gastroesophageal reflux is present. The test is most useful, however, in determining whether atypical symptoms coincide with acid reflux events, and in objectively assessing the response to therapy in patients with refractory symptoms.

5.6 Radionuclide Studies

These assess either gastroesophageal reflux or esophageal transit. In the latter instance, food or fluid labeled with a radioisotope is swallowed and gamma camera scanning is performed over the chest. Computer programs measure transit time in the upper, middle and lower thirds of the esophagus. This has been reported to be a sensitive way of detecting motor dysfunction in patients with dysphagia. It may therefore be a useful screening test, but fails to give reliable information concerning the type of motor disorder present. Gastroesophageal reflux can be quantitated by having the patient ingest the radioisotope and then scanning over the chest and upper abdomen. Binders are placed over the abdomen to increase intra-abdominal pressure; reflux is present if the isotope is seen to travel back up into the esophagus. The role of this test in the assessment of patients with reflux disease remains to be defined, as its sensitivity and specificity are rather poor.

6. ANATOMIC VARIANTS

6.1 Congenital Anomalies

Embryologically the gastrointestinal and respiratory tracts start out as a single tube; however, by the second month of gestation they have completely divided. Problems with this process lead to various congenital anomalies, the most common being tracheoesophageal fistula with esophageal atresia. In 85–90% of cases, the proximal esophagus ends in a blind pouch while the distal esophagus consists of a blind pouch in continuity with the stomach. Neonates with this abnormality develop immediate aspiration with feeding. There is no air in the bowel on x-ray films of the abdomen, contrary to what is observed in those with fistulas involving the distal esophagus. In 1–2% of cases there is an "H-type" fistula with atresia. The patient presents with repeated pulmonary infections and abdominal distention. The latter is caused by air getting into the gastrointestinal tract via the fistula when the infant cries. Because the H-type fistula may be very small, the condition may go unnoticed until adulthood, when it is detected during the investigation of recurrent pulmonary infections. Some of these fistulas may close spontaneously but produce paraesophageal inflammation and ultimately localized esophageal stricture formation.

Treatment of esophageal fistulas (with or without atresia) is surgical. The prognosis is now quite good and mortality is usually related to coexistent congenital malformations. It is important to remember that many of these patients will have gastroesophageal reflux as well as abnormal esophageal peristalsis following surgery, which may cause significant long-term problems.

Congenital esophageal stenosis is a rare anomaly that is also probably related to abnormal differentiation of the gastrointestinal and respiratory tracts, as resected specimens have been found to have pulmonary epithelium and/or bronchial remnants. Sequestered pulmonary remnants with connections to the esophagus but not associated with stenosis have also been described.

6.2 Hiatus Hernia

The majority of hiatus hernias are acquired. Rarely, a hiatus hernia can be caused by a congenitally short esophagus. Hiatus hernias can be divided into two types: (1) sliding and (2) paraesophageal (Figures 3 and 4, respectively). A *sliding hiatus hernia* refers to the condition where a circumferential cuff of cardia and proximal stomach migrates up through the diaphragmatic hiatus and into the thorax. This may reduce and reform spontaneously. These hernias are very common and increase in incidence with advancing age. Generally they are of no clinical significance, despite the fact that many patients and physicians persist in attributing a wide variety of symptoms to them. Large hiatus hernias may be associated with iron deficiency anemia that is presumably caused by recurrent superficial ulcerations at the site where the diaphragm exerts pressure on the herniated stomach. If no other source of GI blood loss is discovered after thorough investigation, and patients continue to be iron-deficient despite supplementation and antiulcer treatment, surgical correction of the hernia should be performed.

The etiology of the sliding hiatus hernia is obscure. Certainly there is laxity and dilation of the diaphragmatic hiatus and associated laxity of the phreno-esophageal ligament; however, these may well be secondary and not primary pathophysiologic factors. In some cases, persistent gastroesophageal reflux may result in inflammation and consequent esophageal shortening, which in turn leads to the development of a hiatus hernia.

A sliding hiatus hernia is often seen in association with GERD; the precise role of the hernia in the pathogenesis of the reflux remains obscure. Certainly the majority of people with hiatus hernias do not have significant reflux dis-

FIGURE 3.   Lateral chest x-ray of a sliding-type hiatus hernia. The fundic air bubble can be clearly seen in the chest, posterior to the cardiac silhouette, indicating that the gastroesophageal junction and upper stomach have slid up through the diaphragmatic hiatus.

FIGURE 4. Barium contrast study of a paraesophageal-type hiatus hernia. Note that the gastro-esophageal junction has maintained its normal position at the hiatus, but a small portion of the gastric fundus has migrated up through the hiatus alongside the esophagus.

ease, and occasionally patients with severe reflux esophagitis will not have a hiatus hernia. It appears that a hiatus hernia may contribute somewhat to gastroesophageal reflux, but it is most unlikely that this is the prime etiologic factor. A hiatus hernia may contribute to GERD by providing a reservoir of gastric acid that has ready access to the distal esophagus whenever the LES relaxes.

Paraesophageal hiatus hernias are uncommon. These consist of the fundus of the stomach migrating through the hiatus alongside the esophagus without any displacement of the gastroesophageal junction. Although these hernias are often asymptomatic, most physicians believe that they should be treated surgically when the diagnosis is made because the herniated portion may become strangulated and infarcted.

7. GASTROESOPHAGEAL REFLUX DISEASE (GERD)

GERD is the most common condition to affect the esophagus. The disease spectrum ranges from patients with heartburn and other reflux symptoms without morphologic evidence of esophagitis (the so-called acid-sensitive esophagus) to patients with deep ulcer, stricture or Barrett's epithelium. Everyone has some degree of gastroesophageal reflux; it becomes pathological only when associated with troublesome symptoms or complications. Fortunately, the vast majority of patients suffering from GERD have an easily controlled disorder. At the other end of the spectrum, there are patients who develop severe damage to the esophagus. Some will develop Barrett's metaplasia as a consequence of gastroesophageal reflux, which in turn predisposes them to adenocarcinoma.

7.1 Pathophysiology
GERD results from the reflux of gastric contents into the esophageal lumen. Early pathogenesis concepts focused on anatomic factors: reflux was considered a mechanical problem, related to the development of a hiatus hernia. We now know, however, that a hiatus hernia can occur without GERD, and conversely, GERD can occur without a hiatus hernia. Many factors are involved in the pathogenesis of GERD.

7.1.1 *BARRIERS TO GASTROESOPHAGEAL REFLUX*
By far the most important barrier to gastroesophageal reflux is the LES. Factors such as the intra-abdominal location of the sphincter, extrinsic compression exerted by the diaphragmatic crura and the angle of His (which forms a "mucosal flap valve") may augment this barrier but play a minor role relative to the LES itself. Some patients developing reflux esophagitis have fee-

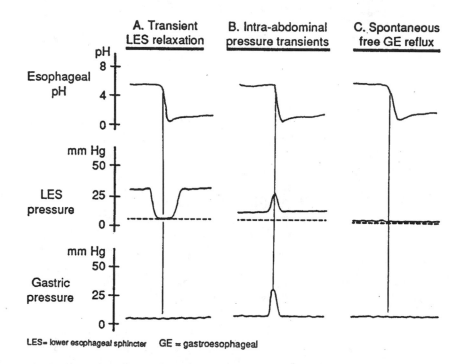

FIGURE 5. Schematic representation of three different mechanisms of gastroesophageal (GE) reflux.

A. Transient LES relaxation refers to the sudden occurrence of LES relaxation that causes obliteration of the gastroesophageal pressure barrier and permits gastric contents to reflux up into the esophagus. The reflux event is marked by the sudden drop in esophageal pH. These transient LES relaxations are sometimes related to incomplete or failed peristalsis but may also occur in isolation.

B. Intra-abdominal pressure transients are sudden increases in intragastric pressure caused by coughing, sneezing or deep inspiration. The increased intragastric pressure overcomes the LES pressure and results in reflux.

C. Spontaneous free reflux occurs when there is very low or nonexistent LES pressure, which permits spontaneous reflux across the gastroesophageal junction. In healthy volunteers without GERD, virtually all reflux episodes are due to transient LES relaxation. In patients with reflux esophagitis, approximately two-thirds of the reflux episodes are due to transient LES relaxation. The remaining one-third are caused by either intra-abdominal pressure transients or spontaneous free gastroesophageal reflux.

SOURCE: Dodds WJ, Dent J, Hogan WJ, et al. Mechanisms of gastroesophageal reflux in patients with reflux esophagitis. N Engl J M 1982; 307:1547–1552. Used with permission.

ble LES tone, but in most, resting LES pressure is nearly normal. Gastro-esophageal reflux occurs by three major mechanisms, as outlined in Figure 5.

7.1.2 ESOPHAGEAL CLEARANCE

Once reflux occurs, the duration of insult to the esophageal mucosa depends on the rapidity with which the esophagus clears this material. Once the initial (primary) peristaltic wave has passed, the bolus (a portion of which frequently remains) is cleared by one or two secondary peristaltic waves. The remaining small adherent acidic residue is then neutralized by saliva, which is carried down by successive swallows. Disorders of salivation or esophageal motor function will impair this clearance mechanism and predispose to the development of GERD.

Patients with severe GERD may have frequent prolonged nighttime reflux episodes because during sleep, peristalsis seldom occurs and salivary flow virtually ceases. Hence the contact time of refluxed material with the esophagus is markedly increased.

7.1.3 GASTRODUODENAL FACTORS

In some patients delayed gastric emptying further predisposes to the development of GERD. Bile salts and pancreatic enzymes, if refluxed back into the stomach, can in turn reflux into the esophagus and may inflict worse damage than when gastric juice is refluxed alone. Such reflux into the stomach and then the esophagus may occur after gastric surgery, when the pylorus is destroyed. Whenever there is increased gastric pressure or an increase in gastric contents, there is greater likelihood that reflux will occur when the sphincter barrier becomes deficient.

7.1.4 MUCOSAL RESISTANCE

The degree of damage to esophageal mucosa depends not only on the composition of the refluxed material and the amount and duration of reflux, but also on defensive factors within the mucosa itself. Certain patients are more susceptible to the development of actual mucosal damage, for reasons that are not clear.

7.2 Clinical Features

Most patients present with heartburn and acid regurgitation that onset after eating certain foods or following various postural maneuvers (e.g., bending over, lying flat). Frequency varies from once a week or less to daily episodes with disruption of sleep. Other presenting symptoms include waterbrash, angina-like chest pain, dysphagia and various respiratory symptoms (hoarse-

TABLE 1.   Diagnostic tests in GERD

Tests to determine the presence of reflux
pH reflux study (short-duration or 24-hour ambulatory)
Barium meal
Radionuclide scintigraphy

Tests to determine whether symptoms are due to reflux
24-hour pH recording
Bernstein (acid perfusion) test

Tests to determine the presence of mucosal damage
Endoscopy
Mucosal biopsy
Barium meal

---

ness, cough, wheezing). The dysphagia may be due to the development of a reflux-induced stricture or to abnormal motility induced by the refluxed acid. Odynophagia is rarely a symptom of GERD and should alert the physician to another diagnosis such as infectious esophagitis.

Reflux symptoms are common during pregnancy because of increased intra-abdominal pressures and the LES-relaxant effect of progesterone.

Physical examination in patients with GERD rarely reveals associated physical signs. In severe cases with stricture formation there may be weight loss secondary to decreased caloric intake, or findings of consolidation, bronchospasm or fibrosis on respiratory examination in patients who have GE reflux with aspiration.

7.3 **Diagnosis**

In the vast majority of patients, GERD can be diagnosed from the history alone and treated without further investigation. Several tests are useful in the assessment of suspected GERD, depending on the information sought: Is there an abnormal degree of reflux? Are symptoms in fact due to reflux? Is there mucosal damage or other complications (Table 1)? Some specialists believe that all patients with symptomatic gastroesophageal reflux should undergo endoscopy. The argument in favor of this approach is that Barrett's esophagus will be found in about 10% of these patients. This identifies those at increased risk for the development of adenocarcinoma (Section 7.5.2). Most physicians, however, feel that in young patients with typical symptoms that are infrequent and relatively mild, empiric therapy should be instituted first without further investigation. In patients with frequent or more severe symptoms but without symptoms that suggest complications, endoscopy is neces-

TABLE 2. Medical therapy of gastroesophageal reflux disease: a pathophysiologic approach

---

Decrease frequency of reflux episodes
Improve LES function (prokinetic drugs; avoid certain drugs and foods, especially alcohol
    and cigarettes)
Elevate head of bed 4–6 inches on blocks
Weight loss

Augment clearing mechanisms; decrease duration of reflux episodes
Prokinetic agents (cisapride, domperidone, metoclopramide)
Agents that stimulate salivation
Gravity (elevate head of bed, avoid bending over)

Decrease irritant quality and volume of gastric juice
Antacids, alginic acid
H_2-receptor antagonists (cimetidine, ranitidine, famotidine, nizatidine)
M_1 antagonists (pirenzepine)
Proton pump inhibitors (omeprazole, lansoprazole)
Prokinetic agents (cisapride, domperidone, metoclopramide)

Augment esophageal mucosal defenses
?Sucralfate

---

sary to rule out other diseases and to document the presence or absence of
mucosal damage or Barrett's metaplasia. Endoscopic biopsy may also detect
microscopic evidence of esophagitis (hyperplasia of the basal zone layer,
elongation of the papillae and inflammatory cell infiltration) when the
esophageal mucosa appears macroscopically normal.

Many patients will have normal endoscopy and biopsy even though significant GERD is present. In these patients or in patients with atypical or multiple symptoms, it is worthwhile to do a Bernstein test and/or a 24-hour pH
reflux study to establish that the symptom(s) are in fact due to acid reflux. It
is important to first rule out ischemic heart disease if the presenting symptom
is angina-like chest pain.

All patients who present with symptoms of complicated GERD (i.e., dysphagia, bleeding or respiratory symptoms) need to be fully investigated. If
dysphagia is present, a barium x-ray study should be performed, followed by
endoscopy. Further investigations will depend on the results of the initial tests.
Esophageal manometry has little role to play in the routine assessment of
patients with GERD. It is useful in the assessment of patients with atypical
symptoms, and can be combined with an acid perfusion (Bernstein) test as
well as with other provocative tests. It is important to perform manometry

TABLE 3.   Agents known to decrease LES tone

Theophylline
Caffeine
Fatty meal
Chocolate
Peppermint
Smoking
Ethanol
Calcium channel blockers
Morphine
Meperidine
Benzodiazepines
β-adrenergic agonists
Nitrates
Anticholinergics (including tricyclic antidepressants)

prior to surgical intervention, because patients with significant underlying primary motor disorders of the esophagus (e.g., scleroderma) often develop severe dysphagia following an antireflux procedure.

7.4 Treatment

7.4.1 MEDICAL TREATMENT

The treatment of GERD is directed toward the abnormal pathophysiology (Table 2). In patients with mild or infrequent symptoms, lifestyle modifications, dietary advice, elevation of the head of the bed and p.r.n. antacids are usually all that is required. If possible, the patient should avoid ingestion of various agents that are known to inhibit LES tone and promote reflux (Table 3). In patients with more severe symptoms or who do not respond to these simple measures, addition of an H_2-receptor antagonist is indicated. Prokinetic agents such as cisapride may also be used alone or in combination with other agents in the treatment of GERD, but are probably best suited to the subgroup of patients who have gastroparesis or coexistent functional, nonulcer dyspepsia (gas-bloat syndrome). Proton pump inhibitors such as omeprazole and lansoprazole represent the most efficacious therapy currently available for GERD. They should be used in patients with complicated GERD (e.g., frank erosive esophagitis, peptic stricture or Barrett's ulcer) or in patients who have not responded to H_2-receptor antagonists.

GERD is a chronic relapsing condition that usually requires long-term treatment. As a general rule the physician should use the simplest, least expensive and least potent therapeutic regime that will keep the patient's symptoms in check.

7.4.2 *SURGICAL TREATMENT*

Antireflux surgery should be considered in patients with reflux esophagitis whose symptoms are not controlled with the aforementioned medical regimen and in younger patients who would prefer to avoid long-term pharmacological therapy. Some patients who develop the complications of GERD (Section 7.5) are also best managed surgically. Several different operative techniques are used for this condition. The most popular are the Nissen fundoplication, the Belsey Mark IV repair and the Hill posterior gastropexy. Currently, many surgeons are doing antireflux surgery via a laparoscopic approach. All procedures adhere to the same basic principles: restoration of the LES to an intra-abdominal position, extrinsic bolstering of the LES pressure and repair of the patulous hiatus.

The results of antireflux surgery depend more on the expertise and experience of the surgeon than on the specific operative procedure. In expert hands, surgery will produce a good-to-excellent result in 85–95% of patients; however, in up to 50% of these patients, objective evidence of recurrent pathological reflux will be present five years after surgery, even though symptomatic benefit is maintained. Overall operative mortality for first-time operations is in the order of 0.5%. Between 10 and 20% of patients develop significant problems with dysphagia and/or gas-bloat symptoms after surgery. In most cases these problems resolve with time.

7.5 Complicated GERD

7.5.1 *PEPTIC STRICTURE*

Chronic GERD may lead to peptic stricture formation. This is a fibrous stricture related to collagen deposition that occurs in the course of repair of esophagitis. Patients are usually asymptomatic until the luminal narrowing has reached 12–14 mm. At this point dysphagia to solids occurs. As the stricture progresses, the dysphagia gradually progresses to semisolids and then liquids. Treatment of peptic strictures involves peroral dilation, using either mercury-filled rubber bougies, rigid dilators passed over guidewires, or balloons passed through endoscopes. In close to 50% of patients one or two dilation sessions prove adequate, and no further dilations are required because ongoing medical treatment of the reflux is successful. In others, the stricture recurs and periodic dilations are required to maintain luminal patency. In patients who are otherwise healthy, consideration should be given to antireflux surgery if frequent dilations are required to maintain luminal patency. The success rate of antireflux surgery is lower in such patients with peptic stricture. Strictures are less likely to recur following dilation if the patient is treated with omeprazole. For this reason, long-term treatment with this agent seems appropriate for patients with peptic stricture.

7.5.2 *BARRETT'S ESOPHAGUS*

In this condition the squamous epithelium of the distal esophagus is replaced by metaplastic columnar epithelium. Deep ulcers as well as strictures at the new squamocolumnar junction may also develop. Severe hemorrhage may complicate the deep ulcers. This condition occurs in approximately 10% of patients with chronic GERD, although recent prospective studies in which careful biopsies were performed from the region of the gastroesophageal junction suggest that the incidence is actually higher.

Barrett's epithelium is a premalignant condition. At the time of initial presentation, up to 10% of patients found to have Barrett's esophagus will have coexistent adenocarcinoma arising in the Barrett's epithelium. This number gives an exaggerated impression of the magnitude of risk, because Barrett's esophagus patients with cancer are more likely to seek medical attention. The true incidence of adenocarcinoma developing in Barrett's epithelium is only about 1 case for every 200 patient-years of follow-up. This nevertheless represents about a 30- to 40-fold increase over the risk faced by the general population. For this reason patients with Barrett's esophagus should be followed periodically with endoscopy and mucosal biopsy in order to detect early cancer. Most patients will develop severe dysplasia before frank invasive carcinoma occurs. Thus, if patients are found to have severe dysplasia or early mucosal carcinoma, esophageal resection should be considered in order to prevent the development of invasive carcinoma. Although there have been case reports of Barrett's esophagus regressing after successful anti-reflux surgery, it is unlikely that such surgery decreases the risk of cancer in the majority of patients. For this reason, Barrett's esophagus per se should not be an indication for antireflux surgery. Surgery should be performed if the patient has symptoms or complications not readily managed by medical therapy.

7.5.3 *RESPIRATORY COMPLICATIONS*

In some patients the refluxed gastric contents may get past the UES and into the larynx and lungs. This produces recurrent chest infections, chronic cough and laryngitis. In addition, gastroesophageal reflux may trigger bronchospasm or cough via a neural reflex. GERD with aspiration is more commonly seen in the pediatric age group; when present, antireflux surgery should be performed unless there is a well-documented response to medical therapy.

8. NONREFLUX-INDUCED ESOPHAGITIS

8.1 Infectious Esophagitis

Bacteria rarely cause primary esophageal infection, although the esophagus can be involved secondarily by direct extension from the lung. The two most common forms of infectious esophagitis are caused by Candida and herpes. Other viruses (e.g., CMV, HIV) and fungi can also cause esophagitis; however, this is uncommon and almost invariably associated with immunosuppression.

8.1.1 CANDIDA ESOPHAGITIS

This is by far the most common form of infectious esophagitis. Usually there is a predisposing cause, such as diabetes mellitus, antibiotic therapy or some form of immunocompromise. The patient may be asymptomatic. Not all patients will have associated oral thrush. More commonly, however, patients present with odynophagia, retrosternal chest pain and/or dysphagia. Severe cases can be complicated by bleeding, a stricture and sinus tract formation with secondary lung abscess. Barium x-rays reveal an irregular granular or even cobblestone appearance to the esophageal mucosa. Approximately 25% of patients will have a normal barium esophagogram; for this reason, endoscopy with biopsy and brushing are required to make the diagnosis. The typical endoscopic appearance is the presence of small raised whitish plaques. When the plaques are removed the underlying mucosa is seen to be erythematous and friable. Specimens obtained by biopsy or brush cytology should be cultured and examined microscopically for the presence of typical Candida yeast with pseudohyphae formation. Most patients can be treated with oral nystatin (luminal treatment); however, more extensive disease, especially if the patient is immunocompromised, may require systemic treatment with either ketoconazole or fluconazole. Amphotericin B is required if there is evidence of systemic spread.

8.1.2 HERPES SIMPLEX ESOPHAGITIS

Next to Candida, this is the most common form of infectious esophagitis. The clinical presentation is much the same as with Candida esophagitis. There may also be constitutional symptoms of a viral upper respiratory tract infection preceding the esophageal symptoms. Herpetic mouth or skin lesions may also develop. This infection occurs most frequently in immunosuppressed patients, but also develops sporadically in healthy young adults. Endoscopy with biopsy and brush cytology is required to confirm the diagnosis. The pathognomonic finding is the eosinophilic "Cowdry's Type A" intranuclear inclusion body. Herpetic esophagitis is self-limiting in immunocompetent individuals; specific treatment is not indicated. Symptoms of odynophagia often respond to a combination of antacids mixed with viscous Xylocaine®. In severely immunocompromised patients, intravenous acyclovir treatment should be instituted.

8.2 Esophagitis Associated with Immune-Mediated Disease

Rarely, esophagitis can occur in association with Crohn's disease or Behçet's syndrome. The typical lesion is scattered aphthous-type ulcerations, although severe transmural involvement with stricture formation can occur. The esophagus can also be severely involved in pemphigoid, in pemphigus and in epidermolysis bullosa.

Esophagitis occurs in as many as one-third of patients who develop chronic graft-versus-host disease after bone marrow transplantation. The typical lesion is a generalized epithelial desquamation of the upper and middle esophagus. There may be associated ring-like narrowings or strictures due to submucosal fibrosis. A nonspecific esophageal motor disorder may also develop and result in superimposed reflux esophagitis because of poor esophageal clearing. Sarcoidosis and eosinophilic gastroenteritis are two other immune-mediated diseases that (rarely) cause esophageal inflammation.

8.3 Chemical-Induced Esophagitis

8.3.1 *CAUSTIC CHEMICAL INGESTION*

Strong acids or alkalis ingested accidentally or as a suicidal gesture cause marked esophagitis. Alkali tends to be more injurious to the esophageal mucosa than acid and produces liquefaction necrosis as well as thermal burns (due to heat release when the alkali is hydrated by gut secretions). Acids tend to produce superficial coagulation necrosis and eschar formation. Typically the patient develops immediate chest pain and odynophagia. Oral burns also may produce local pain and drooling. There may be respiratory symptoms such as stridor, dyspnea and hoarseness if the airway is contaminated. Symptoms alone do not permit accurate prediction of the presence or absence of esophageal injury; therefore early diagnostic endoscopy should be considered in most patients. Clearly, endoscopy should not be performed if there is evidence of esophageal perforation. In the management of these patients, it is imperative to maintain an adequate airway. Oral intake must be stopped and intravenous fluids administered. Empiric treatment classically has involved antibiotics and corticosteroids, but there is no good evidence documenting the efficacy of this approach. Patients who survive the acute phase of the injury are at risk of developing strictures because of the intense collagen deposition associated with healing. This often requires repeated esophageal dilation to maintain luminal patency.

Lye-induced injury increases the risk of developing squamous cell carcinoma of the esophagus. Typically there is a 30- to 50-year lag time before the development of cancer. For this reason any patient with previous lye injury and new esophageal symptoms should be promptly investigated. The extent of the risk is such that periodic endoscopic surveillance is not indicated.

8.3.2 *PILL-INDUCED ESOPHAGITIS*

A large number of oral agents can cause localized esophageal injury. The antibiotic doxycycline and the anticholinergic emepronium bromide are two of the most common culprits. Nonsteroidal anti-inflammatory drugs and slow-release forms of potassium chloride are also frequently implicated. Patients with this type of injury typically take their medication with a small amount of water and then immediately lie down to go to bed. They may then wake up several hours later with severe retrosternal chest pain and odynophagia. Capsules and tablets are notorious for being transported through the esophagus quite poorly unless adequate amounts of fluid are ingested at the same time. This is an important point to remember in counseling all patients who take medicines at bedtime. Rarely, the medication becomes lodged and causes a deep esophageal ulcer with perforation. More commonly the ulceration is superficial and heals in a few weeks. Late stricture formation may occur. Patients with esophageal motility disorders are particularly prone to this complication.

8.4 **Radiation-Induced Esophagitis**

When included in the field of irradiation the esophagus becomes inflamed in up to 80% of patients receiving therapeutic radiation for cancer. The risk of esophagitis is greater if there is concomitant chemotherapy. The patients typically develop chest pain, dysphagia and odynophagia shortly after the initiation of therapy. This can be a serious problem in such patients, who are already often severely malnourished. Late stricture formation is a well-recognized complication.

9. **DISORDERS OF THE OROPHARYNGEAL PHASE OF DEGLUTITION**

A variety of structural and functional disorders can disrupt the oropharyngeal phase of deglutition and result in oropharyngeal or "transfer"-type dysphagia (Table 4). In the assessment of these patients it is important to exclude disorders for which specific treatment is available.

The most important investigation is a carefully performed video fluoroscopic study of the swallowing mechanism. In addition to the usual barium studies, it is helpful to observe deglutition when the patient swallows barium-soaked cookies or bread. Not only will this examination identify and charac-

TABLE 4.   Classification of disorders causing oropharyngeal dysphagia

---

Central nervous system disease
Cerebrovascular accident (brainstem, pseudobulbar palsy)
Wilson's disease
Multiple sclerosis
Amyotrophic lateral sclerosis
Brainstem neoplasm
Tabes dorsalis

Peripheral nervous system disease
Bulbar poliomyelitis
Miscellaneous peripheral neuropathies
Head and neck neoplasms
Post–radical neck surgery

Muscle disease
Muscular dystrophy
Polymyositis and dermatomyositis
Metabolic myopathy (e.g., hypo- and hyperthyroidism)
Amyloidosis
Systemic lupus erythematosus
Myasthenia gravis

Local disorders
Oropharyngeal inflammation
Oropharyngeal neoplasms
Zenker's diverticulum

Idiopathic
Cricopharyngeal achalasia
Idiopathic oropharyngeal incoordination

---

terize disorders of oropharyngeal coordination, it will also help exclude structural lesions. If an inflammatory, neoplastic or other structural lesion is suspected, direct or indirect laryngoscopy is indicated. At present, conventional manometric studies of the pharynx and UES add little to what can be learned from radiologic studies. This is partly because of limitations in recording methods, but also because complex motor events occurring during deglutition (e.g., closure of the nasopharynx, elevation and closure of the larynx – see Section 3, "Physiology") are not amenable to manometric study.

Ideally, treatment of oropharyngeal motor disorders should be directed at the underlying disease. Frequently this is not possible, and nonspecific treatment must be instituted. In some cases reassurance and education are all that is required. Many patients will be able to control their symptoms simply by eating slowly and carefully in a relaxed atmosphere. In patients in whom aspiration develops because of inadequate clearing of the hypopharynx after the initial swallow, it is beneficial to have the patient immediately follow a "bolus" swallow with a second, "dry" swallow. Correcting denture problems and avoiding foods of certain consistency may also help. Most speech pathologists have special expertise as swallowing therapists and can be extremely helpful in the management of these patients.

For patients in whom these simple measures are not helpful and whose symptoms are such that respiratory and nutritional complications are developing, cricopharyngeal myotomy is often performed. This helps patients with true cricopharyngeal achalasia or Zenker's diverticulum (Section 13). Unfortunately, the response to myotomy is inconsistent in most other patients with oropharyngeal dysphagia, because inadequate opening of the UES is rarely due to dysfunction of the cricopharyngeal muscle alone. More often there is associated weakness of the suprahyoid muscles, which actually open the sphincter, and/or associated problems with pharyngeal peristalsis. Cricopharyngeal myotomy does little to improve such altered physiology. Once cricopharyngeal myotomy has been performed, the patient has lost an important defense mechanism against the aspiration of refluxed material. The patient should therefore be instructed to elevate the head of his or her bed on blocks in order to minimize this risk. For this same reason patients with gross GERD should not undergo cricopharyngeal myotomy unless the reflux can be controlled.

When all other measures fail and nutritional and respiratory complications develop, percutaneous endoscopic gastrostomy should be performed. If the problem is so severe that the patient cannot handle salivary secretions, it is sometimes necessary to also perform laryngeal exclusion and tracheotomy.

10. MOTOR DISORDERS OF THE ESOPHAGUS AND LOWER ESOPHAGEAL SPHINCTER

Esophageal motor disorders can be classified as either primary or secondary. Primary disorders refer to those that usually affect the esophagus alone and have no known etiology. Secondary disorders are motility derangements caused by some other systemic or local condition. Examples of secondary disorders include acid-reflux–induced dysmotility, dysmotility related to the neuropathy associated with diabetes or alcoholism, and motor dysfunction secondary to esophageal involvement in scleroderma or other connective tissue disorders. The well-defined primary motor disorders include the hypertensive peristaltic or "nutcracker" esophagus, diffuse esophageal spasm and achalasia

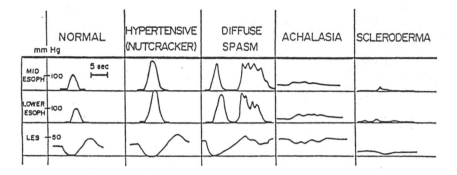

Figure 6.   Manometric features of the major esophageal motor disorders. A *normal* tracing is on the left and depicts sequential "peristaltic" contractions in the esophageal body with full LES relaxation. *Hypertensive peristalsis* or *"nutcracker" esophagus* is characterized by normal peristalsis and LES relaxation, but the amplitude of contraction is the distal esophagus is abnormally high (> 180 mm Hg). In *diffuse esophageal spasm*, normal peristalic waves are interspersed with high-pressure, nonpropulsive (simultaneous) contraction waves are often repetitive. The resting LES pressure may be abnormally high, but swallow-induced LES relaxation is normal. In *achalasia* there is complete absence of normal peristalsis in the smooth-induced LES relaxation is either absent or incomplete. Note also that resting intraesophageal pressures are elevated. *Scleroderma* is characterized by the presence of weak, nonperistaltic esophageal conditions and a markedly hypotensive LES that relaxes normally with swallowing.

(Figure 6). Many cases of primary motility disorders are actually "nonspecific," having a variety of abnormalities that do not fulfill criteria established for the well-defined motor disorders of the esophagus.

Patients with primary motor disorders typically present with dysphagia and/ or chest pain. The pain is often qualitatively similar to angina pectoris and has been classically attributed to smooth-muscle spasm. However, recent studies have suggested that the pain is secondary to a lowered sensory threshold to esophageal stimuli such as distention or acid. Some patients with motor disorders will have secondary GERD because of poor clearing or poor LES function. Here, heartburn and regurgitation may be prominent symptoms.

The diagnosis of a motor disorder can be made on the basis of history and barium swallow x-ray. If there is dysphagia referred to the retrosternal area and no evidence of a structural lesion on x-ray, then by exclusion the patient's dysphagia is related to a motor disorder. As mentioned previously, the quality of the dysphagia (e.g., sporadic, unpredictable dysphagia to both liquids and solids) is also helpful in differentiating motor disorders from structural causes of dysphagia. During fluoroscopy, the radiologist is usually able to detect abnormalities of motor function as the barium is swallowed. The use of a solid bolus, such as a piece of bread soaked in barium, may be helpful in diagnosing esophageal rings or webs. Endoscopy primarily rules out secondary causes of the disorder (i.e., ulcerative esophagitis and neoplasm). In order to define specifically the type of motor disorder present, however, esophageal motility studies are required. The manometric features of the important esophageal motor disorders are depicted schematically in Figure 6.

10.1 "Nutcracker" Esophagus

This motility disorder is characterized by normally propagated but high-amplitude peristaltic waves in the distal esophagus. The duration of the contraction wave is also often prolonged. LES relaxation is normal, although in many patients the resting LES pressure is elevated. Patients often present with angina-like chest pain and usually do not complain of dysphagia. Nutcracker esophagus is the most frequent abnormal manometric finding in patients referred for evaluation of noncardiac angina-like chest pain. The etiology is unknown. Rarely, this disorder progresses to diffuse esophageal spasm or even vigorous achalasia. Reassurance that the pain is not cardiac but is secondary to a benign esophageal condition is the most important part of treatment. Nitrates and calcium channel blockers (to relax smooth muscle) have been used extensively, but have no proven benefit. In some patients with nutcracker esophagus, pain is actually triggered by acid reflux; these patients often respond dramatically to appropriate antireflux therapy.

10.2 Diffuse Esophageal Spasm

This is characterized by normal peristalsis interspersed with frequent high-pressure nonpropagated or "tertiary" waves and multipeaked waves. Patients often present with dysphagia and chest pain. In advanced diffuse esophageal spasm, the x-ray will show a corkscrew pattern as different segments of the esophagus vigorously and simultaneously contract. The etiology is obscure, but may relate to degenerative changes in the intrinsic and extrinsic esophageal nerves. Management involves reassurance and the use of nitrates or calcium channel blocking agents. Patients with severe disease unresponsive to medical measures may benefit from a long esophageal myotomy.

10.3 Achalasia

This uncommon primary motility disorder is characterized by aperistalsis in the body of the esophagus, an elevated LES pressure and absent or incomplete LES relaxation in response to swallowing. Failure of LES relaxation leads to progressive proximal dilation of the esophagus with consequent elevated resting intraesophageal pressures. On x-ray the esophagus is dilated, and retained food and fluid may be present. The distal esophagus narrows in a beak-like fashion (Figure 7A). This "beak" represents the hypertonic, nonrelaxing LES. In some patients there are associated vigorous nonperistaltic contractions in the esophageal body, a condition called *vigorous achalasia*. Achalasia is caused by degeneration of inhibitory neurons within the esophageal and LES myenteric plexus. Nerve damage also occurs in the vagal nerve trunks and the dorsal motor nuclei. The parasite Trypanosoma cruzi, which is endemic in Brazil, can cause achalasia by destroying myenteric neurons (Chagas' disease). Neoplastic disease can also interfere with esophageal and LES nerve function and cause "secondary" achalasia. The cause of the degeneration is unknown in most cases, however.

The cardinal symptom of achalasia is dysphagia, although chest pain and even heartburn may be present. The heartburn is not due to gastroesophageal reflux. It may be caused by lactic acid formed by fermentation of stagnant esophageal contents. Another common symptom of achalasia is regurgitation of esophageal contents.

In mild cases treatment can begin with the use of calcium channel blockers or long-acting nitrates, which have been shown to decrease LES pressure. This is rarely successful in the long term, however. The treatment then usually performed is pneumatic balloon dilation of the LES. This consists of passing a balloon across the sphincter and inflating it rapidly so that the sphincter is forcefully dilated. Pneumatic dilation is successful in alleviating the dysphagia and improving esophageal transport in approximately 70–75% of patients. Patients who do not respond to pneumatic dilation should be treated with Heller myotomy. This consists of a longitudinal incision through the muscle of the LES, which in many centers is now done via a laparoscopic or thoracoscopic approach. Following either pneumatic dilation or Heller myotomy, the patient can develop severe GERD, because the pressure barrier preventing reflux has been destroyed. This tends to be worse after Heller myotomy and has led some surgeons to perform a modified antireflux procedure at the time of myotomy. Because of this problem all patients having successful myotomy or pneumatic dilation should be instructed regarding lifelong antireflux therapy. Usually dietary and posture-type treatment are all that is needed, but in some patients drug therapy is required.

Recent studies have found that injection of botulinum toxin into the muscle of the LES can alleviate dysphagia in approximately two-thirds of patients with achalasia. This therapy is limited because the response is not sustained (average duration is approximately one year), but it may be a useful treatment option in elderly patients who would not tolerate the complications of more invasive therapy. Achalasia patients have an increased risk of developing esophageal cancer and need to be thoroughly investigated if new esophageal symptoms develop.

10.4 Scleroderma Esophagus

Patients with scleroderma frequently have esophageal involvement. This may occur even in the absence of obvious skin and joint involvement, although in such cases, Raynaud's phenomenon is almost always present. The initial event is damage to small blood vessels, which in turn leads to intramural neuronal dysfunction. With time, actual muscle damage and fibrosis occur. This results in a very hypotensive LES, as well as weak nonpropulsive esophageal contractions. Scleroderma may also involve the stomach and cause delayed gastric emptying. As a result, patients develop gross GERD. They present with heartburn and regurgitation, as well as dysphagia. The dysphagia can be due to poor esophageal propulsion and/or reflux-induced stricture (Figure 7B). These patients need very aggressive treatment for GERD. Because they have very poor peristaltic function, increasing the barrier at the LES with antireflux surgery may markedly worsen the dysphagia.

11. THE ESOPHAGUS AS A CAUSE OF ANGINA-LIKE CHEST PAIN

At least one-third of the patients referred to a cardiologist or admitted to a coronary care unit because of angina-like chest pain will have cardiac causes excluded. In most, an alternative etiology is not apparent. Lack of a specific diagnosis may lead to ongoing anxiety, changes in lifestyle and frequent medical consultations if the patient continues to worry that serious heart disease may be present. Such patients should be evaluated for esophageal disease, although the cost-effectiveness of this approach is not known.

Initial investigations include a barium esophagogram and/or upper GI endoscopy to screen for gross esophageal dysmotility and esophagitis. These studies, however, are frequently negative. For this reason, esophageal motility studies with provocative testing (acid perfusion, drug provocation with edrophonium or bethanechol, intraesophageal balloon distention) are usually required to establish an esophageal cause for the pain (Figure 8). In many of these patients, abnormalities of esophageal motility can be documented, suggesting that esophageal dysfunction may be responsible for the pain. Of more diagnostic importance, however, is the demonstration that "provoking" the esophagus with acid perfusion, balloon distention or cholinergic stimulation reproduces the patient's pain.

The pathophysiology of this angina-like chest pain of esophageal origin is poorly understood. In some patients acid reflux is the cause: these patients experience angina-like chest pain under circumstances in which most people would experience heartburn. In others, the pain is caused by abnormal "spastic" contractions of the esophagus that either occur spontaneously or are sec-

FIGURE 7.

A. Typical barium x-ray in a patient with achalasia. Note that the esophagus is dilated and an air-barium level is present, indicating stasis. There is also tortuosity of the distal esophagus, which is often referred to as a "sigmoid" esophagus. At the gastroesophageal junction (lower right) there is a beak-like narrowing, which is caused by the nonrelaxing LES. The mucosal contour at this narrow area appears normal.

B. Barium x-ray of a patient with advanced scleroderma esophagus. The esophagus is dilated, with evidence of retained food debris. Note that the narrowing at the gastroesophageal junction is somewhat irregular on one wall. This is due to an area of structuring caused by gastro-esophageal reflux. This x-ray appearance can be confused with that of achalasia (Figure 7A) and points out the need to confirm a diagnosis of achalasia or scleroderma by performing endoscopy and esophageal manometry.

FIGURE 8. Esophageal motility study in a patient with hypertensive esophageal contractions (nutcracker esophagus) and angina-like chest pain. Calibration (mm Hg) for each "lead" is shown on the left of the record. Zero is set at atmospheric pressure. The uppermost tracing shows respiratory excursion as measured with a belt pneumograph. The lowest tracing is an electromyograph of the neck muscles and indicates the onset of pharyngeal swallowing movement. The lowermost recording lead is positioned in the LES, 41 cm from the incisors. The other leads are recording pressures in the esophageal body 36, 31, 26 and 21 cm from the incisors. The tracing on the left depicts a normal peristaltic sequence; however, the pressures recorded in the distal esophagus are high. The right-hand panel depicts the tracing 16 minutes after the subcutaneous injection of the muscarinic agonist bethanechol. Note that at this time the tracing has become disorganized, with many high-pressure, prolonged and repetitive waves being recorded. During this time the patient experienced reproduction of angina-like chest pain.

SOURCE: Beck IT. Chest pain and the esophagus. Ann RCPSC 1984; 17:13–22. Used with permission.

ondary to acid reflux. In most cases there is a poor correlation between spastic esophageal contractions and the occurrence of pain. Many of these patients appear to have an abnormal esophageal pain threshold; pain episodes may be triggered by multiple different stimuli that in normal subjects would not be perceived as painful.

Both pH and esophageal pressure can be monitored over 24 hours. This method is probably more sensitive and specific than conventional tests, but the equipment is expensive and the test is of limited value in patients with infrequent pain attacks.

Management of angina-like chest pain of esophageal origin should be directed at the specific pathophysiological process. If the pain is triggered by gastroesophageal reflux, then antireflux treatment may be quite helpful. If the pain is due to esophageal spasm, smooth-muscle relaxants such as nitrates, calcium channel blockers, hydralazine and anticholinergics should help, although few controlled clinical trials have demonstrated any significant benefit. Tricyclic antidepressants in relatively low dosage have been shown to be beneficial and should be tried in patients with incapacitating symptoms when other forms of treatment have failed. These are most likely to be useful in patients with abnormal visceral nociception, or the so-called irritable esophagus. Many of these patients will have a significant functional overlay with many other somatic complaints. Simple reassurance is probably the most important part of treatment. Symptoms usually improve once the patient is given a positive diagnosis and no longer fears that underlying heart disease is the cause.

12. ESOPHAGEAL NEOPLASMS

A large number of different tumors can involve the esophagus (Table 5). The vast majority are extremely rare and often do not produce clinical disease. Unfortunately, the most common esophageal neoplasm is squamous cell carcinoma, which has a five-year survival rate (< 10%) that is among the lowest for any neoplastic disease.

12.1 Benign Tumors

Leiomyoma is the most common benign esophageal tumor. Esophageal leiomyomas may produce dysphagia and retrosternal chest pain, but in most cases are asymptomatic. Unlike gastric leiomyomas, they rarely hemorrhage. On barium x-ray a characteristic smooth, round luminal defect is seen projecting from one wall. Its endoscopic appearance is a clearly demarcated projection into the lumen; the overlying mucosa is normal. Endoscopic biopsy is not helpful, as the lesion is submucosal and cannot be reached with biopsy forceps. If leiomyomas are symptomatic, surgical enucleation is indicated.

Squamous cell papillomas consist of frond-like projections of the lamina propria that are covered by squamous epithelium and develop at several sites simultaneously. They rarely grow large enough to produce dysphagia. They occur in association with acanthosis nigricans and tylosis. Except when associated with tylosis, these lesions are not considered to be precursors of squamous cell carcinoma.

Fibrovascular polyps consist of a core of loose fibrous connective tissue, fat and blood vessels covered by a thick layer of squamous epithelium. Such a polyp may become quite large, with a very long stalk that permits the lesions

TABLE 5.   Classification of esophageal tumors

Benign tumors
Epithelial origin
  Squamous cell papilloma
Non-epithelial origin
  Leiomyoma
  Granular cell tumor
  Hemangioma
  Lymphangioma

Malignant tumors
Epithelial origin
  Squamous cell carcinoma
  Adenocarcinoma
  Adenoid cystic carcinoma
  Mucoepidermoid carcinoma
  Adenosquamous carcinoma
  Undifferentiated carcinoma; small-cell carcinoma
Non-epithelial origin
  Leiomyosarcoma
  Carcinosarcoma
  Malignant melanoma
Secondary tumors
  Malignant melanoma
  Breast carcinoma

Tumor-like lesions
  Fibrovascular polyp
  Heterotopia
  Congenital cyst
  Glycogen acanthosis

---

to flop back and forth in the esophageal lumen. Patients with this lesion have presented with regurgitation of the free end of the polyp into the mouth; in other instances, the regurgitated polyp has caused sudden death by obstructing the larynx.

Granular cell tumors are submucosal lesions with intact mucosal covering that are usually picked up incidentally at endoscopy. They may originate from neural elements. They rarely cause symptoms, although there have been occasional reports of dysphagia due to large granular cell tumors. There have also been rare reports of malignant granular cell tumors in the esophagus. Symptomatic tumors need to be removed surgically.

12.2 **Malignant Tumors**

Carcinoma of the esophagus is a relatively uncommon malignancy in Canada, with only 3 to 4 new cases per 100,000 population per year in males and just over 1 new case per 100,000 population per year in females. Nevertheless, because of its poor prognosis, esophageal cancer ranks among the 10 leading causes of cancer death in Canadian men 45 years of age and older.

Although several different types of primary and secondary malignancies can involve the esophagus (Table 5), squamous cell carcinoma and adenocarcinoma are by far the most common esophageal malignancies.

12.2.1 *ADENOCARCINOMA*

Adenocarcinoma used to make up approximately 10% of all esophageal cancers. However, its incidence has been increasing in recent decades such that now it comprises up to 30–40% of esophageal cancers in North America. Rarely, primary esophageal adenocarcinomas arise from embryonic remnants of columnar epithelium or from superficial or deep glandular epithelium. In most instances, adenocarcinoma arises from metaplastic Barrett's epithelium in the distal esophagus. Adenocarcinoma of the cardia of the stomach may also involve the distal esophagus and give the appearance that the cancer arises from the esophagus.

The true incidence of Barrett's-related cancer is uncertain, but most studies suggest that patients with Barrett's esophagus will develop adenocarcinoma at a rate of about 0.5% per year. This is a significant problem given the large number of reflux patients with Barrett's metaplasia. Because dysplasia develops prior to frank carcinoma in Barrett's epithelium, most experts suggest that these patients should undergo surveillance endoscopy with multiple biopsies every one to two years to identify those who are likely to progress to cancer (Section 7).

The clinical presentation and diagnostic evaluation of patients with adenocarcinoma of the esophagus are similar to squamous cell carcinoma (Section 12.2.2). These lesions are not radiosensitive and their response to various chemotherapeutic agents is not very satisfactory. Surgical resection or palliation with laser, photodynamic therapy, peroral dilation and/or stent placement are the preferred treatments. The prognosis is similar to that for gastric adenocarcinoma – i.e., an overall five-year survival rate of < 10%.

12.2.2 *SQUAMOUS CELL CARCINOMA*

The occurrence of squamous cell carcinoma of the esophagus shows striking geographic variability, with high frequencies in certain regions of Iran, Africa, China and the former USSR. This has led to several theories concerning certain environmental agents that may be important etiologically (Table 6). In

TABLE 6.   Esophageal squamous cell carcinoma: possible etiological factors

---

Alcohol
Tobacco
Nutritional exposures
  Nitrosamines; "bush teas" containing tannin and/or diterpene phorbol esters
Nutritional deficiencies (riboflavin, niacin, iron)
Chronic esophagitis
Achalasia
Previous lye-induced injury
Tylosis
Plummer-Vinson (Paterson-Kelly) syndrome

North America, squamous cell carcinoma is associated with alcohol ingestion, tobacco use and lower socioeconomic status. It is also significantly more common in blacks and in males.

Characteristically these cancers extend microscopically in the submucosa for substantial distances above and below the area of the gross involvement. They also have a propensity to extend through the esophageal wall and to regional lymphatics quite early. Furthermore, they usually produce symptoms only when they have become locally quite advanced. For these reasons approximately 95% of these cancers are diagnosed at a time when surgical cure is impossible.

In most studies, the mid-esophagus is the most common site of origin; however, others have reported distal cancers to be most common. The lungs and liver are the most common sites of distant metastases.

Most patients present with progressive, predictable dysphagia and weight loss. Other symptoms include odynophagia, chest pain (which may radiate to the mid-scapular region), hoarseness (due to recurrent laryngeal nerve involvement) and blood loss. Pulmonary complications due to either direct aspiration or esophagorespiratory fistulas are also quite common during the course of the disease. Physical examination is usually negative aside from signs of weight loss. Hepatomegaly or enlarged cervical or supraclavicular lymph nodes may be detected in cases of disseminated metastases.

Barium swallow is usually diagnostic, although small cancers can be missed in up to 30% of cases. Endoscopy with multiple directed biopsies combined with brush cytology is required to confirm the diagnosis. This should be followed by careful attempts to stage the disease prior to deciding on therapeutic intervention. In addition to a careful physical examination, chest x-ray and blood tests for transaminases, alkaline phosphatase and bilirubin, an ultrasound of the abdomen should be performed to look for liver metastasis. If this is negative, one should proceed to a CT scan of the thorax in order to define the extent of local spread. Unfortunately the CT scan lacks sensitivity in this regard. Endoscopic ultrasound appears promising in accurately assessing depth of tumor involvement and presence or absence of enlarged mediastinal lymph nodes. If the above investigations are negative, some experts recommend bronchoscopy, mediastinoscopy and scalene node biopsy prior to attempting surgical resection.

Treatment results of squamous cell carcinoma of the esophagus are discouraging. Although it is traditionally taught that surgical resection is the only chance for a cure, there is no convincing evidence that "curative" surgery is better than "curative" radiotherapy. These tumors are quite radiosensitive; however, most centers give radiotherapy to patients who have advanced unresectable tumors or other health problems that make them poor surgical candidates. This understandably leads to very poor overall survival following radiotherapy. In the few reports where radiotherapy is used as the primary mode of therapy in patients who might otherwise be considered surgical candidates, the five-year survival rate is as high as 17%, which compares quite favorably to surgical results. Both forms of treatment have significant morbidity, and the mortality following esophageal resection is at least 10%. Controlled trials are needed, but in only a small proportion of the total population of esophageal cancer patients is cure a realistic goal. In the majority the disease is too far advanced. New regimens that combine radiotherapy and chemotherapy, with or without surgery, are currently being evaluated.

The goal of treatment has to be palliation in most patients. Both radiotherapy and modified surgery can be used in this setting; however, other modalities are often necessary. The dysphagia can be relieved with peroral dilation, but in many patients this becomes exceedingly difficult as the disease progresses. If this is the case, a prosthetic device can sometimes be placed across the tumor to maintain luminal patency. These stents can work quite well, although tube blockage, tube migration and erosion through the esophageal wall are important complications. These prosthetic devices are the best treatment for an esophagorespiratory fistula. Endoscopic Nd-YAG laser therapy has been used to destroy tumors that obstruct the esophageal lumen. This appears to be a very useful form of palliation, but it is expensive and has not as yet been documented to be superior to dilation and stent placement. Photodynamic therapy has recently been approved for palliation of neoplastic dysphagia. This involves using a photosensitizing compound that accumulates in cancer cells, which leads to their destruction when they are exposed to light of a certain wavelength. The caring physician must also provide emotional support, nutritional support and adequate pain therapy for these unfortunate patients.

13. MISCELLANEOUS DISORDERS OF THE ESOPHAGUS

13.1 Webs and Rings

Webs are thin, membrane-like structures that project into the esophageal lumen. They are covered on both sides with squamous epithelium and are most commonly found in the cervical esophagus. Webs are usually detected incidentally during barium x-rays and rarely occlude enough of the esophageal lumen to cause dysphagia. The etiology of these webs is unclear. Most are probably congenital in origin. In some instances postcricoid esophageal webs are associated with iron deficiency and dysphagia – the so-called *Plummer-Vinson* or *Paterson-Kelly* syndrome. This syndrome is associated with increased risk of hypopharyngeal cancer and should be managed with bougienage, iron replacement and careful follow-up. Esophageal webs may also form after esophageal injury, such as that induced by pills or lye ingestion, and have also been reported in association with graft-versus-host disease.

The lower esophageal or *Schatzki's ring* is also a membrane-like structure, but unlike webs is lined by squamous epithelium on its superior aspect and columnar epithelium inferiorly. Such a ring is quite common, being detected in up to 10% of all upper GI barium x-rays. Few produce sufficient luminal obstruction to cause dysphagia (yet a lower esophageal ring is a common cause of dysphagia). When the lumen is narrowed to a diameter of 13 mm or less, the patient will experience intermittent solid-food dysphagia or even episodic food-bolus obstruction. Treatment of a symptomatic Schatzki's ring involves shattering the ring with a large-diameter bougie or a balloon dilator.

13.2 Diverticula

Pharyngoesophageal diverticula are outpouchings of one or more layers of the pharyngeal or esophageal wall and are classified according to their location.

13.2.1 ZENKER'S DIVERTICULUM (Figure 9)

This diverticulum arises posteriorly in the midline between the oblique and transverse (cricopharyngeal) fibers of the inferior pharyngeal constrictor muscles. As this diverticulum enlarges, it usually shifts to the left of the midline. Zenker's diverticulum forms because of decreased compliance of the cricopharyngeal muscle, which results in abnormally high pressures in the hypophar-

FIGURE 9.   Barium x-ray of a Zenker's diverticulum. Note that barium has filled the diverticulum, which originates posteriorly, just above the cricopharyngeal muscle. Most of these diverticula shift to the left of the midline as they enlarge.

ynx during deglutition. If large, the diverticulum may cause dysphagia secondary to external compression of the cervical esophagus. In addition to oropharyngeal-type dysphagia, Zenker's diverticulum may be associated with effortless regurgitation of stagnant, foul-tasting food, as well as aspiration. A very large diverticulum can produce a neck mass, usually on the left side.

Treatment of a symptomatic Zenker's diverticulum is surgical. Most surgeons will either resect the diverticulum or suspend it (diverticulopexy) so that it cannot fill. This is combined with cricopharyngeal myotomy. In many cases cricopharyngeal myotomy alone will alleviate symptoms. Once the cricopharyngeal myotomy has been performed, the patient has lost an important defense mechanism to prevent the aspiration of refluxed material. The patient should therefore be instructed to elevate the head of the bed in order to minimize this risk. For the same reason patients with gross GERD should not undergo cricopharyngeal myotomy unless the reflux can be controlled either medically or surgically.

13.2.2 MIDESOPHAGEAL DIVERTICULA
Traditionally, midesophageal diverticula have been called "traction" diverticula because of their supposed etiology. They were believed to arise secondary to old mediastinal inflammation, such as tuberculosis, that caused adherence of mediastinal structures to the outer esophageal wall so that outward traction occurred during peristalsis. It now appears likely that very few midesophageal diverticula arise this way. In most there is an associated motility disorder and it is likely that this is actually a "pulsion" diverticulum formed when a peristaltic wave deteriorates into a simultaneous or spastic contraction in the smooth-muscle esophagus. Midesophageal diverticula rarely require specific therapy. Rather, only the associated motor disorder requires treatment if symptomatic.

13.2.3 LOWER ESOPHAGEAL OR EPIPHRENIC DIVERTICULA
These "pulsion" diverticula form just above the LES and are invariably associated with an esophageal motor disorder – usually diffuse esophageal spasm, with or without abnormal relaxation of the LES. Patients with these diverticula usually present with dysphagia and/or angina-like chest pain. In addition, they may complain of nocturnal regurgitation of large quantities of stagnant fluid.

If symptoms are present, treatment with nitrates or calcium channel blockers may be helpful. If this is not successful, surgery is indicated. Any surgical attack on these diverticula should involve a myotomy of the spastic distal esophagus and/or LES. Resection of the diverticula alone seldom affords long-term benefit.

13.2.4 *INTRAMURAL DIVERTICULOSIS*

This disorder has a characteristic radiologic appearance consisting of numerous tiny, flask-shaped outpouchings from the esophageal lumen. There is usually an associated smooth stricture in the proximal esophagus. Patients typically present with dysphagia that responds to peroral dilation. The outpouchings are actually dilated ducts coming from submucosal glands and thus are not true diverticula. The etiology is obscure. Some cases are associated with esophageal candidiasis, but this organism does not appear to be of etiological importance.

13.3 Esophageal Trauma

Blunt or penetrating trauma to the chest can cause esophageal injury. In addition, esophageal instrumentation such as that used in bougienage or endoscopy may cause perforation or mucosal laceration. Severe retching or vomiting can also cause esophageal perforation (*Boerhaave's syndrome*) or mucosal laceration (*Mallory-Weiss tear*). Boerhaave's syndrome is a life-threatening condition that requires immediate surgery to drain the mediastinum and repair the defect in the esophageal wall. Patients, typically alcoholics, present with sudden epigastric and/or chest pain following a bout of vomiting and usually have fever and signs of hypovolemia or shock.

The mucosal laceration of the Mallory-Weiss tear is probably better classified as a disorder of the stomach, because in most cases the laceration starts at the GE junction and extends down into the stomach. These patients present with hematemesis or melena following a bout of retching or vomiting. The bleeding usually stops spontaneously and only supportive therapy is required. If bleeding persists, endoscopically applied hemostasis or surgical intervention may be necessary.

13.4 Food-Bolus Obstruction and Foreign Bodies

A surprising variety of foreign bodies can lodge in the esophagus after being swallowed either inadvertently or deliberately. The three most common sites where foreign bodies become stuck are the piriform sinuses, at the aortic arch and just above the LES. The patient can usually localize the site of the obstruction quite accurately, and this can be confirmed using routine x-rays if the object is radiopaque. (However, as mentioned above, some patients may perceive the obstruction in the throat region when it is really in the distal esophagus.) Otherwise, x-rays using small amounts of water-soluble contrast media may be necessary. Most foreign bodies can be removed by an expert endoscopist. Surgery is rarely required, except when perforation has occurred.

A more common clinical problem is esophageal food-bolus obstruction.

This typically occurs when a patient with a motility disorder, stricture or Schatzki's (lower esophageal) ring swallows a large solid-food bolus. The patient notices immediate chest pain, usually well localized to the site of obstruction. Attempts to swallow anything further are unsuccessful and usually lead to prompt regurgitation.

Many physicians will initially treat these patients with smooth-muscle relaxants such as intravenous glucagon, sublingual nitroglycerin or nifedipine; however, there is little evidence that this approach is efficacious. If the food bolus does not pass on spontaneously within a few hours, endoscopy should be performed, at which time the bolus can either be removed per os or pushed through into the stomach. These patients should not be left too long, as the bolus is capable of causing significant maceration to the esophageal mucosa. Giving the patient meat tenderizer, in an attempt to dissolve the bolus, is probably of no value and may be very harmful; papain can digest the esophageal mucosa and has been reported to cause severe hemorrhagic pulmonary edema when aspirated.

SUGGESTED READING LIST

Beck IT, Connor J, Lemire S, et al. Canadian consensus conference on the treatment of gastrointestinal reflux disease. Can J Gastroenterol 1992; 6(5):277–289.

Clouse RE. Motor disorders. In: Sleisenger MH, Fordtran JS (eds.), Gastrointestinal disease: pathophysiology, diagnosis and management. 4th ed. Philadelphia: WB Saunders, 1989:559–593.

DeVault KR, Castell DO. Guidelines for the diagnosis and treatment of gastroesophageal reflux disease. Arch Intern Med 1995; 155:2165–2173.

Dodds WJ, Dent J, Hogan WJ, et al. Mechanisms of gastroesophageal reflux in patients with reflux esophagitis. N Engl J Med 1982; 307:1547–1552.

Goyal RK, Paterson WG. Esophageal motility. In: Wood JD (ed.), Handbook of physiology: motility and circulation, vol. 4. Washington, DC: American Physiological Society, 1989:865–908.

Helm JF, Dodds WJ, Pelc LR, et al. Effect of esophageal emptying and saliva on clearance of acid from the esophagus. N Engl J Med 1984; 310: 284–288.

McCallum RW, Mittal RK (eds.). Gastroesophageal reflux disease. Gastroenterol Clin North Am 1990; 19(3):501–781.

Wong RK (ed.). Mucosal diseases of the esophagus. Gastroenterol Clin North Am 1991; 20(4):635–890.

ACKNOWLEDGMENT

We would like to acknowledge and thank Dr. I.T. Beck for his contribution of several of the figures for the chapter and valuable editorial advice.

OBJECTIVES

Anatomy and Physiology
1. Know the anatomy and physiology of the normal esophagus and esophagogastric junction.
2. Describe the process of deglutition and esophageal peristalsis.
3. Understand the different physiological control mechanisms between the upper striated-muscle esophagus and distal smooth-muscle esophagus.
4. Understand the mechanisms underlying LES tone and relaxation.

Congenital and Anatomic Abnormalities
1. Define esophageal atresia and tracheoesophageal fistula, and describe how they present.
2. Define hiatus hernia with regard to anatomic type (sliding versus para-esophageal).

Gastroesophageal Reflux Disease (GERD)
1. Outline the clinical symptoms of GERD.
2. Describe the anatomic and physiological factors predisposing to GERD.
3. Discuss the procedures used in the diagnosis of GERD.
4. Discuss medical management of GERD.
5. List the indications for operative management of GERD and discuss the physiological basis for the antireflux procedures.
6. List the complications of gastroesophageal reflux disease.

Nonreflux-Induced Esophagitis
1. List the major infectious causes of esophagitis (Candida, herpetic) and describe how they present.
2. List other causes of esophagitis.

Disorders of the Oropharyngeal Phase of Deglutition
1. Categorize the major causes of oropharyngeal deglutition.
2. Describe how oropharyngeal dysphagia can be differentiated from esophageal dysphagia based on history.
3. Describe the investigations required in the assessment of oropharyngeal dysphagia.
4. What are the complications of oropharyngeal dysphagia?

Motor Disorders of the Esophagus
1. List the major primary and secondary esophageal motor disorders.

  2. Describe the clinical symptoms typically associated with different esophageal motor disorders.

Esophageal Tumors
1. List the symptoms suggestive of an esophageal malignancy.
2. Outline a diagnostic plan for evaluating a patient with suspected esoph ageal tumor.
3. Describe the natural history of malignant esophageal neoplasms.
4. Describe the treatment options for esophageal malignancy.
5. List the common types of benign esophageal tumors.

Miscellaneous Esophageal Disorders
1. Be able to describe the presenting symptomatology and typical x-ray findings of esophageal webs, and Zenker's and esophageal diverticula.
2. Outline the clinical presentation and management of patients presenting with (a) Boerhaave's syndrome and (b) esophageal foreign body or food-bolus obstruction.

Skills
1. Demonstrate the ability to read a barium swallow in patients with sliding and paraesophageal hiatus hernia, esophageal cancer, Zenker's diverticulum, esophageal diverticulum and achalasia.
2. Describe the motility abnormalities in achalasia, diffuse esophageal spasm, "nutcracker" esophagus and scleroderma esophagus.
3. Develop an approach for the diagnostic evaluation of a patient with dysphagia.

6

The Stomach and Duodenum

B.J. Salena and R.H. Hunt

1. INTRODUCTION

Diseases of the GI tract are common, accounting for one out of seven complaints, and disorders of the stomach and duodenum make up a large part of these.

It has been known for many centuries that the gastric juice is acid in nature, but it was not until 1824 that William Prout established that the acid in the stomach is hydrochloric acid. Since then physicians have been fascinated by the ability of the healthy stomach and duodenum to withstand hydrochloric acid and pepsin. In particular they have studied extensively the mechanisms controlling gastric secretion in the hope of finding a satisfactory way of explaining and treating peptic ulcer disease. Recent attention has turned to the role of mucus, bicarbonate and prostaglandins in maintenance and defense of the gastric mucosa against acid injury. This chapter will review the anatomy, physiology and related common disorders of the stomach and duodenum.

2. ANATOMY

2.1 General Anatomy
The stomach is the most capacious part of the GI tract and lies between the distal esophagus and the duodenum. It is situated entirely within the abdomen below the diaphragm (Figure 1). The body of the stomach lies slightly to the left of the midline, the antrum across the spinal vertebrae at the level of T10–L1 and the pylorus to the right of the vertebral column. The duodenum is predominantly retroperitoneal and comprises the cap, descending and distal portions.

The greater curvature is some three or four times the length of the lesser

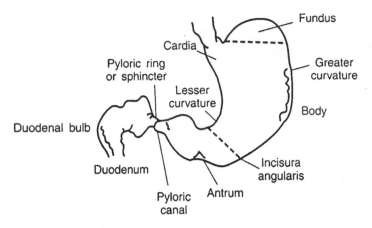

FIGURE 1. Anatomic divisions of the stomach.

curvature. A point known as the angulus or incisura may be defined on the lesser curvature. This point is relatively constant and marks a change from the prominent rugal folds of the body of the stomach to the smoother, less prominent folds of the antrum.

The stomach and duodenum lie in close proximity to a number of important anatomic structures. Anterosuperiorly are the left diaphragm and left lobe of the liver, while the body and tail of the pancreas lie posteriorly. Laterally to the left are the hilum of the left kidney, the left adrenal gland and, above that, the spleen. These organs form the stomach bed and are separated from it by the lesser omentum and the lesser sac. The duodenum, apart from the cap, lies retroperitoneally. The second and distal parts surround the head of the pancreas while the cap, which is attached to the lesser omentum, lies anterior to the head of the pancreas.

2.2 Blood Supply

The main arterial blood supply (Figure 2) arises from the celiac axis. The common hepatic artery gives rise to the gastroduodenal artery and the right gastric artery, which then anastomoses with the left gastric artery. The splenic artery gives rise to the short gastric arteries that supply the body along the greater curvature of the stomach. The right and left gastroepiploic arteries also form an anastomosis along the greater curvature.

Venous drainage essentially follows the arterial supply but passes to the portal venous system and its tributaries, the splenic vein and the superior mesenteric vein. Veins from the fundus communicate with veins draining the

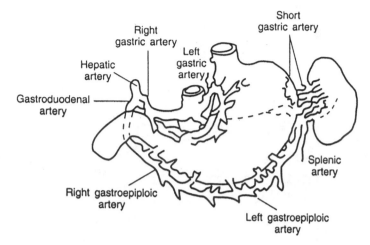

FIGURE 2. Blood supply to the stomach.

lower third of the esophagus and form a connection between the systemic and portal venous systems. This connection assumes clinical importance if portal venous pressure rises, when venous flow is reversed through the esophageal veins, leading to esophageal or fundal varices.

Lymphatic drainage is to the pancreaticosplenic nodes, the left gastric nodes and the pyloric nodes, and then via the celiac group to the preaortic lymph nodes and the cisterna chyli.

2.3 Nerve Supply
The nerve supply is both sympathetic and parasympathetic. The vagal supply arises via the anterior and posterior trunks, which pass through the diaphragm on either side of the esophagus before giving rise to the hepatic and celiac branches. The hepatic branch supplies further branches to the anterior surface of the body of the stomach and to the pyloric region, while the celiac branch passes to the celiac plexus and the posterior aspect of the body of the stomach. The vagal fibers anastomose with ganglion cells of the stomach within the muscle layers, forming Auerbach's plexus or, in the submucosa, forming Meissner's plexus.

The sympathetic nerve supply arises from the spinal cord between T6 and T10 and passes to the sympathetic ganglia. The parasympathetic supply contracts the stomach, relaxes the pylorus and stimulates acid, pepsin and mucus secretion, whereas sympathetic stimulation constricts the blood supply and reduces gastric motor activity and secretion while the pylorus is contracted.

FIGURE 3.   Microscopic appearances of gastric pit and glands.

2.4 Structure of the Stomach and Duodenum

The stomach and duodenum comprise an outer serosal coat, a muscular layer, submucosa and mucus membrane. The mucosal surface is ridged by the rugal folds created by contractions of the muscularis mucosa, especially prominent in the body of the stomach and less obvious in the antrum. The glands of the stomach are of two main types – gastric and pyloric – both of which are closely packed in the columnar epithelium. The gastric glands (known as oxyntic glands) make up 70–80% of the total and are responsible for secreting mucus, pepsinogen, hydrochloric acid and intrinsic factor (Figure 3). The pyloric glands, which secrete mucus and gastrin, make up only about 15%. A line of demarcation can usually be seen between the gastric and pyloric glands in the region of the incisura.

The gastric glands differ in cell type: the chief or peptic cells secrete pepsinogen, while the parietal or oxyntic cells secrete hydrochloric acid and intrinsic factor. The endocrine cells of the antrum secrete gastrin and 5-hydroxytryptamine. In the duodenum the first 4–5 cm of mucosa are smooth, but in the descending duodenum the mucosa is thrown into crescentic folds. The mucosa is lined with columnar, goblet, Paneth's and endocrine cells. The columnar cells line the villi and crypts, which increase in size in the second and third parts of the duodenum. A characteristic feature in the duodenal submucosa is the presence of Brunner's glands, which are similar to pyloric glands.

3. PHYSIOLOGY

The stomach has three major functions: motor, secretory and endocrine (Table 1). The motor functions include temporary storage of food and fluid, mixing of ingested materials with gastric juice and regulated emptying of gastric con-

TABLE 1. Functions of the stomach

Motor
Vagus-mediated and gastrin-induced receptive relaxation
Mixing and emptying

Secretory
Acid, pepsin, intrinsic factor, volume, water, electrolytes

Endocrine
Gastrin, serotonin, somatostatin

---

tents. The most important substances secreted into the lumen of the stomach include hydrochloric acid, pepsin, mucus, bicarbonate, intrinsic factor and water. The stomach releases two hormones into the blood: gastrin and somatostatin. Serotonin-staining (ECL) cells are also present in the gastric fundus and antrum. Gastrin stimulates acid secretion by the stomach, and somatostatin inhibits the release of gastrin.

3.1 Gastric Motility

The motor functions of the stomach include serving as a reservoir, mixing its contents, kneading and churning solid food, and regulating the emptying of its contents into the duodenum. The reservoir function involves temporary storage of ingested and secreted substances. Above a certain threshold volume, the stomach is "full" (whether the volume is large or small); i.e., the intragastric pressure increases very little with the addition of more food and fluid because the walls of the stomach relax to accommodate the load. The stomach also mixes ingested substances with gastric juice to dissolve and dilute food, kneads solid materials to a particle size of less than 1 mm diameter, and finally, empties its contents into the duodenum slowly and in small volumes.

Gastric motility is controlled centrally and by local neurohormonal control of muscle. The muscle layers include the outer longitudinal, middle circular and inner oblique fibers. Neuronal control involves the intrinsic myenteric plexus, the extrinsic postganglionic sympathetic fibers of the celiac plexus, and the preganglionic parasympathetic fibers of the vagus nerve. The vagal afferents are both relaxatory and excitatory. These vagal fibers are neither cholinergic nor adrenergic.

Factors that influence gastric motility may be classified as myogenic, neural and chemical. The resting potential difference of the gastric smooth muscle is 5–15 mV and there is a rhythmic depolarization, with this basic electrical rhythm being set by the gastric pacemaker, which gives rise to slow-wave activity. The action potential produces peristalsis and is influenced by gastrin. The force of the contraction is increased with vagal activity, gastrin and motilin, and is decreased with gastric secretion.

Gastric distention by food or liquid stimulates both intrinsic nerves and vagal afferents. There is increased spike burst activity, more forceful peristaltic contractions and increased gastric emptying. Pyloric sphincter relaxation occurs so that the antral lumen is not occluded by peristaltic waves. Gastric contents are propelled both forward and backward toward the body of the stomach and are thoroughly mixed. Gastrin delays gastric emptying by decreasing gastric motility and at the same time increasing duodenal motility and pyloric tone (events that are mediated by fat, protein or acid in the duodenum). This increase in duodenal motility and pyloric tone is effected by stimulation of duodenal osmoreceptors and by the release of secretin, cholecystokinin (CCK) and gastric inhibitory polypeptide (GIP).

Gastric motility is inhibited for the stomach to accommodate food. Vagal relaxatory fibers are stimulated by swallowing, esophageal or gastric distention, and neurogenic stimulation. Sympathetic and adrenergic fibers influence these cholinergic neurons.

The emptying of the stomach is influenced by the substance, volume, osmolality and composition of the ingested meal. Liquids empty more rapidly than solids. The rate of gastric emptying is related to the square root of the volume, so that a constant proportion of the gastric contents empties per unit time. Stimulation of duodenal osmoreceptors with triglycerides, fatty acids or hydrochloric acid slows gastric emptying.

The gastric body serves as a reservoir, whereas the antrum has the function of mixing, churning and emptying. A high-pressure gradient exists at the gastroduodenal junction, with the pyloric sphincter playing an important role in the coordinated activity of emptying the antral contents into the duodenum.

When the volume of the stomach increases with relaxation, the intragastric pressure does not increase, because of receptive relaxation mediated by way of a vagal reflex and the splanchnic nerves. Receptive relaxation occurs primarily in the gastric fundus and body. Vagotomy, fundoplication and extensive involvement of the stomach by adenocarcinoma result in a loss of this capacity, leading to early satiety. Gastric fundal contractions are infrequent, and of large amplitude and long duration (45 seconds). These contractions propel contents to the body and antrum for mixing to occur.

The distal two-thirds of the stomach is under intrinsic myogenic control. Electrical slow-wave activity can be detected on the greater curvature, with aboral contractions passing from the greater to the lesser curvature at a rate of about 3 per minute. Although antral contractions occur only in response to neural stimulation, the muscle will contract only when a slow wave occurs.

The gastric pacemaker controls the frequency and direction of propagated contractions. This control can be altered by the insertion of an electrical pacemaker, potentially changing the frequency of contraction and reversing its direction. It is possible that some clinical disorders of gastric emptying may give rise to chronic nausea, vomiting, fullness and distention.

As antral contractions pass distally, velocity increases, with near simultaneous contractions of distal antrum and pylorus. A small amount of gastric chyme may enter the duodenum, but most passes back into the stomach, where further mixing and churning takes place.

The pyloric sphincter is recognized macroscopically by thickening of the distal circular antral muscle, forming a muscular ring. However, it is difficult to accept this as a true physiologic sphincter, since in its resting phase it is open, and the rapid closure with antral peristalsis serves more to retard than to facilitate the aboral passage of gastric chyme. The pylorus acts to limit duodenogastric reflux. Duodenal acidification or infusion of secretin results in an increase in pyloric sphincter pressure. Patients with gastric ulcer or bile gastritis experience increased reflux of duodenal contents (including bile and pancreatic enzymes) into the stomach, apparently secondary to a pyloric defect. If the sphincter is ablated by pyloroplasty for duodenal ulcer disease, bile reflux is inevitable.

3.2 Gastric Secretion

Gastric juice contains many substances. The six most important of these are hydrogen ion, pepsin, mucus, bicarbonate, intrinsic factor and water. Hydrochloric acid and the enzyme pepsin participate in the digestion of proteins. Mucus lubricates ingested solids. Mucus and bicarbonate probably protect the mucosal lining against digestion by acid and pepsin. The intrinsic factor is required for normal absorption of ingested cobalamin (vitamin B_{12}). Each day the stomach secretes about 2 L of water in an adult.

3.2.1 GASTRIC ACID SECRETION

It is generally accepted that acid secretion is activated by three separate pathways: the neural, hormonal and paracrinal (local) pathways. The major chemical transmitter substances are acetylcholine, gastrin and histamine.

The vagus and branches from the celiac plexus and ganglia traveling along the celiac artery are the major extrinsic nervous supply to the acid-secreting portion of the stomach. The postganglionic neurons of the vagi that terminate in the oxyntic gland near the oxyntic cells are predominantly cholinergic. These cholinergic fibers are rarely seen in contact with the oxyntic cells, and therefore acetylcholine released by these nerve endings must diffuse a relatively long distance to the cells. There are two types of muscarinic binding sites on oxyntic cells: M_1 and M_2 receptors. The cholinergic binding results in a dose-dependent acid secretory response. Additionally, there may be muscarinic receptors on histamine-containing cells resulting in indirect stimulation by histamine release on paracrine cells.

Histamine has a direct stimulatory action on oxyntic cells via an H_2 receptor. The stimulatory action of histamine on oxyntic cells is competitively antagonized by a group of histamine analogues (such as cimetidine, ranitidine, famotidine, nizatidine and others) that specifically interact with the H_2 receptor. The histamine antagonists binding to the H_1 receptor can decrease gastric histamine, but at much higher doses.

Gastrin, the other major secretagogue, also interacts with oxyntic cells via a gastrin receptor. The weak stimulatory effect of gastrin on acid production can be competitively inhibited by proglumide, a glutamic acid derivative known to antagonize CCK. Since CCK binds with the same affinity and produces a similar weak secretory response, the question has been raised whether the receptor may be a CCK receptor instead of a gastrin receptor, or whether the receptor may be related to the well-known trophic effect of gastrin rather than the acid-secreting effects.

The binding of secretagogues to the oxyntic cell receptors is coupled to at least two possible intracellular messengers, Ca^{++} and cyclic AMP. Cholinergic action controls the influx of extracellular Ca^{++} into the oxyntic cell, with subsequent activation of undefined intracellular events resulting in acid secretion. The weak stimulatory effect of gastrin is also Ca^{++} dependent. Histamine does not require extracellular Ca^{++} for stimulation of acid secretion. Cyclic AMP is the intracellular messenger coupling the effect of histamine to hydrogen ion production and secretion.

After the oxyntic cells have been stimulated, intracellular endoplasmic tubular structures known as tubulovesicles disappear from the cytoplasm, while the microvilli in the secretory canaliculi increase in length to enlarge the secretory surface. The tubulovesicle membranes contain H^+/K^+-ATPase, the enzyme responsible for driving the H^+ pump, exchanging K^+ for H^+. These membranes have a low permeability to K^+ and, at rest, prevent sufficient K^+ from entering the lumen of the tubulovesicles, thus preventing H^+ transport. Stimulatory activity occurs only with a cellular signal from secretagogues.

It is evident that the overall process of acid secretion is controlled by a complex interaction of a number of pathways that will be further elucidated in the future.

3.2.2 *PEPSINOGEN SECRETION*
Pepsinogens are present in the mucous cells of cardiac glands, in the chief and mucous neck cells of oxyntic glands, in the mucous cells of pyloric glands and

in the mucous cells of duodenal Brunner's glands. These proenzymes are secreted and activated by acids to the active form, pepsin. Furthermore, pepsin can activate additional pepsinogen autocatalytically.

The mucosal lining of the stomach contains four types of immunologically distinct pepsinogens with the ability to digest proteins at acid pH. Pepsinogens and hydrochloric acid secretion respond to much the same stimulants. Cephalic-vagal stimulation strongly stimulates pepsinogen secretion. Anticholinergics, histamine H_2-receptor antagonists and vagotomy decrease pepsinogen secretion. Elevated serum type 1 pepsinogen has been associated with duodenal ulcer and gastrinoma, while atrophic gastritis (with or without pernicious anemia) has been associated with low levels of type 1 pepsinogen.

3.2.3 INTRINSIC FACTOR SECRETION

Intrinsic factor (IF) is a glycoprotein secreted by oxyntic cells. It is important in vitamin B_{12} absorption. B_{12} is released from dietary protein by gastric acid and pepsin; it binds to IF and to R protein, which is secreted into saliva. B_{12} binds more efficiently to the R proteins at low pH, so most of the B_{12} is initially complexed with the R proteins. In the upper small bowel, pancreatic enzymes cleave the complexes and the free B_{12} binds to IF, which eventually binds to a specific ileal receptor and is subsequently absorbed and transported to the tissues by another B_{12}-binding protein, transcobalamin II.

Stimulants of acid secretion also stimulate IF secretion. Patients with low or absent acid secretion often have reduced IF secretion. Continued IF secretion is low but the amounts may be adequate to prevent vitamin B_{12} deficiency and pernicious anemia. Rarely, IF secretion can be absent with normal acid secretion. Circulating antibodies to IF and oxyntic cells are found in many patients with atrophic gastritis, achlorhydria or hypochlorhydria, and pernicious anemia.

3.3 Gastric Mucosal Barrier

Healthy gastric mucosa has the ability to resist high intraluminal concentrations of hydrochloric acid and peptic activity. The physiologic basis of this barrier involves several factors.

The tight junctions between the surface epithelial cells seal off the paracellular route for transport between cells. Transport can also occur across the bilipid layer membrane at the apical surface of the mucosal epithelial cells. The fluidity of this membrane can vary and influence permeability to various macromolecules. While there is active and passive transport of H^+, Na^+ and K^+ ions, an electric potential difference exists across the mucosa. With disruption of this barrier, a fall in potential difference occurs.

In the presence of luminal acid, the gastroduodenal pH approaches pH 2, while the immediately adjacent epithelium may be near neutral (pH 7). This pH gradient, which plays some role in protection from acid-peptic digestion, is probably dependent on the combined secretion of mucus and bicarbonate. How the gastric mucosa secretes acid while maintaining a near-neutral pH adjacent to the surface epithelium requires elucidation.

Gastric mucus consists of about 95% water and 5% glycoprotein. It provides lubrication for food particles and its gel-like nature retains water and bicarbonate close to the surface epithelium. Mucus is secreted by exocytosis, apical expulsion and exfoliation, and formed with bicarbonate in the surface epithelial cells, in the epithelial cells of the gastric gland neck and by the Brunner's glands of the duodenum. The mucus layer varies in thickness but averages about 100 μm. The role of mucus in protection against acid-peptic activity is unclear. It does provide a relatively thick unstirred layer adjacent to the mucosa, allowing a rate of diffusion of H^+ ions four times slower than through a similar thickness of unstirred water. This contributes to the maintenance of a hydrogen ion gradient between the gastric lumen and the surface epithelium. That is, when the pH in the gastric lumen is 2, the pH at the gastric membrane will be 6.8 to 7. ASA and nonsteroidal anti-inflammatory agents inhibit mucus synthesis and release, while prostaglandins increase mucus synthesis. Mucus synthesis is decreased after stress and may play a role in stress ulceration. Mucus limits the diffusion of pepsin and other large molecules, thus preventing further injury.

Bicarbonate secretion is an active process dependent on the metabolic integrity of a healthy epithelium. Secretion is stimulated by acetylcholine, prostaglandins, glucagon and cyclic GMP, and inhibited by α-adrenergic agonists and GIP. Luminal acid also appears to stimulate gastric and duodenal bicarbonate secretion. Low concentrations of bile salts in the stomach inhibit gastric bicarbonate secretion.

Prostaglandins probably play an important role in mucosal defense. These saturated, oxygenated fatty acids are derived from arachidonic acid. They may protect the mucosa by maintaining or increasing gastric mucosal blood flow and hence stimulating mucus production and bicarbonate secretion, and increasing protein synthesis (which is necessary for the maintenance and regeneration of cells). It is not known whether prostaglandins play a role in the maintenance of normal membrane function and tight junctions, but they probably maintain sulfhydryl groups, which act as oxidative scavengers.

The development of gastritis and gastric ulcer is thought to arise as a result of defective defense mechanisms. There may be increased degradation of mucus by pepsinogen 1, bile or pancreatic secretions; by infection with Helicobacter pylori; or through mechanical factors. A quantitatively or qualitatively defective secretion of mucus is also possible. Bicarbonate secretion may be reduced or mucosal blood flow and/or mucosal metabolism compromised, as occurs in stress ulceration.

3.4 Gastric Endocrine Secretion

The stomach produces regulatory peptides, such as gastrin and somatostatin. Each agent is a polypeptide; gastrin is known to exist in multiple forms in the body. These peptides are produced by enterochromaffin cells of the gastric mucosa. The cell that produces gastrin is called the "G cell" and is found in large numbers in the antral mucosa.

Gastrin is the most important peptide in the regulation of gastric acid secretion. Under physiologic conditions gastrin is released continually, with increased amounts appearing in the blood at mealtimes. Gastrin is a hormone that increases the rate of oxyntic cell secretion of H^+ and peptic cell secretion of pepsinogen. Gastrin increases contraction of antral smooth muscle and increases mucosal blood flow.

Extragastric actions of gastrin include contraction of the lower esophageal sphincter, stimulation of pancreatic enzyme secretion, gallbladder contraction, increased small intestine motility, and the regulation of glucose-stimulated insulin release. Gastrin is a trophic hormone that stimulates protein synthesis and growth of certain gastrointestinal tissues, such as the mucosal lining of the stomach and gut, and the parenchyma of the pancreas.

Somatostatin inhibits the release of gastrin from the G cells, probably acting as a paracrine substance. In addition, the nerves of the gastric mucosa contain vasoactive intestinal peptide (VIP) and gastrin-releasing peptide (GRP or bombesin). VIP is probably responsible for mediating the relaxation of gastric smooth muscle. Bombesin mediates the release of gastrin in response to vagal stimulation.

3.5 Assessment of Gastric Acid Secretion

Basal acid output (BAO) refers to the quantity of hydrochloric acid (HCl) secreted per hour by the stomach in the unstimulated basal state, expressed in milliequivalents of HCl per hour. The normal range is 1–5 mEq of HCl per hour. The acid output is the product of the volume of gastric juices (in liters) multiplied by the concentration of hydrogen ion (in milliequivalents per liter).

Maximal acid output refers to the total acid output during the hour after stimulation with pentagastrin (6 µg/kg IM or SC) or histamine (40 µg/kg SC). This value is determined by adding the results of either four 15-minute or six 10-minute sample collections after stimulation. The normal range is 25–55 mEq HCl per hour.

Peak acid output reflects the two highest consecutive 15-minute periods of stimulated output, multiplied by a factor of 2 to yield a value for a one-hour output.

Gastric secretory studies may be useful in patients with suspected gastric hypersecretion and in the evaluation of the efficacy of medical and surgical therapy in the reduction of gastric acid output. In suspected Zollinger-Ellison syndrome, elevated basal hypersecretion may point to the diagnosis, but usually gastric acid secretory studies are more useful in establishing the therapeutic response to acid-suppressive pharmacotherapy.

4. PATHOPHYSIOLOGY OF PEPTIC ULCER DLSEASE

4.1 Gastric Ulcer Disease

Acute ulcers may occur in the patient with burns (Curling's ulcer), midbrain disease (Cushing's ulcer) and chronic debilitating disease. ASA-containing analgesics and nonsteroidal anti-inflammatory drugs may also induce acute ulcer bleeding, though the risk of this complication has probably been over-stated. There is epidemiologic evidence suggesting that the incidence and behavior of chronic peptic ulcers vary according to the site at which they occur. Therefore, gastric and duodenal ulcers will be considered separately, although the basic defects that cause either type relate to an imbalance of aggressive and protective factors.

Numerous pathophysiologic defects have been identified in gastric ulcer disease (Table 2A). Not all of these factors are present in each patient. These defects include decreased acid secretion, decreased parietal cell mass and back-diffusion of acid. Many patients with chronic gastric ulcers have associated gastritis. There may be increased concentration of bile acids and pancreatic juice in the stomach as a result of duodenogastric reflux. Delayed gastric emptying has also been identified in some patients with gastric ulcers, and this may accentuate the release of gastrin and the secretion of hydrochloric acid. It has yet to be determined whether delayed gastric emptying is the cause or secondary effect of gastric ulcer disease. However, as a result of back-diffusion of acid, the actual concentration of acid in the gastric lumen may be underestimated. Hypergastrinemia and hyperchloremia are not commonly thought to be associated with gastric ulcers. The pressure of the pyloric sphincter may be inappropriately decreased under basal conditions and may fail to respond normally to acid or fat in the duodenum, thereby predisposing to duodenogastric reflux.

4.2 Duodenal Ulcer Disease

A number of pathophysiologic defects have also been identified in some patients with duodenal ulcer disease (Table 2B). These include increased pari-

TABLE 2. Pathophysiologic defects in some patients with:

A. *Peptic ulcer disease/gastric ulcer disease*
Decreased acid secretion, decreased parietal cell mass (PCM), back-diffusion of acid
Chronic superficial and atrophic gastritis
Increased concentration of bile acids and pancreatic juice in stomach (duodenogastric reflux)
Delayed gastric emptying
Inappropriately decreased pyloric sphincter pressure under basal conditions and in response to
  acid (secretin) or fat (cholecystokinin) in the duodenum

B. *Duodenal ulcer disease*
Increased parietal cell mass
Increased sensitivity of parietal cells to gastrin and secretagogues
Increased secretory drive
Decreased acid-induced inhibition of meal-stimulated gastrin release
Increased gastric emptying
Increased duodenal acid/pepsin loads
Chronic active gastritis

---

etal cell mass (leading to increased maximal and peak acid output); increased sensitivity of the parietal cells to gastrin and other secretagogues; increased secretory drive; decreased acid-induced inhibition of meal-stimulated gastrin release; and increased gastric emptying (leading to increased duodenal acid and pepsin loads).

Apart from an increased parietal cell population (and possibly G-cell hyperplasia), the gastric mucosa is histologically normal in duodenal ulcer. By contrast, in gastric ulcer the nonparietal mucosal area is usually increased, especially on the lesser curvature, and there is often some degree of histologically demonstrable gastritis. Biliary reflux through the pylorus is also a common finding in patients with gastric ulcers, and it has been suggested that the combination of bile and acid may be particularly damaging to the mucosa, probably by causing back-diffusion of hydrogen ions into it and thus disrupting intracellular organelles.

4.3 **Hereditary Factors**

Hereditary factors are important in the pathogenesis of peptic ulcer disease, as suggested by a higher prevalence of peptic ulcer disease in certain genetic syndromes. A number of familial aggregations have been noted in patients with peptic ulcer disease. These include hyperpepsinogenemia 1, normal pepsinogenemia 1, antral G-cell hyperfunction, rapid gastric emptying, childhood duodenal ulcer and immunologic forms of peptic ulcer disease. Heredity also plays a role in the development of ulceration and is associated with the syndrome of multiple endocrine adenomatosis 1 (adenomas of the pancreas, pituitary and parathyroid). Parents, siblings and children of ulcer patients are more likely to have peptic ulcer disease than control individuals. There is greater concordance for ulcer disease in identical than in fraternal twins. Hyperpepsinogenemia 1 appears to be an autosomal dominant trait. Families have been described in which a number of physiologic abnormalities associated with the development of ulcer disease have been noted, including increased meal-stimulated gastrin release and altered gastric emptying. There is increasing evidence to suggest that familial peptic ulcer disease is related to Helicobacter pylori infection amongst family members.

4.4 **Interplay of Acid, Pepsin and Other Factors**

Peptic ulcer disease is thought to occur as a result of an interplay between acid and pepsin. Peptic ulcers occur more commonly in the duodenum and less commonly in the stomach and esophagus. They usually occur near mucosal junctions. Rarely, peptic ulcers occur in the jejunum; this should raise the possibility of the Zollinger-Ellison syndrome. When gastric mucosa is present in a Meckel's diverticulum in the ileum, peptic ulceration and bleeding can occur. The ulceration occurs in the ileum adjacent to the diverticulum.

4.5 **The Patient and the Environment**

When considering the pathogenesis of any disease, we need to examine environmental factors, hereditary associations and pathophysiologic abnormalities. Environmental factors (Table 3) that have been examined include drugs, smoking, alcohol, caffeine-containing beverages and stress. Nonsteroidal anti-inflammatory agents such as ASA are thought to cause ulceration, mostly as a result of damage to the protected mucosal barrier. Smoking is associated with a higher prevalence of peptic ulcer disease and may be associated with impaired healing of duodenal and gastric ulcer disease. Also, death rates from peptic ulcer disease are higher in individuals who smoke. Alcohol and caffeine-containing beverages may affect acid secretion, and have been considered in the pathogenesis of peptic ulcer disease. However, it is fair to say that the role of coffee, alcohol, nonsteroidal anti-inflammatory agents and corticosteroids in the pathogenesis of peptic ulcer disease remains unclear.

Both patients and physicians often express the concern that "stress" is important in the initiation or perpetuation of peptic ulcer disease. Some patients with duodenal ulcer disease may have an exaggerated sense of self-sufficiency and demonstrate overambitiousness and aggressiveness. Some psychiatric views suggest that these attitudes represent a defense against an awareness of dependency. It is possible but unproven that patients exposed to excess stress may have more frequent ulceration, may be more sensitive to the

TABLE 3. Environmental factors in pathogenesis of peptic ulcer disease (PUD)

Infection
Helicobacter pylori

Drugs
NSAIDs

Smoking
Prevalence of PUD
Healing of duodenal ulcer (DU) and gastric ulcer (GU)
Death rates from PUD

Alcohol and caffeine-containing beverages
Acid secretion

---

symptoms of peptic ulcer disease, and may be more likely to develop perforations.

Recent studies from Israel and the United States have identified a number of predictors of duodenal ulcer disease in men. These are psychosocial and biological. The important psychosocial factors include anxiety – stress, brooding (i.e., difficulty coping and difficulty expressing emotions) and inadequate caring, particularly lack of family support. Biological factors include age, lower blood pressure, use of cigarettes and leanness.

4.6 The Molecular Level

At a molecular level, the pathogenesis of ulcer disease is believed to reflect an imbalance between increased aggressive factors and decreased protective factors. In considering the possible aggressive factors, we need to briefly review the normal mechanism of acid secretion. Acid secretion is divided into the cephalic, gastric and intestinal phases. As a result of vagal stimulation arising from the sight, smell, taste or thought of food, acetylcholine is released and acts on the parietal cells to produce acid. In addition, vagal afferents stimulate the antral G cells to release gastrin. Food in the stomach gives rise to antral distention, and this along with peptide breakdown products stimulates the antral G cells to produce gastrin. The gastrin and acetylcholine act directly on the parietal cells or the mast cells. The mast cells in turn release histamine, which stimulates gastric acid secretion.

Once acid secretion has been initiated, how is further acid secretion limited? Clearly, there will be loss of vagal stimulation, loss of antral distention and loss of stimulated release of gastrin as food is virtually digested and emptied from the stomach into the duodenum. Also, the acid released from the parietal cells acidifies the antrum and thereby inhibits the further release of gastrin. The presence of food in the intestine further stimulates the release of a number of gastrointestinal hormones (including secretin, somatostatin, GIP and VIP) that inhibit the secretion of acid by parietal cells.

In health, a basal acid output obtained under unstimulated conditions is 5–10 mmol/hr. Following the administration of 6 mg/kg of pentagastrin, the parietal cell mass will be stimulated to produce hydrochloric acid. The maximal acid output will be less than 35 mmol/hr, and the peak acid output will be less than 60 mmol/hr. In health, the ratio of basal to maximum acid output or basal to peak acid output will be less than 0.25. The peak or maximum acid output reflects the parietal cell mass, whereas the ratio of BAO/PAO reflects the parietal cell function under basal conditions.

In disease, acid secretion may change. With gastric atrophy, both the basal and stimulated acid outputs are reduced. Peak acid output is increased in approximately one-half of patients with duodenal ulcer disease, whereas in patients with the Zollinger-Ellison syndrome, the major change is in the increased basal acid output. In patients with gastric ulcers, basal and peak acid output are usually normal or reduced. It must be stressed that this represents the acid measured in the gastric lumen and does not necessarily reflect the acid-secreting ability of the parietal cells in patients with gastric ulcer disease. That is, as a result of associated gastritis and back-diffusion of acid, these patients may secrete normal amounts of acid, which then diffuse back into the parietal cell. Therefore, the amount of acid measured in the gastric lumen would be normal or reduced.

Gastrin, histamine, acetylcholine and unspecified inhibitors influence the gastric secretory drive. Gastrin concentrations may be increased physiologically following food intake, with an increase of less than 100% above basal or fasting values. Secretory drive may be increased in the Zollinger-Ellison syndrome, G-cell hyperplasia or retained antrum. In the short bowel syndrome, temporary gastric hypersecretion may occur. The pathogenesis of this abnormality is unknown, and may relate to the loss of gastrin inhibitory factor in the small bowel. Gastrin levels are commonly increased in renal failure and pernicious anemia, and more rarely in diabetes mellitus and rheumatoid arthritis. In the latter two conditions, it is presumed that the gastrin levels are increased as a result of hypochlorhydria.

Once the stimulants of acid secretion (gastrin and acetylcholine) have been released, parietal cells are stimulated to secrete acid. The receptor for acetylcholine and gastrin may be on the mast cells, which are then stimulated to release histamine, which acts directly on the parietal cells to produce acid. Alternatively, there may be three separate receptors on the parietal cell: those for gastrin, acetylcholine and histamine. The histamine acts on adenylate cyclase in the parietal cell membrane to increase the production of cyclic AMP. In the presence of calcium, a protein kinase is stimulated, which then acts on the H^+/K^+-ATPase to secrete hydrochloric acid. This H^+/K^+-ATPase is known as the "proton pump." It represents the final common pathway for hydrogen ion secretion. Acetylcholine may act on the mast cells to release histamine, but may also act on the parietal cells to increase the influx of calcium ions, which then stimulate the protein kinase. The intracellular mechanism of gastric-mediated acid secretion is not known, although gastrin may stimulate the mast cells to release histamine, which further stimulates acid secretion.

This discussion of the mechanism of acid secretion provides the basis for understanding the pathogenesis of peptic ulcer disease. The parietal cell mass may be increased, and this may be reflected by an increase in the peak acid output or in serum pepsinogen 1. Secretory drive may be increased, and this is reflected by an increase in the ratio of BAO/PAO. Stimulated secretion is abnormal, as reflected by an increased parietal cell sensitivity to gastrin and possibly to histamine. Finally, the acid load in the duodenum is increased (as a result of increased acid secretion, as well as an increased rate of gastric emptying) in duodenal ulcer disease.

4.7 Diagnosis

Radiology for the diagnosis of peptic ulcer disease is being increasingly replaced by upper gastrointestinal endoscopy (esophagogastroduodenoscopy, or EGD). A chronic lesser-curve ulcer is usually seen as a distinct niche or pocket of barium projecting out from the line of the barium-filled stomach. The crater has a clean, smooth outline, and often its upper part contains a fluid level between the barium below and gastric juice or gas above. A posterior-wall gastric ulcer is often best seen *en face* as a barium-filled niche after a small amount of the barium suspension has been drunk, and when the abdomen has been compressed. A spastic notch on the greater curvature opposite the ulcer is a common feature of chronic gastric ulcer. Occasionally, a gross horizontal fibrous contracture in association with long-standing ulceration can cause a permanent hourglass constriction, or the lesser curvature can shorten longitudinally. Antral or prepyloric ulcers present special diagnostic difficulties to the radiologist, because the associated spasm or inflammatory swelling cannot always be distinguished from the appearance of gastric cancer. Greater-curvature ulceration is uncommon, and is seldom malignant. Lesser-curvature ulcers above the angulus can usually confidently be separated from malignant disease by their regularity and relative absence of mucosal distortion within the line of the barium-filled viscus (except by the classical appearances of fibrous contracture). The size of a gastric ulcer is not a guide to the presence of malignancy or to the severity of symptoms; furthermore, large

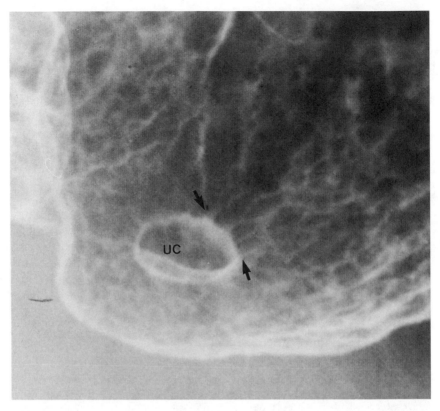

FIGURE 4A. Benign gastric ulcer. Barium meal showing an ulcer crater (UC) situated on the greater curvature of the stomach, in the gastric antrum. The ulcer is visualized *en face* with a slightly oblique projection. Smooth mucosal folds radiating from the edge of the crater (arrows) in a regular fashion are a pathognomonic sign of a benign gastric ulcer. (Courtesy of Dr. J. Rawlinson.)

gastric ulcers often respond better to medical treatment than small ones (Figure 4A, 4B).

The radiologic diagnosis of duodenal ulcer is complicated by the problem of distinguishing simple deformity (scarring) in the duodenal bulb (due to previous and now healed ulceration) from deformity with active ulceration. Ulceration in an undeformed cap is relatively uncommon. It may be seen either as a niche in profile on one border of the bulb (Figure 5A, 5B) or *en face* through the bulb when the bulb contains a small quantity of barium suspension and is compressed or examined in air contrast films (e.g., in a posterior view with the patient lying slightly on the left side). Scarring of the bulb

FIGURE 4B.   Malignant gastric ulcer. Barium meal demonstrating an ulcer crater (UC) on the lesser curvature of the stomach, also visualized *en face*. In this case the radiating mucosal folds are irregularly thickened (e.g., between closed arrows) and do not extend to the edge of the crater (open arrow) – features indicating a local infiltrative, malignant process. (Courtesy of Dr. J. Rawlinson.)

can induce a number of deformities, such as trefoil deformity following ulceration at the base of the bulb, and pseudodiverticulum formation. A minority of ulcers occur in the immediate postbulbar region of the duodenum. Close attention to this region is needed if they are to be found.

4.8 **Endoscopy**

Modern fiberoptic instruments used in endoscopic examination have greatly

FIGURE 5A. Duodenal ulcer. Situated at the base of the duodenal cap, the ulcer crater is filled with barium (arrow). The surrounding inflammatory process has considerably distorted the normal bulbar configuration of the proximal duodenum. (Courtesy of Dr. J. Rawlinson.)

FIGURE 5B. Duodenal ulcer. Endoscopic view of the duodenal cap ulcer.

increased its safety and diagnostic range, and the patient's comfort. The available instruments are either end- or side-viewing. The former are good general-purpose instruments that allow an adequate view of the esophagus, stomach and upper duodenum. Distal duodenal lesions can be viewed using an enteroscope or pediatric colonoscope through the upper gastrointestinal tract.

4.9 Therapy of Peptic Ulcer Disease

Medications used in the treatment of peptic ulcer disease can be classified into those that inhibit or neutralize acid secretion and those that are cytoprotective (Figure 6). Acid that has already been secreted can be neutralized with antacids, or the synthesis of acid can be inhibited by the use of H_2 blockers (such as ranitidine and cimetidine), anticholinergics (such as pirenzepine) or antigastrin agents (such as proglumide). The cytoprotective agents include licorice extracts, sucralfate and prostaglandins. Recent attention has turned to combining various therapeutic agents with antibiotic therapy to treat both the peptic ulcer and the Helicobacter pylori–associated gastritis in an attempt to prevent ulcer recurrence (see Section 8.2.3 for a further discussion).

The medications that inhibit acid secretion act either on the three receptors on the parietal cell or on the acid pump. These include H_2-receptor antagonists (cimetidine and ranitidine), muscarinic-receptor antagonists (pirenzepine, propantheline), gastrin-receptor antagonists (proglumide) and H^+/K^+-ATPase inhibitors (omeprazole).

Cimetidine is structurally similar to histamine, with an imidazole ring. The side structure of ranitidine is vaguely similar to that of cimetidine, but there is a furan rather than an imidazole ring. This difference in ring structure may account for the differences in side effects of these two H_2-receptor antagonists. Many side effects have been ascribed to H_2 blockers (Table 4). It must be stressed, however, that these side effects are rare with H_2 blockers. Cimetidine is metabolized by the cytochrome P-450 system, as are a number of cardiovascular, anorexic, CNS, analgesic and anesthetic medications. Those in common use include diazepam, warfarin, theophylline, propranolol, phenytoin and lidocaine. As a result of this interaction, patients receiving cimetidine must have a reduction in the dose of any medication that is also metabolized by the cytochrome P-450 system. Ranitidine is not metabolized to the same degree by this hepatic oxidative system; therefore no adjustment in the dosage of other medications is necessary in patients on this H_2-receptor antagonist. Furthermore, antiandrogenic effects, particularly gynecomastia, are exceedingly rare in patients taking ranitidine.

The basic aluminum salt of the sulfated disaccharide sucralfate enhances mucosal defense, possibly by providing a protective barrier at the ulcer base,

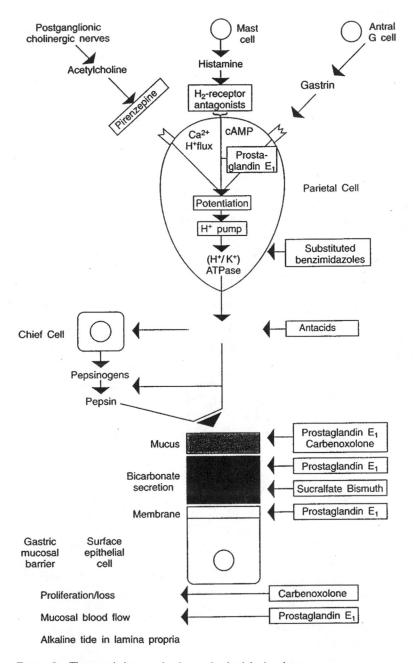

FIGURE 6.   Therapeutic intervention in a pathophysiologic scheme.

TABLE 4.   Side effects of anti-secretory therapy

	H₂ blockers	*Proton pump inhibitors*
CNS	Confusion, dizziness	Headache
CVS	Bradycardia	—
Endocrine	Gynecomastia	Gynecomastia
	Antiandrogenic	
	Prolactinemia	
Blood	Neutropenia	—
	Immune system	
Liver	Blood flow	Hepatitis
	Increased serum transaminases	
	Cytochrome P-450 (cimetidine)	
Kidney	Increased plasma creatinine	—
	(1–2% of patients)	
Intestine	Diarrhea	Nausea, diarrhea, constipation
Skin	Rash	Rash, alopecia, urticaria
Muscle	Pain	Pain

inhibiting the action of pepsin and bile, and blocking the back-diffusion of acid, as well as increasing mucosal prostaglandins.

What is the practical approach to the management of patients with ulcer disease? Based on the history and physical examination, peptic ulcer disease may be suspected. If the patient's symptoms are mild and of short duration, then the use of antacids and avoidance of obviously irritating agents should be undertaken. If the antacids are ineffective or if the symptoms are severe or prolonged, then either an upper gastrointestinal series or an endoscopy should be performed. Because of the approximately 20% false-positive and false-negative rate of an upper GI series, many family physicians prefer to refer a patient for endoscopy. In this way the diagnosis is confirmed, and if a gastric ulcer is demonstrated, then biopsies and cytology can be performed to exclude gastric malignancy. Although the new potent antacids have a high neutralizing effect, they must be taken in large volumes frequently throughout the day, are generally unpalatable, and cause side effects (e.g., diarrhea). Therapy of gastric and duodenal ulcer disease is now recommended to begin with an H_2-receptor antagonist. If the patient is elderly or on multiple-drug therapy, the agent of choice is ranitidine 150 mg b.i.d. or 300 mg h.s. Alternatively, in the majority of patients cimetidine may be given as an 800 mg h.s. dose. If the ulcer does not heal after six weeks of therapy with one of these agents, and if the diagnosis is certain, then the H_2-receptor antagonist can be stopped and the patient switched to sucralfate 2 g b.i.d. As long as there is no evidence of gastric outlet obstruction, metoclopramide 10 mg q.i.d. one-half hour before meals and at night can be used in a patient with mild nausea and bloating. If the patient's ulcer still has not healed, then a fasting gastrin concentration must be obtained to exclude hypergastrinemia, endoscopy must be performed or repeated to exclude malignancy, and every effort must be taken to ensure that the patient is not taking nonsteroidal anti-inflammatory agents. Patients over the age of 40 years complaining of dyspepsia should be investigated with endoscopy.

4.10 **Other Agents**

A number of tricyclic agents are available to reduce acid secretion. The tricyclic antidepressants have been shown to be modestly useful in the treatment of acid-peptic disorders. The non-antidepressant tricyclic agent pirenzepine is efficacious in the healing of duodenal ulcer disease when given in a dose of 50 mg b.i.d., but this dose is associated with prevalent side effects (including bradycardia, dry mouth and difficulty in focusing the eyes). Because of its anticholinergic effects, this medication is contraindicated in patients with glaucoma or with GI or genitourinary obstruction. The tricyclic agents are generally not considered to be the first line of therapy.

Omeprazole is the first agent of a class of substituted benzimidazoles that are able to specifically block the H^+/K^+-ATPase enzyme that is unique to the secretory canaliculus for the parietal cell. Inhibition of this final common pathway of gastric acid secretion is able to abolish the secretory response to all known secretagogues. Omeprazole is a weak base absorbed from the proximal small intestine at the highly acidic compartment of the secretory canaliculus, leading to activation of a sulfoxide metabolite, which is either rapidly inactivated or binds to the H^+/K^+-ATPase enzyme. Binding to the H^+/K^+-ATPase inactivates the enzyme and profoundly inhibits gastric acid secretion. Omeprazole will act in the stimulated parietal cell only when the drug can be trapped and converted to its active form in the highly acidic compartment. Peak absorption occurs 3 to 4 hours after oral administration, and the plasma levels are undetectable by about 11 hours after a single dose of the drug. The bioavailability of omeprazole increases with repeated doses up to about four days, probably as a result of increasing drug absorption as intragastric acidity decreases. Gastric acid inhibition approaches 98% following omeprazole 30 mg daily for one week.

The powerful antisecretory effects of omeprazole result in an elevation of serum gastrin concentrations, which in humans appear to be related to the degree of acid suppression. However, toxicologic studies in the rat in which massive doses of omeprazole have been used have shown markedly elevated gastrin levels associated with ECL-cell hyperplasia and gastric carcinoid tumors, which have been found after long-term treatment. Omeprazole at present is approved for short-term clinical use. It is an effective agent in the treatment of peptic ulcer disease and reflux esophagitis. Omeprazole inhibits the hepatic microsomal P-450 mono-oxygenase system, and the plasma half-life of drugs metabolized by this route may be extended.

Another therapeutic approach to the patient with peptic ulcer disease, based on different pathophysiologic mechanisms, includes the use of drugs that enhance mucosal defense. Colloidal bismuth compounds (e.g., tripotassium dicitrato bismuthate [De Nol®]) are used in the United Kingdom to treat peptic ulcer disease. Licorice extracts have been used for many years for the treatment of peptic ulcer disease, but the active agent, carbenoxolone, is unfortunately associated with significant aldosterone-like side effects and this compound has not gained wide acceptance. We have already considered the potential application of prostaglandins for the treatment of gastric and duodenal ulcer disease, current clinical studies have shown that methylated prostaglandins E_2 given by mouth may be as effective as H_2-receptor antagonists in the rapid healing of peptic ulcers.

It is likely that in the future, prostaglandins will become the drug of choice for the treatment of gastritis and gastric ulcer. Since the side effects from these medications are few, prostaglandins may in time replace H_2-receptor antagonists or sucralfate in the treatment of peptic ulcer disease. Because of their frequent side effects, anticholinergics are generally avoided except in the patient with nighttime pain despite maximal doses of H_2-receptor antagonists. Depression, both overt and masked, occurs in patients with peptic ulcer disease. These individuals may improve with an antidepressant; trimipramine has been shown to accelerate the healing of duodenal ulcer disease.

4.11 General Recommendations

What therapeutic recommendations can be made? The proportion of patients whose ulcers heal after six weeks of cimetidine, ranitidine, sucralfate or prostaglandin is comparable. Recommendations must therefore be made on other factors, including convenience, side effects, cost and maintenance of healing. Liquid antacids are inconvenient to take, and patient compliance is poor. Side effects from the anticholinergics are frequent, and cimetidine should be avoided in the older patient or in the individual taking multiple drugs. A therapeutic dose of each of these agents – that is, a dose necessary to obtain ulcer healing – is comparable and expensive (about $60 to heal an ulcer).

Peptic ulcer disease has a natural history of recurrence. Once an ulcer has healed, there is a 75% chance that the ulcer will recur in 12 months; 50% will be symptomatic, whereas 25% will be asymptomatic. If patients are maintained on low-dose H_2-receptor antagonists, then only 25% of the patients will have an ulcer recurrence in 12 months. There is no widely accepted practice advised for maintenance therapy. The general rule of thumb would be to advise maintenance therapy for the patient with severe aggressive recurrent ulcer disease.

More recently, attention has turned to the role of Helicobacter pylori in ulcer recurrence. In particular, Helicobacter pylori is associated with an antral gastritis seen in 95% of duodenal ulcer patients. Eradication of Helicobacter pylori infection associated with duodenal ulcer disease through antibiotic therapy may eliminate ulcer recurrence (see Section 8.2.3).

4.12 Failure of Medical Therapy

If the ulcer fails to heal with medical therapy, the patient may have taken inadequate doses of medication for an inadequate duration, or the medication may have been taken improperly. For example, an antacid must be taken one and three hours after meals; sucralfate must be taken one hour before meals and concurrent antisecretory therapy and antacid use must be avoided; and H_2-receptor antagonists must be taken with meals. The possibility of malabsorption of the medication must be considered. An ulcer complicated by penetration or pancreatitis may be associated with continued symptoms. The continuation of the environmental factors responsible for the initial development of the ulcer may be responsible for lack of healing. The adequacy of the diagnosis must be questioned, and it is for this reason that endoscopy is generally recommended for the proper diagnosis of peptic ulcer disease. Finally, concurrent infection of the stomach or duodenum with Helicobacter pylori may be a factor in a resistant ulcer (see Section 8.2.3).

An additional cause of failure of medical therapy and failure of ulcer healing is the presence of a hypersecretory state, possibly due to hypergastrinemia. It is disputed whether G-cell hyperplasia occurs in patients with duodenal ulcer disease. Clearly, however, a small proportion of patients with ulcer disease would have a hypersecretory state due to the presence of a gastrinoma (which will lead to basal and/or stimulated hypergastrinemia). Other conditions leading to basal hypergastrinemia include retained antrum, pyloric obstruction, pernicious anemia, hypercalcemia, renal failure, massive small bowel resection and portacaval anastomoses (Table 5). Peptic ulcer disease does not occur in patients with pernicious anemia, because they lack parietal cells. However, these other conditions associated with basal hypergastrinemia may also be associated with hyperchlorhydria and associated peptic ulcer disease. It is unclear whether hypergastrinemia also occurs in patients with diabetes mellitus or rheumatoid arthritis.

For the complications of hemorrhage, obstruction, perforation or intractability, surgery will be necessary. There is no consensus regarding the procedure of choice, but generally some form of vagotomy (e.g., truncal, selective

TABLE 5.   Causes of hypergastrinemia

With acid hypersecretion
Gastrinoma
Isolated retained gastric antrum
Antral G-cell hyperplasia
Massive small bowel resection
Pyloric outlet obstruction
Hyperparathyroidism

With variable acid secretion
Hyperthyroidism
Chronic renal failure
Pheochromocytoma

With acid hyposecretion
Atrophic gastritis
Pernicious anemia
Gastric cancer
Postvagotomy and pyloroplasty

---

or parietal cell) with a drainage procedure (pyloroplasty or antrectomy) is advised.

In general, a vagotomy is performed with a gastric draining procedure (pyloroplasty/gastroenterostomy) and/or a gastric resection to avoid gastric stasis (Figure 7). Three forms of vagotomy are in vogue: truncal, selective and parietal cell. A Billroth I or Billroth II anastomosis may also be performed, particularly when the antrum or portions of the body of the stomach are resected. A drainage procedure is needed to avoid the gastric atony resulting from the vagotomy and associated delayed gastric emptying.

4.13 **Gastrinoma**

The Zollinger-Ellison (ZE) syndrome is characterized by autonomous gastrin production by an adenoma or adenocarcinoma of the pancreas or duodenum. Patients may present either with severe acute ulcer disease or recurrent ulcer disease; the ulcers will often occur in unusual sites and be associated with diarrhea. The Zollinger-Ellison syndrome is distinguished from peptic ulcer disease by the demonstration of fasting hypergastrinemia. There are many causes of fasting hypergastrinemia (gastritis, vagotomy and pyloroplasty, the short bowel syndrome, rheumatoid arthritis, retained antrum, G-cell hyperplasia), but only two conditions – atrophic gastritis and renal failure – are associated with gastrin levels increased several times above the upper limit of the normal range. However, in a patient with peptic ulcer disease and

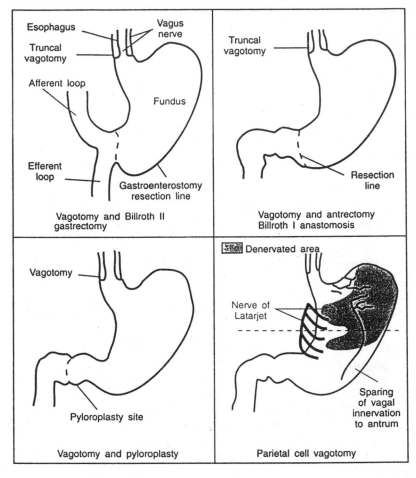

FIGURE 7.   Some surgical procedures for peptic ulcer disease.

hypergastrinemia, it is important to exclude the Zollinger-Ellison syndrome. Gastric analysis may be helpful: the finding of a dramatically increased basal output relative to a modestly increased maximal acid output (i.e., BAO/MAO greater than 0.6) is suggestive of this syndrome. Ingestion of a protein-containing meal normally produces a doubling of the gastrin concentration (a.c. versus p.c.), but an exaggerated response is seen in G-cell hyperplasia rather than in gastrinoma syndrome. Infusion of calcium intravenously results in an increase in gastrin concentration in normal individuals and an exaggeration of this response in patients with the Zollinger-Ellison syndrome. However, the most useful diagnostic test is the secretin infusion. In normal individuals or those with G-cell hyperplasia, injection of secretin results in a rapid decline in plasma gastrin concentrations, whereas in patients with the Zollinger-Ellison syndrome, the gastrin concentration will increase in response to secretin.

The Zollinger-Ellison syndrome arises from a gastrinoma, a tumor in the pancreas. This may be a localized or diffuse tumor. The presence of hypergastrinemia leads to hypersecretion; while the maximal acid output may be increased, the major defect is basal hypergastrinemia and a marked increase in the basal acid output. The patient will have aggressive peptic ulcer disease with ulceration in unusual sites, or multiple ulcers that fail to heal on medical therapy. Hypertrophic gastric folds and diarrhea may be prominent features (see Section 6.5). The presence of a gastrinoma should be suspected from the history, and confirmed with provocative tests. A protein meal will increase the serum gastrin concentration in patients with G-cell hyperplasia; a calcium infusion will markedly increase the gastrin concentration in patients with gastrinoma, and have a lesser effect in normal patients and patients with G-cell hyperplasia. The best test to diagnose a gastrinoma is a secretin test in which the basal gastrin concentration increases dramatically, in contrast to the reduction in gastrin concentration that occurs following secretin infusion in patients with G-cell hyperplasia or a normal stomach. A CT scan or an angiogram may be useful in identifying the gastrinoma, although these tumors are often small and difficult to identify. A laparotomy will be necessary to determine whether there is a localized tumor. Since one-half of these tumors are malignant, it is worthwhile to undertake surgery in the hope that resection of the tumor will produce a cure.

If the high dose of H_2-receptor antagonists does not sufficiently relieve the patient's pain, then nighttime anticholinergics can be used. A trial of parietal cell vagotomy is under way, but this is not yet accepted therapy.

5. POSTGASTRECTOMY PROBLEMS

Numerous problems follow peptic ulcer surgery. These postgastrectomy problems may occur early after surgery or many months later. The early problems relate to the surgery itself. There are many late postgastrectomy syndromes (Table 6); these may be more disabling than the dyspeptic symptoms that led to the surgery in the first place.

5.1 Esophageal Symptoms

The incidence of gastroesophageal reflux after vagotomy or partial gastric resection is unknown, although it is a common symptom even in unoperated

TABLE 6.   Complications of gastric surgery

Esophagus
Gastroesophageal reflux
Dysphagia

Stomach
Delayed gastric emptying
Bezoars
Outlet obstruction
Stomatitis
Recurrent ulcers
Stump carcinoma
Afferent loop syndrome

Small intestine
Diarrhea
   Dumping syndrome
   Bacterial contamination syndrome
   Unmasked celiac disease, unmasked pancreatic
      insufficiency or unmasked lactase deficiency
Weight loss and malabsorption
   Iron
   Folate
   Vitamin B_{12}
   Calcium
   Fats
Anemia

Gallbladder
Cholelithiasis

---

patients. The effect of vagotomy on lower esophageal sphincter pressure is uncertain, but operations involving mobilization and manipulation of the proximal stomach can damage the sphincter. Operations that involve the antrum and pylorus may allow duodenal juice to reflux into the stomach. From there it may enter and damage the esophagus, an additional factor that may contribute to therapeutic problems. Assessment of patients with symptoms of gastroesophageal reflux should include a barium swallow and endoscopy. If the patient's acid output is low, then the esophagitis may be due to the reflux of bile and pancreatic juice from the duodenum into the stomach and esophagus. If the bile-induced esophagitis does not respond to bile acid binding agents (cholestyramine, sucralfate, aluminum hydroxide antacid), then surgical revision with a Roux-en-Y anastomosis may be necessary.

One of the more troublesome postgastrectomy syndromes is that of dysphagia. This usually occurs in the early postoperative period. Although spontaneous improvement is the rule, occasionally esophagitis and stricture may occur. This dysphagia may result from trauma to the esophagus at the time of surgery, the development of a periesophageal hematoma, or a vagotomy.

5.2 Delayed Gastric Emptying

Delayed gastric emptying may result from recurrent ulceration, stomal edema, fibrosis or decreased gastric tone and motility, and may lead to bezoar formation. The patient may suffer early satiety or postprandial fullness. Gastric bezoars are secretions of food or foreign material in the stomach. Vegetable bezoars are called phytobezoars; those composed of hair are called trichobezoars. These develop following antrectomy and vagotomy, and probably relate to inadequate chewing, hypochlorhydria, and a high-fiber diet. Bezoars may be suspected on plain film of the abdomen or upper GI series and may be confirmed at endoscopy. It is occasionally possible at endoscopy to fragment the bezoar, but therapy with papain (an enzyme that digests protein, and thus helps dissolve either type of bezoar) is usually necessary.

If stomal fibrosis is present, surgery is usually indicated. Intravenous therapy may be required if the obstruction is severe, but if the outlet is patent, metoclopramide or domperidone may improve gastric emptying. Alternatively it may be necessary to revise the surgical anastomosis.

5.3 Recurrent Ulcers

Ulcers that recur following gastric surgery bear many names (e.g., stomal ulceration, recurrent ulcers, postgastrectomy ulcers). These recurrent ulcers may be due to incomplete vagotomy, incomplete resection of G cells or acid-producing cells, retained antrum, delayed gastric emptying, duodenogastric reflux, ulcerogenic drugs or gastrinoma. Naturally, these benign conditions must be excluded from a stump ulcer. Recurrent ulceration with edema and partial obstruction may benefit from a trial of an H_2-receptor antagonist.

5.4 Carcinoma

Carcinoma of the gastric stump may develop 20 or more years following gastric surgery for benign peptic ulcer disease. Stump carcinoma appears to be more common following a Billroth II anastomosis. The carcinoma develops at the anastomosis, or in the gastric body or fundus. The pathogenesis is thought to be related to the development of chronic atrophic gastritis. Initially, there may be metaplasia of the Paneth's and goblet cells, and then subsequent dysplasia. These morphologic changes seem to relate to chronic bile and alkaline reflux.

5.5 Afferent Loop Syndrome

In patients with a gastrojejunostomy or a Billroth II anastomosis, obstruction of the afferent loop may occur. Symptoms may be acute or chronic and due to the presence of an internal hernia, kinking, the formation of adhesions or stenosis of the stoma. The acute afferent loop syndrome occurs in the early postoperative period. There may be partial or complete obstruction of the afferent loop, giving rise to pain, nausea, vomiting of nonbilious material, the palpation of an abdominal mass, and occasionally elevation in the serum amylase and liver function tests. The chronic afferent loop syndrome is due to partial obstruction of the afferent loop. The patient will complain of postprandial bilious vomiting without food. This vomiting will be intermittent, severe and painful.

5.6 Diarrhea

Diarrhea commonly occurs immediately after truncal vagotomy; various mechanisms have been suggested, including the dumping syndrome, the bacterial overgrowth syndrome, use of excessive amounts of magnesium-containing antacids, the Zollinger-Ellison syndrome, unmasked celiac disease, unmasked lactose intolerance and unmasked pancreatic insufficiency. Other causes of diarrhea seen in patients without previous gastric surgery or vagotomy also need to be considered.

Most cases of postvagotomy diarrhea improve with time. Antidiarrheal agents such as loperamide and diphenoxylate may improve symptoms; in those patients who do not respond, cholestyramine or antibiotics are sometimes helpful. More persistent diarrhea should be fully investigated to rule out infection, malabsorption or gastrin-secreting tumors. In extreme cases, surgical intervention may be necessary.

"Early dumping" occurs 10 to 20 minutes after meals and has three components: gastrointestinal, vasomotor and cardiovascular. The patient may develop pain, nausea, vomiting, fullness and diarrhea. Vasomotor symptoms include weakness, dizziness, faintness, pallor and sweating; cardiovascular symptoms include palpitations and tachycardia. The early dumping syndrome is caused by rapid emptying of gastric contents with osmotic fluid shifts, abdominal distention and release of vasoactive substances. The intestinal distention produces the pain, nausea and vomiting, whereas the vasomotor and cardiovascular symptoms are due to the release of serotonin and bradykinin.

The "late dumping" syndrome occurs 1 to 3 hours after meals, particularly meals containing large amounts of carbohydrate. The late dumping syndrome is characterized by evidence of sympathetic discharge due to hypoglycemia. These symptoms include weakness, sweating, hunger and confusion. The pathophysiologic basis for this dumping syndrome is straightforward: rapid gastric emptying, rapid absorption of glucose, release of large amounts of insulin, rapid decline in blood sugar levels due to the rapid cessation of glucose absorption, and excessively high insulin levels.

The dumping syndrome may be treated with dietary therapy: six small meals per day containing high-protein, low-carbohydrate foods, and the ingestion of liquids between rather than with meals. This is effective for most patients, but in some individuals anticholinergics will be necessary before meals, or the serotonin antagonist cyproheptadine may be prescribed. Tolbutamide or pectin may be useful in some individuals. When all else fails, a Billroth II anastomosis will need to be converted into a Billroth I. If the patient already has a Billroth I, then in rare cases an antiperistaltic loop of small bowel will need to be inserted.

5.7 Weight Loss and Malabsorption

Weight loss occurs after surgery in 30–60% of patients; it is less common with vagotomy alone than with vagotomy and antrectomy. The most common cause is decreased caloric intake because of early satiety, but in patients with severe malnutrition or persistent diarrhea, an investigation of malabsorption should be undertaken.

5.8 Anemia

Anemia is common following gastric surgery. Iron deficiency may be due to a preoperative iron deficiency, surgical blood loss inadequately replaced during or following surgery, postoperative GI or GU losses, or malabsorption of iron resulting from reduction in gastric acid (necessary for the absorption of food iron) or bypassing of the duodenum (the optimal site for the absorption of all forms of iron). In some patients, an associated malabsorption syndrome unmasked by the gastric surgery will result in folate deficiency from inadequate intake or malabsorption of folate. B_{12} deficiency may occur if a sufficient number of intrinsic-factor–producing cells have been resected. B_{12} deficiency may also occur if there is associated bacterial overgrowth syndrome, and rarely if there is pancreatic insufficiency. In patients with pernicious anemia, the urinary excretion of vitamin B_{12} (Schilling test) will increase to normal when the intrinsic factor is given together with a low dose of vitamin.

5.9 Cholelithiasis

Cholelithiasis occurs more frequently following a truncal than other types of vagotomy. The mechanism is thought to be decreased bile flow and gallbladder contraction, associated with increased gallbladder size and the development of lithogenic bile.

TABLE 7.   ABC classification of gastritis

Autoimmune	Congenital pernicious anemia
Bacterial	Helicobacter pylori
Chemical	Bile reflux
Drug-induced	NSAIDs, alcohol
Eosinophilic	Eosinophilic gastroenteritis
Follicular	Helicobacter pylori
Granulomatous	Tuberculosis, Crohn's disease
Hypertrophic	Ménétrier's disease

6. GASTRITIS

6.1 Acute Gastritis

Acute gastritis is an acute self-limiting syndrome caused by irritation of the gastric mucosa by alcohol, corrosive poisons, and the various bacterial and oral causes of food poisoning. It is characterized by anorexia, nausea and vomiting. In some patients, the same causal agents produce acute ulcers that may bleed or perforate. The role of analgesics is not clear.

6.2 Chronic Gastritis

Three main types of gastritis are recognized by histological examination: superficial gastritis, atrophic gastritis and gastric atrophy. Chronic gastritis is characterized by mononuclear and polymorphonuclear cell infiltration of mucosa, glandular atrophy and intestinal metaplasia. In superficial gastritis inflammation is marked and glandular atrophy is minimal, whereas in gastric atrophy inflammatory cells are few and glandular atrophy is extensive. These represent different degrees of gastritis, though not necessarily all cases that progress to atrophy must be preceded by the two lesser lesions.

With progressive degeneration of the mucosa, gastric secretion progressively fails. Hydrochloric acid secretion fails first, followed by pepsinogen secretion and finally by the secretion of intrinsic factor. As intrinsic factor secretion fails, the body becomes depleted of vitamin B_{12} and pernicious anemia develops. Antibodies to parietal cells and intrinsic factor appear in the serum. The presence of these antibodies together with a partial response to steroids suggests that autoimmunity may play an etiologic role.

The cause of chronic gastritis is unknown, but it is probably due to a combination of genetic and acquired factors (Table 7). Among the latter may be included repeated minor trauma due to alcohol and analgesics, reflux of duodenal contents and gastric irradiation. Deficiencies of vitamin B_{12}, folic

TABLE 8.   Causes of hypochlorhydria

Chronic gastritis (Table 7)
Gastric ulcer or cancer or polyposis
Resection

---

acid and iron interfere with the regenerative and functional capacity of the gastric mucosa.

Predisposition to gastric cancer is probably due to an unknown biochemical lesion within the cell that leads to secretory failure, cellular degeneration and in some cases gastric carcinoma. While most of the causes of hypochlorhydria are associated with gastritis, it remains disputed whether gastritis is necessarily associated with an increased risk of gastric cancer. Gastric cancer is 5 to 10 times as common as expected in those with chronic atrophic gastritis; the same increased incidence is also found in first-degree relatives of patients with gastric cancer and pernicious anemia.

It is uncertain whether chronic gastritis causes symptoms. Chronic gastritis can be diagnosed only by gastric biopsy of body or fundic mucosa. Marked gastric hyposecretion or anacidity is present if the lesion is diffuse.

6.2.1 COMPLETE GASTRIC ATROPHY AND PERNICIOUS ANEMIA

There are many causes of hypochlorhydria (Table 8). The ability to produce acid, pepsin and intrinsic factor is lost altogether in patients with complete gastric atrophy. However, vitamin B_{12} deficiency – which leads to pernicious anemia or (much more rarely) to subacute combined degeneration of the spinal cord – takes several years to supervene because of the large liver stores of the vitamin. In the complete atrophy of pernicious anemia, gastric glandular and all parietal cells are lost, and the mucosa is infiltrated by large numbers of plasma cells and lymphocytes. Pentagastrin stimulation will demonstrate that the patient is achlorhydric. Studies will demonstrate antibodies to intrinsic factor and to parietal cells in serum, gastric secretions and mucosa in most patients. Though the presence of such antibodies is a useful marker, it is not diagnostic: intrinsic factor antibodies can be demonstrated occasionally (and parietal cell antibodies frequently) in patients with simple atrophic gastritis or chronic superficial gastritis without vitamin B_{12} malabsorption.

Hydroxocobalamin has replaced cyanocobalamin for the treatment of pernicious anemia, because it is better retained in the body. A dose of 100 µg by injection every month is more than sufficient to maintain body stores after loading treatment with 200 µg on three alternate days.

6.2.2 *CONGENITAL PERNICIOUS ANEMIA*

Congenital pernicious anemia is a rare condition, inherited as a Mendelian recessive, and is due to an inherited inability to secrete intrinsic factor in adequate amounts. It presents as megaloblastic anemia in infancy and is associated with normal acid secretory potential. The specific failure of intrinsic factor synthesis in this condition must be distinguished from congenital ileal receptor deficiency for the vitamin B_{12}-intrinsic factor complex (the Imerslund-Graesbeck syndrome) and from vitamin B_{12} deficiency due to gastric failure in the hypoparathyroidism-candidiasis syndrome.

The cause of pernicious anemia is unknown. The presence of auto-antibodies, mucosal infiltration by plasma cells and reversibility of the gastric lesion by corticosteroids suggest an autoimmune process. There is also a small but definite genetic predisposition; like gastric cancer, the disease is slightly more common in individuals of group A than in those of the remaining ABO groups. Exogenous factors that predispose to gastric cancer also seem likely to predispose to pernicious anemia. It is unclear why most patients present with pernicious anemia while a few develop the neurological condition of subacute degeneration of the spinal cord without anemia.

6.3 **Chronic Superficial Gastritis**

In this form of gastritis, inflammatory cells, mainly polymorphonuclear, infiltrate the superficial mucosa but gastric glands are well preserved. It has been found with increased frequency in those who smoke excessively or who consume large amounts of alcohol or hot beverages. No specific symptom pattern has been correlated with it, and it does not seem necessarily to predispose to gastric atrophy. Chronic superficial gastritis is commonly found in patients with chronic gastric ulcer, but is not a universal concomitant.

6.4 **Chronic Atrophic Gastritis**

With chronic atrophic gastritis, in addition to cellular infiltration, predominantly lymphocytic and plasma cell in pattern, there is a loss of gastric glands, and acid and pepsin secretory capacity is reduced in parallel. It does not cause symptoms, but in a minority of patients there is progression to the complete atrophy of pernicious anemia. Patients with atrophic gastritis probably develop eventual gastric cancer approximately as often as those with pernicious anemia.

6.5 **Giant Mucosal Rugal Hypertrophy**

Giant mucosal rugal hypertrophy is a histologic change occurring in association with the Zollinger-Ellison syndrome and rarely as an isolated entity. Ménétrier's disease (giant hypertrophic gastritis), a rare condition associated

TABLE 9.   Differential diagnosis for intrinsic causes of thickened gastric folds

---

Lymphoma
Mucosa-associated lymphoid tissue (MALT) syndrome
Gastric adenocarcinoma
Linitis plastica
Ménétrier's disease
Acute H. pylori gastritis
Lymphocytic gastritis
Eosinophilic gastritis
Gastric varices
Gastritis cystica profunda
Gastric antral vascular ectasia
Kaposi's sarcoma
Zollinger-Ellison syndrome
Gastric Crohn's disease

---

with mucosal hypertrophy, involves reduced acid secretion. Hypertrophic-hypersecretory gastropathy, another associated condition, involves increased acid secretion. In giant mucosal rugal hypertrophy, as a result of protein loss into the gastric lumen, the serum albumin concentration will be reduced. The condition usually occurs in males between the ages of 30 and 50, and the patient will present with pain, nausea, vomiting, weight loss, bleeding, or edema as a result of hypoalbuminemia. The condition is suspected from the presence of large rugal folds identified on upper GI series or at endoscopy. A biopsy will demonstrate hyperplasia of the parietal, chief and mucus cells. There may be cystic structures in the mucosa and submucosa as well. The condition must be distinguished from giant hypertrophic gastritis, the Zollinger-Ellison syndrome, gastric carcinoma, lymphoma and amyloidosis (Table 9). The protein loss may be reduced with anticholinergics. If gastric hypersecretion occurs, as in the case of hypertrophic-hypersecretory gastropathy, H_2 blockers will prove useful. If pain, bleeding and protein loss persist, then a vagotomy and pyloroplasty or subtotal gastrectomy is necessary.

6.6 Granulomatous Gastritis
Chronic inflammatory changes in the gastric mucosa may occur in Crohn's disease, tuberculosis, syphilis and sarcoidosis, and granulomas may be present. These diseases are all uncommon.

6.7 Eosinophilic Gastritis
The cause of eosinophilic gastritis is unknown. There is extensive infiltration

of the gastric and often the small intestinal mucosa by eosinophils, in association with peripheral eosinophilia. The disease produces nonspecific dyspeptic symptoms, and antral distortion is radiographically visible. Spontaneous cure is common, but some patients require steroid therapy and in a few the disease is progressive.

6.8 Bile Gastritis

The common occurrence of gastritis following gastric surgery is thought to be due to the effect of bile and alkaline duodenal secretion damaging the gastric mucosal barrier and giving rise to an inflammatory reaction. Some patients will respond to medical treatment with cholestyramine, aluminum hydroxide or sucralfate. Cholestyramine and aluminum hydroxide act by binding bile acids and pepsin, and providing a protective surface to the gastric mucosa. When the condition persists and is associated with pain or bleeding, a surgical procedure (Roux-en-Y) will be necessary.

6.9 Miscellaneous

There are two forms of gastritis that fall outside the classifications listed above. One is intestinal metaplasia, where a large number of cells with the histochemical properties of intestinal mucosal cells are found in the stomach. This is commonly associated with chronic gastritis. The second is Ménétrier's disease or giant hypertrophic gastritis, where the giant mucosal folds may be confused with neoplastic disease (Table 9); excess protein loss from the folds may cause a syndrome of protein depletion (protein-losing enteropathy). Erosive gastritis and hyperplastic atrophic gastritis are less well defined entities.

7. PREMALIGNANT CONDITIONS OF THE STOMACH AND GASTRIC CANCER

7.1 Premalignant Conditions

Possible premalignant gastric conditions include pernicious anemia, atrophic gastritis, polyps and previous gastric surgery. People with a family history that is positive for gastric cancer also have an increased risk of developing this disease. Benign gastric ulcer is not a premalignant condition, but can appear so because of the long natural history of some ulcerating cancers. At present, regular endoscopy is not necessary for most patients with conditions predisposing to gastric ulcer. A high index of suspicion for cancer, however, must be maintained. If endoscopy and biopsy have been performed and distinct dysplastic changes are found in the epithelium, regular follow-up endoscopy and biopsy are advised.

7.1.1 *PERNICIOUS ANEMIA*

Patients with pernicious anemia have long been considered at risk for gastric cancer, but the risk is likely to be low and does not justify intensive endoscopic screening. Pernicious anemia is invariably associated with fundal gland atrophy, usually with intestinal metaplasia and sometimes with polyps. When cancer develops, it tends to occur in the body or fundus of the stomach.

7.1.2 *ATROPHIC GASTRITIS*

There are two main types of atrophic gastritis: fundal gland (type A), and pyloric (antral) gland (type B). These occur in older people. Antral gastritis increasingly involves the fundal gland area with advanced age. Both types A and B are associated with intestinal metaplasia and a predisposition to gastric cancer. Type A gastritis is less common and its distribution in the stomach resembles that of pernicious anemia. Type B gastritis is predominant in those areas of the body where gastric cancer is common and appears to be a risk factor mainly for the intestinal type of gastric cancer. Helicobacter pylori, which is the cause of type B gastritis, has been implicated as a risk factor for gastric cancer.

7.1.3 *GASTRIC POLYPS*

There are two main types of gastric polyps: hyperplastic and adenomatous. Hyperplastic polyps are small, often multiple, and do not become malignant. Adenomatous polyps are uncommon and are usually larger than 2 cm in diameter. They are premalignant, and a substantial minority show areas of cancer at the time of detection. Endoscopic or surgical excision is recommended.

7.1.4 *PREVIOUS GASTRIC SURGERY*

Patients who have had a partial gastrectomy for peptic ulcer disease may have an increased probability of developing gastric cancer some 15 to 20 years after the operation. Endoscopic surveillance of these patients does not appear to be justified in North America, since the risk is low.

7.2 Other Conditions

Individuals with a parent or sibling with gastric cancer are three times as likely to develop gastric cancer as the general population. People born in a country where gastric cancer is common (e.g., Japan or Eastern Europe) are also at increased risk, even if they have lived in North America for many years. Although regular screening is not warranted in either case, minor symptoms should be promptly and thoroughly investigated.

Barrett's epithelium (columnar cell lining of the lower esophagus) is a proven precursor of esophageal adenocarcinoma, and there is increasing suspicion that lesser degrees of Barrett's epithelium may predispose to the much more common adenocarcinoma of the gastric cardia.

·7.3 Gastric Cancer

Adenocarcinoma is the most common gastric cancer, but lymphoma and leiomyosarcoma also occur. The frequency of gastric cancer has decreased considerably over the past 50 years in North America, but it still ranks as the second most common GI malignancy (after colon cancer). Most patients are over 60 years of age. Men are affected about twice as often as women. The cancer usually involves the antrum, body or cardia with about equal frequency. The three main macroscopic types are polypoid, ulcerative and infiltrative. The two main microscopic types are intestinal and diffuse. The intestinal type is often associated with atrophic gastritis and intestinal metaplasia; the diffuse type is often manifest as a linitis plastica.

Most patients have advanced incurable disease by the time they have significant complaints, but some patients with early gastric cancer may have mild epigastric discomfort or ulcer-like symptoms. Physical examination is usually normal but may reveal a mass or a succussion splash in a minority of patients. There may be evidence of metastases, such as a supraclavicular node, hepatomegaly, ascites, a "shelf" on a rectal examination, an ovarian mass or an umbilical node. Iron deficiency anemia is found in about 50% of patients and occult blood is present in the stool in about 75% of cases. Occasionally, the neurological signs of subacute combined degeneration of the spinal cord from associated pernicious anemia will be found. Measurement of gastric acid secretion or carcinoembryonic antigen (CEA) is not helpful. Barium radiograph is usually the first diagnostic procedure. Experienced radiologists can show some abnormality in up to 90% of patients, particularly if double contrast techniques are used. While there are distinguishing clinical and radiological features, every patient with a presumed benign gastric ulcer should have biopsies obtained to exclude a malignant ulcer. Endoscopy and biopsy, with or without brush cytology, are required to establish the diagnosis.

The diffuse type of gastric cancer often manifests itself as a linitis plastica. It is harder to diagnose than the intestinal type, particularly in the earlier stages. Thus, although diagnostic techniques have improved, some gastric cancers are still missed on the initial investigation. Although routine endoscopic screening is not feasible in North America, minor symptoms should be thoroughly investigated in people with predisposing conditions. It is also important to ensure that only benign gastric ulcers are treated medically; if a gastric ulcer fails to heal after three months of intensive medical therapy, surgery is generally recommended.

Early surgery offers the only hope for cure, but is not performed if there is evidence of metastatic disease, unless the patient suffers from gastric outlet obstruction. Cancers of the distal and mid-stomach are treated by subtotal gastrectomy. In order to remove the regional lymph nodes, the lesser and greater omenta are resected and, if necessary, the spleen is removed. Cancers of the proximal stomach are usually treated by esophagogastrectomy. With the increased proportion of diffusely infiltrating cancer, total gastrectomy with biliary diversion is being performed more often. Palliative resection, bypass, surgery or laser photoablation is justified in those patients with gastric outlet obstruction. Palliative esophagogastrectomy or total gastrectomy is not recommended. The prognosis after surgical treatment is related to the depth of the tumor's penetration. Overall, about 10–15% of patients survive five years. Occasionally, patients have a long course without treatment or with only palliative surgery.

Therapy includes chemotherapy with 5-fluorouracil, doxorubicin and mitomycin (FAM). This approach achieves a response rate of up to 40% but gives a disappointing median survival of less than one year. Occasionally, good responses are obtained, and a trial is recommended for patients in good condition and with advanced disease. Adjuvant chemotherapy or radiotherapy remains of unproven value, but palliative radiotherapy is useful to control bleeding, to alleviate pain from bone metastases and to relieve dysphagia. Esophageal dilation and endoscopically placed plastic tubes can also help dysphagia caused by persistent spread of a cardia tumor.

General supportive care is important, including dietary advice, replacement of iron and vitamin B_{12}, judicious use of analgesics, antiemetics, and antacid support. Emotional support is particularly important and increasingly includes guidance in interpreting the common, overoptimistic "breakthroughs" reported in the press.

8. OTHER GASTRIC DISEASES

8.1 Acute

Partial (antral) or total gastric volvulus is a rare cause of acute upper abdominal pain and vomiting. These obstructions can arise by themselves, or as torsion within a hiatus hernia. Volvulus within a hernia is not uncommon in the elderly, when there may be no symptoms. The belief that twisting obstruction poses an important risk to the blood supply is probably unjustified. Gastric aspiration is followed by surgical relief of the volvulus in those who present with obstruction.

Sudden gross gastric distention and acute dilation of the stomach can arise after any form of upper abdominal surgery, including cholecystectomy, and especially after vagotomy, after childbirth and in diabetic coma. The causes are uncertain. Vomiting of relatively clear gastric contents is succeeded by the production of dirty brown or feculent material and the development of abdominal distention. Prompt decompression with a large-bore stomach tube and intravenous fluid replacement are required. After a variable interval the condition should then resolve spontaneously.

8.1.1 *GASTRIC RUPTURE*

Acute, nontraumatic, spontaneous rupture of the stomach is a rare, catastrophic and poorly understood event. The majority of ruptures occur on the lesser curvature. They have also been reported to occur during upper gastrointestinal radiography using barium, sodium bicarbonate ingestion, nasal oxygen therapy, cardiopulmonary resuscitation and labor, and during the postpartum period.

8.2 **Chronic**

Hypertrophic pyloric stenosis is an idiopathic condition that may occur in infants or adults. The muscle of the pyloric canal is unduly hypertrophied. Infantile hypertrophic pyloric stenosis is more common in boys than in girls (the sex ratio is approximately 10:1), is a frequent anomaly (its incidence is about 3 per 1,000 live births) and is thought to be due to a combination of genetic predisposition and some abnormality of fetal or early postnatal development. Symptoms usually develop in the first few weeks after birth and characteristically consist of copious projectile vomiting of the gastric contents after feeding. On examination there is usually visible gastric peristalsis; a lump can be felt abdominally in the region of the pylorus. Barium-meal examination is not usually necessary but will confirm the presence of a narrow segment, 1–2 cm long, at the pylorus. The condition must be distinguished clinically from esophageal atresia (which involves onset at birth of difficulties with swallowing) and duodenal obstruction/atresia (which involves bile-stained vomitus). A minor proportion of all cases settle in the first two to three months with conservative management with anticholinergic drugs, but most patients will require early surgery with Ramstedt's procedure (pyloromyotomy).

Occasionally, adult patients present with obstructive symptoms resulting from pyloric stenosis associated with muscular hypertrophy. This is rarely if ever caused by recurrence of infantile pyloric stenosis; it is usually associated with juxtapyloric peptic ulceration, but sometimes the problem seems to be due to primary hypertrophic stenosis arising in adult life. The differential also includes pyloric mucosal diaphragm and annular pancreas. Pyloric obstruction requires pyloroplasty together with a procedure such as vagotomy if there is an associated ulcer.

8.2.1 *GASTRIC DIVERTICULA*

Gastric diverticula occur most commonly near the cardia on the lesser curve, but occasionally are found in the prepyloric region. They seldom cause symptoms. Their principal importance lies in the likelihood of confusion with gastric ulceration.

8.2.2 *PSEUDOLYMPHOMA*

Localized lymphoid hyperplasia of the stomach is also known as pseudolymphoma. The lesions are raised, flat or nodular folds, and are often associated with gastric ulceration. The etiology of this condition remains unclear, but Helicobacter pylori infection has been implicated. It is difficult to exclude lymphoma using radiology or endoscopic biopsy; thus, a resected specimen is required for diagnosis.

8.2.3 *GASTRIC INFECTIONS AND INFESTATIONS*

Gastric acid provides a bactericidal barrier against infection. Acid-suppressive pharmacotherapy, hypochlorhydria or gastric surgery may increase the risk of bacterial infection. Recent attention has been turned to Helicobacter pylori, a spiral bacillus found in the upper gastrointestinal tract, particularly the gastric antrum. H. pylori has been associated with chronic gastritis in addition to peptic ulcer disease.

Helicobacter pylori infection is now recognized to be a major causative factor associated with a spectrum of gastroduodenal disease. It is found in about 95% of patient with gastritis and 100% with chronic active gastritis. It is found in 90–95% of patients with duodenal ulcer and 60–80% of patients with gastric ulcer. It is also highly associated with gastric carcinoma and gastric lymphoma. The association of H. pylori infection with nonulcer dyspepsia is more controversial and as yet not convincingly substantiated.

Viral infections such as cytomegalovirus (CMV) and herpes simplex virus are very often found in immunocompromised hosts. They are associated with gastric erosions, although CMV has been found in intact mucosa. Cultures or endoscopic biopsies and smears demonstrating intranuclear inclusions are helpful in establishing a diagnosis. Candida albicans is commonly found in the gastric ulcers or erosions of immunocompromised hosts. Candidal infection should be a consideration in an ulcer that fails to heal. In the immunocompromised host, parasites such as Strongyloides stercoralis may become overwhelmingly disseminated. Histoplasmosis and mucormycosis involving the stomach are rare causes of gastric ulceration and bleeding.

8.2.3.1 *Helicobacter pylori gastritis*

Helicobacter pylori (H. pylori) is a small (3×0.5 μm) gram-negative, micro-

FIGURE 8. Helicobacter pylori. (Courtesy of McMaster University Medical Centre Electron Microscopy Lab.)

aerophilic urease-producing rod-shaped bacillus, which has been closely linked to both acute and chronic active type B gastritis, especially of the antrum (Figure 8). H. pylori is an important pathogenic factor in peptic ulcer disease.

H. pylori is present in almost all cases of chronic active gastritis, which most commonly involves antral inflammation but may spread to the whole stomach over time. H. pylori does not colonize areas of intestinal metaplasia, but has been seen in the distal esophagus of some patients with Barrett's esophagus.

The source of H. pylori is unknown, although person-to-person spread is probably demonstrated by intrafamilial clustering and a high prevalence of seropositivity in institutionalized persons, those of low economic status, and populations in less developed countries. The prevalence of H. pylori infection increases with age; in Western countries it is uncommon before the third decade but thereafter increases with seropositivity at the rate of approximately 1% per year of age.

Most people with H. pylori–associated gastritis are asymptomatic and have normal-appearing gastric mucosa at endoscopy. The histologic spectrum of H. pylori–associated gastritis ranges from minimal to severe inflammation, but the organisms noted in the mucous layer are associated with severe depletion of mucus and an intense inflammation, which most often is chronic, although neutrophils can be noted in some instances. Eradication of H. pylori with antibiotics has resulted in a marked lessening in the severity of the gastritis.

8.2.3.1.1 *Diagnosis* The organism can be identified on histology with conventional hematoxylin- and eosin-stained sections at high-power magnification, but is more easily seen with the Warthin-Starry or the modified Giemsa stains. The enzyme-linked immunosorbent assay (ELISA) is the most widely employed serologic method; its sensitivity and specificity are greater than 90%. Rapid urease tests can be performed on tissue biopsies in the endoscopy unit since H. pylori produces large amounts of urease, which can convert urea into ammonia and carbon dioxide. Rapid urease tests involve urease and pH indicator gel, into which the biopsy is placed. The presence of H. pylori results in an alkaline pH of the medium and a color change when the pH rises. Approximately 75% of the positive tests occur between 20 minutes and 1 hour, and 90% are positive between 6 and 24 hours. Carbon-urea breath tests using carbon ^{13}C and ^{14}C employ carbon-labeled urea that is fed to the patient and is subsequently hydolyzed by the H. pylori urease, resulting in the formation of ammonia and carbon dioxide. This labeled carbon dioxide in the breath is then measured.

8.2.3.1.2 *H. pylori association with peptic ulcer disease* Numerous studies have established the close association of antral H. pylori and peptic ulcer disease. Over 90% of patients with duodenal ulcer have H. pylori identified in gastric antral biopsies. The association for gastric ulcer and H. pylori is up to 80%. Although ulcers can be healed with a variety of agents that do not eradicate H. pylori, in these cases relapse is common. However, when the H. pylori organism is eradicated the impact on the subsequent course of duodenal ulcer is dramatic. The recurrence rate in patients in whom H. pylori is eradicated ranges from 0–4% per year. This is in marked contrast to those who remain H. pylori–positive, whose recurrence rates vary from 40–80% per year.

H. pylori infection is associated with doudenal ulcer by way of an antral-predominant gastritis that is accompanied by a decrease in somatostatin and an increase in gastrin. This may augment gastric acid secretion, which may already be high as a result of genetic factors. Increased gastric acid secretion leads to gastric metaplasia in the duodenum, which can be colonized by H. pylori leading to duodenal bulb inflammation, duodenitis and duodenal ulcer. The ulcer diathesis may reflect more damaging strains of the organisms,

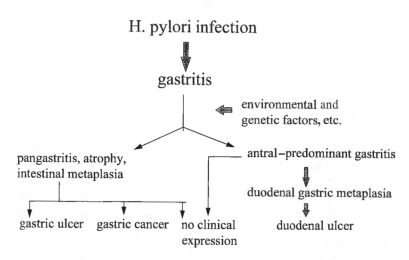

FIGURE 9.   Possible mechanisms of H. pylori–associated disease.

greater density of the infecting organisms or an exaggerated host inflammatory response (Figure 9).

The therapy for the eradication of H. pylori has evolved over the past decade (Table 10). The early regimen of bismuth triple therapy included a bismuth compound (Pepto-Bismol®) plus metronidazole and tetracycline or bismuth plus metronidazole and amoxicillin. The therapy is effective in patients with metronidazole-sensitive H. pylori infection but not very effective in those with metronidazole-resistant strains. This regimen has limited compliance because of dosing frequency and adverse effects.

Therapy later evolved to combinations of a proton pump inhibitor (PPI) and one antibiotic, usually clarithromycin. Eradication rates with a PPI plus clarithromycin are usually between 70 and 85%. The addition of a second antibiotic to the regimen, usually metronidazole, has led to much higher eradication rates, such as 88–94% for a PPI plus metronidazole and clarithromycin. With amoxicillin and clarithromycin the eradication rates are between 75 and 96%; the rates decrease about 10% with amoxicillin and metronidazole compared to the previous two combinations.

8.2.3.1.3 *Nonulcer dyspepsia and H. pylori*   The role of H. pylori infection in nonulcer dyspepsia remains an important question. There may be a subset of patients with nonulcer dyspepsia whose symptoms are due to H. pylori infection. However, many patients harboring H. pylori are symptom-free.

TABLE 10.   Eradication rates for H. pylori

Bismuth triple therapy (2 weeks)	PPI + 1 antibiotic (2 weeks)	PPI + 2 antibiotics (1 week)
90–98% (metronidazole-sensitive)	70–85% (clarithromycin)	88–94% (metronidazole/clarithromycin)
31–63% (metronidazole-resistant)	55–70% (amoxicillin)	75–96% (amoxicillin/clarithromycin)
		79–90% (amoxicillin/metronidazole)

Acute infection with H. pylori is associated with belching, pyrosis and malaise, and may be associated with decreased gastric acid secretion. At present, there is no evidence to suggest that the presence of H. pylori is associated with any particular symptom cluster related to functional dyspepsia.

SUGGESTED READING LIST

Marshall BJ, Warren JR. Unidentified curved bacilli in the stomach of patients with gastritis and peptic ulceration. Lancet 1984; 1(8390):1311–1315.

Walsh JH, Peterson WI. The treatment of Helicobacter pylori infection in the management of peptic ulcer disease. N Engl J Med 1995; 333:984–991.

Antonioli DA. Chronic gastritis: classification. In: Bayless TM (ed.), Current therapy in gastroenterology and liver disease. 4th ed. St. Louis: CV Mosby, 1994.

Correa P, Fox J, Fontham E, et al. Helicobacter pylori and gastric carcinoma: serum antibody prevalence in populations with contrasting cancer risks. Cancer 1990; 66: 2569–2574.

Hughes R. Diagnosis and treatment of gastric polyps. Gastrointest Endosc Clin North Am 1993; 2:457–467.

Yamada T, Alpers DH, Owyang C, et al. (eds.). Textbook of gastroenterology. Philadelphia: JB Lippincott, 1995.

OBJECTIVES

Anatomy and Physiology
1. Describe the arterial and nerve supply to the stomach.
2. List the three major functions of the stomach.
3. Describe the factors that determine gastric motility and emptying.

Peptic Ulcer Disease
1. What is Helicobacter pylori?
2. How is infection transmitted?

3. Where in the gastrointestinal tract does H. pylori live?
4. What is the best method to detect H. pylori in clinical practice?
5. Describe the mechanism(s) by which H. pylori causes damage.
6. Describe the association of H. pylori with histologic gastritis, gastric ulcer and duodenal ulcer.
7. List the causes of ulcer other than H. pylori.
8. What treatment regimens have been used to eradicate H. pylori?
9. List the indications for H. pylori eradication.

Gastritis
1. List 10 causes of thickened gastric folds.
2. What are the cardinal symptoms of gastritis?
3. List the causes of acute gastritis.
4. List the complications of gastric surgery.

Gastric Cancer
1. List the premalignant conditions associated with gastric cancer.
2. Describe the relationship of Helicobacter pylori to gastric cancer.
3. Which radiologic features distinguish a benign from a malignant gastric ulcer?

7
The Small Intestine
A.B.R. Thomson, P. Paré and R.N. Fedorak

1. GROSS ANATOMY OF THE SMALL INTESTINE

1.1 Duodenum

The term *duodenum* (a Latin derivation from the Greek *dodekadaktulon*, "12 fingers") is applied to the most proximal segment of the small intestine because of its length – 12 fingers' breadth. The duodenum is subdivided into four portions: the first portion, which corresponds to the radiologic designation of duodenal bulb or cap; the second (descending) portion; the third (transverse) portion; and the fourth (ascending) portion.

Situated immediately above the first portion of the duodenum are the quadrate lobe of the liver and the gallbladder. The gallbladder normally can impinge on the lesser curve of the duodenal cap to produce the smooth concavity seen in radiographs. Behind the first portion of the duodenum is the head of the pancreas. Because of this relationship, the pancreas is the commonest site of penetration by a duodenal ulcer.

The second portion of the duodenum is concave; it hugs the head of the pancreas. A carcinoma or inflammatory mass in the head of the pancreas can occasionally affect the mucosal pattern along the medial aspect of the second portion of the duodenum. Congenital duodenal diverticula are commonly seen extending from the medial aspect of the second portion.

The third portion of the duodenum lies horizontally at the level of the third lumbar vertebra. The superior mesenteric artery, vein and nerve run anterior to its middle segment. In a thin individual or a person with recent massive weight loss, the superior mesenteric vessel sheath may impinge on the third portion of the duodenum, which is associated with chronic, intermittent obstruction of the duodenum.

The fourth portion of the duodenum as it ascends to the level of the second lumbar vertebra is in intimate contact with the aorta. This intimacy of duodenum and aorta can lead to fatal complications of aortic grafting when the graft erodes the duodenal wall, resulting in hemorrhage. Bleeding may be either catastrophic (due to a tiny connection between the aortic lumen and the duodenal lumen) or chronic with iron deficiency and fever (due to erosion of the duodenal mucosa by the exterior of the graft).

The mucosal pattern of the first portion (the duodenal cap or bulb) can be distinguished radiologically and endoscopically from the remaining duodenum. In the cap, shallow folds run longitudinally and are obliterated as the cap is distended. Beginning at the junction between the first and second portions of the duodenum, permanent transverse conniventes, characteristic of the small intestine, begin.

1.2 Jejunum and Ileum

The length of the small intestine is approximately 6 m; the length can vary from 4 to 7 m according to the technique used to make the measurement. The proximal 40% of the small intestine is referred to as the *jejunum* (from the Latin, meaning "empty"), and the distal 60% is designated as the *ileum* (from the Greek *eilein*, "to roll or twist"). The wall of the jejunum is thicker and its lumen wider than are those of the ileum. There is also a gradual diminution in the caliber of the lumen from duodenum to ileum. Because of its narrower lumen, the ileum is more prone to obstruction. There is a characteristic difference in the mesentery between jejunum and ileum. The fat is thicker in the ileal mesentery and extends fully to the intestinal attachment. In Crohn's disease, the thickened mesenteric fat encroaches further beneath the serosa of the small intestine. On x-ray, the mucosa in the proximal and ileal segments of the small intestine also differs. In the jejunum, the valvulae conniventes (also known as plicae circulares) are thick, tall and numerous, giving a feathery mucosal pattern on x-ray. This contrasts with the sausage-shaped ileal loops, where the valvulae conniventes are progressively fewer and less prominent but are more clearly seen as transverse folds on x-ray.

2. SMALL INTESTINAL MOTILITY

The main function of the small intestine is digestion and absorption of nutrients. In this process, the role of small bowel motility is to mix food products with the digestive enzymes, to promote contact of chyme with the absorptive cells over a sufficient length of bowel and finally to propel remnants into the colon. Well-organized motility patterns occur in the small intestine to accomplish these goals in the fed as well as the fasting state. During fasting, a migrating motor complex (MMC) exists. This complex is characterized by a front of intense spiking activity (phase III activity) that migrates down the entire small intestine; as the front reaches the terminal ileum, another front develops in the gastroduodenal area and progresses down the intestine. The purpose of this phase III myoelectric and contractile activity is to sweep remnants of the previous meal into the colon and prevent stagnation and bacterial overgrowth. The MMC often starts in the lower esophagus. Sweeping through the stomach, it removes debris and residual material not emptied with the last meal. Absence of phase III activity is associated with bacterial overgrowth and diarrhea. Thus, the small bowel is active even during fasting.

During meals, this cycle is interrupted and the motility pattern in the small bowel becomes an irregular spiking activity called the fed pattern. This fed pattern of motility does not seem to move intestinal contents forward to any great extent but does mix these contents with digestive juices, spreading them again and again over the absorptive surface of the brush border. Diarrhea can thus occur when this normal fed pattern is replaced by aggressive propulsive contractions.

3. PRINCIPLES OF ABSORPTION

Understanding the pathophysiology of diarrhea and malabsorption is based on understanding the normal steps in the digestion and absorption of food. The normal gastrointestinal tract is a finely integrated system geared to carry out the assimilation of ingested foodstuffs. Assimilation (the process by which ingested foods reach body fluids and cells) consists of two stages: (1) digestion (the breakdown of large molecules in the lumen of the intestine into their component small molecules) and (2) absorption (the transport across the intestinal mucosa to systemic body fluids).

Many disease processes directly or indirectly alter gastrointestinal physiology in such a manner that normal absorptive mechanisms are compromised, resulting in maldigestion or malabsorption of one or more dietary constituents. Too simplistic an approach to these diseases may be confusing because of the large number of illnesses involved and because of the plethora of diagnostic tests. This chapter will (1) present a classification of malabsorption and (2) outline the usefulness and potential pitfalls of common tests of intestinal function.

4. ABSORPTION OF VITAMINS AND MINERALS

4.1 Folic Acid (Pteroylglutamic Acid, PteGlu$_1$)

4.1.1 *FOOD SOURCES*
Dietary folates (folacins) are synthesized by bacteria and plants. They occur mostly as polyglutamates, which are not absorbed intact. All folacins, or poly-

pteroylglutamates (PteGlu$_n$), are hydrolyzed to folic acid, or pteroylglutamic acid (PteGlu$_1$), during absorption. Pteroylglutamic acid (PteGlu$_1$) is absorbed at a faster rate than larger polymers (PteGlu$_n$). Only 25–50% of dietary folacin is nutritionally available; boiling destroys much of folate activity. Therefore, uncooked foods with a large portion of the monoglutamate form (PteGlu$_1$) – e.g., bananas, lima beans, liver and yeast – contain the highest availability of folacin. Average Canadian diets contain about 240 μg of folate a day. The daily requirement for folate is approximately 100 μg, although the recommended dietary allowance is 400 μg. Tissue stores of folate are only about 3 mg; therefore, malabsorption can deplete the body of folate within one month.

4.1.2 HYDROLYSIS AND ABSORPTION OF POLYGLUTAMATE FOLATES

Polyglutamate forms of folate (PteGlu$_n$) hydrolyze sequentially down to the monoglutamate form (PteGlu$_1$). This hydrolysis takes place at the brush border by the enzyme folate conjugase (Figure 1). Folic acid (PteGlu$_1$) is absorbed from the intestinal lumen by a sodium-dependent carrier. Once in the intestinal epithelial cell, folic acid is methylated and reduced to the tetrahydro form (CH$_3$H$_4$PteGlu$_1$).

Interference with folic acid absorption at the brush-border carrier site occurs with drugs such as phenytoin and sulfasalazine. In addition, folic acid deficiency itself can impair folic acid absorption by producing "megaloblastic" changes in columnar epithelial cells of the gut – an abnormal epithelium.

4.2 Cobalamin (Vitamin B$_{12}$)

4.2.1 FOOD SOURCES

Cobalamin refers to cobalt-containing compounds with a corrin ring: these have biological activity for humans. Vitamin B$_{12}$ is the generic term for all of these compounds with bioactivity in any species. Cobalamin is therefore the preferred term to distinguish those compounds that are active in humans from the many analogues produced by bacteria. Cobalamin enters animal tissues when the animal ingests bacteria-containing foods or from production in the animal's rumen. Microorganisms in the human colon synthesize cobalamin, but it is not absorbed. Thus, strict vegetarians who do not eat cobalamin-containing meats will develop cobalamin deficiency. The average Western diet contains 10–20 μg per day. The daily requirement for cobalamin is 1 μg. The human liver is the repository of approximately 5 mg of cobalamin. These large hepatic stores account for the delay of several years in the clinical appearance of deficiency after cobalamin malabsorption begins.

INTESTINAL   INTESTINAL   MESENTERIC
LUMEN   EPITHELIUM   CIRCULATION

FIGURE 1. Proposed scheme of the digestion and absorption of dietary pteroylglutamates. Hydrolysis of polypteroylglutamates (shown here as $PteGlu_7$) probably occurs outside the intestinal epithelial cell. The overall rate of absorption into the mesenteric circulation is governed by the rate of transport of the monoglutamyl product ($PteGlu_1$). At physiologic doses, a substantial amount of $PteGlu_1$ is reduced and then methylated to $CH_3H_4PteGlu_1$ in the intestinal cell before release to the circulation.

SOURCE: Rosenberg IH. Folate absorption and malabsorption. N Engl J Med 1975; 293:1303.

4.2.2 ROLE OF THE STOMACH, PANCREAS AND ILEUM

Once cobalamin is liberated from food, it is bound at acid pH to R proteins (so called because of their rapid movement during electrophoresis). R proteins are glycoproteins present in many body secretions, including serum, bile, saliva and gastric and pancreatic juices. Most of the gastric R protein is from swallowed saliva. The R proteins cannot mediate the absorption of cobalamin alone, and their physiologic function is incompletely understood. Rare cases of complete R-protein deficiency have occurred without obvious clinical effect on the patient.

The cobalamin/R protein complex leaves the stomach along with free intrinsic factor (Figure 2). In the duodenum, pancreatic proteases in the presence of bicarbonate (i.e., neutral pH) hydrolyze the R protein, thereby liberating free cobalamin. The cobalamin now combines with gastric intrinsic fac-

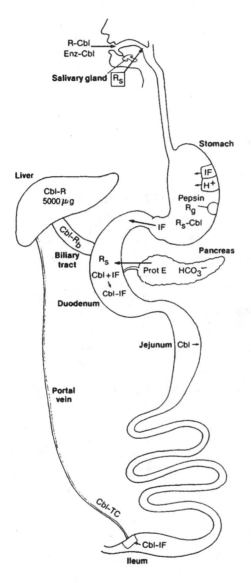

FIGURE 2.   Absorption of cobalamin (Cbl) requires proteolysis and intrinsic factor (IF). The intrinsic factor secreted is far in excess of that needed for binding the available cobalamin. R protein derived from saliva is also present in great abundance. Note that Cbl binds initially to R protein in the stomach at acid pH. Only after R protein is degraded by protease does Cbl bind to IF. After Cbl is absorbed in the ileum, it is bound to transcobalamin II.

SOURCE: Kalser MH. Absorption of cobalamin (vitamin B_{12}), folate, and other water-soluble vitamins. In: Berk JE (ed.), Bockus gastroenterology, vol. 3. 4th ed. Philadelphia: WB Saunders, 1985:1556.

TABLE 1. Abnormalities of cobalamin absorption that produce deficiency

Physiologic step	Disorder
Decreased IF secretion	Pernicious anemia, gastrectomy, achlorhydria
Impaired transfer to IF (acidic pH)	Pancreatic insufficiency
Competition for uptake	Bacterial overgrowth
Impaired attachment to ileal receptor	Ileal disease or resection
Impaired passage through the ileal cell wall	Familial cobalamin malabsorption
Impaired uptake into blood	Transcobalamin II deficiency

tor. A conformational change takes place, allowing the cobalamin/intrinsic-factor complex to be resistant to proteolytic digestion. This resistance allows the complex to safely traverse the small intestine and reach the ileum, its site of active absorption.

Since transfer of cobalamin from R protein to intrinsic factor depends upon pH, pancreatic insufficiency (with deficient bicarbonate production) or the Zollinger-Ellison syndrome (with excess hydrogen ion production) interferes with this process and may result in cobalamin deficiency.

In the ileum, the cobalamin/intrinsic-factor complex binds to a specific receptor located on the brush border. Free cobalamin does not bind to the ileal receptor. After passage across the enterocytes, cobalamin is transported in blood bound to circulating proteins known as transcobalamins.

Understanding the normal absorptive processes allows a classification of cobalamin malabsorption and deficiency (Table 1).

4.3 Iron

4.3.1 *FOOD SOURCES*
Iron is available for absorption from vegetables (nonheme iron) and from meats (heme iron). Heme iron is better absorbed (10–20%) and is unaffected by intraluminal factors or its dietary composition. Nonheme iron is poorly absorbed, with an efficiency of 1–6%, and absorption is largely controlled by luminal events. The average dietary intake of iron is 10–20 mg/day. Men absorb 1–2 mg/day, while menstruating women and iron-deficient patients absorb 3–4 mg/day. In acute blood loss, increased absorption of iron does not occur until three days later. Nonheme iron (in the ferric, Fe^{+++} state), when ingested into a stomach unable to produce acid, forms insoluble iron complexes, which are not available for absorption (Figure 3). In the presence of gastric acid and such agents as ascorbic acid, however, ferrous iron (Fe^{++}) forms. The ferrous iron complexes bind to a mucopolysaccharide of about 200,000 MW_r and are transported as an insoluble complex into the duodenum

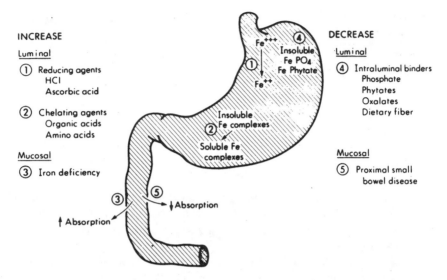

INCREASE

Luminal

① Reducing agents
HCl
Ascorbic acid

② Chelating agents
Organic acids
Amino acids

Mucosal

③ Iron deficiency

↑ Absorption

DECREASE

Luminal

④ Intraluminal binders
Phosphate
Phytates
Oxalates
Dietary fiber

Mucosal

⑤ Proximal small
bowel disease

Fe⁺⁺⁺ ④ Insoluble
Fe PO₄
① Fe Phytate
Fe⁺⁺
Insoluble
② Fe complexes
Soluble Fe
complexes

③ ⑤
↓ Absorption

FIGURE 3. Factors that affect iron absorption. Nonheme iron absorption is affected both by intra-luminal factors (1, 2 and 4) and by the total iron body content (3) as well as by small bowel disease (5). Heme iron absorption is altered only by those factors that affect the mucosa itself (3 and 5).

SOURCE: Alpers DH. Absorption of water-soluble vitamins, folate, minerals, and vitamin D. In: Sleisenger MH, Fordtran JS (eds.), Gastrointestinal disease: pathophysiology, diagnosis, management. 3d ed. Philadelphia: WB Saunders, 1983:835.

and proximal jejunum. Here, with the assistance of ascorbic acid, glucose and cysteine, the iron is absorbed. Dietary factors such as phosphate, phytate and phosphoproteins can render the iron insoluble and so inhibit nonheme iron absorption.

Heme iron (ferrous, Fe^{++}) is ingested as myoglobin and hemoglobin. In the presence of gastric acid, the globin molecule is split off, and ferrous iron is liberated and transported with its phosphorin ring from the stomach into the duodenum and jejunum for absorption.

Both heme and nonheme iron are absorbed most rapidly in the duodenum. Some of the iron taken up is deposited as ferritin within the enterocyte, and the remainder is transferred to the plasma-bound transferrin. When the entero-cyte defoliates, iron deposited as ferritin is lost into the intestinal lumen. This mechanism for loss is probably overwhelmed by the large amounts of iron ingested. The amount of iron entering the body depends largely upon two factors: (1) total body iron content and (2) the rate of erythropoiesis.

5. ABSORPTION OF WATER AND ELECTROLYTES

5.1 Passive Permeability to Ions and Water

The epithelium of the small intestine exhibits a high passive permeability to salt and water that is a consequence of the leakiness of the junctions between epithelial cells. Osmotic equilibration between plasma and lumen is fairly rapid; therefore, large differences in ion concentration do not develop. These intercellular junctions are more permeable to cations than anions, so that lumen-to-blood concentration differences for Na^+ and K^+ are generally smaller than those for Cl^- and HCO_3. The colonic epithelium displays lower passive permeability to salt and water. This ionic permeability diminishes from cecum to rectum. It also decreases from duodenum to ileum. One consequence of this lower passive ionic permeability (higher electrical resistance) is that electric potential differences across the colonic epithelium are an order of magnitude greater than those in the small intestine (remember Ohm's law, $E = IR$, where E is electrical potential, I is electrical current, and R is electrical resistance). Active Na^+ absorption, which is the main transport activity of the distal colon, generates a serosa-positive charge or potential difference (PD). Under the influence of aldosterone (i.e., salt depletion), this PD can be 60 mV or even higher. A 60 mV PD will thus sustain a 10-fold concentration difference for a monovalent ion such as K^+. Most of the high K^+ concentration in the rectum is accounted for, therefore, by the PD. Despite the high fecal K^+ level, little K^+ is lost in the stool, since stool volume (about 200–300 mL per day) is normally so low. In contrast, during high-volume (several liters per day) diarrhea of small bowel origin, the stool K^+ concentration is considerably lower (10–30 mmol) but stool K^+ loss is nonetheless great because of the large volumes involved. In such states, the stool K^+ concentration is low (and the Na^+ concentration relatively high) because diarrheal fluid passes through the colon too rapidly to equilibrate across the colonic epithelium.

5.2 Active Electrolyte Absorption along the Intestine

The intestine, especially the small intestine, has the largest capacity for secreting water and electrolytes of any organ system in the body. In both the small bowel and the colon, secretion appears to arise predominantly, if not exclusively, in crypts; the more superficial villous tip epithelium is absorptive. Disease processes that result in damage to the villus or to superficial portions of the intestinal epithelium (e.g., viral enteritis) inevitably shift the overall balance between absorption and secretion toward secretion. This is especially important in patients with celiac disease, where there is villous atrophy as well as hypertrophy of the crypts of Lieberkühn.

FIGURE 4. Na$^+$-coupled sugar(s) absorption.

In the small intestine, active electrolyte and fluid absorption can be conceived of as either *nutrient-dependent* or *nutrient-independent*.

5.2.1 *NUTRIENT-DEPENDENT TRANSPORT*

The absorptive processes for the nutrients glucose and neutral amino acids are Na$^+$-dependent – i.e., one Na$^+$ molecule is translocated across the brush border with each glucose or amino acid molecule (Figure 4). The sodium pump (Na$^+$/K$^+$-ATPase), which is located exclusively in the basolateral membrane of the enterocyte, extrudes Na$^+$ that has entered the cell from the lumen, thereby maintaining a low intracellular Na$^+$, a high intracellular K$^+$ and a negative intracellular electric potential. This Na$^+$/K$^+$ pump provides the potential energy for uphill sugar and amino acid absorption. Glucose is cotransported with sodium. Patients in intestinal secretory states such as cholera can absorb glucose normally. Na$^+$ (and thus water) are also absorbed, accompanying the transport of glucose. As a consequence, the fluid losses incurred by these patients can be replaced by oral glucose-electrolyte solutions[1] and do not require intravenous fluids unless the patient is comatose or too nauseated to

---

[1] The WHO oral rehydration solution contains in mmol/L: glucose, 111; Na$^+$, 90; K$^+$, 20; Cl$^-$, 80; HCO$_3^-$, 30.

FIGURE 5.   Electrogenic Na⁺ absorption and Cl⁻/HCO₃⁻ exchange.

drink the necessary large volumes of fluid to correct the dehydration. Application of this knowledge has had a major impact on world health, and especially on that of children, since the parts of the world where cholera-like diarrheas are prevalent generally have very limited hospital facilities and insufficient supplies of sterile electrolyte solutions.

5.2.2 NUTRIENT-INDEPENDENT TRANSPORT

Nutrient-independent active absorption of electrolytes and water by intestinal epithelial cells occurs through several specific mechanisms, located at different levels of the mammalian intestinal tract (Figures 5 and 6). All of these mechanisms have in common the Na^+/K^+-ATPase pump, located on the basolateral membrane, and also a requirement for luminal Na^+.

In the distal colon (Figure 5), the luminal membrane contains Na^+ channels, which can be blocked by low concentrations of the pyrazine diuretic amiloride. The Na^+ entering through these channels in the luminal membrane is then extruded across the basolateral membrane by the Na^+/K^+-ATPase pump. Aldosterone increases the number of these channels and also, more slowly, increases the number of Na^+/K^+-ATPase pumps. Aldosterone therefore enhances active Na^+ absorption in the distal colon. To a more limited extent, aldosterone also causes the appearance of Na^+ channels more proximally in the colon and even in the distal ileum. Cl^- is absorbed along with Na^+ and traverses the epithelium by both cellular and paracellular routes. Its transcellular route involves a Cl^-/HCO_3^- exchanger in the luminal membrane and Cl^- chan-

FIGURE 6.   Electroneutral Na^+/H^+ and Cl^-/HCO_3^- exchanges.

nels in the basolateral membrane. Intracellular mediators such as cyclic AMP (cAMP) do not appear to affect these Na^+ channels. Thus, patients with secretory diarrheas, especially those who are salt-depleted and therefore have elevated blood levels of aldosterone, are able to reabsorb some of the secreted fluid in their distal colon. Spironolactone, which inhibits the action of aldosterone, can increase the severity of diarrhea in such patients.

In the more proximal colon and in the ileum, the luminal membrane contains Na^+/H^+ exchangers that permit net Na^+ entry (Figure 6). The colon and the ileum (but not the jejunum) also have Cl^-/HCO_3^- exchangers in their luminal borders. Cell pH adjusts the relative rates of these two exchangers. Thus, H^+ extrusion by Na^+/H^+ exchange can cause cell alkalinization, which then stimulates Cl^- entry and HCO_3^- extrusion by this Cl^-/HCO_3^- exchange. The latter exchanger increases cell H^+, thereby sustaining Na^+/H^+ exchange. Increases in cell concentrations of cAMP and free Ca^{2+} inhibit the Na^+/H^+ exchange. Cyclic AMP and its agonists thereby cause cell acidification – which, in turn, inhibits Cl^-/HCO_3^- exchange. Therefore, electrolyte absorption in small and large intestinal segments (except the distal colon) can be down-regulated by hormones, neurotransmitters and certain luminal substances (bacterial enterotoxins, bile salts, hydroxylated fatty acids) that increase cell

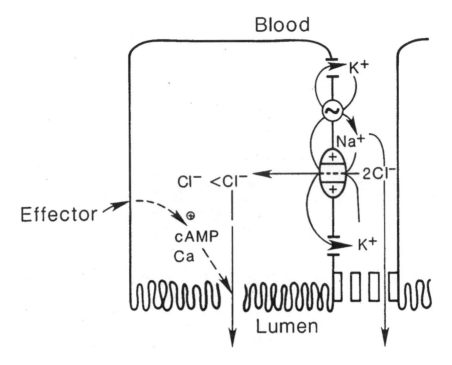

FIGURE 7. Secretory cell.

concentrations of cAMP or free Ca^{2+}. For this reason, body fluid secreted in response to these stimuli cannot be effectively reabsorbed in the absence of amino acids and sugars, except in the distal colon. In the jejunum, where Cl^-/HCO_3^- exchange does not appear to be present, Na^+/H^+ exchange can be well sustained by anaerobic glycolysis, which generates H^+ as well as some ATP.

There is also some evidence for a direct cotransport of Na^+ and Cl^-, although this is difficult to separate experimentally from dual exchangers. This entry mechanism may exist in the ileum and proximal colon.

5.3 Active Electrolyte Secretion along the Intestine

In the secretory cell, the entry of Cl^- from the contraluminal bathing medium (blood or serosal side of the enterocyte) is coupled to that of Na^+ and probably also K^+ by a triple cotransporter with a stoichiometry of 1 Na^+, 1 K^+ and 2 Cl^-. Na^+ entering in this fashion is then recycled to the contraluminal solution by the Na^+/K^+ exchange pump (Figure 7). K^+, entering via the pump and

TABLE 2.   Hormones and neurotransmitters that stimulate intestinal secretion

| | Intracellular mediator | |
cAMP	Ca^{2+}	Unknown
Vasoactive intestinal peptide	Bradykinin	Bombesin
Prostaglandins	Acetylcholine	Lipoxygenase products
Bradykinin	Substance P	Thyrocalcitonin
	Neurotensin	Histamine
	Serotonin	Vasopressin

Only agents found effective in vitro have been listed. Several other hormones have been found to stimulate secretion in vivo, but it is unclear whether they act directly on the intestinal mucosa. The latter include glucagon and pentagastrin.

also the triple cotransporter, diffuses back to the contraluminal side through K^+ channels. Owing to the Na^+ gradient, Cl^- accumulates above electrochemical equilibrium and can either (1) recycle back to the contraluminal solution through the $Na^+/K^+/2\ Cl^-$ cotransporter or through basolateral membrane Cl^- channels, or (2) be secreted into the lumen through luminal membrane Cl^- channels. When Cl^- is secreted into the lumen it generates a serosa-positive electric potential difference, which provides the driving force for Na^+ secretion through the paracellular pathway between cells. In the resting secretory cell, the luminal Cl^- channels are closed. When secretion is stimulated by a hormone or neurotransmitter, these channels open. Secretion is initiated, therefore, by opening the Cl^- "gate" in the luminal membrane of the secretory cell.

The known intracellular mediators of secretion are cAMP, cGMP and Ca^{2+} (Table 2). These can arise from the blood; nerve endings; endocrine cells in the epithelium (APUD cells); mesenchymal elements such as lymphocytes, plasma cells and mast cells; or the enterocytes themselves. Except for the cAMP agonists, lipoxygenase products and calcitonin, the actions of the other agonists are short-lived; desensitization rapidly develops. They operate to fine-tune electrolyte transport rather than invoke persistent secretion.

Predictably, since there are hormones and neurotransmitters that stimulate active electrolyte secretion in the gut, there are also agonists that inhibit secretion and/or stimulate absorption. These include adrenocorticosteroids, norepinephrine, somatostatin, enkephalins and dopamine. Glucocorticoids enhance electrolyte absorption throughout the intestinal tract, but the mechanisms involved are less well understood than for aldosterone. They may act in part by inhibiting phospholipase A_2 and therefore the arachidonic acid cascade.

The adrenergic receptors on enterocytes are almost exclusively α2 in type. The sympathetic nervous system in the intestinal mucosa releases norepinephrine (an α2 antagonist) and so inhibits electrolyte secretion and stimulates absorption. Sympathectomy, whether chemical or surgical, leads to diarrhea, at least transiently. Chronic diabetics with autonomic neuropathy sometimes develop persistent diarrhea that is associated with degeneration of adrenergic nerve fibers to the gut. Somatostatin and endogenous enkephalins are also antisecretory.

6. ABSORPTION OF FAT

The overall process of fat digestion and absorption consists of four distinct phases, related to the respective functions of the pancreas, liver, intestinal mucosa and lymphatics (Figure 8). Physiologically, these involve (1) lipolysis of dietary triglyceride (TG) to fatty acid (FA) and β-monoglyceride (MG); (2) micellar solubilization with bile acid; (3) uptake into the mucosal cell, with re-esterification of the MG with FA to form TG, and chylomicron formation in the presence of cholesterol, cholesterol esters, phospholipids and protein; and (4) delivery of chylomicrons in lymphatics to the body for utilization of fat.

The average North American diet contains 60–100 g of fat each day, mostly in the form of neutral fat or triglycerides. In the proximal intestine, TG comes under hydrolytic attack by lipases, producing glycerol, FA and MG. These products of lipolysis first form an emulsion and later a micellar solution.

Following the entry of food and particularly fat into the duodenum, cholecystokinin (CCK) is released from mucosal cells, causing gallbladder contraction. Bile acids, along with other biliary constituents, are released into the proximal small intestine. Bile acids chemically resemble detergent molecules, in that a portion of the molecule is polar and water-soluble, while another portion of the molecule is nonpolar and fat-soluble. When the bile acids are present in sufficient amounts, known as the critical micellar concentration (CMC), they form negatively charged spheres, called simple micelles. Incorporation of FA and MG forms a larger, polymolecular aggregate, a mixed micelle. All this is necessary to solubilize fat and disperse it in small packets more effectively, setting the stage for further digestion by pancreatic lipase. This enzyme acts only at oil–water interfaces and requires a large surface area. Pancreatic lipase is secreted into the duodenunal lumen where it acts on ingested food.

Adequate concentrations of bile acid must be present within the jejunal lumen for effective micellar solubilization and lipolysis by pancreatic lipase,

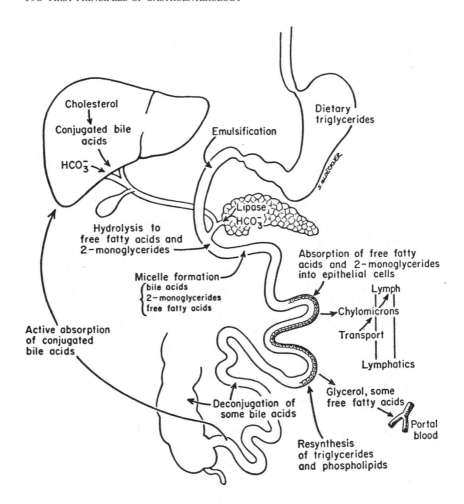

FIGURE 8.   Diagram of the major steps in the digestion and absorption of dietary fat. These include (1) the lipolysis of dietary triglyceride (TG) by pancreatic enzymes; (2) micellar solubilization of the resulting long-chain fatty acids (FA) and β-monoglycerides (βMG; shown in figure as 2-monoglycerides) by bile acids secreted into the intestinal lumen by the liver; (3) absorption of the fatty acids and β-monoglycerides into the mucosal cell with subsequent re-esterification and formation of chylomicrons; and, finally, (4) movement of the chylomicrons from the mucosal cell into the intestinal lymphatic system. During the process of chylomicron formation, small amounts of cholesterol (C), cholesterol ester (CE), and phospholipid (PL) as well as triglyceride are incorporated into this specific lipoprotein fraction.

SOURCE: Wilson FA, Dietschy JM. Differential diagnostic approach to clinical problems of malabsorption. Gastroenterology 1971; 61:912.

a preliminary to esterification and uptake. Such adequate concentrations of bile acids are maintained by the constant reutilization of a relatively small pool of bile acid. In the liver, about 0.6 g of new bile acid is produced daily from cholesterol. This is added to the total bile acid pool of 3.0 g, which cycles 6 to 10 times daily from passive absorption in the jejunum and active absorption in the ileum. Approximately 96% of the bile acid is absorbed through these mechanisms with each cycle; the remainder is lost in the stool. Bile acids return to the liver via the portal vein and are excreted once more. This recirculation of bile acid between the intestine and the liver is called the enterohepatic circulation.

The principal role of the bile salt micelle is to facilitate lipid absorption by maintaining the lipid in a water-soluble form, overcoming the resistance of the unstirred water layer and maintaining a high concentration of a local source of fatty acid and cholesterol, which leave the micelle and enter the mucosal cell.

The lipid-containing bile acid micelle is now ready for mucosal uptake. Two important events occur within the mucosal cell: re-esterification and chylomicron formation. The fatty acids are first reattached to the monoglycerides through re-esterification, and the resultant triglyceride is then combined with small amounts of cholesterol and coated with phospholipids and proteins to form a specific class of lipoproteins known as chylomicrons. The chylomicrons are then released from the basal portion of the columnar epithelial cell and find their way into the central lacteal of the intestinal villus. From there, chylomicrons travel in lymph up the thoracic duct and eventually reach the general circulation. Chylomicrons are then transported in the blood to the sites of disposal and utilization in the periphery (e.g., liver, muscle and adipose tissue).

From these physiological considerations, malabsorption of fat due to impaired lipolysis or micellar solubilization would be expected to occur in the following circumstances: (1) rapid gastric emptying and improper mixing – e.g., following vagotomy or postgastrectomy; (2) altered duodenal pH – e.g., the Zollinger-Ellison syndrome, where excessive duodenal acidification inhibits the action of lipase; (3) pancreatic insufficiency; (4) cholestasis – e.g., biliary obstruction, liver disease; and (5) an interrupted enterohepatic circulation – e.g., ileal disease or loss, and bile salt deconjugation due to the bacterial overgrowth syndrome.

Fat malabsorption due to impaired mucosal uptake, assembly or delivery would be expected to occur following (1) generalized impaired enterocyte function – e.g., celiac disease, Whipple's disease; (2) failure of the packaging process – e.g., abetalipoproteinemia, which represents a genetic defect of lipoprotein B synthesis with consequent impairment of chylomicron forma-

FIGURE 9.   The action of pancreatic α-amylase on linear (amylose) and branched (amylopectin) starch. Circles indicate glucose residues and the reducing glucose unit.
SOURCE: Gray GM. Mechanisms of digestion and absorption of food. In Sleisenger MH, Fordtran JS (eds.), Gastrointestinal disease: pathophysiology, diagnosis, management. 3d ed. Philadelphia: WB Saunders, 1983:851.

tion; (3) disorders of lymphatics – e.g., intestinal lymphangiectasia, retroperitoneal fibrosis or lymphoma; and (4) loss of mucosal surface area – e.g., the short bowel syndrome.

7. ABSORPTION OF CARBOHYDRATES

Starch, sucrose and lactose constitute the main carbohydrates in the human diet. All are inexpensive sources of food. Together they constitute the major source of calories when considered worldwide. People in the Western world consume about 400 g of carbohydrates daily: 60% as starch, 30% as sucrose and 10% as lactose (milk contains 48 g of lactose per liter).

Starch present in wheat, rice and corn is a polysaccharide whose molecular weight ranges from 100,000 to greater than 1,000,000. The straight chain of glucose molecules in starch is bridged by an oxygen molecule between the first carbon (C_1) of one glucose unit and the fourth carbon (C_4) of its neigh-

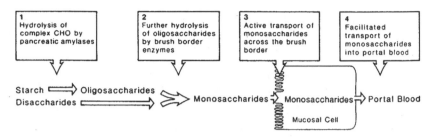

FIGURE 10. Major steps in the digestion and absorption of dietary carbohydrate.

bor (α1,4 glucose link). This type of starch is called amylose and makes up as much as 20% of the starch in the diet. The glucose-to-glucose bridge is of the alpha type – in contrast to the beta type, which connects glucose units in cellulose, an indigestible saccharide. The remaining 80% of the starch that humans ingest has a branch point every 25 molecules along the straight α1,4 glucose chain. This starch is called amylopectin. These branches occur via an oxygen bridge between C_6 of the glucose on the straight chain and C_1 in the branched chain (α1,6 branch points), which then continues as another α1,4 glucose-linked straight chain (Figure 9).

Salivary and pancreatic α-amylases act on interior α1,4 glucose–glucose links of starch but cannot attack α1,4 linkages close to a 1,6 branch point. The products of amylase digestion are therefore maltose and maltotriose. Since α-amylase cannot hydrolyze the 1,6 branching links and has relatively little specificity for 1,4 links adjacent to these branch points, large oligosaccharides containing five to nine glucose units and consisting of one or more 1,6 branching links are also produced by α-amylase action. These are called α-limit dextrins, and represent about 30% of amylopectin breakdown.

The responsibility for digesting the oligosaccharides, including α-limit dextrins, and the amylose and amylopectin rests with the hydrolytic enzymes on intestinal epithelial cells (Figures 10 and 11). These hydrolytic enzymes are called disaccharidases, but most are in fact oligosaccharidases: they hydrolyze sugars containing three or more hexose units. They are present in highest concentration at the villous tips in the jejunum and persist throughout most of the ileum, but not in the colon. Lactase breaks down lactose into glucose and galactose. Glucoamylase (maltase) differs from pancreatic α-amylase since it sequentially removes a single glucose from the nonreducing end of a linear α1,4 glucose chain, breaking down maltose into glucose. Sucrase is a hybrid molecule consisting of two enzymes – one hydrolyzing sucrose and the other, the α1,6 branch points of the α-limit dextrins. This enzyme is commonly called sucrase-isomaltase, because the isomaltase moiety hydro-

Disaccharides ⟶ Monosaccharides

FIGURE 11. Disaccharides are split into monosaccharides at the brush border.

lyzes isomaltose, the α1,6 glucosyl disaccharide. However, the only products containing α1,6 linkages after amylase action on starch are the α-limit dextrins. Thus no free isomaltose is presented to the intestinal surface and the term "isomaltase" is a misnomer. The sucrase moiety thus breaks down sucrose into glucose and fructose.

Humans normally are born with a full complement of brush-border-membrane disaccharidases. Intake of large amounts of sucrose results in an increase in sucrase activity, probably as the substrate stabilizes the enzyme and reduces its rate of breakdown. In contrast, there is no evidence that dietary manipulation can regulate the activities of human lactase or maltase.

Once the disaccharides are broken down, how are the monosaccharides absorbed? Sodium facilitates glucose uptake by binding to the brush-border membrane carrier (SGLT1) along with glucose. Since intracellular Na^+ concentration is low, the Na^+ ion moves down its concentration gradient into the cell, to be pumped out subsequently at the basolateral membrane by Na^+/K^+-ATPase, an active process that utilizes energy derived from the hydrolysis of ATP. The electrochemical gradient thus developed by Na^+ provides the driving force for glucose entry. Glucose accompanies Na^+ on the brush-border carrier and is released inside the cell, where its concentrations may exceed those in the intestinal lumen. Glucose then exits from the basolateral membrane of the cell into the portal system by a non–Na^+-dependent carrier (GLUT2).

Fructose, released from the hydrolysis of sucrose, is transported by facilitated diffusion, a carrier-mediated process in the brush-border membrane (GLUT5) that is independent both of Na^+ and of the glucose transport mechanism.

From these physiological considerations, carbohydrate malabsorption can occur in the following circumstances: (1) severe pancreatic insufficiency; (2) selective deficiencies of brush-border disaccharidases – e.g., lactase deficiency; (3) generalized impairment of brush-border and enterocyte function – e.g., celiac disease, tropical sprue, gastroenteritis; and (4) loss of mucosal surface area – e.g., the short bowel syndrome.

Although infants often have a deficiency of amylase, starch is not usually fed for the first few months of life. In the adult, there is a great excess of pancreatic amylase secreted into the intestinal lumen, so that even in patients with severe fat malabsorption due to pancreatic exocrine insufficiency, residual salivary and pancreatic amylase output appears to be sufficient to completely hydrolyze starch to the final oligosaccharides by the time a meal reaches the mid-jejunum. Hence, maldigestion of starch rarely, if ever, occurs in humans.

Secondary deficiency of disaccharidases results from anatomic injury of the small intestine, as in celiac disease, tropical sprue and gastroenteritis. When disaccharidase levels are sufficiently low, the particular oligosaccharide or disaccharide remains unhydrolyzed within the intestinal lumen and augments intraluminal fluid accumulation by virtue of its osmotic effect. Bacterial fermentation of disaccharides that reach the colon produces fatty acids (butyric, formic, acetic and propionic acids), alcohols and gases (H_2 and CO_2) (Figure 12). The benefits of this bacterial fermentation to the host are twofold. First, the bulk of the caloric value present in carbohydrates remains in the fermentative products. Reabsorption of fatty acids and alcohols in the colon "salvages" calories from malabsorbed carbohydrates. Second, this colonic "salvage" reduces the number of osmoles in the lumen and hence lessens the water lost in feces. During the fermentation of carbohydrates to organic acids, colonic bacteria liberate H_2 and CO_2 gas. In general, the passage of large quantities of rectal gas suggests that excessive carbohydrates are reaching the colon. (Remember your beer-drinking days!)

Primary (congenital) deficiencies of disaccharidases are unusual. Such entities can be differentiated from a secondary defect, since general tests of absorption and mucosal histology are normal; however, assay of an intestinal biopsy reveals the absence of hydrolytic activity for a single disaccharide. Lactase deficiency (even when secondary) is very common.

FIGURE 12.   Intermediate and end products of anaerobic bacterial fermentation of carbohydrates. Minor pathways are depicted by dashed lines.

SOURCE: Soergel KH. The role of the colon in case of inhibition of carbohydrate absorption. In: Creutzfeldt W, Fölsch UR (eds.), Delaying absorption as a therapeutic principle in metabolic diseases. Stuttgart and New York: Thieme Verlag, 1983:854.

8. ABSORPTION OF PROTEIN

8.1 Intraluminal Digestion

Digestion of protein begins in the stomach under the influence of pepsin. This lasts for only one to two hours, while the pH is acidic following meal-stimulated acid secretion. Most dietary protein, however, is hydrolyzed by pancreatic proteases secreted into the proximal duodenum in inactive form. Activation of each protease is initially catalyzed by the duodenal mucosal surface enzyme enterokinase and by activated trypsin (Figure 13). Activation is virtually instantaneous in the first and second portions of the duodenal lumen. Intraluminal digestion of dietary protein occurs in the duodenum by sequential action of pancreatic endopeptidases and exopeptidases. The endopeptidases trypsin, chymotrypsin, elastase, DNAase and RNAase act on the peptide at the interior of the protein molecule. These peptides are then acted upon by the exopeptidases carboxypeptidase A and B, which remove a single amino

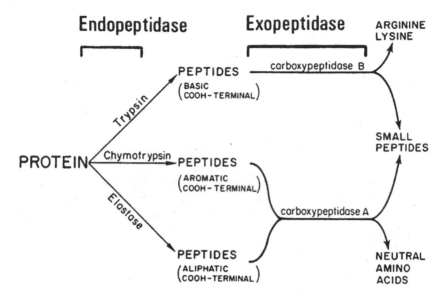

FIGURE 13. Sequence of events leading to hydrolysis of dietary protein by intraluminal proteases.

SOURCE: Gray GM. Mechanisms of digestion and absorption of food. In Sleisenger MH, Fordtran JS (eds.), Gastrointestinal disease: pathophysiology, diagnosis, management. 3d ed. Philadelphia: WB Saunders, 1983:854.

acid from the carboxyl terminal end of the peptide, yielding basic and neutral amino acids (AAs) as well as small peptides.

8.2 Cellular Digestion

Peptidases in the brush border then hydrolyze the residual di-, tri- and tetra-peptides that contain neutral AAs. Peptides consisting primarily of glycine, proline, hydroxyproline or dicarboxylic AA appear to be hydrolyzed inside the cell. AA and dipeptides are then transported into the mucosal cell interior. The transport system for neutral AA absorbs aromatic (phenylalanine, tyrosine, tryptophan) and aliphatic (valine, leucine, isoleucine, methionine) AAs. The basic AAs (arginine, lysine) are absorbed by a separate mechanism. There is a third mechanism for glycine, proline and hydroxyproline, and a fourth for dicarboxylic AAs (aspartic and glutamic AA).

From these physiological considerations, protein malabsorption would be expected in diseases causing (1) pancreatic insufficiency; (2) generalized impaired enterocyte function – e.g., celiac disease; and (3) loss of mucosal surface – e.g., the short bowel syndrome.

9. MALDIGESTION AND MALABSORPTION: THE MALASSIMILATION SYNDROMES

Normal digestion and absorption of foods is essential for life and well-being. Given the length of the gastrointestinal tract, the number of organs involved in digestion, and the large number of nutrients that must be taken into our bodies, it is not surprising to find a large number of disease states that impair the processes of food digestion and absorption. Clinical malassimilation occurs in only one of two ways: (1) through intraluminal disorders (maldigestion of food) and (2) through intramural disorders (malabsorption of food).

9.1 Clinical Manifestations

The list of diseases that can cause malassimilation is long (Table 3), necessitating logical history-taking.

Clinical suspicion, as always, comes from the patient's history and physical examination. A patient with malassimilation may have symptoms and signs of specific nutrient deficiencies or those of the underlying disease process itself (e.g., Crohn's disease). Furthermore, considering that malassimilation usually involves multiple nutrients, the symptoms and signs of a malassimilation state can vary from a straightforward presentation to myriad symptom complexes (Tables 4 and 5).

The patient who gives a history of progressive weight loss, polyphagia, excessive flatus, diarrhea, bulky and foul-smelling stools, food particles or fat in the stool, abdominal distention, muscle wasting, bone pain, bleeding, weakness, tetany, paresthesia, glossitis, cheilosis or dermatitis is giving you the "classical" history of severe intestinal malassimilation. Rarely will you hear such a history from a patient in North America. It is far more common to see patients who will have vague symptoms for which there is some abnormality in their blood chemistry that alerts you to the presence of disease.

Early symptoms of the disease may easily be overlooked, and a severely malnourished state may come to exist. Often a patient will have noticed "early" symptoms, which will become apparent only when questioned directly. Hence, the physician must inquire about minor changes in bowel habits occurring before the onset of weight loss, hyperphagia, pain, anorexia or gross changes in bowel habits. Subtle changes in stool volume or bulk (manifested by a slight increase in the number of bowel movements per day), consistency or odor are early manifestations of malassimilation. A slight increase in the frequency of stools occurring at a time when the patient is mildly anorexic

TABLE 3. Classification of malassimilation syndromes

Defective intraluminal digestion	*Defective intramural absorption*
Mixing disorders	Inadequate absorptive surface
Postgastrectomy	Intestinal resection or bypass
	Mesenteric vascular disease with massive intestinal resection
Pancreatic insufficiency	Regional enteritis with multiple bowel resections
Primary	Jejunoileal bypass
Cystic fibrosis	Mucosal absorptive defects
Secondary	Biochemical or genetic abnormalities
Chronic pancreatitis	Celiac disease
Pancreatic carcinoma	Disaccharidase deficiency
Pancreatic resection	Hypogammaglobulinemia
	Abetalipoproteinemia
Reduced intestinal bile salt concentration	Hartnup disease
Liver disease	Cystinuria
Hepatocellular disease	Monosaccharide malabsorption
Cholestasis (intrahepatic or extrahepatic)	Inflammatory or infiltrative disorders
Abnormal bacterial proliferation in the	Regional enteritis
small bowel	Amyloidosis
Afferent loop stasis	Scleroderma
Strictures	Lymphoma
Fistulas	Radiation enteritis
Blind loops	Eosinophilic enteritis
Multiple diverticula of the small bowel	Tropical sprue
Hypomotility states (diabetes, scleroderma, intestinal pseudo-obstruction)	Infectious enteritis (e.g., salmonellosis)
Interrupted enterohepatic circulation of	Collagenous sprue
bile salts	Nonspecific ulcerative jejunitis
Ileal resection	Mastocytosis
Ileal inflammatory disease (regional ileitis)	Dermatologic disorders (e.g., dermatitis herpetiformis)
Drugs (by sequestration or precipitation of	Lymphatic obstruction
bile salts)	Intestinal lymphangiectasia
Neomycin	Whipple's disease
Calcium carbonate	Lymphoma
Cholestyramine	

occurs a long time before disease becomes clinically apparent. An early increase in bulk of the stool is caused by increased water and gas content and leads to an inability to flush the stool easily. It is not uncommon for the patient to think the toilet is malfunctioning because several flushings are needed to remove the stool. A greasy character and truly rancid odor are indicative of increased stool fat, but are often absent until late. These complaints are often readily passed over by the busy physician. At such time, physical findings are

TABLE 4. Clinical signs and symptoms of malassimilation

	Clinical sign or symptom	*Deficient nutrient*
General	Weight loss	Calorie
	Loss of appetite, amenorrhea, decreased libido	Protein energy
Skin	Psoriasiform rash, eczematous scaling	Zinc
	Pallor	Folate, iron, vitamin B$_{12}$
	Follicular hyperkeratosis	Vitamin A
	Perifollicular petechiae	Vitamin C
	Flaking dermatitis	Protein energy, niacin, riboflavin, zinc
	Bruising	Vitamin K
	Pigmentation changes	Niacin, protein energy
	Scrotal dermatosis	Riboflavin
	Thickening and dryness of skin	Linoleic acid
Head	Temporal muscle wasting	Protein energy
Hair	Sparse and thin, dyspigmentation Easy to pull out	Protein
Eyes	History of night blindness	Vitamin A
	Photophobia, blurring, conjunctival inflammation	Riboflavin, vitamin A
	Corneal vascularization	Riboflavin
	Xerosis, Bitot's spots, keratomalacia	Vitamin A
Mouth	Glossitis	Riboflavin, niacin, folic acid
	Bleeding gums	Vitamin C, riboflavin
	Cheilosis	Riboflavin
	Angular stomatitis	Riboflavin, iron
	Hypogeusia	Zinc
	Tongue fissuring	Niacin
	Tongue atrophy	Riboflavin, niacin, iron
	Scarlet and raw tongue	Niacin
	Nasolabial seborrhea	Pyridoxine
Neck	Goiter	Iodine
	Parotid enlargement	Protein
Thorax	Thoracic "rosary"	Vitamin D

(cont'd)

TABLE 4. Clinical signs and symptoms of malassimilation (cont'd)

	Clinical sign or symptom	Deficient nutrient
Abdomen	Diarrhea	Niacin, folate, vitamin B_{12}
	Distention	Protein energy
	Hepatomegaly	Protein energy
Extremities	Edema	Protein, thiamine
	Softening of bone	Vitamin D, calcium, phosphorus
	Bone tenderness	Vitamin D
	Bone ache, joint pain	Vitamin C
	Muscle wasting and weakness	Protein, calories
	Muscle tenderness, muscle pain	Thiamine
	Hyporeflexia	Thiamine
Nails	Flattening, brittleness, luster loss, spooning	Iron
	Transverse lines	Protein
Neurologic	Tetany	Calcium, magnesium
	Paresthesias	Thiamine, vitamin B_{12}
	Loss of reflexes, wrist drop, foot drop	Thiamine
	Loss of vibratory and position sense, ataxia	Vitamin B_{12}
	Dementia, disorientation	Niacin
Blood	Anemia	Iron, vitamin B_{12}, folate
	Hemolysis	Phosphorus

usually absent, but hyperactive bowel sounds may be noted, especially in small intestinal disease. If symptoms are intermittent or if they progress slowly over many years, patients may exhibit vague, seemingly unrelated symptoms such as chronic fatigue and depression, long before the physician considers the possibility of serious organic disease.

9.2 Manifestations of Carbohydrate Malassimilation
Carbohydrate malassimilation will result in both specific and generalized symptoms. Specific to the maldigestion and malabsorption of carbohydrates are diarrhea and excess flatus. Unfortunately, everyone has flatus, and a definition or measure of excessive "wind" is lacking. Malabsorbed carbohydrates that enter the colon are fermented by colonic bacteria to gases (CO_2, H_2 and CH_4) and organic acids (Figure 12). These organic acids produce diarrhea by acting directly on colonic epithelium to stimulate fluid secretion and by their

TABLE 5. Specific vitamin and mineral deficiencies

Vitamin/mineral		Clinical manifestation
Vitamin A	Eyes	Night blindness
		Xerosis (dry bulbar conjunctiva)
		Bitot's spots (conjunctiva plaques)
		Keratomalacia (corneal ulceration)
	Skin	Hyperkeratosis
Vitamin B$_{12}$	Hematologic,	Anemia
	neurologic systems	Nonreversible loss of vibratory and position sense
		Paresthesia
	Gastrointestinal	Diarrhea
Vitamin C	Skin	Perifollicular papules (brittle hair)
		Perifollicular hemorrhages
		Gum bleeding
		Skin purpura, ecchymosis
Vitamin D	Bone	Bone pain and softening
		Joint pain
		Rickets
		Proximal myopathy
Vitamin K		Bruising
		Bleeding
Vitamin B$_6$	Skin	Seborrheic dermatitis
(Pyridoxine)		Cheilosis
		Glossitis
Niacin		Dermatitis
		Diarrhea
		Dementia
Thiamine	CVS	Congestive heart failure
	CNS	Wernicke's encephalopathy
		Wernicke-Korsakoff syndrome
Zinc	Skin	Acrodermatitis enteropathica
		Alopecia
	Taste	Hypogeusia
Folate	Hematologic,	Anemia
	neurologic systems	Reversible loss of position and vibratory sense

CVS = cardiovascular system; CNS = central nervous system

osmotic effect, which further draws water into the lumen. The presence of organic acids in the stool reduces the pH below 6 and suggests carbohydrate malassimilation. The gas produces flatulence, with associated borborygmi and abdominal distention. The presence of intraluminal H_2 gas, eventually absorbed into the circulation and exhaled, forms the basis of the hydrogen breath test to detect carbohydrate malabsorption. Physical examination often reveals a distended tympanitic abdomen with hyperactive bowel sounds. Stools seem to float on the water because of their increased gas content (not because of their fat content).

Generally, lack of carbohydrate as an energy source will result in decreased plasma insulin levels, increased plasma glucagon and cortisol levels and decreased peripheral T_4-to-T_3 conversion. Given sufficient time, the body will enter a state of oxidative metabolism: fat and muscle will be catabolized. Physical examination may reveal signs of weight loss from both fat stores and lean body mass. The patient will be weak and will easily develop fatigue. Fat loss will generally be noted as sunken cheeks and flat buttocks, with wrinkled or loose skin indicative of loss of subcutaneous fat stores. The loss of muscle mass is easily noted as thenar mass reduction and sunken soft tissues between the extensor tendons on the dorsum of the hands. There may be direct evidence of a reduced metabolic rate secondary to decreased T_3 conversion. The patient will often be mentally slowed.

9.3 Manifestations of Fat Malassimilation

Failure to digest or absorb fats results in a variety of clinical symptoms and laboratory abnormalities. These manifestations are the result of both fat malassimilation per se and a deficiency of the fat-soluble vitamins. In general, loss of fat in the stool deprives the body of calories and contributes to weight loss and malnutrition. More specific is the action of unabsorbed long-chain fatty acids, which act on the colonic mucosa to cause diarrhea by an irritant effect on the colon. In addition, fatty acids bind calcium, which would normally be available to bind oxalate. In fat malabsorption, oxalate is not bound to calcium and remains free (undissociated) within the colonic lumen, where it is readily absorbed. This results in oxaluria and calcium oxalate kidney stones. This occurs in Crohn's disease more readily than in other cases of fat malabsorption (steatorrhea).

Failure to absorb the fat-soluble vitamins A, D, E and K also results in a variety of symptoms. Vitamin K deficiency presents as subcutaneous, urinary, nasal, vaginal and gastrointestinal bleeding. Deficiencies in factors II, VII, IX and X produce defective coagulation. Vitamin A deficiency results in follicular hyperkeratosis. Vitamin E deficiency leads to a progressive demyelination of the central nervous system. Malabsorption of vitamin D causes rickets and osteopenia, as discussed later.

9.4 Manifestations of Protein Malassimilation

Severe loss of body protein may occur before the development of laboratory abnormalities. Impaired protein synthesis from liver diseases and excessive protein loss in renal disease can further aggravate protein deficiencies. Clinically, protein deficiency results in edema and diminished muscle mass. Since the immune system is dependent upon adequate proteins, protein deficiency can manifest as recurrent or severe infections. Protein deficiency in children results in growth retardation, mental apathy and irritability, weakness and muscle atrophy, edema, hair loss, deformity of skeletal bone, anorexia, vomiting and diarrhea. Protein-calorie malnutrition is known as marasmus, whereas protein malnutrition by itself is known as kwashiorkor.

9.5 Manifestations of Iron Deficiency

Hypochromic microcytic anemia characterizes iron deficiency. Since malassimilation may result in folate or B_{12} deficiency (producing megaloblastic red cells), the microcytosis of iron deficiency may be obscured with automated cell counters; a dimorphic picture is present. Rarely accompanying the development of anemia may be symptoms of pica and dysphagia. Pica originally referred to the eating of clay or soil; however, the commonest "pica" in North America is the eating of ice. Dysphagia may be due to the Plummer-Vinson (Paterson-Kelly) syndrome (with atrophic papillae of the tongue and postcricoid esophageal webs), and/or cheilosis (reddened lips with angular fissures, also known as cheilitis or angular stomatitis). Weakness, fatigue, dyspnea and edema also can occur. Physical examination often reveals pallor, an atrophic tongue and koilonychia (brittle, flat or spoon-shaped fingernails).

The clinical picture of vitamin B_{12} and folic acid deficiency includes the nonspecific manifestations of megaloblastic anemia and its sequelae – i.e., anemia, glossitis, megaloblastosis, and elevated serum lactate dehydrogenase (LDH). In addition, deficiency of B_{12} may induce neurologic abnormalities consisting of symmetrical paresthesias in the feet and fingers, with associated disturbances of vibration sense and proprioception, progressing to ataxia with subacute combined degeneration of the spinal cord. This subacute combined spinal cord degeneration includes cortisospinal as well as dorsal column damage. Neurologic manifestations are not part of folic acid deficiency alone.

9.6 Manifestations of Calcium, Vitamin D and Magnesium Malabsorption

Impaired absorption of calcium, magnesium and vitamin D may lead to bone pain, fractures, paresthesias, tetany, Chvostek's sign and Trousseau's sign. Osteomalacia resulting from vitamin D deficiency principally affects the spine, rib cage and long bones with or without fractures (Milkman's fractures), and may cause extreme pain, particularly in the spine, pelvis and leg bones. A child with calcium or vitamin D malabsorption will present with classical rickets. Hypomagnesemia may cause seizures and symptoms identical to those of hypocalcemia. In addition, hypomagnesemia may reduce the responsiveness of the parathyroids to calcium and impair parathyroid regulation of calcium homeostasis.

9.7 Investigation of Maldigestion and Malabsorption

To avoid embarking on the shotgun approach to investigation, there are several questions one must ask. First, does malassimilation exist? And second, if so, is it due to a disorder of intraluminal digestion or a disorder of intramural absorption? Physicians should attempt to restrict the use of laboratory tests to those that establish the presence of malassimilation and the cause of the malassimilation (Figure 14).

To determine if malassimilation exists, one begins, as always, with the simplest, least invasive tests. A complete blood count (CBC) and differential might reveal a macrocytic or microcytic anemia. A peripheral smear may demonstrate megaloblastosis, microcytosis and/or lymphopenia. Serum calcium, phosphorus and alkaline phosphatase will detect the presence of osteomalacia. Serum albumin can assess protein stores. Serum cholesterol, carotene and prothrombin time (vitamin K) indirectly assess fat assimilation. Iron stores from serum iron, total iron binding capacity (TIBC) and ferritin assess proximal intestinal integrity. Serum B_{12} is an index of ileal integrity. Red cell folate measures folate stores.

If their results are abnormal, the above tests suggest the presence of malassimilation and may indicate the deficient nutrient(s). Steatorrhea is the most important feature in the diagnosis of generalized malassimilation. Accurate measurement of fecal fat is important. Qualitative Sudan stain for fat globules on suspension of stool will give an indication of possible steatorrhea. However, this test cannot substitute for a quantitative fecal fat determination for a definitive diagnosis.

Quantitative fecal fat determination is the most reliable measure of steatorrhea. In the normal individual, the amount of fat appearing in the stool is relatively constant despite small changes in the quantity of dietary fat. Even when the daily fat intake is zero, the fecal fat output equals about 2.9 g/day. Presumably this is the amount of fat that is derived from endogenous sources, such as sloughed mucosal cells, excreted bile lipids (cholesterol and bile acids) and bacterial lipids. As the dietary intake of fat is increased, the fecal fat will

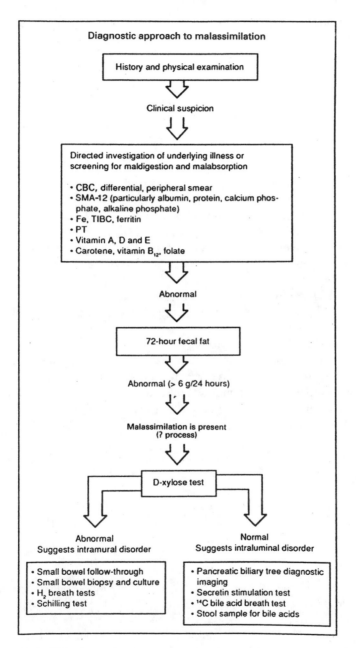

FIGURE 14.   Diagnostic approach to malassimilation.

SOURCE: Fedorak RN. Maldigestion and malabsorption. Medicine North America 1988; 3:3400.

increase to about 5 g/day on a 100 g fat diet. Fecal fat (FF) bears some relation to dietary fat: normally, the fecal fat loss is usually less than 5% of dietary intake. A defect at one of the four steps in the overall process of fat assimilation dramatically increases this fat loss. In disease the absolute value of the quantitative fecal fat output may depend on the dietary load, which must be carefully assessed prior to adequate evaluation of the test. Thus a number of conditions should be met in order to obtain a reliable quantitative stool fat output. The patient should be on a steady dietary intake of a known 60–100 g fat, there must be a regular pattern of stooling, and all stool must be collected for 72 hours.

There are numerous possible artifacts for this test. Poor food intake, interrupted food intake, constipation or incomplete stool collection all give rise to a spuriously low value for the 24-hour fecal fat output. An artifactually high value will be seen when castor oil or nut oils have been consumed, but not petroleum mineral oils. The Van de Kamer method is the most commonly used procedure to chemically determine fecal fat output. This method, however, may lead to incomplete extraction and quantitation of medium-chain triglycerides (MCT) and thus may underestimate (by 10%) the quantity of fecal fats in patients whose diet has been supplemented with MCT. Steatorrhea does not indicate into which category of malassimilation the patient falls. An elevated fecal fat may be due to intraluminal maldigestion or intramural malabsorption. Therefore, further investigations are required to fully characterize the problem (Figure 15).

9.8 Intraluminal Maldigestion

Intraluminal maldigestion will occur with (1) inadequate mixing; (2) pancreatic insufficiency; and (3) reduced bile salt concentration. If the D-xylose absorption test and small bowel x-rays are normal, then it is likely but not absolutely certain that malassimilation is due to an intraluminal disorder. Pancreatic function is assessed by the secretin stimulation test used to measure secretory capacity of the exocrine pancreas. A tube placed in the duodenum adjacent to the ampullae of Vater collects pancreatic juice to measure volume, bicarbonate and enzyme (amylase) output. Maximal secretion should reach 2 mL/min at 90 minutes after injection of 2 units of secretin/kg of body weight, and bicarbonate concentration is normally 90 mEq/L. Both enzyme and bicarbonate secretion are diminished in chronic pancreatitis. Partial duct obstruction resulting from pancreatic cancer often reduces the volume of secretion without reducing bicarbonate concentration. The test is cumbersome and not very sensitive.

Assessment of biliary disease includes liver biochemistry, abdominal ultrasound and, where indicated, transhepatic or endoscopic cholangiography to

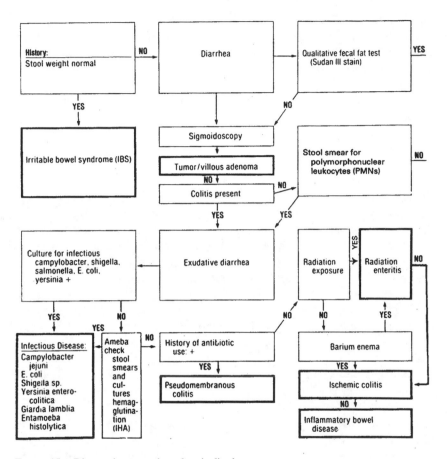

FIGURE 15.   Diagnostic approach to chronic diarrhea.
SOURCE: Knapp AB, Farkas PS. Diagnostic diagrams: gastroenterology. Baltimore: Williams and Wilkins, 1985:54–55.

ensure patency of the ductal system. In the bacterial overgrowth syndrome, bile acids are deconjugated and rapidly absorbed in the small intestine, and are not available or active for micellar solubilization. With bacterial overgrowth, the Schilling test for vitamin B_{12} is abnormal, even with the addition of intrinsic factor. Bile salt concentration may be diminished as a result of failure of reabsorption in a diseased ileum, adding to the malabsorption from gut loss. A ^{14}C-labeled bile acid breath test detects bile acid deconjugation in the bacterial overgrowth syndrome; an isotope scan with a radiolabeled bile acid analogue measures bile acid absorption.

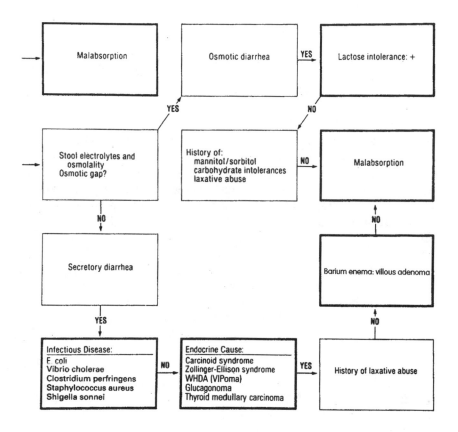

The bile acid breath test is used if one suspects bile acid malabsorption due to ileal dysfunction (decreased absorption) or bacterial overgrowth (deconjugation and thus diminished absorption). The basis of the test is that the amino acid (glycine) part of the bile salt is labeled with ^{14}C-glycine. Bacteria deconjugate the glycine and metabolize this amide to $^{14}CO_2$, which is then exhaled. With ileal dysfunction, an excess of bile salts reaches the colon, where colonic bacteria split off the glycine, producing $^{14}CO_2$. With bacterial overgrowth, the excess coliform bacteria in the jejunum metabolize these bile salts to $^{14}CO_2$. The bile acid breath test is beginning to be replaced by the hydrogen breath test, which assesses the presence of an abnormal increase in the concentration of breath H_2 after the subject has ingested a nonabsorbable sugar such as lactulose. This is an inexpensive and sensitive test for bacterial overgrowth. The type of sugar used in the breath test may be changed to test for malabsorption of various carbohydrates. The H_2 breath test is not used to test for bile salt malabsorption.

Disordered mixing of ingested food with endogenous enzymes results from the rapid transit in postgastrectomy syndromes. Small bowel x-rays with transit times sometimes help in the diagnosis.

9.9 Intramural Malabsorption

Malabsorption from an intramural defect occurs as a result of (1) inadequate absorptive surface – e.g., the short gut syndrome; (2) mucosal absorptive defects – e.g., celiac disease; or (3) lymphatic obstruction. Since the pentose sugar D-xylose does not require intraluminal digestion, D-xylose absorption tests serve to separate patients with intramural malabsorption from those with intraluminal maldigestion. An abnormal result points toward intramural malabsorption, while a normal result points toward intraluminal maldigestion. Remember that patients with renal impairment (who cannot excrete the sugar), delayed gastric emptying, bacterial overgrowth (who metabolize the sugar in the lumen) and advanced age may have spuriously low measurements of D-xylose absorption. Aspirin (ASA) or nonsteroidal anti-inflammatory drugs (NSAIDs) inhibit the renal excretion of xylose and may lead to a false-negative test. The presence of ascites may also lead to a false-negative test by increasing the volume of distribution of the sugar and thereby decreasing its renal clearance. Measurement of the serum level of xylose may be a better test of xylose absorption because it avoids these issues of renal function. Indeed, clinicians may elect to omit a xylose test and advance to specific intramural or intraluminal investigations (Figure 14).

Following an abnormal D-xylose test, the next evaluation should be barium contrast x-rays of the small intestine. They may demonstrate structurally abnormal bowel patterns, dilation of bowel lumen, segmentation of barium or a dilution of barium because of increased intraluminal fluid. Although segmentation and flocculation of barium have been used as indications of malassimilation in the past, the use of nondispersible barium sulfate in recent years rarely allows us to observe such signs. Additionally, x-ray films may demonstrate diverticula as sites of bacterial overgrowth or thickening of folds resulting from infiltration or edema.

Following the x-ray, endoscopic or suction biopsy of the small intestine will identify evidence of specific mucosal disease. If there is a high clinical suspicion of a small bowel disorder such as celiac disease, the patient may be referred at a much earlier stage for a small bowel biopsy to be performed. Once the position and/or etiology of the intramural disease is known, further tests can be carried out to determine the extent of functional derangement.

TABLE 6. Therapy for malassimilation syndromes

Site of defect	Therapy
Pancreas	Enzyme supplements; insulin; dietary counseling; surgery for pancreatic duct obstruction or cancer
Hepatobiliary	Surgery for obstruction of biliary tree
Mucosa	Diet, such as gluten withdrawal or milk-free diet; nutrient supplements; steroids for Crohn's disease; antibiotics for bacterial overgrowth or Whipple's disease
Lymphatics	Low-fat diet; medium-chain triglycerides (MCTs)

Tests can help define unabsorbed carbohydrate as a result of disaccharidase deficiency, generalized mucosal damage, inadequate surface area or bacterial overgrowth. Unabsorbed carbohydrate produces stool with an acid pH, easily tested on pH paper strip. The hydrogen breath test will detect an increase in exhaled hydrogen, which might result when an ingested carbohydrate is not absorbed. This test is used to diagnose suspected disaccharidase deficiencies or bacterial overgrowth. The basis of the test is that bacteria ferment sugars to fatty acids and H_2, which is exhaled. Normally, sugars are absorbed as monosaccharides in the small intestine and no H_2 is exhaled. In lactase deficiency, exhaled H_2 is elevated after ingestion of the test sugar lactose, since the unabsorbed sugar reaches colonic bacteria and is catabolized. In bacterial overgrowth, bacteria in the jejunum ferment the sugar before it can be absorbed and H_2 is exhaled. The hydrogen breath test is reliable, noninvasive and helpful in establishing the diagnosis of carbohydrate malabsorption and/or the bacterial overgrowth syndrome.

Vitamin B_{12} absorption is tested by the Schilling test. Radiolabeled vitamin B_{12} with intrinsic factor (labeled with ^{58}Co) and without intrinsic factor (labeled with ^{57}Co) are simultaneously administered orally. The excretion of both compounds is then measured in the urine over a 24-hour period. Excretion of both radiolabeled compounds is normal. Failure to excrete ^{57}Co-labeled vitamin B_{12} indicates absent gastric intrinsic factor – e.g., pernicious anemia or gastrectomy, while failure to excrete ^{58}Co- and ^{57}Co-labeled vitamin B_{12} indicates ileal disease or loss, or absent ileal B_{12} receptors.

9.10 Treatment

The specific treatments for malabsorption or maldigestion are given in Table 6. The nutritional therapies necessary for any associated deficiencies are given in Table 7.

TABLE 7.   Representative doses for agents used in replacement therapy in patients with malassimilation syndromes

---

Minerals

Calcium	PO:	requires at least 1,200 mg elemental calcium daily as: (a) Calcium gluconate (93 mg Ca^{2+}/500 mg tablet) (b) Calcium carbonate (200 mg Ca^{2+}/500 mg tablet)
	IV:	Calcium gluconate, 10 mL (9.3 mg Ca^{2+}/mL) of 10% soln over 5 min

Magnesium	PO:	Magnesium gluconate (29 mg Mg^{2+}/500 mg tablet), 2–6 g/day
	IV:	Magnesium sulfate (50% soln, 1 mL contains 2.03 mmol Mg^{2+})

Iron	PO:	Ferrous fumarate (65 mg elemental Fe/200 mg tablet), 200 mg tid Ferrous gluconate (35 mg elemental Fe/300 mg tablet), 600 mg tid Ferrous sulfate (60 mg elemental Fe/300 mg tablet), 300 mg tid
	IM:	Iron dextran 1 mL once daily (calculated from existing Hb)*
	IV:	Iron dextran approx. 30 mL (calculated from existing Hb)* in 500 cc 5% D/W over 4 hrs, beginning with slow observed infusion
		*NOTE: IM/IV Fe for deficit replacement only

Zinc	PO:	Zinc sulfate (89 mg elemental zinc/220 mg capsule), 220 mg tid

Vitamins

Vitamin A	Water-miscible vitamin A (25,000 IU/capsule), 25,000 IU daily
Vitamin B_{12}	100 µg/IM monthly
Vitamin D_2	(Ergocalciferol) (50,000 IU/capsule), 50,000 IU 3 times per week
Vitamin E	Water-miscible vitamin E (100 IU/capsule), 400 IU daily
Vitamin K_1	(Phytonadione) has caused fatal reactions, thus should be avoided

Vitamin K_3		(Menadione) water-soluble
	PO:	5–10 mg/day
	IV:	5–10 mg/day

Folic acid	PO:	1 mg/day

Other water-soluble	Multiple vitamin 1/day

(cont'd)

TABLE 7.   Representative doses for agents used in replacement therapy in patients with malassimilation syndromes (cont'd)

Pancreatic supplements

Preparation	Type	Enzyme activity (IU/unit)			
		Lipase	*Trypsin*	*Proteolytic*	*Amylase*
Ku-Zyme HP®	Capsule	2,330	3,082	6,090	594,048
Festal®	Enteric-coated	2,073	488	1,800	219,200
Cotazym®	Capsule	2,014	2,797	5,840	499,200
Viokase®	Tablet	1,636	1,828	440	277,333
Pancrease®	Micro-encapsulated	>4,000	>25,000		

4–18 g/day at meals, with antacid or cimetidine (to prevent HCl inactivation of the supplement)

Bile salt binding agents
Cholestyramine 4 g (1 scoop), 3–6 times daily, according to response
Psyllium and aluminum hydroxide gel may also be effective
Colestipol 1 g 3–6 times daily, according to response

(cont'd)

10. ACUTE DIARRHEA

With a complaint of "diarrhea," the physician must establish if this represents a change in the patient's bowel habit and if the complaint arises from a perception of increased frequency of stool, increased volume or both.

If the diarrhea is acute (i.e., lasting less than two weeks), the malabsorption of fluid and electrolytes probably has an infectious or toxic cause (Table 8). When diarrhea lasts for a longer period of time, other explanations need to be considered. In the absence of prior gastric surgery, the four most common causes of chronic diarrhea are (1) the irritable bowel syndrome; (2) inflammatory bowel disease; (3) malabsorption; and (4) carcinoma of the colon. The physician also must consider altered bowel function due to drug or alcohol abuse (see Section 11). Associated tenesmus, urgency or a sense of incomplete evacuation suggests involvement of the rectum or sigmoid colon. The passage of blood, pus and mucus suggests bowel inflammation, ischemic bowel disease or cancer. Malassimilation syndromes (discussed in the previous section) are suspect if there is passage of food and oil droplets, or if the patient develops symptoms suggestive of nutrient deficiency, particularly weight loss.

In Western societies, stool weight is approximately 200 g/day. Since stools are 70–90% water, regardless of their consistency, excess fecal water must

TABLE 7. Representative doses for agents used in replacement therapy in patients with malassimilation syndromes (cont'd)

Caloric supplements

Medium-chain triglyceride oil: (8 cal/mL), 60 mL/day po, 480 cal/day
Portagen®: medium-chain triglyceride + other oils: (1 cal/mL), 1 L/day
Enteral supplements:

Product	Kcal*/ 1,000 mL	Grams of protein/ 1,000 mL	Na mg/L	K mg/L	Osmolality mOsm/kg Water
Ensure®	1,060	37	740	1,270	450
Isocal®	1,040	34	530	1,320	300
Osmolite®	1,060	37	540	1,060	300
Precision Isotonic Diet®	960	29	800	960	300
Precision LR Diet®	1,110	26	700	810	525
Travasorb STD® (unflavored)	1,000	45	920	1,170	450
Standard Vivonex® (unflavored)	1,000	21	470	1,170	550
High-Nitrogen Vivonex® (unflavored)	1,000	44	530	1,170	810
Meritene Powder® in milk	1,065	69	1,000	3,000	690
Compleat B®	1,000	40	1,200	1,300	390
Formula 2®	1,000	38	600	1,760	435–510

*When prepared in standard dilution
Parenteral supplements: Intralipid® 1 L/day IV (10 mL/kg/day)
                         Travasol® 2 L/day IV (mix as per patient's protein requirements)

accompany diarrheal diseases with elevated stool weight. This concept leads directly to consideration of the mechanisms responsible for the malabsorption or stimulated secretion of water.

Two caveats need to be remembered. First, fecal bulk varies with the diet, being influenced most notably by the content of indigestible carbohydrates (dietary fiber). Stools are smaller in developed countries than they are among societies whose members regularly ingest large amounts of dietary fiber. Second, disease of the distal colon or rectum can lead to the frequent, often painful passage of small stools (due to limited capacity as a reservoir), yet there may be little fecal water and no increase in stool weight. In fact, "constipation" may be common in patients with proctitis.

TABLE 8. Common causes of acute diarrhea

Drugs	*Bacteria (toxin-mediated, cytotoxic)*
Laxatives	Clostridium difficile
Antacids	Staphylococcus aureus
Antibiotics	Shigella dysenteriae
Cholinergic drugs	Campylobacter jejuni
Lactose	Yersinia enterocolitica
Guanethidine	
Quinidine	*Bacteria (invasive)*
Digitalis	Salmonella
Colchicine	Enteroinvasive Escherichia coli
Potassium supplements	
Lactulose	*Bacteria (unknown mechanism)*
	Enteropathogenic Escherichia coli
	Enteroadherent Escherichia coli
	Viruses
Bacteria (toxin-mediated, cytotonic)	Parvovirus (Norwalk agent)
Enterotoxigenic Escherichia coli	Reovirus (rotavirus)
(both heat-labile and heat-	
stable toxins)	*Protozoa*
Vibrio cholerae	Cryptosporidia
Vibrio parahaemolyticus	Giardia lamblia
Clostridium perfringens	Entamoeba histolytica
Bacillus cereus	
	Parasites
	Strongyloides
	Trichuris

Acute diarrhea is thus defined as stool weight > 200 g/day for less than 14 days' duration. It always will represent a change in bowel habit for the individual and will often be associated with an increased frequency of bowel movements.

10.1 **Bacterial Diarrhea**

Most enteric infections are self-limiting and resolve in less than two weeks. Acute bacterial diarrheas can be classified into *toxigenic types*, in which an enterotoxin is the major pathogenic mechanism, and *invasive types*, in which the organism penetrates the enterocyte as a primary event, although an enterotoxin may be produced as well. Enterotoxins are either *cytotonic* (producing intestinal fluid secretion by activation of intracellular enzymes, without damage to the epithelial surface) or *cytotoxic* (causing injury to the enterocyte as well as inducing fluid secretion). Three major clinical syndromes caused by bacterial infections are (1) food poisoning, (2) infectious gastroenteritis and (3) traveler's diarrhea.

10.1.1 *FOOD POISONING*

The food poisoning syndrome characteristically features the development of a brief but explosive diarrheal illness in subjects following exposure to a common food source contaminated with bacteria or bacterial toxins. Staphylococcus aureus, Salmonella, Clostridium perfringens and Bacillus cereus are responsible for 90% of these outbreaks.

Staphylococcus aureus produces a heat-stable, odorless and tasteless enterotoxin that is generated in poorly refrigerated desserts and seafoods. Ingestion of the preformed enterotoxin causes nausea, vomiting and profuse diarrhea within 4 to 8 hours. Spontaneous resolution occurs within 24 hours. No specific therapy is available or necessary.

Clostridium perfringens produces a preformed toxin from spores that germinate in contaminated meats cooked to less than 50°C. Symptoms are diarrhea and crampy abdominal pain without vomiting, beginning 8 to 24 hours after the meal. The illness lasts less than 24 hours. No specific therapy is indicated.

Bacillus cereus produces either a diarrheal syndrome or a vomiting syndrome, depending upon the enterotoxin. The vomiting syndrome is always associated with ingestion of rice and is caused by a preformed toxin that is elaborated when rice is left to cool unrefrigerated. Flash-frying later does not generate enough heat to destroy the toxin. The diarrheal syndrome occurs after ingestion of the organism itself. Both illnesses are short-lived and require no specific therapy.

The diagnosis of food poisoning is usually made by history. Except in special circumstances (e.g., botulism), isolation of the toxin is not cost-effective.

10.1.2 *GASTROENTERITIS*

The organisms responsible for bacterial gastroenteritis exert their predominant effects by invading and destroying the intestinal epithelium or by producing various enterotoxins.

10.1.2.1 *Toxin-mediated, cytotoxic bacterial gastroenteritis*

Vibrio cholerae is the prototypic cause of toxigenic diarrhea. The Vibrio cholerae organisms elaborate a toxin that attaches to the inner cell membrane and activates adenylate cyclase (formerly "adenyl cyclase"). The presence of adenylate cyclase then elevates cyclic AMP (cAMP) levels. Cyclic AMP then stimulates the enterocyte to secrete fluid and electrolytes while at the same time impairing their absorption. Stool output can exceed 1 L/hour. Treatment

TABLE 9.   Types of Escherichia coli intestinal pathogens

Name	Toxin	Mechanism
Enteropathogenic (EPEC)	Shiga-like toxin	Adherence
Enterotoxigenic (ETEC)	Labile toxin (LT)	Activates adenylate cyclase
	Stable toxin (ST)	Activates guanylate cyclase
Enteroinvasive (EIEC)	Shiga-like toxin	Penetrates epithelium
Enteroadherent (EAEC)	—	Adherence
Enterohemorrhagic (EHEC)	Shiga-like toxin (verotoxin)	Unknown

is based on restoring fluid and electrolyte balance and maintaining intravascular volume. Even though fluid and electrolyte transport is impaired, glucose transport is intact. Since glucose absorption carries Na^+ (and thus water with it), an oral rehydration solution containing glucose, sodium and water will enhance water absorption during the profound dehydration stage of cholera.

Several types of Escherichia coli (E. coli) are intestinal pathogens. Each exerts its effects through different mechanisms (Table 9). Invasive forms of E. coli may cause colitis that resembles colitis from other bacterial infections and also may resemble ischemia clinically, endoscopically and histologically.

Enterotoxigenic E. coli (ETEC) colonizes the upper small intestine after passing through the acid barrier of the stomach. The organisms colonize the surface without penetrating the mucus layer. Like cholera, ETEC causes no mucosal damage and no bacteremia. Two types of enterotoxins are produced by ETEC: the heat-labile toxin (also called "labile toxin" or LT) and the heat-stable toxin (also called "stable toxin" or ST). ETEC can elaborate LT only, ST only, or both toxins. ST produces diarrhea by stimulating intestinal secretion through guanylate cyclase and subsequently cyclic GMP. LT produces diarrhea by a similar mechanism, except that it acts through adenylate cyclase and cyclic AMP. After a 24- to 48-hour incubation period, the disease begins with upper abdominal distress followed by watery diarrhea. The infection can be mild (with only a few loose movements) or severe (mimicking cholera). Treatment is symptomatic. Antibiotic therapy is ineffective and favors the emergence of resistant ETEC strains.

Vibrio parahaemolyticus causes acute diarrheal disease after consumption of seafood: raw fish or shellfish. The common factor in most outbreaks appears to be storage of the food for several hours without proper refrigeration. Explosive, watery diarrhea is the cardinal manifestation, along with abdominal cramps, nausea and vomiting. Fever and chills occur in 25% of cases. The duration of illness is short, with a median of three days. Treatment is symptomatic; there is no role for antimicrobial therapy.

After ingestion, Shigella dysenteriae organisms attack the colon, sparing the stomach and small bowel. Shigella organisms adhere to the mucosal surface, penetrate the mucosal surface, and then multiply within epithelial cells, moving laterally through the cytoplasm to adjacent cells by filopodium-like protrusions. Shigella organisms rarely penetrate below the intestinal mucosa and almost never invade the bloodstream. Both attached and intracellular organisms elaborate toxic products.

Even a small inoculum of 200 organisms (as contrasted with Salmonella, which requires greater than 10^7 organisms) will lead to crampy abdominal pain, rectal burning and fever associated with multiple small-volume bloody mucoid bowel movements. Intestinal complications include perforation and severe protein loss. Extraintestinal complications include respiratory symptoms, meningismus, seizures, the hemolytic uremic syndrome, arthritis and rashes. Ampicillin 500 mg q.i.d. or co-trimoxazole 2 tablets b.i.d. for 5 days is the treatment of choice. Amoxicillin, interestingly, is not effective therapy for shigellosis.

Salmonella food poisoning has been attributed to an enterotoxin similar to that of Staphylococcus aureus, but none has been clearly identified. Within 12 to 36 hours after ingestion of contaminated foods (usually poultry products), there is a sudden onset of headaches, chills and abdominal pain, with nausea, vomiting and diarrhea. These symptoms may persist for one to four days before subsiding. Antibiotic therapy of nontyphoidal Salmonella gastroenteritis fails to alter the rate of clinical recovery. In fact, antibiotic therapy will increase the duration of intestinal carriage of the Salmonella and is thus contraindicated.

Campylobacter jejuni–induced diarrhea is more common than diarrhea from either Salmonella or Shigella. Infection is from consumption of improperly cooked or contaminated foodstuffs. Campylobacter attaches to the mucosa and releases an enterotoxin that destroys the surrounding epithelia. Clinically, there is often a prodrome of constitutional symptoms along with headache and generalized malaise. A prolonged diarrheal illness follows – often with a biphasic character, with initial bloody diarrhea, slight improvement, then increasing severity. The illness usually lasts less than one week, although symptoms can persist for a longer period, and relapses occur in as many as 25% of patients. Erythromycin 500 mg q.i.d. for 7 days is optimal therapy.

Yersinia enterocolitica is often transmitted to humans from pets or food sources. The organism invades epithelial cells and produces an enterotoxin. Clinically, the spectrum of illness ranges from simple gastroenteritis to invasive ileitis and colitis. This organism causes diarrheal illness most frequently in children less than 5 years of age. Children over 5 years of age develop mesenteric adenitis and associated ileitis, which mimic acute appendicitis. Yersinia is less likely to cause disease in adults; if it does, the illness is an acute diarrheal episode that may be followed two to three weeks later by joint symptoms and a rash (erythema nodosum). Treatment is symptomatic. There is no evidence that antibiotics alter the course of the gastrointestinal infection.

Clostridium difficile causes antibiotic-associated colitis (Section 10.4).

10.1.2.2 *Invasive bacterial gastroenteritis*

Certain strains of E. coli are invasive, producing an illness indistinguishable from shigellosis. Isolates of E. coli 0157:H7 have been identified in the stools of patients with a diarrheal illness clinically designated as "hemorrhagic colitis." Infection has been traced to contaminated hamburger meat obtained from a variety of sources, including large national restaurant chains.

Ingestion of this organism results in severe crampy abdominal pain and fever, followed within 24 hours by bloody diarrhea that lasts five to seven days. Since the organism is shed in the stool for only a short period of time, early stool collections are critical for the diagnosis. Treatment is symptomatic, as antibiotics do not appear to alter the disease course. In severe cases with possible toxic megacolon, systemic antibiotics may be in order.

Approximately 1,700 serotypes and variants of Salmonella are potential pathogens for humans. A dose of approximately 10^7–10^9 organisms is required to produce a clinical illness. Salmonella organisms invade the mucosa of the small intestine and (particularly) the colon. This form of gastroenteritis produces nausea and vomiting followed by abdominal cramps and diarrhea that lasts three to four days and then gradually subsides. In 10% of the cases bacteremia of the Salmonella organism occurs, and in approximately 5% there are disseminated infections to bones, joints and meninges. Certain conditions increase the risk of salmonellosis: hemolytic anemia, malignancy, immunosuppression, achlorhydria and ulcerative colitis. With uncomplicated Salmonella gastroenteritis, treatment is symptomatic. In fact, antibiotic therapy increases the duration of intestinal carriage of these organisms. Patients with complicated Salmonella gastroenteritis (e.g., those with predisposing conditions or sepsis, or who are very young or very old) should be treated with ampicillin or co-trimoxazole.

10.1.2.3 *Bacterial gastroenteritis of unknown mechanism*

Enterohemorrhagic E. coli–induced diarrhea tends to occur in neonates and

TABLE 10.   Traveler's diarrhea: recommendations for treatment

---

General
Avoid ice cubes, raw vegetables and fruits, raw fish and shellfish, unrefrigerated food.
Drink canned pop and beer, boiled water.
Drink oral replacement solutions for acute attacks.
Avoid over-the-counter preparations sold locally for acute attacks.

Specific
To provide symptomatic relief of acute attack:
    Diphenoxylate 1 tab, 2.5 mg, after each bowel movement to max 9 tab/day
    Loperamide 1 cap, 2.0 mg, after each bowel movement to max 8 cap/day
    Pepto-Bismol® 30 mL q 30 min × 8 doses

To decrease severity of acute attack:
    Co-trimoxazole 1 tab bid po × 3 days
    Doxycycline 100 mg bid po × 3 days

Prophylaxis:
Not recommended except for persons who are immunosuppressed or suffer chronic illness. If
indicated, then:
    Co-trimoxazole 1 tab bid po × 3 days
    Doxycycline 100 mg bid po × 3 days
    Ciprofloxacin 500 mg bid po × 7 days

---

young children. Only occasionally does it affect older children and adults. The pathogenic mechanism of this diarrhea is unclear; adherence of the organism to the intestinal epithelial cell seems to cause intestinal damage. There is no indication for specific treatment except for neonates in a nursery epidemic. In this case, oral nonabsorbable aminoglycosides should be used.

10.1.3 *TRAVELER'S DIARRHEA*

Traveler's diarrhea is a syndrome characterized by an increase in frequency of unformed bowel movements, typically four to five loose stools per day. Associated symptoms include abdominal cramps, nausea, bloating, urgency, fever and malaise. Traveler's diarrhea usually begins abruptly, during travel or soon after returning home, and is generally self-limiting, lasting three to four days. Ten percent of cases persist longer than one week, approximately 2% longer than one month and very few beyond three months. Enterotoxigenic E. coli (ETEC) is the most common causative agent of traveler's diarrhea. These organisms adhere to the small intestine, where they multiply and produce an enterotoxin that causes fluid secretion and hence diarrhea. Salmonella gastroenteritis, Shigella dysentery, and viral enteric pathogens (rotavirus and Norwalk-like virus) are less common causes of traveler's diarrhea.

Since traveler's diarrhea is usually mild and self-limiting, with complete recovery even in the absence of therapy, therapy should be considered optional (Table 10). The value of prophylaxis for travelers is unclear. Bismuth preparations are helpful, but their use is limited by the large volumes necessary and by their taste. Antibiotic prophylaxis can reduce the likelihood of developing diarrhea, but carries its own risks.

10.2 Viral Gastroenteritis
At least two groups of viruses are capable of producing an acute diarrheal illness.

10.2.1 *NORWALK VIRUS*
The Norwalk virus causes a self-limiting syndrome that affects children and adults, mainly in winter. An incubation period of 24 to 48 hours is followed by a variable combination of fever, anorexia, nausea, vomiting, myalgia, abdominal pain and diarrhea. Spontaneous recovery occurs two to three days later. Immune electron microscopy of fecal filtrates demonstrates a characteristic 27 nm viral particle (the Norwalk agent). No specific treatment is available. The vomiting represents delayed gastric emptying; there are no morphologic features of gastritis.

10.2.2 *ROTAVIRUSES*
Rotaviruses are the most common causes of acute nonbacterial gastroenteritis in infancy and childhood. Rotaviruses invade mucosal epithelial cells. The resulting illness is more severe than that caused by the Norwalk virus. Rotavirus infection commonly requires hospital admission and intravenous fluids. Infection occurs mainly in children from 6 to 24 months old, and almost always in winter. Virus excretion is maximum three to four days after the onset of symptoms and disappears after a further three to four days. The stability of the virus and the large number of viral particles excreted make environmental contamination inevitable, with a high risk of secondary infection in susceptible contacts. For example, 20% of the rotavirus infections diagnosed in pediatric hospitals are acquired in the hospital. Most older children and adults have antibodies to rotaviruses, so any subsequent infection is generally mild.

10.3 Parasitic Enteritis
The parasites that infect the intestine may be divided into three broad groups. These include protozoa, roundworms and flatworms. The flatworms may be further divided into cestodes (tapeworms) and trematodes (flukes). This chapter will focus upon only a few relevant protozoa.

10.3.1 *GIARDIA LAMBLIA*

Giardia lamblia is endemic in many areas of the world, including Canada. Some patients with giardiasis present with an abrupt, self-limiting illness that develops one to three weeks after infection and lasts three to four days. Others may develop chronic and episodic diarrhea associated with bloating and, at times, steatorrhea and a malabsorption syndrome clinically like celiac disease. Diagnosis is made by recovery of the organism; it is found in the stool of approximately 50% of patients and in 90% of histologically examined smear preparations obtained from small bowel biopsy specimens. The treatment of choice in both asymptomatic and symptomatic patients is metronidazole 250 mg t.i.d. for 7 days. Repeat therapy will occasionally be needed to totally eradicate the organism. Quinacrine 100 mg t.i.d. for 7 days also is effective.

10.3.2 *AMEBIASIS*

This is an acute and chronic disease caused by the organism Entamoeba histolytica. Although there are numerous species of ameba that inhabit the human intestinal tract, E. histolytica seems to be the only variety that is pathogenic for humans. Its manifestations vary from the asymptomatic carrier state to a severe fulminating illness with mucosal inflammation and ulceration. Asymptomatic patients harbor only cysts in their stools and have no evidence of tissue invasion. Since the cysts are resistant to the outside environment, the disease can be transmitted by individuals unaware of their infective potential. This is in contrast to patients with acute or chronic invasive disease, who harbor a trophozoite that cannot survive outside the host.

The acute illness is characterized by diarrhea with the passage of blood and mucus, and by variable degrees of abdominal pain. In its most severe form it may mimic fulminating ulcerative colitis and may progress to a toxic dilation (toxic megacolon) and perforation of the colon. During the acute illness, trophozoites may be recovered in the stool, from biopsies of shallow ulcers in the rectum, or from smears of rectal mucus.

Chronic infectious features may develop many years after the patient has left an endemic area. Patients present with nonspecific bowel complaints and may show radiologic changes in the distal small bowel and colon that mimic Crohn's disease, cancer or tuberculosis. Diagnosis necessitates recovering trophozoites from the stool. As an adjunct, the indirect hemagglutination test can help detect patients with invasive disease.

Intestinal complications of amebiasis include massive intestinal hemorrhage, which is rare; ameboma formation in any part of the colon, which may lead to obstruction or intussusception; permanent stricture formation during the healing stage; and postdysenteric colitis, which usually resolves over several weeks or months without specific therapy.

Systemic dissemination of the ameba may involve other organs, such as the brain, lung, pericardium and liver. Liver abscess is the most common extraintestinal infection by the ameba.

Therapeutic agents used for the treatment of amebiasis act at selected sites: intraluminally, intramurally or systemically. Treatment must therefore be individualized to the location of the disease. Asymptomatic carriers are treated with iodoquinol 650 mg t.i.d. for 20 days; this effective agent acts against amebas located intraluminally. Acute or chronic intestinal disease is treated with metronidazole 750 mg t.i.d. for 10 days. However, because metronidazole is less effective against organisms within the bowel lumen, iodoquinol (650 mg t.i.d. for 20 days) must be added.

10.3.3 CRYPTOSPORIDIA

Cryptosporidia are a genus of protozoa classified within the subclass Coccidia. Cryptosporidia infection has been recognized as a diarrheal disease in humans only since 1979. In immunocompetent persons it presents as a transient, self-limiting diarrheal state lasting from one to seven days. Adults are less commonly affected than young children. In most, the illness is mild and medical help is not sought. With immunological incompetence (e.g., AIDS, neoplasia, hypogammaglobulinemia or concurrent viral infection), a persistent chronic watery diarrhea may occur. Diagnosis is made by demonstrating Cryptosporidia oocysts in the stool or, better still, by mucosal biopsy and examination of the microvillus border for embedded Cryptosporidia oocysts.

A successful treatment for Cryptosporidia has not yet been found. Spiramycin and hyperimmune bovine colostrum remain experimental.

10.4 Drug-Related Diarrhea

Since almost every drug can cause diarrhea, the first question to ask a patient is "What medications, both prescribed and over-the-counter, are you currently taking?" Discontinuing the drug is often the only therapeutic move required in nonantibiotic diarrhea; even in patients with antibiotic-associated diarrhea, with or without colitis, this may be the only step necessary. Although many drugs can cause diarrhea, little is understood about the ways in which they do so. The common causes of drug-induced diarrhea with pathogenic mechanisms follow.

10.4.1 ANTIBIOTIC-ASSOCIATED DIARRHEA AND PSEUDO-
MEMBRANOUS COLITIS

Antibiotics are the most common cause of drug-induced diarrhea. In many cases, the condition is self-limiting. The development of pseudomembranous colitis (PMC) in association with antibiotics may be a serious and sometimes life-threatening condition.

PMC secondary to antibiotics was first recognized during the 1950s. Initially, it was thought to be caused by overgrowth with Staphylococcus aureus, but later research revealed that the colitis was usually caused by an entero-toxin produced by Clostridium difficile.

PMC can follow virtually any antibiotic use. It may occur months after antibiotic exposure, and may rarely occur without a past history of antibiotic use. The frequency of diarrhea or colitis does not appear to be related to dose or route of administration. Symptoms can occur while the patient is on the antibiotic or within six weeks following its discontinuation. Only increasing age is clearly identifiable as a risk factor. The diarrhea is usually loose with a blood-streaked mucus. Frank bleeding is uncommon. The diarrhea can be devastating, with up to 30 bowel movements in a 24-hour period. The diarrhea may be associated with varying degrees of abdominal pain and low-grade fever. Depending on the severity of the diarrhea and the amount of fluid loss, hypotension, shock and even death have been reported. In many patients the problem is self-limiting and resolves spontaneously with discontinuation of the antibiotic. Further investigation is required in those patients who have severe diarrhea associated with systemic symptoms and those whose diarrhea persists despite discontinuing the implicated antibiotic.

An accurate history is usually sufficient to suggest the diagnosis of PMC, and a sigmoidoscopy may be all that is required for confirmation. The presence of copious amounts of mucus and typical raised white pseudomembrane plaques are characteristic features on sigmoidoscopy. Biopsies help confirm the diagnosis. The distal colon is involved in most cases so that sigmoidoscopy is usually adequate. Lesions may be restricted to the right colon, necessitating colonoscopy.

Isolation of C. difficile plus toxin in the stools provides the diagnosis. If it is certain that there can be no other cause for the diarrhea, treatment can be undertaken while awaiting assay results. Treatment depends upon the condition of the patient. If symptoms are resolving with discontinuance of the antibiotic, no further therapy may be indicated. In mild cases, metronidazole 250 mg p.o. t.i.d. for 14 days is effective. In severe hospitalized cases the drug of choice is vancomycin 125 mg p.o. q.i.d. for 14 days. Vancomycin is poorly absorbed and central nervous system and renal toxic effects are uncommon. The high cost of this medication limits its use, even though the eradication rate is quite high. If oral therapy cannot be used, as with severe ileus or recent surgery, parenteral metronidazole is preferred. Some 20% of treated patients will have a recurrence of symptoms, PMC or C. difficile, usually within 4 to 21 days of stopping treatment. In this case, another course of metronidazole or vancomycin should be given. Cholestyramine (Questran®) binds the toxin and can provide symptomatic relief even though it will not eliminate the microorganism.

10.4.2 MAGNESIUM-CONTAINING ANTACIDS
Usually, the osmotic diarrhea produced by Mg^{++} is mild; it may even be welcomed by previously constipated patients. A change to a magnesium-free aluminum-containing antacid is all that is required to control the situation in some. (Magnesium can be used to induce diarrhea by the rare patient with the Münchausen syndrome seeking medical attention for self-induced problems.)

10.4.3 ANTIARRHYTHMIC DRUGS
The antiarrhythmic drugs most commonly associated with diarrhea include quinidine, procainamide and disopyramide. The mechanism involved is unknown. Changing the antiarrhythmic drug may halt the diarrhea.

10.4.4 OTHER MEDICATIONS
Colchicine, often administered for acute gout, produces diarrhea as a common side effect. It resolves with discontinuance of the medication. The mechanism of the diarrhea is unknown, but may relate to an intestinal cytotoxic effect of colchicine. Antimetabolites (e.g., methotrexate) often cause diarrhea as a result of damage to the small or large bowel mucosa. This type of diarrhea can be devastating and difficult to control. Except for rehydration and stopping the drug, little can be done.

11. CHRONIC DIARRHEA

11.1 Pathogenesis
The four basic mechanisms that cause chronic diarrhea are osmotic, secretory and exudative factors, and abnormal intestinal transit (Table 11).

If the diarrhea ceases when fasting, or if there is a significant osmotic gap in the stool water, then an osmotic cause for the diarrhea is suspect. Examples include diarrhea after ingesting milk (a result of lactase deficiency) or drugs such as laxatives and antacids, or the excessive use of artificial sweeteners such as sorbitol and mannitol, which contain polycyclic alcohols.

If the patient's diarrhea persists when fasting (such as may occur at nighttime when the diarrhea awakens the person from sleep), a secretory diarrhea is likely. Secretory diarrhea usually arises from infection or inflammation associated with toxigenic and invasive bacteria. Secretory diarrhea may also result from the spillage of excess bile acids into the colon (choleretic enteropathy) or from the cathartic effect of hydroxy fatty acids arising from

TABLE 11.   Pathophysiologic mechanisms of chronic diarrhea

Major disturbance	Probable mechanisms	Examples/Associated conditions
Osmotic*	Ingestion	Antacids, laxatives
	Maldigestion	Pancreatic insufficiency, disaccharidase deficiency
	Malabsorption	Carbohydrate malabsorption, congenital chloridorrhea
Disorders of intestinal transit	*Slow* transit ("blind loop syndrome") – excessive contact time	Fistulas, strictures (such as in the patient with Crohn's disease), diabetic neuropathy
	Rapid transit – insufficient contact time	Intestinal resection, hyperthyroidism, irritable bowel
Secretory**	Bacterial enterotoxins	Vibrio cholerae, enterotoxigenic E. coli
	Secretagogues	Bile acids, fatty acids, ethanol, prostaglandins, phenolphthalein, dioctyl sodium sulfosuccinate, VIP, gastrin, calcitonin
Exudative	Increased passage of body fluids into lumen	Ulcerative colitis, Crohn's disease

*See Table 12. **See Table 13.

the colonic bacterial action on malabsorbed fat. Very rarely, secretory diarrhea can arise from a tumor producing an intestinal secretagogue (e.g., pancreatic islet cell tumor producing vasoactive intestinal peptide or gastrin).

Exudative diarrhea results from mucosal damage to the small or large bowel, which interferes with absorption of salt and water, and may be associated with the exudation of serum proteins, blood, and mucus and sloughed cells. This mechanism is seen in infectious, inflammatory and neoplastic disorders.

Disorders of intestinal transit may give rise to diarrhea secondary to abnormal intestinal motility in hyperthyroidism or diabetic neuropathy. Scleroderma leads to bacterial overgrowth and steatorrhea (as can the rapid transit in hyperthyroidism). The mechanism of diarrhea in these conditions relates to a combination of bacterial overgrowth, bile salt wastage and disorders of motility (slow or rapid intestinal transit).

TABLE 12.   Causes of osmotic diarrhea

Carbohydrates
Specific disaccharidase deficiencies
Glucose–galactose malassimilation
Fructose malassimilation
Mannitol, sorbitol ingestion ("chewing gum diarrhea")
Lactulose therapy

Divalent ions
Magnesium sulfate (Epsom salts)
Sodium sulfate
Sodium phosphate
Sodium citrate
Magnesium-containing antacids

11.1.1 *OSMOTIC DIARRHEA*

Retention of solute molecules within the bowel lumen generates osmotic forces that retard the normal absorption of water (Table 12). Practical examples include poorly absorbed carbohydrates or a divalent ion. Poorly absorbed divalent ions (e.g., phosphate, sulfate and magnesium) are the laxative constituents of several common antacids and saline purges. Since the "pores" through which ions are absorbed are highly charged, these polyvalent ions tend to be absorbed slowly. Thus, they accumulate within the intestinal lumen, raise the osmolality, and so retard the normal absorption of water or even act to draw water from the circulation into the intestinal lumen.

Carbohydrates constitute the other major group of osmotic agents. Some are poorly absorbed by everybody; lactulose, for example, was developed to be a nonhydrolyzable, nonabsorbable disaccharide that would act as a cathartic. The action of lactulose mimics the effects of *primary lactase deficiency*. This condition normally develops after weaning in the majority of African-, Caribbean- or Asian-Canadians and occurs in 30% of persons with southern European ancestry. The unabsorbed lactose acts osmotically to retain water in the small intestine. In fact, any disease that interferes with carbohydrate absorption (e.g., impaired intraluminal digestion due to pancreatic disease, primary disaccharidase deficiencies, and secondary disaccharidase deficiencies due to small bowel disease) will lead to osmotic diarrhea. Since carbohydrates are not inert in the colon, their metabolism leads to further osmotic forces. Once carbohydrate reaches the fecal flora, anaerobic fermentation occurs (Figure 12). Intermediary products are ethanol and formic, succinic and lactic acids. These products are further consumed to varying degrees. CO_2

and H_2 are rapidly absorbed, and CO_2 rises in exhaled air. (Exhaled H_2 is the basis for the hydrogen breath test described earlier.) Excess gas production causes borborygmi and flatus rich in H_2. Short-chain fatty acids (SCFAs) are also produced (acetic acid, propionic acid and butyric acid) and account for the acidic stool pH noted in diarrhea of carbohydrate malabsorption. The caloric loss due to carbohydrate malabsorption is diminished to the extent that short-chain fatty acids can be absorbed from the colon (where they may be used as nutrients by the colonocytes), thus "salvaging" some of the malabsorbed carbohydrates that enter the colon.

The consequences of malabsorption are as follows: With minor impairment of sugar absorption, colonic fermentation is complete and only small amounts of excess solute are present in stool water. Stool volume and stool pH do not initially change much, and up to three-quarters of the glucose energy is returned to the body in the form of short-chain fatty acids (colonic "salvage"). As the extent of carbohydrate malabsorption increases, more short-chain fatty acids are formed than can be reabsorbed. This results in diarrhea due to the presence of osmotically active short-chain fatty acids. The stool pH consequently begins to fall, which further decreases colonic salvage.

Clinically, osmotic diarrhea should stop when the patient stops ingesting the poorly absorbed solute. Stool analysis should not reveal fat, RBC or WBC. There should be a positive osmotic gap – that is, stool osmolality minus stool Na^+ plus stool K^+ times 2 (multiplied by 2 to account for anions) is greater than 50, the size of the osmotic gap being approximately equivalent to the concentration of poorly absorbed solutes in fecal water.

11.1.2 INTESTINAL TRANSIT AND DIARRHEA

The basal electrical rhythm of the small intestine alters the excitability of the muscle cells. The motility patterns of the small intestine consist of three essential patterns: (1) migrating motor complex (MMC), periodic bursts of contractile activity lasting at least 5 minutes that are succeeded by periods of quiescence and appear to migrate down the small intestine at a slow rate of less than 5 cm/min; (2) minute rhythm, regular groups of between 3 and 10 contractions that occur at intervals of 1 to 2 minutes, separated by periods of quiescence, and appear to migrate down the small intestine at a rapid rate of 60–120 cm/min; (3) migrating action potential complex, a single ring contraction or single burst of spike potentials that migrates down the intestine at a rate exceeding 90 cm/min.

These forms of small intestinal motility control the rate at which material travels along the intestine and hence arrives at the anus. Gastrointestinal motor activity also determines the time and thus the degree of contact between gut contents, the digestive enzymes and the absorptive epithelium. Accelerated transit of material through the gut produces diarrhea by limiting digestion and absorption.

Understanding of motility-associated diarrhea remains limited, and only rudimentary measures of intestinal myoelectrical activity exist for humans. The oral–anal transit times of radiolabeled markers, radiopaque tubing, or nonabsorbable carbohydrate markers provide the only clinical assessments. Even small intestinal motility, unlike esophageal motility, remains a research tool.

The ileocecal valve is important to gut function. The ileocecal sphincter extends over a 4 cm length of distal small intestine and produces a high-pressure zone of about 20 mm Hg. Distention of the ileum results in a decrease in the ileocecal sphincter pressure, whereas distention of the colon results in an increased pressure in this area. The ileocecal valve slows down intestinal transit and prevents backwash from the colon. By this mechanism the ileocecal valve is important in regulating intestinal transit. Removal of the ileocecal valve during surgery will result in marked intestinal hurry as well as the potential for bacterial overgrowth from fecal "backwash." Disorders that impair peristalsis in the small gut allow bacterial overgrowth, resulting in diarrhea. Lastly, premature evacuation of the colon because of an abnormality of its contents or because of intrinsic colonic "irritability" or inflammation results in a reduced contact between luminal contents and colonic mucosa and, therefore, in more frequent, liquid stools.

11.1.3 SECRETORY DIARRHEA

The small intestine normally secretes as well as absorbs fluid and electrolytes; the secretion rate is lower than the absorption rate. Therefore, the net effect of small bowel transport is absorption of fluid. This is an important concept, because it means that a pathophysiologic event may reduce the absorption rate in either of two ways: by stimulating secretion or inhibiting absorption. Either or both can result in what is clinically recognized as secretory diarrhea. It is usually difficult, if not impossible, to ascertain which of the two events is predominant. For clinical purposes, it seems best to consider inhibition of ion absorption and stimulation of ion secretion together.

The prototype of secretory diarrhea is Vibrio cholerae; its clinical description first aroused interest in the secretory process as a mechanism for diarrhea (Table 13).

Bacterial secretagogues fall into two major classes. The first class comprises large (MW 84,000), heat-labile proteins, of which cholera enterotoxin is the prototype. These toxins appear to stimulate secretion by activating mucosal adenylate cyclase and thus increasing cyclic AMP levels in the mucosa. The intracellular "messenger" for secretion is less well defined;

TABLE 13. Causes of secretory diarrhea

Pathophysiologic mechanisms
Enterotoxins
Circulating secretagogues (VIP, calcitonin, prostaglandins, serotonin)
Increased hydrostatic pressure and tissue pressure
Gastric hypersecretion (Zollinger-Ellison syndrome)
Pancreatic hypersecretion
Laxatives (ricinoleic acid, bisacodyl, phenolphthalein, oxyphenisatin, dioctyl sodium sulfo-
    succinate, aloe, senna, danthron)
Bile salts
Fatty acids

Clinical syndromes
Acute secretory diarrhea
Chronic secretory diarrhea
    Surreptitious laxative ingestion
    Pancreatic cholera syndrome (VIP)
    Medullary carcinoma of the thyroid (calcitonin)
    Ganglioneuroma, ganglioneuroblastoma, neurofibroma
    Zollinger-Ellison syndrome (gastrin)
    Malignant carcinoid syndrome (serotonin)
    Idiopathic secretory diarrhea
    Congenital chloridorrhea (some cases)
    Secreting villous adenoma
    Total villous atrophy of small bowel mucosa
    Niacin deficiency
    Intestinal lymphoma
Miscellaneous
    Intestinal obstruction
    Intestinal distention/ileus

---

cyclic AMP is considered important, though there are additional steps that might also involve intracellular levels of Ca^{++} and the calcium regulatory protein, calmodulin. A second class of secretagogues comprises smaller proteins that are heat-stable. The best studied is the ST (heat-stable toxin) of E. coli, which stimulates secretion by activating mucosal guanylate cyclase, leading to higher levels of cyclic GMP in the mucosa.

Bacterial toxins, however, are only part of the story. Secretion is also stimulated experimentally by hormones, peptides acting locally (paracrine hormones), luminal factors (e.g., dihydroxy bile acids and fatty acids), neurotransmitters, prostaglandins and physical factors (e.g., distention). Bile acids and fatty acids not absorbed in the small intestine evoke secretion of electrolytes and water by the colon. The exact mechanism(s) for this are uncertain. Both groups have multiple effects on the bowel, including stimulation of secretion, increased intestinal permeability and transient alterations in morphology.

One or more humoral stimuli can elicit a massive secretion of water and electrolytes from the small bowel. The colon is usually not involved directly, but it may be unable to adequately reabsorb the fluid load imposed on it. A key question, difficult to answer, is "What is the responsible hormone?" Putative secretagogues include vasoactive intestinal peptides in the pancreatic cholera syndrome, calcitonin in medullary carcinoma of the thyroid, gastrin in the Zollinger-Ellison syndrome, serotonin in the malignant carcinoid syndrome, and glucagon in glucagonomas. Prostaglandins are also potent stimulators of intestinal secretion. Diarrhea secondary to prostaglandin-stimulated intestinal secretion is a common side effect.

The intestinal distention that occurs with obstruction or ileus also produces a local secretory state proximal to the obstruction. The mechanism is not entirely clear and may be related to changes in permeability (as tight junctions are stretched and broken) as well as to direct, perhaps neural, stimulation of secretory mechanisms.

Secretory diarrhea is recognized clinically by four features: (1) the stools are large-volume, watery and often >1 L/day; (2) the diarrhea persists during fasting; (3) there is a measured stool osmolar gap of <50 mOsm/L; and (4) patients with secretory diarrhea do not have excessive fat, blood or pus in their stools, but often develop depletion in fluid, Na^+ and K^+.

Therapeutically, the offending agent must be removed. A variety of empirical therapies that influence the secretory process (e.g., somatostatin, prostaglandin inhibitors, phenothiazines, calcium channel blockers, $\alpha2$-adrenergic agonists and lithium) may be effective but should be reserved for use in a research center. Oral glucose-saline replacement therapy is useful for maintenance of hydration. For bile acid–induced diarrhea, cholestyramine works well unless there has been a greater than 100 cm resection of the terminal ileum.

11.1.4 *EXUDATIVE DIARRHEA*

Exudation is a far simpler concept. Structural disruption of the intestinal wall by diffuse ulceration, inflammation, infiltrations and tumors will add cellular debris, mucus, serum proteins and blood to the lumen. The effects on stool volume will be most pronounced when the lesions also involve the colon, since there will be little opportunity for normal mechanisms of colonic fluid and electrolyte absorption to compensate for the increased volume of chyme.

11.1.5 *SELF-INDUCED DIARRHEA*

The possibility that the diarrhea is self-induced must be considered when a patient complains of chronic diarrhea and when the routine investigations are negative. In general, abusing laxatives, diuretics and sometimes thyroid hormones will induce diarrhea. Often the diarrhea is sufficiently severe to cause electrolyte disturbances, acid-based problems and dehydration. The diagnosis can be extremely difficult since the history is often misleading or not obtained. The usual investigations (including sigmoidoscopy and radiographs) will be negative, unless the patient is taking a drug that can cause melanosis coli (brown-black pigmentation of the colonic mucosa), such as the anthracene laxatives senna or aloe. Stool analysis for Mg^{++}, sennas or phenolphthalein may reveal the culprit. Finding packages of laxatives and other drugs in room searches is often the only method that permits the diagnosis; this approach has been criticized because of ethical considerations, but may be the only way to uncover the problem. Ethical issues and respect for the patient's privacy must be carefully considered before embarking on a room or locker search.

11.2 Investigation of the Patient with Chronic Diarrhea

For a patient with chronic diarrhea, a careful history and physical examination can help define the site in the intestinal tract responsible (Table 14). This may avoid the expense and frustration of the unproductive "shotgun" approach. One possible diagnostic approach appears in Figure 15.

12. DISACCHARIDASE DEFICIENCIES

Disaccharide intolerance is a characteristic symptom complex resulting from the ingestion of ordinary dietary quantities of disaccharides, which produces a symptomatic diarrhea. The cause is a deficiency of one or more disaccharidases, but not all people with such a deficiency will experience symptoms.

Dietary carbohydrates are presented to the surface of the jejunal mucosa in the form of isomaltose, maltotriose and three major disaccharides – maltose, sucrose and lactose. Trehalose, a disaccharide contained in young mushrooms and in certain insects, is a minor component of modern Western diets. Deficiencies of disaccharidases may be *primary* (hereditary) or *secondary* (acquired) deficiencies. Characteristically in primary deficiencies, which are rare, only one enzyme is involved; the deficiency is present at birth (with the exception of the adult-onset form of lactase deficiency), not associated with intestinal disease, and irreversible. Secondary deficiencies usually involve all the disaccharidases, may occur at any age, are associated with a disorder of the small intestinal mucosa, and may be reversed if the intestinal disorder (e.g., celiac disease, stasis syndromes or acute enteritis) heals. Because primary lactase deficiency is uncommon in Canadians with northern European

TABLE 14. Anatomic approach to the causes of chronic diarrhea

---

Gastric
Excessive use of antacids*
Hypergastrinemia/Zollinger-Ellison syndrome
Postoperative unmasked celiac disease, lactase deficiency or pancreatic
   insufficiency
Postoperative dumping syndrome*

Small intestine
Crohn's disease*
Celiac disease*
Lymphoma
Whipple's disease
Bacterial, viral or parasitic infection*
Abnormal intestinal integrity: scleroderma, amyloidosis, diabetes

Large bowel
Colon neoplasia*
Irritable bowel syndrome*
Inflammatory bowel disease: ulcerative colitis, Crohn's disease*

Drugs
Antacids*
Antibiotics*
Alcohol*
Antimetabolites
Laxatives
Digitalis
Colchicine

Metabolic
Hyperthyroidism
Hypoparathyroidism
Addison's disease
Diabetes*
Carcinoid syndrome
VIPoma syndrome

---

*Common

ancestors, the appropriate tests need to be performed to exclude secondary causes such as celiac disease.

The clinical manifestations of enzyme deficiency result from the osmotic diarrhea following ingestion of the disaccharide. The affected individual develops crampy, abdominal distress and distention, relieved by the expulsion of liquid stool and flatus. The severity of the diarrhea varies with the disaccharide load, the degree of deficiency of enzyme activity and any associated/ causal intestinal disease. The clinical diagnosis can be confirmed by direct enzyme assay of jejunal mucosal biopsies or by indirect methods for detecting disaccharide malabsorption (e.g., the breath hydrogen test). Treatment of hereditary deficiencies is usually by elimination diets. For children and adolescents (who have high nutritional requirements) and for adults who enjoy milk, low-lactose milk is available in some localities. It can also be prepared by adding yeast lactase (available in commercial form) to milk and refrigerating it for 24 hours; 80% lactose hydrolysis can be obtained with this method.

Delayed-onset (adult-onset) hereditary lactase deficiency is extremely common and probably "normal" for humans. Beginning as early as age 2 years in some racial groups, and as late as adolescence in others, the activities of lactase in the majority of the world's populations drop sharply. This is the result of the genetically controlled "switching off" of lactase synthesis by intestinal cells. Individuals of northern European ancestry and certain groups in Africa and India, however, maintain lactase activity throughout adulthood.

13. GLUTEN-INDUCED ENTEROPATHY (CELIAC DISEASE)

In celiac disease (gluten-induced or gluten-sensitive enteropathy) the mucosa of the small intestine is damaged by gluten-containing foods (i.e., those containing wheat, rye, barley and possibly oats). This causes a characteristic though nonspecific lesion and subsequent malabsorption of most nutrients. The precise mechanism of gluten toxicity is unknown. Fractionation of cereal proteins reveals that the component that is toxic to the intestinal mucosa is a portion of the gluten molecule called gliadin. Although gliadin can be inactivated in a test tube by enzymatic degradation, digestion to smaller peptides by pepsin and trypsin does not alter its toxicity in humans. In susceptible people, symptoms and pathologic changes occur within 12 hours of gluten intake. The immune system is also involved. The small intestine in patients with untreated celiac disease shows an increase in lamina propria lymphocytes, plasma cells and intraepithelial lymphocytes. Immunocytochemical studies indicate that cells producing IgA, IgG and particularly IgM are increased. Increased levels of serum IgA and decreased levels of serum IgM have also been reported and appear to revert toward normal with treatment.

Genetic studies indicate that about 10% of the patient's first-order relatives have asymptomatic disease. HLA-B8 and HLA-DW3, generally associated through linkage disequilibrium, are present in 80% of patients (compared to 20% of the general population). In addition, a specific antigen is present on the surface of B lymphocytes in approximately 80% of celiac disease patients (compared to 10–15% of controls). It is found in all parents of affected indi-

TABLE 15. Symptoms of celiac disease

Manifestations	Probable causes or deficiencies
Common	
Anemia	Iron, folate, B_{12}, pyridoxine
Glossitis	Iron, folate
Weight loss/weakness	Malassimilation – Negative nitrogen balance
Diarrhea/flatulence	Fat and carbohydrate malassimilation
Abdominal pain	Increased intestinal gas production secondary to carbohydrate malassimilation
Occasional	
Follicular hyperkeratosis and dermatitis	Vitamin A, folate
Pigmentation	Associated adrenal insufficiency
Edema	Hypoproteinemia
Tetany	Vitamin D, calcium, magnesium
Osteomalacia	Vitamin D, calcium
Purpura	Hypoprothrombinemia (vitamin K)
Rare	
Spinal cord degeneration	B_{12}
Peripheral neuritis	B_{12}, vitamin E, thiamine, pyridoxine
Psychosis	B_{12}
Malignancy (usually small bowel lymphoma)	Unknown

viduals, which suggests that this antigen is inherited by an autosomal recessive method. Celiac disease is also present in about 2% of insulin-dependent diabetics.

13.1 Clinical Features

13.1.1 *CHILDHOOD PRESENTATION*
In children, onset of symptoms suggestive of celiac disease is gradual with failure to thrive after the introduction of cereals in the diet (Table 15). The affected infant is irritable, anorexic, pale and wasted. Physical examination discloses generalized hypotonia and abdominal distention. The stools are soft, bulky, clay-colored and offensive. In the slightly older child, abdominal pain may be the presenting complaint. It may be sufficiently severe to simulate an intestinal obstruction. Older children may also present with anemia, rickets and failure to grow normally. Quite often, adolescents have a clinical quiescence of the disease. Even if relatively asymptomatic in childhood, affected

people often do not attain their normal growth potential, being shorter than their sibs.

13.1.2 ADULT PRESENTATION

Celiac disease can present at any age, even after 70 years, but in adults it usually occurs between 20 and 60 years. In adult and adolescent patients, presentations with classical features of diarrhea, weight loss and malnutrition, or bone pain (osteomalacia) have become much less common. Mild and subclinical forms are frequent, occurring in more than 50% of patients. The sole presentation may be an otherwise unexplained hematologic abnormality (iron deficiency with or without anemia, folate deficiency, macrocytosis), constitutional symptoms or fatigue with minimal weight loss and no intestinal symptoms, or mild abdominal or digestive complaints. The entity is most common in those of Irish and Scottish background or those who have a family history.

Diarrhea is common but many patients experience normal bowel habits, alternating diarrhea and constipation, and even constipation. The diarrhea is usually mild, with fewer than three bowel movements per day in most. Floating stools, also common in healthy subjects excreting high amounts of stool gas, are often not reported. Indeed, stools suggesting steatorrhea (i.e., unformed, bulky and hard to flush, greasy, sticky, pale and foul-smelling) are quite uncommon. Flatulence, abdominal distention, abdominal cramps and borborygmi are common complaints. Fatigue is the most frequent symptom at presentation. Weight loss is usually moderate (averaging 10 kg) and may be absent in mild cases. Clinically overt metabolic (tetany) and bone (osteomalacia) diseases have become uncommon with our generous Western diets, but these situations are hallmarks of celiac disease. A clue to the diagnosis of celiac disease is the development of lactose intolerance in person whose heritage is northern European.

Patients with dermatitis herpetiformis have gluten enteropathy but often without clinical impact. Overall, mucosal involvement in celiac disease progresses from duodenum to jejunoileum and is most severe proximally; the length of bowel involved determines to a great extent the clinical picture of the disease.

13.2 Laboratory Findings

Laboratory findings, as clinical signs and symptoms, vary widely. The definitive diagnosis of celiac disease requires the demonstration of small bowel mucosal villous atrophy that improves upon gluten withdrawal. In practice, several tests can be used to strengthen the suspicion of celiac disease and/or evaluate the possible biochemical consequences.

13.2.1 *HEMATOLOGIC TESTS*

Anemia is present in less than 50% of adult patients and may be secondary to iron, folate or (very rarely) vitamin B_{12} deficiency. Since celiac disease involves the proximal small bowel (i.e., the duodenum, where iron absorption occurs) most severely, iron deficiency is the most common laboratory abnormality. Folate deficiency also occurs, providing two laboratory screening tests for celiac disease. Decreased absorption of B_{12} and malabsorption of vitamin K (with prolonged prothrombin time) are uncommon.

13.2.2 *STOOL EXAMINATION*

Steatorrhea can be confirmed by a 72-hour fecal fat study. It is usually mild (10–20 g/24 hours) and may be absent in some patients. Its severity correlates with the extent of the intestinal lesion, so that patients whose disease is limited to the proximal small intestine often have normal stool fat excretion.

13.2.3 *BLOOD CHEMISTRY TEST*

Depletion of minerals (zinc, magnesium) and ions (potassium) occurs only with severe disease. Plasma proteins are often within normal limits but this protein-losing enteropathy (leakage of serum protein into gut lumen) and possible malnutrition may result in decreased serum albumin. A low serum carotene (and sometimes cholesterol) level may be a clue to the presence of the disease.

13.2.4 *CARBOHYDRATE TOLERANCE TEST*

Approximately two-thirds of patients with celiac disease exhibit an abnormal D-xylose test. D-xylose is an aldopentose that is absorbed in the upper small intestine and is excreted in the urine almost completely within the first five hours after ingestion. Abnormal D-xylose absorption is best evaluated by the serum concentration after ingestion and points specifically to small bowel disease or luminal bacterial overgrowth. Similarly, the absorptive cell lesion also results in secondary lactase deficiency; thus, the H_2-lactose breath test may be abnormal in celiac disease.

13.2.5 *RADIOGRAPHIC STUDIES*

Barium studies of the small bowel may show dilation of the bowel and slight thickening of the mucosal folds. Intraluminal signs of malabsorption with flocculation, segmentation and clumping of the barium (features due to excess amount of fluid present within the lumen) are variable and not common. (The new barium suspensions now used have made this a rare finding.) Radiographic findings in celiac disease are not specific for this syndrome of malabsorption.

13.2.6 *PERMEABILITY TESTS*

The intestine of patients with celiac disease may be "leaky" and allow passage from the lumen into the blood and then into the urine of sugars such as mannitol or lactulose. The finding of increased amounts of these sugars in the urine after an oral dose suggests an abnormal intestinal permeability barrier. Such a finding of increased permeability may suggest the presence of celiac disease or other small intestinal disorders.

13.2.7 *SEROLOGICAL TESTS*

The demonstration of antibodies in the serum to gliadin, reticulin or endomysium suggests the presence of celiac disease. Anti-endomysial IgA antibody measurement has proved to be a sensitive test for celiac disease, even in screening studies of asymptomatic children.

13.2.8 *SMALL BOWEL BIOPSY*

Small intestinal biopsies can be obtained endoscopically from the distal duodenum (at least four forceps biopsies). Rarely, when diagnostic uncertainty persists, a larger mucosal specimen may be needed and obtained from the duodenojejunal area using the peroral Rubin tube or the Crosby capsule.

A flat mucosal biopsy from a white adult in the Western world is almost certain to indicate celiac disease, although other disorders can be associated with similar changes (e.g., tropical sprue, diffuse lymphoma of small bowel, immunoglobulin deficiency syndromes and the Zollinger-Ellison syndrome with gastric hypersecretion). In infants, soy protein intolerance, cow's milk protein intolerance and viral gastroenteritis produce a similar appearance. Therefore, to establish unequivocally the diagnosis of celiac disease, clinical improvement with a gluten-free diet is needed. Proving this improvement with a second biopsy is usually not necessary in adults. Mucosal small bowel atrophy improves similarly, although reversion of histology toward normal requires months or even years of gluten withdrawal and often is not complete in the duodenum.

Microscopically the characteristic "flat" lesion of celiac disease will demonstrate absence of villi, an abnormal cuboidal surface epithelium, markedly lengthened crypts and increased numbers of plasma cells and lymphocytes in the lamina propria. The lesion may be very subtle and include increased intraepithelial lymphocytes and a change in the normal position of the nuclei in the enterocyte. In a subtle lesion with shortened villi, proper orientation of the specimen is important in order to correctly estimate the height of the villi. The proximal small bowel is most severely involved, while the lesion decreases in severity toward the distal small intestine. The lesion may be patchy. Celiac disease will not spare the proximal small intestine while involving the distal small intestine, however. Sometimes the gross appearance of the mucosa observed at the time of an upper endoscopy may alert the physician to the possibility of celiac disease and direct her/him to obtain a duodenal biopsy.

13.3 Treatment

The mainstay of therapy for celiac disease is the gluten-free diet, which requires avoiding wheat, rye, barley and oats but allows widely diversified foods. Expert dietetic counseling is a major determinant of successful treatment. Supplements of iron and folic acid are often needed. If milk products cause diarrhea, commercially available lactase enzymes may be used for the first few months. Usually, clinical symptoms improve within weeks, but drastic changes may be seen in sicker patients after a few days.

13.4 Complications and Prognosis

A primary failure to respond to treatment is usually due to incomplete (often involuntary) exclusion of gluten from the diet. Revision of the diet is necessary. A dietary consultation may help to identify sources of unsuspected gluten such as medications, candies or toothpaste. Motivation for continuing with the gluten-free diet is provided by contacts with the physician and dietitian. Other causes of primary failure include diagnostic error (tropical sprue, lymphoma, etc.), dysgammaglobulinemia syndromes, "functional" associated pancreatic insufficiency and so-called refractory sprue. Deterioration after a period of clinical improvement suggests dietary indiscretions, malignancies (there is increased risk of lymphoma) or rare instances of refractory sprue, collagenous sprue and nongranulomatous ulcerative jejunoileitis.

13.4.1 *REFRACTORY SPRUE*

Refractory sprue is a disease in which malabsorptive symptoms and mucosal small bowel atrophy persist or recur while the patient remains on a strict gluten-free diet. Corticosteroids, total parenteral nutrition and cyclosporine therapy have been used in treatment, but their value is not clear. The prognosis is serious.

13.4.2 *NONGRANULOMATOUS ULCERATIVE JEJUNOILEITIS*

This very rare complication presents with abdominal pain, intestinal bleeding and diarrhea. Ulcers may lead to small bowel perforations or strictures. The mortality rate for this condition is very high.

13.4.3 *COLLAGENOUS SPRUE*

This rare disorder is generally associated with severe malabsorption. In addition to the characteristic small intestinal biopsy of untreated celiac disease, a striking trichrome-positive band of collagen is seen beneath the surface epithelium. Changes may be patchy, necessitating multiple biopsies from different sites to confirm the diagnosis. There is no effective therapy other than nutritional supportive care.

13.4.4 *MALIGNANCIES*

Incidence of malignancies is increased in patients with celiac disease. Most of these are small bowel lymphomas and carcinomas of the esophagus and colon. A strict gluten-free diet decreases this risk – another reason to reinforce a lifetime commitment to gluten avoidance. Overall, the vast majority of patients with celiac disease have a normal life expectancy.

14. **SHORT BOWEL SYNDROME**

The severity of symptoms following resections of large segments of the small bowel relates to the extent of the resection, to the specific level of the resected small bowel and to the reason for which the resection was undertaken. The level of resection is important because absorption of nutrients is most effective in the proximal small bowel (iron, folate and calcium). Resection of up to 40% of the intestine is usually tolerated provided the duodenum and proximal jejunum and distal half of the ileum and ileocecal valve are spared. In contrast, resection of the distal two-thirds of the ileum and ileocecal valve alone may induce severe diarrhea and significant malabsorption even though only 25% of the total small intestine has been resected. Resection of 50% of the small intestine results in significant malabsorption, and resection of 70% or more of the small intestine will result in severe malnutrition sufficient to cause death unless the patient's malnutrition is aggressively treated.

The most common cause of massive resection of the small bowel is small bowel ischemia, due to thrombosis or embolism of the superior mesenteric artery, thrombosis of the superior mesenteric vein, or low flow in the splanchnic vessels. Less commonly, volvulus, strangulated hernias, Crohn's disease, neoplasm and trauma necessitate massive resection.

Two major types of diarrhea can develop after massive ileal resection. One is induced primarily by malabsorbed bile acids, and the other by malabsorbed fat. When the ileal resection is small (less than 100 cm), hepatic synthesis of bile acids is sufficient to compensate for increased fecal losses. The luminal concentrations of bile acids are maintained within the micellar range, and significant steatorrhea does not occur. However, with inadequate absorption in the terminal ileum, bile acids enter the colon, impairing electrolyte and water absorption. Thus the term "bile acid diarrhea" is applied to this circumstance.

When the ileal resection is extensive (greater than 100 cm), hepatic compensation for wastage of bile acids is incomplete and the concentration of bile acids in the lumen is too low for adequate micellar solubilization of fat. Steatorrhea results. Here the malabsorbed fat is primarily responsible for the diarrhea. With excessive amounts of fatty acids now in the colon, electrolyte and water absorption are further impaired.

Consistent with these proposed pathogenic mechanisms are the therapeutic observations that a reduction in the dietary intake of long-chain fats will reduce the severity of diarrhea in the second instance (extensive resection and steatorrhea), whereas a sequestrant of bile acids such as cholestyramine, colestipol or aluminum hydroxide is needed for effective therapy of bile acid diarrhea.

Additional metabolic complications arise from the short bowel syndrome. These include hyperoxaluria and subsequent nephrolithiasis. Normally dietary oxalate is excreted in the feces, bound to calcium as an insoluble complex. However, in a patient with steatorrhea, fatty acids in the intestine preferentially bind to calcium, leaving the oxalate soluble and available for absorption in the colon. The short bowel syndrome may also give rise to cholelithiasis. If bile acid malabsorption is extensive, a lithogenic bile will be produced, predisposing to gallstone formation.

15. POSTGASTRECTOMY MALABSORPTION

Postgastrectomy malabsorption frequently follows gastric surgery. The small size of the gastric remnant causes inadequate mixing of food with digestive juices, particularly after a gastroenterostomy. With the loss of the pylorus, there may be rapid gastric emptying, poor mixing of bile and pancreatic secretions, and rapid transit down the small intestine. Incoordinated secretion and poor mixing of bile and pancreatic juice leads to fat maldigestion. Bacterial contamination in a blind loop (with gastroenterostomy) results in maldigestion of fat, carbohydrate, protein, vitamins and minerals. Gastric surgery that allows food to enter into the upper small intestine without dilution and with minimal digestion may "unmask" mild and subclinical celiac disease, lactase deficiency or pancreatic insufficiency.

16. NORMAL SMALL INTESTINAL FLORA

The concentration and population of microorganisms that constitute the normal intestinal flora vary with the location along the intestine. Flora in the stomach, duodenum, jejunum and proximal ileum are sparse, usually less than 10^5/mL. The distal ileum represents a transitional zone between the sparse flora of the proximal small intestine and the luxuriant flora of the lower bowel, where microorganism concentrations reach 10^{11}/mL. The predominant species are strict anaerobes, including bacteroides, anaerobic streptococci, bifidobacteria and Clostridium. The commonest aerobic organisms are E. coli; however, their concentration (10^8/mL) is only 1/1,000 of the usual concentration of anaerobes in the colon.

Normally, bacterial flora are present in the intestinal lumen and in the mucus layer overlying the epithelium, and attached to the mucosal cells themselves. There is a specific tissue or cell type to which each microbial species attaches. For example, Streptococcus mutans, the oral organism that causes tooth decay, attaches only to the enamel surface of teeth; removal of the teeth leads to the disappearance of S. mutans from the oral microflora. This phenomenon of adherence may play an important role in the establishment and maintenance of a normal flora.

What are the mechanisms controlling normal small intestinal flora? First, in the stomach, acid suppresses the growth of most organisms that enter from the oropharynx. Bile added in the duodenum has additional antibacterial properties. Second, small intestinal motility mechanically sweeps bacteria downstream, helping to maintain a low concentration of organisms in the proximal small intestine. Third, the ileocecal valve plays an important role in preventing reflux of large amounts of colonic organisms. Additionally, mucus secreted by goblet cells and immunoglobulins has antibacterial properties.

Whereas the small intestine regulates the number of organisms present, in the colon the microorganisms themselves are responsible for maintaining their own population levels. Volatile fatty acids (e.g., acetic, butyric and propionic acid) are produced by anaerobes as well as by some coliforms. These short-chain fatty acids reduce the intraluminal pH and suppress the growth of certain organisms, thereby serving to control proliferation. In addition, some organisms produce other substances that inhibit bacterial growth, called bacteriocins.

Thus far we have considered what the microorganisms are, where they are located, and how their numbers are controlled. We next examine the concept that the normal flora exert a profound influence on intraluminal constituents, including food, urea, bilirubin, bile salts, drugs and potential toxins. Bacteria ferment dietary carbohydrates, yielding short-chain fatty acids, hydrogen and carbon dioxide. Fatty acids from carbohydrates and those from fat in the diet are hydroxylated by the intestinal flora. The hydroxy fatty acids formed stimulate fluid secretion and are thus cathartics.

Similarly, bacteria alter protein and amino acids. Tryptophan is converted to indole compounds, glycine to ammonia, and methionine to hydrogen sulfide. Urea is converted to ammonia, a reaction that may contribute to hepatic

TABLE 16. Etiology of the bacterial overgrowth syndrome

Breakdown of normal defense mechanisms
Achlorhydria
Stasis: Anatomic (Crohn's disease, diverticula, lymphoma, strictures)
　　　Functional (scleroderma, diabetic autonomic neuropathy, pseudo-obstruction)
Loss of ileocecal valve

Contamination
Postinfection
Enteroenteric fistulas, gastrocolic fistulas

---

encephalopathy. Bilirubin is metabolized to urobilinogen; bile salts may be deconjugated (removing glycine and taurine) and dehydroxylated (cholic acid becomes deoxycholic acid, and chenodeoxycholic acid becomes lithocholic acid). This deconjugation and dehydroxylation renders bile acids more insoluble and less capable of forming micelles. Bacteria also can affect vitamin synthesis and metabolism. Vitamin B_{12} may be bound, thereby becoming unavailable for absorption (hence the abnormal Schilling test in bacterial overgrowth) and vitamin K and folic acid produced.

The normal flora also affect drugs and other ingested materials. Sulfasalazine, a drug used in ulcerative colitis, is unabsorbed in its native form. Intestinal bacteria, however, convert the substance into two moieties, a therapeutically active aminosalicylic acid and an inactive sulfapyridine. The sulfa drug succinylsulfathiazole is itself inactive, but is converted by intestinal bacteria to sulfathiazole, which is an active antimicrobial agent. Another example is cyclamate, unabsorbed and inert in its native form. Intestinal bacteria produce cyclohexylamine, a potential carcinogenic agent. Thus, bacteria can activate pro-drugs and produce carcinogens.

17. BACTERIAL OVERGROWTH SYNDROME

The bacterial overgrowth syndrome can result from any disease that interferes with the normal balance (ecosystem) of the small intestinal flora and brings about loss of gastric acidity; alteration in small bowel motility or lesions predisposing to luminal stasis; loss of the ileocecal valve; or overwhelming contamination of the intestinal lumen (Table 16).

The bacterial overgrowth syndrome gives rise to clinical abnormalities arising from the pathophysiological effects on the luminal contents and the mucosa. Bacteria can consume proteins and carbohydrates. In bacterial overgrowth there may be defective transport of sugars, possibly related to the toxic

TABLE 17.   Diagnosis of the bacterial overgrowth syndrome

Jejunal culture

Tests of bile salt deconjugation
^{14}C-glycocholate breath tests
In vitro deconjugation assessment

Tests of malassimilation
Vitamin B_{12} (Schilling test)
D-xylose, glucose, lactulose
H_2 breath tests

---

effect of deconjugated bile acids. Steatorrhea results from the deconjugation and dehydroxylation of bile acids; lithocholic acid is precipitated and free bile acids are reabsorbed passively, making them unavailable and incapable of performing micellar solubilization. There may also be mucosal damage. Fats, cholesterol and fat-soluble vitamins are malabsorbed. Vitamin B_{12} is also malabsorbed as a result of the binding and incorporation of this vitamin into the bacteria. Folate deficiency, however, is not a common occurrence in bacterial overgrowth; unlike vitamin B_{12}, folate synthesized by microorganisms in the small bowel is available for host absorption. In patients with small bowel bacterial overgrowth, serum folate levels tend to be high rather than low. The enteric bacteria also produce vitamin K, and patients with bacterial overgrowth who are on the anticoagulant warfarin may have difficulty in maintaining the desired level of anticoagulation. In addition to steatorrhea, patients with bacterial overgrowth frequently complain of watery diarrhea. Important mechanisms in producing this diarrhea include (1) disturbances of the intraluminal environment with deconjugated bile acids, and hydroxylated fatty and organic acids; and (2) direct changes in gut motility.

In some patients, symptoms of the primary disease predominate, and evidence of bacterial overgrowth may be found only on investigation. In others, the primary condition is symptomless, and the patient presents with a typical malabsorption syndrome due to bacterial overgrowth (Table 17). Once diagnosis of bacterial overgrowth is suspected a careful history should be performed to identify possible causes. Physical examination may be normal or may demonstrate signs related to specific nutrient deficiencies.

A small bowel biopsy is of value in excluding primary mucosal disease as the cause of the malabsorption. Histologic abnormalities of the jejunal mucosa are usually not seen in patients with bacterial overgrowth. The sine qua non for the diagnosis of bacterial overgrowth is a properly collected and appropriately cultured aspirate of the proximal small intestine. Specimens should be obtained under anaerobic conditions and quantitative colony counts determined. Generally, bacteria concentrations of greater than 10^5 organisms per mL are highly suggestive of bacterial overgrowth. Such methods are difficult and usually undertaken only in a research setting. Alternatively, one can attempt to demonstrate a metabolic effect of the bacterial overgrowth, such as intraluminal bile acid deconjugation by the bile acid or ^{14}C-glycocholate breath test. Cholylglycine-^{14}C (glycine-conjugated cholic acid with the radio-labeled ^{14}C on the glycine moiety) when ingested circulates normally in the enterohepatic circulation without deconjugation. Bacterial overgrowth within the small intestine splits the ^{14}C-labeled glycine moiety and subsequently oxidizes it to ^{14}C-labeled CO_2, which is absorbed in the intestine and exhaled. Excess $^{14}CO_2$ appears in the breath. The bile acid breath test cannot differentiate bacterial overgrowth from ileal damage or resection where excessive breath $^{14}CO_2$ production is due to bacterial deconjugation within the colon of unabsorbed ^{14}C-labeled glycocholate. This creates clinical difficulties, since bacterial overgrowth may be superimposed on ileal damage in such conditions as Crohn's disease.

Breath hydrogen analysis allows a distinct separation of metabolic activity of intestinal flora of the host, since no hydrogen production is known to occur in mammalian tissue. Excessive and early breath hydrogen production has been noted in patients with bacterial overgrowth following the oral administration of either 50 g of glucose or 10 g of lactulose.

Another hallmark of bacterial overgrowth is steatorrhea, detected by the 72-hour fecal fat collection.

The Schilling test also is abnormal. ^{57}Co-B$_{12}$ is given with intrinsic factor following a flushing dose of nonradioactive B$_{12}$ given parenterally to prevent tissue storage of the labeled vitamin. In healthy subjects, ^{57}Co-B$_{12}$ combines with intrinsic factor and is absorbed and >8% excreted in the urine within 24 hours. In patients with bacterial overgrowth, the bacteria combine with or destroy intrinsic factor, the vitamin or both, causing decreased vitamin B$_{12}$ absorption. Following treatment with antibiotics the B$_{12}$ absorption returns to normal.

Treatment of bacterial overgrowth involves removing the cause, if possible. The addition of a broad-spectrum antibiotic (tetracycline 250 mg q.i.d., often accompanied by metronidazole 250 mg q.i.d., for 10 days) will often induce a remission for many months. If the cause cannot be eliminated and symptoms recur, good results can be achieved with intermittent use of antibiotics (e.g., one day a week, or one week out of every six).

18. PROTEIN-LOSING ENTEROPATHY

Protein-losing enteropathy describes a wide range of gastrointestinal disorders that are associated with an excessive loss of plasma protein into the gut lumen. Normal daily enteric loss of plasma protein corresponds to less than 1–2% of the plasma pool. The route of plasma protein loss across the normal mucosa is not well defined. It is likely that rapid shedding of epithelial cells from the mucosal surface is accompanied by loss of plasma proteins from the lamina propria at the site of cell extrusion.

In virtually any small intestinal disease, excessive transmural loss of plasma proteins may result from several mechanisms: in mucosal disease without ulceration but with increased permeability; in mucosal disease with erosion or ulceration (loss of inflammatory exudate that contains protein occurs); and in lymphatic obstruction with direct leakage of intestinal lymph from obstructed lacteals. Protein-losing enteropathy may also occur as a result of colonic inflammation, ischemia or tumor. Adaptive changes in endogenous synthesis of individual plasma proteins may compensate partially for excessive enteric loss.

Clinically, albumin loss may be manifested by dependent edema. A depression of the levels of thyroid and cortisol binding proteins will lower the total plasma level of these hormones, although normal levels of free hormone will maintain normal hormone function. Excessive enteric loss of plasma proteins other than albumin rarely leads to clinical problems; secondary hypogammaglobulinemia in these patients does not predispose them to infection, and the loss of blood clotting factors is rarely sufficient to impair hemostasis.

Patients with protein-losing enteropathy due to lymphatic obstruction, however, lose not only albumin and other plasma proteins but also intestinal lymph, with loss of long-chain triglycerides, fat-soluble vitamins and small lymphocytes.

Protein-losing enteropathy is considered in patients who exhibit hypoproteinemia and in whom other causes for hypoproteinemia (e.g., proteinuria, protein malnutrition and liver disease) are excluded. Fecal protein loss can then be quantitated using ^{51}Cr-labeled albumin or α_1-antitrypsin clearance into stool.

Management of protein-losing enteropathy involves the appropriate treatment of the disease(s) causing the protein loss. Enteral or parenteral feeding can be used to improve nutrition while the underlying disease is being treated. Enteric protein loss in patients with intestinal lymphangiectasia usually decreases with a low-fat diet. The normal absorption of long-chain triglycerides stimulates intestinal lymph flow; in their absence there is a decrease in the pressure within intestinal lymphatic vessels and hence a diminished loss of lymph into the lumen. Medium-chain triglycerides, which do not require intestinal lymphatic transport, can be substituted for the long-chain triglycerides and further decrease intestinal lymphatic pressure, with subsequent reduction in enteric lymph and protein loss.

19. MECKEL'S DIVERTICULUM

Meckel's diverticulum, an omphalomesenteric duct remnant, is a congenital outpouching usually located in the distal 100 cm of the ileum. Such diverticula are present in 1–3% of the general population. Of these, 30–40% are asymptomatic. Complications of Meckel's diverticulum include hemorrhage, intestinal obstruction, diverticulitis, umbilical discharge, perforation and peritonitis. Bleeding is the most common complication, resulting from ulceration of the ileal mucosa adjacent to ectopic gastric mucosa located within the diverticulum. (However, in the patients with a Meckel's diverticulum but without ectopic gastric mucosa, bleeding does not usually occur.) This bleeding is often painless and is usually encountered in children and young adults. Meckel's diverticulum accounts for nearly 50% of all lower gastrointestinal bleeding in children. Technetium-99m pertechnetate is normally taken by the ectopic gastric mucosa, providing the basis for the Meckel scan. Since only 60% of Meckel's diverticula contain ectopic gastric mucosa, false negative results occur. If the scan is positive, increased sensitivity can be achieved by repeating the scan after a short course of an H_2-RA: the H_2-RA releases acid secretion by the ectopic parietal cells in the Meckel's diverticulum and may thereby convert a positive into a negative scan.

20. CARCINOID SYNDROME

Over 90% of carcinoid tumors originate in the gastrointestinal tract. The most frequent sites are the appendix, terminal ileum and rectum. In general, non-metastasized carcinoid tumors are asymptomatic. The carcinoid syndrome is associated only with carcinoid tumors that have metastasized extensively to the liver or are extraintestinal (e.g., lung tumors). Metastasis is infrequent in carcinoids of the appendix, but is common in extra-appendiceal carcinoids.

Although carcinoid tumors differ in their ability to produce and store 5-hydroxytryptamine (5-HT), the excessive production of this substance and its metabolite 5-hydroxyindoleacetic acid (5-HIAA) remains their most characteristic chemical abnormality. Production of this hormone (as well as histamine, catecholamines, kinase and prostaglandins) causes the majority of symptoms. The symptom complex comprises diarrhea, flushing, wheezing, cluster headache, valvular heart disease (particularly pulmonary stenosis) and a pellagra-like skin rash. The carcinoid syndrome can be suspected clinically and confirmed biochemically by the demonstration of increased urinary 5-HIAA or platelet 5-HT.

Once the carcinoid syndrome is apparent, cure is usually impossible, since the tumor has metastasized by this time. Nevertheless, the intestinal origin of the tumor should be removed if it is causing obstruction. Serotonin antagonists (e.g., methysergide and cyproheptadine) can sometimes reduce symptoms. The somatostatin analogue octreotide may prove to be very effective in reducing the patient's symptoms; interferon may also prove to be useful. It is prudent to delay initiation of chemotherapy or radiation in the early metastatic stage of the disease, since the course is often indolent and patients survive many years with diffuse metastatic disease.

21. WHIPPLE'S DISEASE

Whipple's disease characteristically occurs in middle-aged men, who present with weight loss, fever, abdominal pain, arthralgias and intestinal symptoms of diarrhea and malabsorption. Small bowel biopsy characteristically demonstrates PAS-positive macrophages and bacilliform bodies plus an enteropathy with villous atrophy. Treatment improves the fever and joint symptoms within a few days; the diarrhea and malabsorption disappear within two to four weeks. Because some patients with Whipple's disease may develop CNS involvement with the recently identified organism, trimethoprim-sulfamethoxazole antibiotics are recommended; treatment is continued for one year. Relapses may occur up to one or two years later and require repeat therapy.

22. IDIOPATHIC INTESTINAL PSEUDO-OBSTRUCTION

Idiopathic intestinal pseudo-obstruction is a disease of the muscular layer or of the enteric nervous system of the intestine. The myogenic form of idiopathic intestinal pseudo-obstruction is an autosomal dominant disease characterized by thinning of the intestinal musculature due to degeneration, fibrosis, malaligned smooth fibers and abnormal contractile filaments. All parts of the intestinal tract may be involved, but usually the small intestine, esophagus and colon are the most severely affected.

The neurogenic form of this disease is characterized by abnormal neuronal and glial cells. The damage may be in the spinal cord or in the splanchnic ganglia. When the splanchnic ganglia are involved, intranuclear inclusion bodies can be identified. The condition is characterized by abnormal systemic neural function, with an inappropriate blood pressure response to phenylephrine,

Valsalva's maneuver, or achieving the upright posture. There is a lack of sweating on warming of the skin, pupillary denervation hypersensitivity, and lack of intestinal spike activity after small intestinal distention.

Treatment of both the myogenic and neurogenic forms of idiopathic intestinal pseudo-obstruction is generally unsuccessful. Various promotility agents have been tried with only transient success. The somatostatin analogue octreotide may be useful in some patients. Associated bacterial overgrowth may worsen bloating and diarrhea, and should be treated with antibiotics. Surgery only aggravates the disorder and provides long intervals of severe ileus. Home parenteral nutrition may be the only alternative to maintain the patient's nutritional status, reduce the frequency and severity of the associated intestinal complaints, and improve the quality of the patient's life.

23. SMALL INTESTINAL VASCULAR DISORDERS

23.1 Acute Mesenteric Ischemia

The major causes of acute mesenteric ischemia are embolic obstruction thrombosis of the superior mesenteric artery (SMA), mesenteric venous thrombosis and nonocclusive ischemia. The congenital hypercoagulable states due to protein C or S antithrombin III deficiency can also cause thrombosis of the superior mesenteric vein. Embolic obstruction of the superior mesenteric artery is usually associated with cardiac arrhythmias, valvular disease, recent myocardial infarction or mycotic aneurysm. When an embolus lodges at the origin of the superior mesenteric artery, the entire small bowel and proximal colon are affected. Mesenteric venous thrombosis usually involves the superior mesenteric vein or its branches and the portal vein. It can be "primary" or "secondary" to a variety of hypercoagulable states (e.g., polycythemia rubra vera, carcinomatosis, oral contraception); to intra-abdominal sepsis (e.g., cholangitis, diverticular abscess); or to a condition in which blood flow is impaired (e.g., cardiogenic shock).

Nonocclusive bowel ischemia is the most common and lethal form of intestinal vascular insufficiency, accounting for at least 50% of all cases, with a mortality rate approaching 100%. It is commonly associated with reduced cardiac output, intra-abdominal sepsis and advanced malignant neoplasms. Digitalis constricts the splanchnic circulation and may aggravate or even precipitate mesenteric ischemia.

The typical patient is over 50 years of age, with arteriosclerotic or valvular heart disease, poorly controlled long-standing congestive heart failure, hypotension, recent myocardial infarction or cardiac arrhythmias. Abdominal pain is characteristically periumbilical and crampy. In the early stages, physical signs are often minimal. The abdomen is soft, sometimes slightly distended, with mild tenderness on palpation. Abdominal pain of any degree of severity associated with minimal abdominal findings and a high WBC (often over 20,000/mm^2) is an important early clue to the correct diagnosis. Signs of advanced ischemia include nausea, vomiting, peritoneal irritation, leukocytosis and a progressive metabolic acidosis. In a minority, unexplained abdominal distention or gastrointestinal bleeding, or the rapid onset of confusion and acidosis in an elderly patient, may be the first manifestation of small bowel ischemia.

Initial resuscitation is directed at correcting the predisposing or precipitating cause(s). Restoration of cardiac output with IV fluid is paramount. Digitalis, diuretics and vasoconstrictors should be discontinued if possible. Plain radiographs, ultrasound or CT scans as appropriate should exclude other radiologically diagnosable causes of acute abdominal pain. After volume repletion, the key step in the management of acute mesenteric ischemia is abdominal angiography. Remember that angiography in a hypovolemic or hypotensive patient frequently shows mesenteric vasoconstriction; for such patients the technique loses its usefulness as a diagnostic tool. Also, angiography in a volume-depleted patient may precipitate renal failure. If the angiogram is normal, the patient should be carefully observed, and a diagnostic laparotomy performed only if peritoneal signs develop. If the angiogram shows a minor arterial occlusion and clinically there is no peritoneal irritation, papaverine can be infused into the superior mesenteric artery through the catheter used for angiography at a rate of 60 mg/hour. (The role of angioplasty or other angiographic techniques remains unproven.) If peritoneal signs occur at any time, a laparotomy with resection of the ischemic segment is indicated. If the angiogram shows a major obstruction at the origin of the superior mesenteric artery, laparotomy should be carried out immediately. An embolus can usually be easily removed, while thrombotic obstruction requires a bypass graft from the aorta to an area of the artery distal to the site of obstruction. After revascularization, any nonviable bowel should be resected. It is advisable to save all bowel that may be viable and to re-explore the patient 24 hours later. The decision to perform a "second look" operation is made at the initial laparotomy and should not be changed on the basis of a favorable postoperative course. Since acute occlusion of the superior mesenteric artery is associated with prolonged vasospasm, the artery should be perfused with papaverine for 24 hours postoperatively.

If nonocclusive splanchnic vasoconstriction is present, intra-arterial papaverine infusion should be started. If, in spite of the infusion, abdominal pain persists and signs of peritoneal irritation appear, a laparotomy must be performed without delay.

Venous thrombosis is characterized on the angiogram by a prolonged arterial phase and a lack of opacity in the venous system. If a firm diagnosis of venous thrombosis has been made, anticoagulants are appropriate. However, if the patient develops peritoneal signs, immediate laparotomy and resection are indicated.

This systemic approach to the management of ischemia originating in the superior mesenteric artery results in earlier diagnosis and avoidance of surgery. The overall mortality rate has been reduced to about 50%; 90% of the patients who have no peritoneal signs at the time of angiography survive.

23.2 Chronic Mesenteric Ischemia

This uncommon condition occurs in elderly patients with partial occlusion of at least two of the three principal mesenteric vessels (the celiac axis and the superior and inferior mesenteric arteries). Epigastric or periumbilical abdominal pain beginning after a meal and lasting for one to three hours ("*intestinal angina*") is the most characteristic clinical feature, although it is not often elicited. The pain may lead to a reduction in food intake (sitophobia) and secondarily a significant loss of weight. Bloating, flatulence and diarrhea are common, and steatorrhea is present in 50% of patients. This is the case because chronic mesenteric ischemia can cause mucosal damage. The physical examination is usually not diagnostic. A systolic abdominal bruit is present in 50% of patients but is not pathognomonic. (Epigastric bruits are common in normal persons.) Patients in whom the syndrome is suspected, and who have no other demonstrable abnormality to explain their symptoms, should have abdominal angiography. If angiography shows greater than 90% occlusion of at least two vessels, aorto-SMA graft is the procedure of choice. The mortality rate for this procedure is less than 10% and the majority of patients will be relieved of their postprandial intestinal angina. It is important to identify and to treat chronic mesenteric ischemia because of the high risk of thrombosis of the SMA.

24. SMALL BOWEL TUMORS

24.1 Benign Small Bowel Tumors

Adenomas, leiomyomas and lipomas are the three most frequently discovered primary tumors of the small intestine. Hamartomas, fibromas, angiomas and neurogenic tumors are much less common. As a general rule, benign tumors are least common in the duodenum and increase in frequency toward the ileum. Benign tumors often remain asymptomatic and are usually found incidentally.

Symptomatic benign tumors present primarily with obstructive features, giving rise to intermittent colicky abdominal pain or complete bowel obstruction. Bleeding may occur, particularly from leiomyomas that ulcerate central-ly. Intussusception occurs with polypoid distal lesions.

24.2 Malignant Neoplasms of the Small Intestine

Adenocarcinomas, lymphomas, leiomyosarcomas and carcinoids are the most common primary small bowel malignant tumors. Metastatic cancer to the small intestine occurs rarely in patients with melanoma, breast cancer and lung cancer. Primary adenocarcinomas occur in the duodenal and proximal jejunum as annular lesions, narrowing the lumen and presenting with the signs and symptoms of obstruction. Leiomyosarcomas are evenly distributed along the small bowel. Symptoms are similar to those of adenocarcinoma – i.e., crampy abdominal pain and bleeding. Lymphoma of the small bowel must be carefully evaluated to determine whether the tumor has originated in the small intestine (primary lymphoma) or whether the small bowel is involved by a dif-fuse systemic lymphoma. Primary lymphoma of the small intestine is usually a histiocytic lymphoma. The lymphoma is most often proximal and presents with abdominal pain, weight loss, malabsorption, perforation and anemia. There is an increased incidence of primary lymphoma in patients with long-standing celiac disease or immunodeficiency states and in renal transplant patients receiving chronic immunosuppressive therapy.

A specific form of malignant lymphoma called immunoproliferative small intestinal disease occurs in people of Mediterranean descent. It is character-ized by proliferation of mucosal B cells and has a high incidence of α-heavy chain paraproteinemia. It typically involves the duodenum and proximal jejunum, presenting with diarrhea and malabsorption.

OBJECTIVES

1. Discuss the intestinal fluid and electrolyte transport mechanisms.
2. Explain the normal digestion and absorption processes of fat, protein and glucose.
3. Describe the normal pathway of vitamin B_{12}, folate and iron absorption.
4. Locate the absorption sites of Fe, folate and B_{12}.
5. Utilize proper malabsorption screens in patients with chronic diarrhea.
6. Discuss normal enterohepatic circulation of bile acids.
7. Discuss normal assimilation of fat-soluble vitamins (A, D, E and K).

Diarrhea
1. Define diarrhea.
2. Classify the causes of diarrhea.
3. Discuss the pathogenic mechanisms of diarrhea.

4. Review diarrhea as altered fluid and electrolyte transport.
5. Differentiate between large and small bowel diarrhea.
6. Discuss diagnostic plans in patients with chronic diarrhea.
7. List conditions that are associated with typical small bowel lesions on biopsy.
8. List the complications of celiac disease.
9. List extraintestinal manifestations of celiac disease.
10. Outline the diagnosis and dietary management of celiac disease.
11. Give the differential diagnosis of "unresponsive" sprue.
12. Discuss the immunologic basis of celiac disease.
13. Recognize the principal manifestation of the carcinoid syndrome.
14. Discuss pharmacologic agents used in the carcinoid syndrome.
15. List biochemical tests used in diagnosing the carcinoid syndrome.
16. Discuss the management of traveler's diarrhea.
17. List the common causes of traveler's diarrhea.
18. Discuss the mechanisms of E. coli–induced diarrhea.
19. List the infectious causes of diarrhea and their management.
20. Discuss the use and mechanisms of antidiarrheal agents.
21. Give the differential diagnosis of abnormal terminal ileum.
22. Describe the radiographic features of small bowel obstruction.
23. Outline the etiology of vitamin B_{12} deficiency with the bacterial overgrowth syndrome.
24. List the underlying conditions associated with bacterial overgrowth.
25. Discuss the mechanisms of steatorrhea associated with the bacterial overgrowth syndrome.
26. Recognize the clinical presentations of the bacterial overgrowth syndrome.
27. Outline the management of the bacterial overgrowth syndrome.
28. Utilize appropriate diagnostic tests for the bacterial overgrowth syndrome.
29. Recognize complications of the short bowel syndrome and their mechanisms.
30. Discuss the adaptive mechanisms of the small bowel following resection.
31. Discuss the management of the short bowel syndrome.
32. Give the indications for the use of medium-chain triglycerides.
33. Outline the diagnosis and treatment of giardiasis.
34. Recognize the clinical presentations and treatment of amebiasis.
35. Describe typical features of Whipple's disease.
36. List the causes of protein-losing enteropathy.
37. List the possible mechanisms of diarrhea in patients with diabetes mellitus.

38. List the possible mechanisms of diarrhea in the Zollinger-Ellison syndrome.
39. List mechanisms of diarrhea following gastric surgery.
40. Discuss diagnostic tests for lactase deficiency/lactose intolerance.
41. List conditions associated with protein-losing enteropathy.
42. Recognize the features of intestinal lymphangiectasia and outline its treatment.

Skills

1. Give the indications for gastroscopy, small bowel biopsy, sigmoidoscopy and colonoscopy.
2. Arrange the proper sequences of GI diagnostic procedures, including radiographic examination (ultrasound, CT scan), and the appropriate order of investigational tests.
3. Utilize proper tests – including malabsorption screen, ^{14}C breath test, H_2 breath test, Schilling test, 72-hour stool collection, x-ray, small bowel biopsy and jejunal aspiration – in the investigation of chronic diarrhea.

8

Ischemic Disease of the Intestine

P.H. MacDonald and I.T. Beck

1. INTRODUCTION

Intestinal ischemia occurs when, as a result of inadequate systemic blood flow or local vascular abnormalities, the metabolic demand of the tissue supersedes the delivery of oxygen. In older patients inadequate vascular supply is frequent, and thus ischemic bowel disease occurs most often in the elderly. It may also be seen in young patients suffering from vascular abnormalities – e.g., collagen diseases, vasculitis, diabetes – or in those taking vasoconstrictor drugs. Clinical manifestations are varied, depending on the site of the vascular occlusion and the extent of the bowel necrosis.

2. CLASSIFICATION OF INTESTINAL ISCHEMIA

Many clinicians broadly classify intestinal ischemia into acute or chronic disease. However, because certain acute events may change to a chronic condition, a clear-cut classification of ischemic bowel disease using this two-category system is not always applicable. Since the extent of intestinal ischemia and the pathological consequences depend on the size and the location of the occluded or hypoperfused intestinal blood vessel(s), we find it useful to classify ischemic bowel disease according to the size and type of the vessel(s) that are hypoperfused or occluded (Figure 1). Accordingly, intestinal ischemia may result from occlusion/hypoperfusion of a large mesenteric vessel (mesenteric artery or vein) or from occlusion/hypoperfusion of smaller intramural intestinal vessels. In each of these situations the resultant intestinal ischemia may be acute or chronic. In addition, it is important to point out that vessel occlusion/hypoperfusion may be the result of a mechanical intralumi-

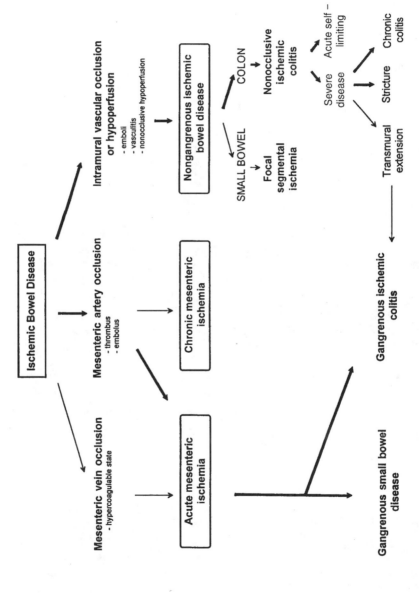

FIGURE 1. Classification of ischemic bowel disease. The more common pathways are indicated by heavier arrows.

nal obstruction (i.e., embolus or thrombus) or the result of decreased blood flow due to vasospasm, increased blood viscosity, hypotension or other similar conditions. The latter is referred to as *nonocclusive ischemia*. Therefore, the etiology of vessel occlusion/hypoperfusion may be the basis for subclassification of ischemic bowel disease. A clinically important further classification is whether the ischemia-induced necrosis is transmural (*gangrenous ischemia*) leading to peritonitis, or remains intramural (*nongangrenous ischemia*) resulting in localized disease. Figure 1 attempts to combine these different aspects of subdivision in a comprehensive classification.

3. MESENTERIC VASCULATURE

3.1 Anatomy

The blood flow to the splanchnic organs is derived from three main arterial trunks: the celiac, the superior mesenteric artery and the inferior mesenteric artery. The celiac artery supplies blood to the foregut (stomach and duodenum), the superior mesenteric artery supplies blood to the midgut (duodenum to transverse colon), and the inferior mesenteric artery is responsible for blood to the hindgut (transverse colon to the rectum). Each of these three arterial trunks supplies blood flow to its specific section of the gastrointestinal tract through a vast arcade network. This arcade system is an effective collateral circulation and is generally protective against ischemia, since blood can reach a specific segment of gut via more than one route. As shown in Figure 2, additional vascular protection is obtained from vascular connections between the three arterial systems. Communication between the celiac system and the superior mesenteric system generally occurs via the superior pancreaticoduodenal and the inferior pancreaticoduodenal arteries. The superior mesenteric and inferior mesenteric systems are joined by the arch of Riolan and the marginal artery of Drummond, vessels that connect the middle colic artery (a branch of the superior mesenteric artery) and the left colic artery (a branch of the inferior mesenteric artery). In addition, communication also exists between the inferior mesenteric artery and branches of the internal iliac arteries via the rectum. The caliber of these collateral connections varies considerably depending on the existence of vascular disease, but it is important to realize that in chronic states of vascular insufficiency, blood flow to an individual system can be maintained through these collateral connections even when an arterial trunk is completely obstructed. It is not uncommon to find one or even two arterial trunks completely occluded in the asymptomatic patient with chronic vascular disease. In fact, there are reports of occlusion of all three trunks in patients who are still maintaining their splanchnic circulation. However, in up to 30% of people, the collateral connections between the superior

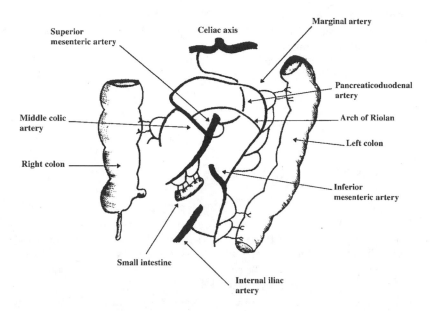

FIGURE 2.   Schematic representation of splanchnic circulation.

and inferior mesenteric arteries, via the arch of Riolan and the marginal artery of Drummond, can be weak or nonexistent, making the area of the splenic flexure particularly vulnerable to acute ischemia. This region of poor collateral circulation is often referred to as a "watershed area."

3.2 Physiology of Splanchnic Blood Flow

The mesenteric circulation receives approximately 30% of the cardiac output. Mesenteric blood flow is less in the fasting state and is increased with feeding. Blood flow through the celiac and superior mesenteric trunks is about equal (approximately 700 mL/min in the adult) and is twice the blood flow through the inferior mesenteric trunk. Blood flow distribution within the gut wall is not uniform, and it varies between the mucosa and the muscularis. The mucosa has the highest metabolic rate and thus it receives about 70% of the mesenteric blood flow. If one compares gut segments of equal weight, the small bowel receives the most blood, followed by the colon and then the stomach.

Much has been written on the control of gastrointestinal blood flow. Many factors are involved. A few important highlights of mesenteric vascular resistance will be discussed here. Vascular resistance is proportional to $1/r^4$ (where r = the radius of the vessel). Thus the smaller the artery, the greater its ability to effect vascular resistance. It is known that the majority of blood flow control occurs at the level of the arterioles, the so-called resistance vessels. Very little control of blood flow occurs at the level of the large arterial trunks. In fact, the diameter of these large arterial trunks can be compromised by 75% before blood flow is reduced. Additional control of blood flow occurs at the level of the precapillary sphincter. In the fasting state only one-fifth of capillary beds are open, leaving a tremendous reserve to meet increased metabolic demands.

Among the most important control mechanisms of splanchnic blood flow are the sympathetic nervous system, humoral factors and local factors. The sympathetic nervous system through α-adrenergic receptors plays an important role in maintaining the basal vascular tone and in mediating vasoconstriction. Beta-adrenergic activity appears to mediate vasodilation, and it appears that the antrum of the stomach may be particularly rich in these β receptors. Humoral factors involved in the regulation of GI blood flow include catecholamines, the renin-angiotensin system and vasopressin. These humoral systems may play a particularly important role in shock states and in some patients may play a role in the pathogenesis of nonocclusive ischemia. Local factors appear to be mainly involved in the matching of tissue blood flow to the metabolic demand. An increased metabolic rate may produce a decreased pO_2, increased pCO_2 and an increased level of adenosine, each of which can mediate a hyperemic response.

More recent and exciting research has identified the vascular endothelium as a source for potent vasoactive substances, such as nitric oxide (vasodilator) and endothelin (vasoconstrictor). Although these endothelial-derived substances may act systemically, it would appear that their major effect is local in a paracrine hormonal fashion. Although these vasoactive substances have the potential to dramatically alter mesenteric blood flow, their exact role in health and disease remains to be elucidated.

The integration of these control systems and their alteration by factors such as vascular disease, motor activity, intraluminal pressure and pharmaceuticals remains poorly understood. The key to our understanding and successful treatment of intestinal ischemia lies in a better knowledge of this physiology.

3.3 Pathophysiology of Intestinal Ischemia

Intestinal ischemia occurs when the metabolic demand of the tissue supersedes the oxygen delivery. Obviously, many factors can be involved in this mismatch of oxygen need and demand. These include the general hemodynamic state, the degree of atherosclerosis, extent of collateral circulation, neurogenic/humoral/local control mechanisms of vascular resistance and abnormal products of cellular metabolism before and after reperfusion of an ischemic segment. Acute occlusion/hypoperfusion of a large mesenteric vessel usually results in transmural (gangrenous) ischemia of the small bowel and/or colon. On the other hand, acute occlusion of the intramural vessel(s) usually results in intramural (nongangrenous) ischemia. However, there are exceptions in both cases, depending on the severity of occlusion/hypoperfusion. As previously mentioned, the mucosa is the most metabolically active gut wall tissue layer and thus it is first tissue layer to demonstrate signs of ischemia. The earliest form of intestinal ischemia produces changes at the tip of the intestinal villi. With ongoing ischemia ultrastructural changes begin within 10 minutes and cellular damage is extensive by 30 minutes. Sloughing of the villi tips in the small bowel and the superficial mucosal layer of the colon is followed by edema, submucosal hemorrhage and eventual transmural necrosis.

The intestinal response to ischemia is first characterized by a hypermotility state. It is this intense motor activity that results in the patient experiencing severe pain, even though the ischemic damage may be limited to the mucosa at this stage. As the ischemia progresses, motor activity will cease and gut mucosal permeability will increase, leading to an increase in bacterial translocation. With transmural extension of the ischemia, the patient will develop visceral and parietal inflammation resulting in peritonitis.

An important factor often responsible for or aggravating intestinal ischemia is the phenomenon of vasospasm. It has been well demonstrated that both occlusive and nonocclusive forms of arterial ischemia can result in prolonged vasospasm, even after the occlusion has been removed or the perfusion pressure restored. This vasospasm may persist for several hours, resulting in prolonged ischemia. The mechanism responsible for this vasospasm is not clearly defined, but there is preliminary evidence that the potent vasoconstrictor endothelin may be involved. To date, many of the interventional techniques used in the treatment of acute mesenteric ischemia have been directed at counteracting this vasospasm.

A second factor that may be responsible for accentuating ischemic damage is reperfusion injury. This phenomenon has been well demonstrated in the laboratory, where it has been shown to be responsible for a greater degree of cellular damage than that brought about during the actual ischemic period. Parks and Granger have shown in an animal model that the injury after one hour of ischemia and three hours of reperfusion is more severe than that observed after four hours of continuous ischemia. The mechanism responsible for this reperfusion injury appears to be related to the release of harmful reactive oxygen metabolites, which are thought to be released from adhering polymorphonuclear leukocytes. It is not known what role ischemia reperfusion injury plays in humans with occlusive and nonocclusive disease.

4. ACUTE MESENTERIC ARTERIAL OCCLUSION

4.1 Clinical Presentation

Several intra-abdominal disease processes can present in a fashion identical to that of mesenteric ischemia; thus, the key to diagnosis lies in a high index of suspicion. Patients with advanced ischemia present with diffuse peritonitis, shock and severe metabolic derangements. In these patients it is clear that a catastrophic event has occurred. However, ischemia is only one of a few possible diagnoses. In most situations these patients will come to surgery, and in those where the diagnosis was not confirmed preoperatively, the diagnosis will become obvious at the time of surgery. Often these patients can not be salvaged; the mortality is reported to be between 70 and 90%. It must be stressed that the patient with early ischemia is far more challenging to diagnose. Given that the mortality rate is extremely high in advanced ischemia, the best chance of successfully treating a patient with this condition depends on early diagnosis and treatment.

The typical patient is usually over 50 years of age and often has a history of cardiac and peripheral vascular disease. In the early stage of ischemia the patient complains of severe abdominal pain (due to vasospasm) in the absence of peritoneal findings. This scenario has been described by clinicians as "pain out of proportion to the physical findings." Other nonspecific symptoms such as nausea, vomiting and altered bowel habit may be present, but they are usually not particularly helpful in the diagnosis.

4.2 Investigation

4.2.1 LABORATORY

Unfortunately, there is no serum marker that can reliably predict early intestinal ischemia. Many studies have attempted to identify such a biochemical marker. Creatinine kinase, alkaline phosphatase, lactate dehydrogenase, diamine oxidase and inorganic phosphate are among those biochemical markers that have been examined. Although all of these will eventually become altered with advanced disease, their alteration with early ischemia is too varied to provide any clinical usefulness.

Although biochemical changes with advanced intestinal ischemia are nonspecific, one can expect to find a leukocytosis. Due to third-space loss of fluid into the abdomen, electrolyte and renal function abnormalities secondary to dehydration are also often seen. Hyperamylasemia may occur secondary to amylase leaking from the infarcted bowel into the abdominal cavity, which may then enter the systemic circulation. In some situations this hyperamylasemia can be misinterpreted as an indication of pancreatitis. Finally, in advanced ischemia blood gas analysis will usually show a metabolic acidosis.

4.2.2 *RADIOLOGICAL*

Initial radiological investigations are aimed at ruling out other causes of abdominal pain and peritonitis. All patients should have an upright and supine plain film of the abdomen. Although these films may support a diagnosis of ischemia, as indicated by bowel wall thickening and "thumb-printing," the main purpose of the films is to rule out visceral perforation or bowel obstruction. In many centers CT scan is being used as a first-line investigation in patients with abdominal pain. Several markers of intestinal ischemia have now been described by radiologists with expertise in CT scans. These include bowel wall thickening, mucosal edema, pneumatosis and mesenteric and portal vein gas. Using large injections of peripheral venous contrast, mesenteric arterial and venous occlusion can now also be identified in some patients. Of course, many of these findings are not specific, and thus we do not at present advocate the CT scan as a diagnostic test for intestinal ischemia. However, the CT scan can play a role in ruling out other intra-abdominal disease processes. For example, differentiating acute pancreatitis from abdominal ischemia on clinical grounds can sometimes be difficult. Both can present with hyperamylasemia and/or peritonitis. This is one situation where an abdominal CT scan may be useful to rule out retroperitoneal inflammation.

Ultrasonography combined with Doppler assessment of blood flow in the splanchnic arterial and venous system is now being used in some centers to screen for mesenteric ischemia. Our personal experience with this technique is limited and the exact role this technique will play is not clearly defined. There is experimental evidence, using a rabbit model of ischemia, that magnetic resonance (MR) scanning may also be of significant use in the diagnosis of mesenteric ischemia. Certainly, both arterial and venous abnormalities as well as the extent of the collateral circulation can be identified in some patients using MR technology; however, further clinical experience is required before this technique can be completely evaluated.

Angiography remains the gold standard in the diagnosis of mesenteric ischemia (Figure 3), and as will be discussed, it may play a significant role in the treatment of such patients. It is our belief that all patients with suspected mesenteric intestinal ischemia should undergo angiography to confirm the diagnosis and plan treatment. Wherever possible this approach should include even those patients presenting with peritonitis. Often there is a tendency to take patients with peritonitis straight to the operating room without perform-

FIGURE 3.   Mesenteric arteriogram (lateral view). In this patient the origin of the superior mesenteric artery (SMA) is completely thrombosed and is barely visible (arrow). Normally the SMA comes off the aorta at an oblique angle and is easily visualized on a lateral film.

ing angiography. These patients need to be treated in an expedient fashion. However, the short delay to obtain an angiogram may prove to be beneficial. Not only will it identify those patients who may require embolectomy or vascular reconstruction, but it will also provide a means to treat vasospasm in the perioperative period. This type of treatment policy has two implications: First, in order for management to be effective, an invasive radiologist must be available at all times and a system must be in place that will allow the angiography suite to be functioning with a short lead time. Second, the physician must realize that an appreciable number of negative angiograms should be expected with this low angiography threshold.

4.3 Treatment

4.3.1 RESUSCITATION AND ASSESSMENT

It must be strongly stressed that if a diagnosis of mesenteric ischemia is being questioned, the subsequent investigation and management must proceed in an efficient and aggressive fashion if morbidity and mortality are to be reduced. Initial management of all patients consists of resuscitation. The degree of resuscitation required varies widely with the degree and extent of ischemia. Patients with early ischemia will require very little resuscitation, whereas those with infarcted intestine may require admission to a critical care unit for invasive monitoring. Insertion of a Swan-Ganz catheter with central pressure monitoring can be very useful in resuscitating the shocked patient with underlying cardiac disease. It must be kept in mind that in patients with extensive and advanced infarction, complete "stability" may never be obtained and thus investigation and treatment should proceed without extensive delay. However, ongoing patient "instability" is no doubt an ominous sign. As a general rule vasopressors to support blood pressure should be avoided, as they may further increase the degree of intestinal ischemia. The role of antibiotics is not clear-cut. Our policy is to administer broad-spectrum antibiotic coverage as soon as possible to those patients presenting with peritonitis. In those without peritonitis, antibiotics are used in the perioperative period, should surgery be required.

The treatment algorithm we recommend is outlined in Figure 4. Essentially, patients are divided into two groups: those with peritonitis and those without. Although all patients with peritonitis will require laparotomy, the exact treatment plan for both groups of patients will be dictated by the angiographic findings. Angiographic findings fall into four major categories:

Thrombotic occlusion. This finding is usually identified with an aortic flush of contrast dye; however, it can sometimes be difficult to differentiate from a proximal arterial embolus. The other pitfall with this finding is that sometimes

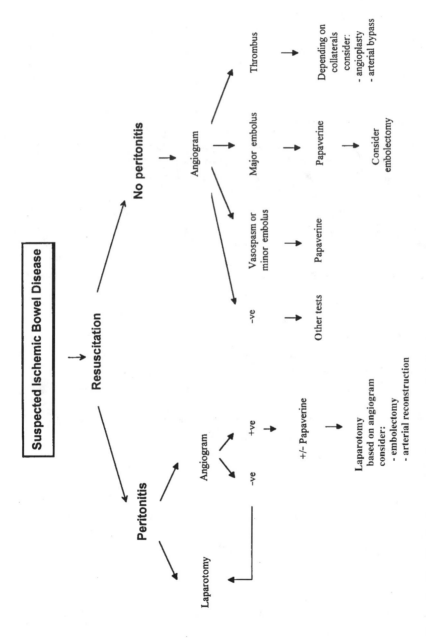

FIGURE 4. Algorithm for the treatment of acute mesenteric ischemia.

it represents a chronic obstruction that is not necessarily related to the patient's present symptoms and findings. In most cases, these patients require arterial reconstruction, although the final treatment plan will be based on the exact vascular anatomy and degree of collateral circulation. Patients with peritonitis will almost always require a bowel resection. Perioperative papaverine infusion in these patients may indeed be useful; however, depending on the site of vascular obstruction, it may not be possible to secure a catheter for infusion.

Major embolus. Major emboli are usually located in the proximal portion of the superior mesenteric artery. The majority of these patients should be referred to surgery for consideration of embolectomy regardless of the presence or lack of peritoneal findings. Papaverine infusion in the perioperative period should be used to reduce vasospasm-induced ischemia.

Minor embolus. These emboli are limited to the branches of the superior mesenteric artery or to that portion of the vessel distal to the origin of the ileocolic artery. Unless peritoneal signs are present, these patients should be managed with papaverine infusion and observation.

Vasospasm (nonocclusive ischemia). This finding may occur in response to a mechanical arterial obstruction; however, when it represents the sole finding it is diagnostic of nonocclusive ischemia. The recommended management is papaverine infusion.

4.3.2 *PAPAVERINE INFUSION*

Papaverine infusion has been recommended as a major component of the medical therapy for mesenteric ischemia. Although we support its use, it must be stressed that the efficacy has not been absolutely proven by proper clinical trials.

Papaverine is a smooth-muscle relaxant. Administered systemically it will nonspecifically dilate the vascular tree. However, since it is virtually completely metabolized by a single pass through the liver, selective administration into the mesenteric circulation results in very few systemic effects. This allows vasodilation in the mesenteric circulation to occur without a drop in the systemic blood pressure. Typically, papaverine is infused into the mesenteric circulation (usually the superior mesenteric artery) after angiographic-guided selective catheterization of an arterial trunk. Papaverine is dissolved in normal saline to a concentration of 1mg/mL, although a higher concentration can be used. Heparin should not be added to the solution, as it will crystallize. The infusion is started at 30 mg/hour and may be increased to 60 mg/hour. In most cases the papaverine infusion is maintained for 24 hours. The catheter is then flushed with normal saline for 30 minutes and the angiogram is then repeated. If vasospasm persists, the cycle should be repeated every 24 hours for a maximum of 5 days. During the papaverine infusion the patient's systemic vital signs must be monitored. A sudden drop in the blood pressure usually suggests that the catheter has slipped out of the mesenteric circulation into the aorta. A repeat angiogram at the bedside can be performed to confirm this. Generally, papaverine infusion is quite safe and major complications are usually related to the initial passage of the arterial catheter. Complications include injury to the femoral artery, dislodgement of atherosclerotic plaques with embolic accidents in the lower extremities and the formation of a false aneurysm after the catheter is removed.

4.3.3 SURGERY

The role of surgery is to evaluate the viability of ischemic bowel, to resect if necessary and if possible to alleviate or bypass a vascular obstruction. If at all possible the vascular surgery should be performed first so that its effect on intestinal viability can be assessed.

One of the most difficult decisions the surgeon has to make is to decide if the bowel injury is reversible or not. Subjective criteria such as the bowel wall color, the presence of peristalsis and the presence of palpable mesenteric pulses are often used. Unfortunately, these criteria can lead to an inaccurate assessment in over 50% of cases. This has led surgeons to adopt a second-look approach. With this approach only the most obviously infarcted gut is resected and any questionable bowel is left in situ. A second look within 24 hours is then used to decide on the necessity for further resection. More recently, several objective measurements have been employed in the assessment of bowel viability. These include fluorescence staining, laser Doppler flowmetry, surface oximetry and intramural pH measurements. At present, no single technology has been widely adopted, but as these techniques are further refined they may eventually play a valuable role in the assessment of intestinal viability.

A second difficult situation for the surgeon is the management of patients with near-total intestinal infarction. Even with resection, the mortality rate in this group of patients is very high, and survivors will be dependent on total parental nutrition indefinitely. In elderly patients with other underlying medical problems, many surgeons elect to close without resections. The approach in a younger patient with a catastrophic vascular accident tends to be more aggressive, particularly in the hope that with increasing advances in bowel transplantation, in some years the resected bowel can be replaced.

5. ACUTE MESENTERIC VENOUS OCCLUSION

Ischemia of mesenteric arterial origin is far more frequent than that of venous disease. It is now recognized that many reported cases of mesenteric vein thrombosis in actuality represented incorrectly diagnosed cases of nonocclusive ischemia. The true incidence of mesenteric vein thrombosis is quite low. Although the etiology of acute mesenteric vein thrombosis may be idiopathic, the thrombosis is usually secondary to another disease process. Conditions that predispose to mesenteric vein thrombosis are (1) severe intra-abdominal sepsis, (2) hypercoagulable state (i.e., polycythemia vera) and (3) portal venous stasis (secondary to portal hypertension associated with hepatic cirrhosis, or to extrinsic compression of the venous system secondary to a tumor mass).

Thrombosis of the superior or inferior mesenteric vein alone is usually not sufficient to produce intestinal ischemia. However, acute thrombosis in a large mesenteric vein has the potential to cause retrograde propagation of the clot up into the venous tributaries within the bowel wall. This resultant venous occlusion within the bowel wall will usually produce ischemia, possibly with infarction. In many cases of venous intestinal ischemia the thrombosis does not begin in a large mesenteric vein. In these situations it appears that the venous thrombosis begins primarily in the small venous intramural tributaries. In either case, if the venous thrombosis becomes extensive, arterial thrombosis may follow, making it very difficult to determine the exact etiology of the intestinal ischemia.

The clinical presentation of patients with venous intestinal ischemia is often similar if not identical to that of patients with acute mesenteric artery occlusion. Accordingly, the diagnosis is often made only at the time of surgery or by the pathologist who examines the resected specimen.

The treatment of this disease is generally surgical, with the infarcted segment of intestine being resected. The surgeon should be aware that the venous thrombosis may extend beyond the limits of the gross infarction. Since any residual thrombosis has the potential to propagate, the resection should include adjacent bowel and mesentery until all grossly involved thrombosed veins are removed. It has been shown that mortality from this disease can be reduced if patients are anticoagulated as soon as possible after surgery.

6. CHRONIC MESENTERIC ISCHEMIA

Because of the extensive collateral arterial network of the gut, chronic mesenteric ischemia is relatively uncommon. It is usually related to extensive mesenteric atherosclerosis. Patients classically present with postprandial abdominal pain, "fear of eating" and weight loss. However, most patients do not present with "classic" symptomatology and are frequently misdiagnosed for other diseases. Until patients with a high index of suspicion proceed to angiography, these patients may be treated for prolonged periods for suspected peptic ulcer, functional dyspepsia, irritable bowel syndrome, etc. Unfortunately, angiographic evidence of thrombosis of large vessels is not always diagnostic, as two or even three of the major arteries may be thrombosed in apparently asymptomatic patients. Once the diagnosis is clearly established, the treatment is surgical. Many surgical procedures have been described with various results. Endarterectomy and aortovisceral bypass have been employed. More recently balloon angioplasty has appeared to provide good results with a less invasive approach.

7. NONGANGRENOUS ISCHEMIC BOWEL DISEASE

7.1 Etiology
In contrast to mesenteric ischemia, where the cause of the disease is occlusion of major vessels, in nongangrenous ischemic bowel disease the hypo-oxygenation is caused by hypoperfusion of the gut wall microcirculation. Only occasionally is there secondary occlusion of intramural vessels. Many causes may precipitate this disorder. Hypoperfusion is most commonly caused by vascular diseases – e.g., collagen disease, vasculitis, diabetes, atherosclerosis – or by increased viscosity of the blood in sickle cell disease or polycythemia vera. Acute hypotension due to hemorrhage, myocardial infarct, congestive heart failure, sepsis or vasoconstricting drugs may precipitate local ischemia in patients who already have impaired local circulation. Because of an adequate collateral circulation, localization is usually segmental. The necrosis of the gut wall is rarely transmural, and as a result, peritonitis is a rare complication. In the small bowel nongangrenous ischemic bowel disease manifests as "focal segmental ischemia" and in the colon as "nongangrenous ischemic colitis." A list of the more common causes of nonocclusive ischemic bowel disease is provided in Table 1.

7.2 Focal Segmental Ischemia of the Small Intestine
Ischemia to short segments of the small bowel results in a variable clinical course that depends on the severity of the infarct. For short segment involvement there is usually appropriate collateral circulation, and thus the disease involves only the mucosa and submucosal tissues. Limited necrosis may heal completely. Ongoing repeated injury may cause chronic enteritis, almost indistinguishable from Crohn's disease. In some patients the necrotic ulcer may lead to late stricture formation. Occasionally the process may become transmural, resulting in peritonitis. Diagnosis is difficult, as the symptoms may be those of chronic recurrent abdominal pain, bowel obstruction or frank peritonitis. Unless there is complete spontaneous resolution, the treatment of strictures and persistent ulcers is usually surgical. The diagnosis is often made only on histology of the resected small bowel.

TABLE 1.   Causes of nonocclusive ischemic bowel disease

A. Acute diminution of intramural blood flow

1. Small vessel disease
Cholesterol embolus
Diabetes
Rheumatoid arthritis
Amyloidosis
Chronic radiation injury
Systemic vasculitis
Collagen diseases
Allergic granulomatosis
Behçet's syndrome

2. Nonocclusive hypoperfusion
Hypercoagulable states and increased viscosity
   Oral contraceptives
   Polycythemia vera
   Sickle cell disease
   Acute leukemia
   Antithrombin C disease
Shock
   Hemorrhage
   Hypovolemia
   Cardiopulmonary bypass
   Abdominal aortic reconstruction
   Sepsis
   Pancreatitis
   Anaphylaxis
   Cardiogenic shock
   Multiple organ dysfunction syndrome
Congestive heart failure
Portal hypertension
Medications
   Digitalis
   Diuretics
   Catecholamines
   Estrogens
   Nonsteroidal anti-inflammatory agents
   Neuroleptic agents
   Verapamil overdose
   Cocaine abuse
Long-distance running

(cont'd)

TABLE 1.   Causes of nonocclusive ischemic bowel disease (cont'd)

B. Increased demand on marginal blood flow

1. Increased motility
Mass lesions
   Carcinoma
   Diverticular disease
Obstruction

2. Increased intraluminal pressure
Obstruction
Fecal impaction
Colonoscopy
Barium enema

C. Idiopathic (spontaneous)

7.3 Nongangrenous Ischemic Colitis

7.3.1 *PATHOGENESIS*

There are two major forms of colonic ischemia: gangrenous (transmural) and nongangrenous colitis (disease contained within the colonic wall). These are in fact two different diseases, with different etiologies and clinical courses, and require different approaches to their management. Gangrenous ischemic colitis is caused by obstruction of the major mesenteric vessels and is discussed in Section 4 (see Figure 1). Occasionally, transmural gangrene may develop when nongangrenous ischemic colitis slowly progresses to transmural necrosis. The recognition and management of this complication of the originally nongangrenous disease is crucial, and as discussed below, depends on careful ongoing observation of the patient with nongangrenous ischemic colitis.

   In contrast to the rarity of nonocclusive ischemia of the small bowel is the relative frequency of local vascular hypoperfusion of the colon. The cause of this relative frequency may be related to the following factors: In comparison to the small intestine, the colon receives less blood, has fewer vascular collaterals, has susceptible "watershed areas" and possesses an ongoing forceful motor activity. Elevated intramural pressure during increased motility in patients with constipation, diverticular disease and cancer of the colon may lead to diminished gut wall blood flow. Similarly, distention with air during colonoscopy or barium enema may temporarily reduce blood flow to the colon. The large bowel also has a different neuroendocrine control. Evidence in our laboratory has indicated that the vessels of the canine colon respond more vigorously to hypotension than those of the small intestine and that contrary to the latter, in the colon the major local vasoconstrictory substance is angiotensin.

7.3.2 CLINICAL PRESENTATION

The classic clinical presentation is characterized by a sudden onset of severe crampy abdominal pain, diarrhea mixed with bright red blood, and occasionally melena. Physical examination may reveal a distended abdomen. Bowel sounds are present and there are no signs of peritoneal involvement. The patient is usually elderly and may show signs of one of the associated diseases such as hypotension, congestive heart failure and atherosclerosis. Under specific conditions, nongangrenous ischemic colitis can also occur in the young. This is often due to iatrogenic or patient-induced causes such as contraceptive medication, nonsteroidal anti-inflammatory agents, cocaine abuse, verapamil overdose, etc. (for details see Table 1). In the elderly, the specific event that precipitated the attack occasionally cannot be determined. The early clinical presentation may be so similar to that of infectious colitis, ulcerative colitis, Crohn's colitis and pseudomembranous colitis that the diagnosis can be established only by exclusion of infection, including Clostridium difficile, and by demonstrating the classic radiographic (Figures 5 and 6) and/or colonoscopic (Figure 7) findings of ischemic colitis. Because large vessels are never involved, angiography has no place in the diagnosis of nongangrenous ischemic colitis.

Radiographic and colonoscopic investigations have to be carried out within 24–48 hours of the onset of the disease, as the typical findings tend to disappear and are rapidly replaced by nonspecific signs. The first radiologic examination should be an abdominal survey film (Figure 5), which may demonstrate the classic intramural hemorrhage-induced thumb-printing in an air-filled segment of the colon. This finding, however, may not always be diagnostic, because occasionally it can be mimicked by mucosal and submucosal edema caused by severe inflammatory processes. Colonic involvement is usually segmental in ischemic colitis. Although any part of the colon may be affected, the "watershed" areas of the splenic flexure and of the rectosigmoid junction are most commonly involved. Thumb-printing can be demonstrated by barium enema (Figure 6), but differentiation between edema and submucosal hemorrhage can be done only by colonoscopy, where hemorrhage can be recognized as large dark red submucosal blebs (Figure 7). Because distention of the colon with air may compress intramural blood vessels and thus further decrease blood flow, barium enema and colonoscopy must be carried out carefully with minimal air insufflation. After 24–48 hours, the hemorrhage resolves and the mucosa becomes necrotic. If colonoscopy is

FIGURE 5. Abdominal survey film demonstrating ischemic colitis. This film was taken five hours after the onset of acute hematochezia and severe abdominal pain. Note the air-containing transverse colon exhibiting the classic picture of thumb-printing.

done at this stage, the endoscopist may be unable to differentiate the necrosis and ulcerations resulting from ischemic colitis from those caused by Crohn's disease or pseudomembranous enterocolitis. The pathologist reviewing biop-

FIGURE 6.   Single contrast barium enema. To avoid increased intraluminal pressure the examination was carried out without preparation and no air was insufflated. Closely adjacent small soft indentations of a normal mucosa are caused by submucosal hemorrhage. The multiple adjacent areas of indentations provide the appearance of thumb-printing.

sies taken a few days after the onset of the disease may have similar difficulties. Not infrequently, only time will tell whether the patient has inflammatory bowel disease (IBD) or ischemia. It is not impossible that some elderly patients with what is thought to be late-onset IBD or young women on contraceptive medication who are thought to have Crohn's are actually suffering from ischemic colitis.

The disease can progress in four different ways (Figure 1). Mild disease may resolve spontaneously. In patients with involvement of only small seg-

ID. NO:　　　NAME:
SEX: AGE:
D. O. BIRTH:

07/31/94
13:38:22

VTR
SCV————23

COMMENT:

FIGURE 7. Colonoscopic view of a recent-onset ischemic colitis of the splenic flexure. Note the normal mucosa on the left and the dark hemorrhagic mucosal indentation at the top and bottom of the image. These blood-filled submucosal blebs in the absence of mucosal damage are diagnostic of the initial stage of ischemic colitis.

ments, the symptoms and physical findings subside within 24–48 hours and complete resolution can occur within two to three weeks. In some, the disease does not resolve and may progress to ongoing or recurrent chronic colitis. As the pathological response of colonic tissue to chronic injury is restricted to a very few modalities, such as infiltration with leukocytes, crypt abscess, hemorrhage, necrosis, ulceration and regeneration of crypts, the pathologist may also have difficulty in differentiating ongoing ischemic colitis from Crohn's disease. Hemosiderin, a sign of previous bleeding, is often considered a typical manifestation of ischemic colitis (Figure 8). Unfortunately, this finding is not restricted to ischemic colonic disease, as it can be found in any type of colitis, including IBD, if hemorrhage has occurred sometime in the past.

Once ischemic colitis has become chronic, it may resolve, relapse or progress to deeper intramural inflammation and necrosis. In severe disease the patient may exhibit toxic symptoms with chills, fever, severe bloody diarrhea and abdominal distention with diminished bowel sounds. The patient may

FIGURE 8.   Photomicrograph of mucosal biopsy in patient with ischemic colitis taken five days after onset of disease.

A. Routine HPS stain showing ischemic necrosis of the mucosa and submucosa.

B. Prussian blue stain. Arrows indicate dark blue iron-laden macrophages in the mucosa and submucosa.

develop leukocytosis, anemia, elevated platelet count and electrolyte disturbances. If the necrosis does not progress further, the process will heal first with granulation tissue, which is replaced by fibrous tissue, scarring and finally a stricture. In some instances the disease progresses to toxic megacolon, and if the intramural necrosis becomes transmural, acute peritonitis will ensue. This progression may take only a few hours or several days to develop, and as the patient must be surgically treated well before peritonitis develops, this process must be detected early by careful, sometimes hourly, follow-up of the patient.

7.3.3 *TREATMENT*

Infectious enteropathies, IBD and other precipitating causes such as diverticulitis, cancer, etc. have to be detected and appropriately treated. Therapy for ischemic colitis can be considered under the following three categories: (1)

nonspecific supportive therapy, (2) specific medical treatment and (3) surgical therapy.

Nonspecific supportive therapy. Fluid and electrolyte balance must be carefully maintained. Oral intake should be restricted according to the severity of disease. Well-nourished patients can be maintained for a few days without specific nutritional support, except for what they receive in intravenous solutions. Severely undernourished patients may require enteral nutrition, or if this is poorly tolerated, total parenteral nutrition (TPN). Bleeding is rarely severe enough to require blood transfusion, but if anemia is present it may have to be corrected even in elderly patients with poor cardiovascular reserve. This requires careful balancing, so that an already precariously maintained circulation is not overloaded. Usually, the patient will request medication to relieve diarrhea and abdominal pain. However, the use of analgesics, antispasmodic or antidiarrheal agents is contraindicated, because they may lead to an inert bowel, which may result in a toxic megacolon.

As the patient improves, a low-residue diet may be slowly started. If this is not well tolerated, enteric feeding may be required. However, in some patients the diarrhea and abdominal pain may become worse on enteric nutrition. This may be overcome with the use of an iso-osmotic product, dilution of the solution and constant slow administration over 24 hours.

Patients have to be carefully followed to detect deterioration, as they may progress to toxic megacolon or perforation. In patients who show signs of deterioration, the use of antibiotics may be justified. If there is further progression and the patient develops increasing peritoneal signs, surgery becomes imperative, even in an elderly patient who appears to be a poor surgical risk.

Specific medical treatment. There is no need for specific therapy for mild self-limiting disease. For chronic ongoing disease there is no proven specific therapy and no experimental data exist to assess the usefulness of any of the drugs utilized in IBD. Because of the relatively low incidence of ischemic colitis, up to now it has not been possible to design a valid prospective double-blind study to assess the efficacy of these drugs. However, patients with long-standing progressive disease have been treated with variable results using 5-aminosalicylic acid (5-ASA) by oral and/or (depending on the location of the disease) rectal administration. For patients who do not respond to 5-ASA, a trial with oral or local steroids may be attempted. There is no experience with metronidazole or immunosuppressive agents. In contrast to acute mesenteric arterial occlusion, there is no evidence in nongangrenous ischemic colitis that vasodilators (papaverine, ACE inhibitors, nitrites, etc.) are useful. By the time the patient is seen the intramural ischemic injury has already occurred and vasodilators cannot reverse the pathological changes. Treatment of heart disease, change of digitalis to other medication, discontinuation of estrogens, management of diabetes, recognition and treatment of vasculitis, polycythemia, etc., may not necessarily alter the outcome of already established chronic disease, but may prevent future recurrences.

Surgical therapy. Indications for immediate surgery are toxic megacolon and transmural necrosis leading to peritoneal signs. Usually within six months after onset of the disease a considerable number of patients with severe ischemic colitis will develop strictures. They present with symptoms of partial obstruction. One should attempt colonoscopic dilation, but if this fails stricturoplasty or surgical resection may be necessary.

SUGGESTED READING LIST

Haglund U. Gut ischaemia. Gut 1994; 35(Suppl 1):S73–76.

Levine JS, Jacobson ED. Intestinal ischemic disorders. Dig Dis 1995; 13:3–24.

Gandhi SK, Hanson MM, Vernava AM, Kaninski DL, Longo WE. Ischemic colitis. Dis Colon Rectum 1996; 39:88–100.

Howard TJ, Plaskon LA, Wiebke EA, Wilcox MG, Madura JA. Nonocclusive mesenteric ischemia remains a diagnostic dilemma. Am J Surg 1996; 171:405–408.

Pastores SM, Katz DP, Kvetan V. Splanchnic ischemia and gut mucosal injury in sepsis and the multiple organ dysfunction syndrome. Am J Gastroenterol 1996; 91: 1697–1710.

OBJECTIVES

1. Understand the anatomy and physiology of splanchnic circulation.
2. Understand the pathophysiology of ischemic bowel disease.
3. Realize the importance of differentiating superficial (mucosal and submucosal) from deep (transmural) necrosis.
4. Be aware of the risk factors that may lead to intestinal ischemia.
5. Develop a high index of suspicion for the possibility of acute mesenteric ischemia in an emergent patient with extremely severe abdominal pain.
6. Learn to act immediately when this condition is suspected, as delay may lead to rapid necrosis of the bowel.
7. Understand the value of the different imaging techniques used in acute mesenteric ischemia.
8. Learn the methods of management of acute mesenteric ischemia.
9. Become aware of the possibility of chronic mesenteric ischemia in a certain group of patients who present with unexplained postprandial abdominal pain.
10. Learn to consider nongangrenous ischemia in localized small bowel disease.

11. Suspect nongangrenous ischemic colitis in patients with severe crampy abdominal pain and hematochezia.
12. Learn the risk factors that can lead to nongangrenous ischemic colitis.
13. Understand the differences between imaging techniques used in non-gangrenous ischemic colitis and those used in acute mesenteric ischemia.
14. Learn the problems involved in differentiating nongangrenous ischemic colitis from inflammatory bowel disease or infectious colitis.
15. Understand the natural history and evolution of nongangrenous ischemic colitis.
16. Learn to be aware of possible progression of acute ongoing non-gangrenous disease to toxic megacolon and occasionally to transmural necrosis.
17. Understand the problems involved in managing nongangrenous ischemic colitis during its acute and chronic phases.

9

Gastrointestinal Manifestations of Human Immunodeficiency Virus Infection

G.R. May

1. INTRODUCTION

Infection with the human immunodeficiency virus (HIV) and the development of the acquired immunodeficiency syndrome (AIDS) represents a significant problem worldwide. As of the end of 1994 it was estimated that over 17 million persons worldwide were infected with the HIV. In Canada, it is estimated that over 30,000 persons are infected with the HIV, giving an approximate prevalence of 191/100,000. The clinical manifestations of HIV infections and AIDS are varied and can involve all organ systems. The gastrointestinal (GI) tract is a common site for opportunistic infections and neoplasms in patients with HIV infection. Over 75% of patients will have significant symptoms related to the gastrointestinal tract at some point during the course of their infection. In many patients GI involvement represents the major manifestation of their HIV infection.

2. BASIC PRINCIPLES OF HIV INFECTION

HIV is a human retrovirus that is acquired predominantly through contact of infected body fluids with the bloodstream, a situation similar to the transmission of hepatitis B virus. It mainly infects the CD4 population of lymphocytes, which perform a helper cell function; immunodeficiency develops as the number of CD4 lymphocytes decreases. Cell-mediated immunity is mainly affected, but there is also impairment in the ability to mount new B-cell–mediated responses. As a result, the patient becomes susceptible to infections and neoplasms. Normal individuals usually have approximately 600–800 × 10^6/mL CD4 lymphocytes. Patients with HIV infection slowly lose their CD4 cells.

Opportunistic infections and neoplasms rarely occur until the number of CD4 lymphocytes drops below 300×10^6/mL. Certain infections are not seen until CD4 counts are below 100×10^6/mL. HIV is also known to infect other cell populations such as macrophages, nerve cells and possibly enterocytes, where it may be clinically latent and act as a reservoir of virus.

Persons recognized to be at high risk for acquiring HIV infection include homosexual or bisexual men, intravenous drug users, hemophiliacs and others who received blood or blood products prior to universal testing of blood in approximately 1985. Heterosexuals who have unprotected intercourse with infected partners are also at risk and at present represent the group with the fastest-rising incidence of HIV infection in North America. In Africa, where HIV infection is endemic, heterosexual transmission through unprotected intercourse is the commonest mode of HIV transmission. When seeing patients with suspected HIV infection, it is important to get an accurate history of risk factors including sexual orientation and practices, history of intravenous drug use, past exposure to blood and blood products and travel to endemic areas.

Many physicians find it difficult to discuss sexual orientation and sexual practices with patients. It is often best to ask the patient directly whether he or she is heterosexual, homosexual or bisexual. For male patients the question can also be addressed by asking the patient if he has ever had sexual relations with other men. Many persons may classify themselves as heterosexual but may have had same-sex sexual experiences. Sexual activity and practices should be ascertained by inquiring about the number of sexual partners in the past and whether the patient has had anal intercourse. Unprotected receptive anal intercourse represents the highest-risk sexual practice for HIV transmission. A history of other sexually transmitted diseases is also important as it suggests high-risk activity, and the presence of open lesions during unprotected intercourse may increase the risk of HIV transmission. It is important to address these issues in a clinical and nonjudgmental way, as negatively phrased questions or judgmental attitudes toward sexual orientation and practices can interfere with the doctor–patient relationship. Patients who perceive a judgmental or negative attitude are less likely to discuss these issues truthfully with the physician.

The acquired immunodeficiency syndrome (AIDS) results from infection with the HIV and the resultant immunodeficiency. The diagnosis of AIDS is usually made on the basis of demonstrating positive serology for HIV with the presence of an opportunistic infection, neoplasm or a CD4 lymphocyte count less than 200×10^6/mL. At present it appears that most patients with HIV infection will eventually progress to AIDS; however, the rate of progression is variable. It has been well documented that therapy with antiretroviral drugs slows the progression of HIV infection to AIDS and prolongs the life of patients with established AIDS. The common antiretroviral drugs in use are the nucleoside reverse transcriptase inhibitors zidovudine (AZT), dideoxyinosine (ddI), dideoxycytidine (ddC), stavudine (d4T) and lamivudine (3TC). New drugs showing promise and currently under evaluation include protease inhibitors (siquinavir, ritonivir and indinavir) and the non-nucleoside reverse transcriptase inhibitors. It appears that combination therapy with two or three antiretroviral drugs is better than single-drug therapy and reduces the incidence of drug resistance. Current recommendations for antiretroviral therapy are that therapy with AZT alone or in combination should be started once the CD4 lymphocyte count falls below 500×10^6/mL. The best combination of antiretroviral drugs has yet to be determined. With advancing immunosuppression, the common occurrence of certain opportunistic infections such as Pneumocystis carinii pneumonia, Mycobacterium avium-intracellulare and toxoplasmosis has also prompted recommendations for prophylactic therapy.

3. GASTROINTESTINAL INVOLVEMENT IN HIV INFECTION

3.1 General Considerations
The GI tract represents a common site of involvement of opportunistic infection and neoplasms in HIV infection. GI symptoms such as dysphagia, abdominal pain, diarrhea and weight loss are common and affect over 75% of patients with HIV infection at some time during the course of their disease. It is important to remember that HIV-infected patients may also have common gastrointestinal problems unrelated to the HIV infection. The approach to HIV-infected patients with gastrointestinal symptoms should be guided by the CD4 count. In patients with counts greater than 300×10^6/mL an opportunistic infection or neoplasm is very unlikely, and the approach to investigation of these patients should be similar to that in immunocompetent individuals. Once the CD4 count falls below 300×10^6/mL the risk for opportunistic problems increases, and they must be considered in the differential diagnosis.

Other issues that must be considered in the evaluation of HIV-positive patients with gastrointestinal symptoms are drug side effects and problems specific to risk factor groups. Many of the antiretroviral drugs and antimicrobials used in HIV infection have prominent GI side effects, which are often overlooked in the differential diagnosis of GI problems in these patients. Homosexual males are also at risk for a variety of gastrointestinal problems as a result of their sexual practices. This includes an increased risk of gastrointestinal parasitic infections and proctitis resulting from gonorrhea, syphilis or Chlamydia. Patients having receptive anal intercourse are at risk for rectal trauma manifesting as lacerations, fissures, perianal infections and rarely, bowel perforations. Intravenous drug users are also at risk for infection with hepatitis B and hepatitis C viruses.

3.2 Bacterial Infections

Typical enteric bacterial pathogens such as nontyphoidal strains of Salmonella, Shigella species and Campylobacter jejuni occur with only a slightly increased frequency in HIV-infected patients. When they do occur in immunocompromised patients the presentation is often atypical with a high incidence of bacteremia in addition to the typical symptoms of enteritis or colitis. Immunocompromised HIV patients also appear to be unable to effectively eradicate these organisms so that recurrent infection is common, often necessitating the use of chronic antibiotic suppression. Diagnosis is made with stool cultures. Because of the high incidence of bacteremia, blood cultures should also be done in patients presenting with acute diarrhea and fever.

The principles of treatment for acute bacterial enteritis or colitis in HIV-infected patients are generally the same as for other patients, with supportive care and intravenous fluids as required. Immunocompetent patients will usually clear the infection, and indications for antibiotic therapy are the same as for other patients. Immunocompromised patients and those with bacteremia should be treated with appropriate antibiotics (Table 1). Chronic suppressive therapy is often required as a result of the high incidence of recurrent infection.

3.3 Mycobacterial Infections

3.3.1 MYCOBACTERIUM AVIUM-INTRACELLULARE

Mycobacterium avium-intracellulare (MAI) is an atypical mycobacterium of environmental origin that is a common opportunistic infection in immuno-compromised HIV-infected patients (CD4 lymphocyte counts $< 100 \times 10^6$/mL) and is an AIDS-defining illness. It usually presents as a chronic systemic illness including fever, night sweats, weight loss and lymphadenopathy in addition to diarrhea. The diarrhea is often mild to moderate in severity and may have features to suggest malabsorption. Hepatosplenomegaly is a common finding on examination, as the liver and spleen are also commonly involved in MAI infection. The organism commonly infects the small bowel mucosa where it causes thickening and blunting of the villi as a result of an increased number of macrophages in the lamina propria. The appearance on hematoxylin and eosin stains is strikingly similar to Whipple's disease. With mycobacterial stains the macrophages can be seen to be filled with acid-fast organisms. In addition to the liver and spleen, the intra-abdominal lymph nodes and bone marrow are also commonly involved with MAI. Diagnosis can usually be made with blood and stool cultures. Blood cultures will usual-

TABLE 1. Treatment regimens for HIV-related gastrointestinal infections

Organism	Drug of first choice	Alternative treatments
Bacteria Salmonella	Ceftriaxone 1–2 g IV q12–24h	Ciprofloxacin 500 mg q12h Trimethoprim-sulfamethoxazole 160 mg/800 mg po bid
Shigella	Ciprofloxacin 500 mg po bid	Trimethoprim-sulfamethoxazole 160 mg/800 mg po bid Ceftriaxone 1–2 g IV q12–24h
Campylobacter	Ciprofloxacin 500 mg po bid or Erythromycin 500 mg po qid	Tetracycline 500 mg po qid
Mycobacteria Mycobacterium tuberculosis	Isoniazid 300 mg po qd + Rifampin 600 mg po qd + Pyrazinamide 15–25 mg/kg po qd + Ethambutol 15–25 mg/kg po qd or Streptomycin 15 mg/kg IM qd	Depends upon sensitivity patterns
Mycobacterium avium-intracellulare	Clarithromycin 500–1,000mg po bid + one or more of: Ethambutol 15–25 mg/kg po qd Clofazimine 100–200 mg po qd Ciprofloxacin 750 mg po bid Amikacin 7.5–15 mg/kg IM qd	Rifabutin 450–600 mg po qd + one or more of the other agents
Fungi Candida albicans (oral)	Clotrimazole troches 100 mg po 1–3 times/day Fluconazole 100 mg po qd	Ketoconazole 200 mg po qd Itraconazole 200 mg po qd
(esophageal)	Fluconazole 100–200 mg po qd	Ketoconazole or itraconazole 200 mg po qd Amphotericin B 0.3 mg/kg IV qd × 7 days
Histoplasmosis	*Initial therapy:* Amphotericin B 0.5–0.6 mg/kg IV qd for 4–8 weeks *Chronic suppression:* Itraconazole 200 mg po bid	Itraconazole 200 mg po bid Amphotericin B 0.5–0.8 mg/kg IV weekly

(cont'd)

TABLE 1.   Treatment regimens for HIV-related gastrointestinal infections (cont'd)

Organism	Drug of first choice	Alternative treatments
Parasites		
Giardia lamblia	Metronidazole 250 mg po tid	Quinacrine hydrochloride 100 mg po tid
Entamoeba histolytica	Metronidazole 750 mg po tid × 10 d followed by Iodoquinol 650 mg po tid × 20 d	
Cryptosporidium	Supportive fluid therapy Loperamide 2–24 mg po qd	Paromomycin 500–750 mg po qid Octreotide 50–500 µg sq tid
Microsporidium	Supportive fluid therapy Loperamide 2–24mg po qd	Albendazole 400 mg po bid Octreotide 50–500 µg sq tid
Isospora belli	Trimethoprim-sulfamethoxazole 160 mg/800 mg po qid × 10 d then bid × 21 d	Pyrimethamine 50–75 mg qd × 21 d
Viruses		
Herpes simplex virus	*For active lesions:* Acyclovir 200 mg po 5 times/day *For maintenance therapy:* Acyclovir 400 mg po bid	Foscarnet 40 mg/kg IV q8h × 21 d Foscarnet 40 mg/kg IV qd
Cytomegalovirus	*For active disease:* Ganciclovir 5 mg/kg IV q12h × 14–21 d *For maintenance therapy:* Ganciclovir 5 mg/kg IV qd or 6 mg/kg IV qd 5 times/week	Foscarnet 60 mg/kg IV q8h × 14–21 d Foscarnet 90–120 mg/kg IV qd

ly be positive within 3–4 weeks, as this is a rapidly growing mycobacterium. Barium radiographs of the small bowel will often show dilation of the small bowel and irregular thickening of the small bowel folds. Ultrasound or CT scan of the abdomen will document hepatosplenomegaly, and there will often be enlarged intra-abdominal lymph nodes. Small bowel biopsy showing typical histology can also be used to establish a diagnosis.

Therapy for MAI is difficult and requires combinations of 4–6 antituberculous drugs, and the results are generally poor (Table 1). The organism usually cannot be eradicated; the goal of therapy is chronic suppression. Drug side effects are common, and many patients are unable to tolerate full therapy. Despite treatment, many patients have progressive symptoms and wasting. Because of the difficulty in treating established MAI infection, prophylactic therapy is recommended, and recent studies have shown some benefit to using rifabutin 300 mg p.o. daily once the patient's CD4 cell count falls below 100×10^6/mL.

3.3.2 *MYCOBACTERIUM TUBERCULOSIS*
Pulmonary Mycobacterium tuberculosis (TB) is being seen with increased frequency in HIV-infected patients and is especially common in IV drug users. The incidence of multiple-drug-resistant tuberculosis is increasing at an alarming rate. In HIV infection the GI tract may be involved with extrapulmonary TB either as direct extension from pulmonary lesions, where the esophagus is usually involved, or from systemic spread, where any part of the GI tract including liver and pancreas may be involved. Isolated involvement of the GI tract is unusual. Diagnosis should be made with biopsy and culture of the most readily accessible lesions. It is important to culture and do sensitivities on isolates of TB because of the rising incidence of multiple drug resistance. Initial therapy should include three or four antituberculous drugs. Choice of drugs should be determined on the basis of local sensitivity patterns.

3.4 **Fungal Infections**

3.4.1 *CANDIDA ALBICANS*
Candida albicans is one of the most common opportunistic infections in HIV-infected patients. Oropharyngeal candidiasis occurs frequently and is often one of the earliest clinical signs of immune impairment. When limited to the oropharynx it is often asymptomatic or associated with mild discomfort. Esophageal involvement is usually associated with dysphagia; however, many patients may have only vague epigastric discomfort during meals. Odynophagia can occur with esophageal candidiasis, but severe pain with swallowing is unusual and suggests other infections such as cytomegalovirus (CMV), herpes simplex virus (HSV) or nonspecific HIV-associated esophageal ulceration. Patients with esophageal involvement usually have evidence for oropharyngeal Candida, commonly seen as whitish plaques on the buccal mucosa and posterior oropharynx. Esophageal involvement may occasionally occur in the absence of oral Candida, but this is unusual.

Candidal esophagitis can be demonstrated with a barium swallow that shows abnormalities ranging from small filling defects on the mucosal surface representing mucosal plaques to thickening of the mucosal folds with a shaggy outline to the wall. Severe or deep ulcerations may be seen but are unusual. Diagnosis is best made with endoscopy, which shows typical white adherent pseudomembranous plaques. In severe cases the entire esophageal mucosa may be covered with a confluent white membrane. The diagnosis is confirmed by brush cytology or mucosal biopsy showing invasion of the candidal pseudohyphae into the squamous epithelium. Cultures are not routinely done, as these organisms are commonly present in normal individuals and tissue invasion should be demonstrated to confirm the diagnosis.

Oropharyngeal candidiasis can be treated with either local therapy using clotrimazole troches 100 mg p.o. 1–3 times/day or with systemic antifungals such as ketoconazole 200 mg p.o. daily, fluconazole 100 mg p.o. daily or itraconazole 200 mg p.o. daily. Esophageal involvement should be treated with one of the oral antifungal agents, as topical agents are generally not effective. Higher doses may be required for initial treatment in symptomatic patients (Table 1) . Initial therapy should continue for approximately 14 days. Recurrence is common, and many patients require ongoing therapy with an oral antifungal agent. Resistance to oral antifungal agents is starting to emerge. Intravenous amphotericin B can be used in low doses for those who fail therapy with oral antifungal agents. Esophageal candidiasis is so common in HIV infection that many experts recommend empiric therapy in patients with esophageal symptoms, especially if oral Candida is present. Further investigation with endoscopy can be reserved for those who do not respond to empiric antifungal therapy or for those with atypical symptoms. Disseminated infection with Candida may occur in HIV infection but is unusual, as the infection usually remains mucocutaneous. Disseminated infection has a poor prognosis and is often fatal.

3.4.2 OTHER FUNGAL INFECTIONS

Other fungal infections seen in HIV infection include cryptococcosis, histoplasmosis and coccidioidosis. Disseminated infection of any of these fungi establishes a diagnosis of AIDS when present with a positive HIV antibody test. The incidence of these infections varies, and they are usually seen in patients who have lived in or have visited endemic areas. Clinically, patients usually present with prominent systemic symptoms such as fevers, night sweats and weight loss. Neurologic involvement is usually seen with cryptococcosis. With histoplasmosis, the liver is often involved as part of a disseminated infection producing abnormalities of liver chemistry. Diagnosis of these infections generally depends on the demonstration of fungi through examination or culture of clinical specimens. Serologic tests are not dependable in the immunocompromised patient. Therapy usually requires intravenous amphotericin B in high doses. The response to therapy is generally poor, with a high rate of relapse and a poor overall prognosis.

3.5 Intestinal Parasitic Infections

3.5.1 *GIARDIASIS*
Giardia lamblia is a common intestinal parasitic infection that is commonly seen in homosexual or bisexual males. Its increased frequency in HIV patients is likely due to the high frequency in homosexual men rather than as a direct result of the HIV infection, as it does not appear to have a significantly higher incidence in other risk groups. Transmission occurs via the fecal–oral route. It usually infects the small bowel mucosa where it may be asymptomatic but usually causes diarrhea with abdominal cramping, bloating and nausea. In severe cases it may produce malabsorption and steatorrhea. Dissemination is rare and does not appear to be a significant problem in HIV infection.

The diagnosis depends upon demonstrating Giardia in the stool with an examination for ova and parasites. It may also be diagnosed on a duodenal aspirate or duodenal biopsy taken at the time of endoscopy. Treatment with metronidazole 250 mg p.o. t.i.d. for 5 days is usually effective in eradicating the organism even in HIV-infected patients; alternatively, quinacrine 100 mg p.o. t.i.d. for 5 days can be used.

3.5.2 *ENTAMOEBA HISTOLYTICA*
Entamoeba histolytica is an intestinal ameba that is also seen with increased frequency in HIV-infected patients as a result of its increased frequency in homosexual and bisexual males. It usually causes colitis with bloody diarrhea and abdominal cramps. Asymptomatic carriage is seen more commonly in HIV-infected patients than in patients with amebiasis who are not infected with the HIV. Dissemination is rare and is not seen more frequently in HIV-infected patients than in other Entamoeba histolytica patients. Diagnosis is made by demonstrating ameba on a stool examination for ova and parasites. Sigmoidoscopy may show evidence for colitis, and typically Entamoeba histolytica infection causes punched-out "flask-shaped" ulcers. Diagnosis can be confirmed by demonstrating organisms on biopsy or from a fresh stool aspirate.

Therapy for symptomatic Entamoeba histolytica infection is with metronidazole 750 mg p.o. t.i.d. for 10 days followed by iodoquinol 650 mg p.o. t.i.d. for 20 days. Asymptomatic carriers may just be treated with iodoquinol. Patients should have follow-up stool studies to confirm the eradication of the infection.

3.5.3 *CRYPTOSPORIDIUM*

Cryptosporidium is a protozoal parasite that is now recognized as a cause of self-limited diarrhea in immunocompetent persons. Several epidemic outbreaks have been identified. In immunocompromised patients it causes chronic watery nonbloody diarrhea that can be severe, leading to significant dehydration with electrolyte disturbances and death. Patients may have associated abdominal cramps and bloating, but these are not usually severe. Cryptosporidiosis is an AIDS-defining illness in HIV-infected patients.

The diagnosis of Cryptosporidium infection is based upon the demonstration of cryptosporidial oocysts in stool or on mucosal biopsy from the small intestine or colon. Involvement of the bowel may be patchy and involve the ileum, so intestinal biopsy from the duodenum or distal colon is not reliable and examination of the stool is the best diagnostic test. Recently, special stains have been developed, which have increased the yield of diagnosis from stool tests. Therapy in immunocompromised patients usually is supportive with the use of intravenous fluids as necessary to correct volume depletion and antidiarrheal agents such as loperamide 2–24 mg per day to keep diarrhea under control. In severe cases where diarrhea cannot be controlled with antidiarrheal agents, the somatostatin analogue octreotide has been used successfully in doses ranging from 50 µg to 500 µg s.q. t.i.d. to control the diarrhea. To date, there is no proven therapy to specifically treat and eradicate Cryptosporidium. Trials using spiramycin and paromomycin have been reported, but the results have been disappointing.

3.5.4 *MICROSPORIDIUM*

Microsporidia are a group of intracellular protozoans that measure 1–2 µm in size and have been described in HIV-infected patients. The commonest organisms of this group identified are Enterocytozoon bieneusi and Septata intestinalis. They are believed to be pathogenic in most patients, but asymptomatic carriage in HIV patients has been documented. When symptomatic, infection with Microsporidium resembles that of Cryptosporidium, usually with watery nonbloody diarrhea of variable severity, mild abdominal cramps and bloating.

When these organisms were initially described, the diagnosis required electron microscopy of a small bowel biopsy to see the small intracellular parasites. More recently, special stains have been developed to detect Microsporidia in stool samples. Experienced pathologists can usually see the organisms with high-power microscopy of thin plastic sections of mucosal biopsies. Therapy of symptomatic microsporidial infection is similar to that of Cryptosporidium, with the use of supportive therapy and antidiarrheal agents. Octreotide has also been used successfully for severe watery diarrhea.

Metronidazole and albendazole have been used to try to eradicate Microsporidium, but neither has been shown to be reliably effective.

3.5.5 ISOSPORA BELLI

Isospora belli is another intestinal protozoal parasite that has been identified as causing infection in the setting of HIV, and infection with Isospora belli is also an AIDS-defining illness. Uncommon in North America, it has been seen in up to 15% of Haitian patients with AIDS. Clinically it causes a nonspecific nonbloody watery diarrhea similar to that of Cryptosporidium. Diagnosis is usually easily made by examination of stool for ova and parasites. Unlike infection with Cryptosporidium and Microsporidium, isoporiasis can usually be treated successfully with trimethoprim-sulfamethoxazole 160 mg tmp/800 mg smx p.o. q.i.d. for 10 days, then b.i.d. for 3 weeks. Recurrence is common (approximately 50%), and some patients may need chronic therapy.

3.5.6 STRONGYLOIDES STERCORALIS

Strongyloides stercoralis is a nematode endemic in tropical areas. It usually infects a host by penetrating the skin as filariform larvae. The larvae then travel via the bloodstream to the lungs where they leave the alveolar capillaries, are coughed up and swallowed. Once they reach the small intestine they release eggs that develop into infective filariform larvae that burrow into the small bowel mucosa. Pruritus, papillary rashes and edema may occur at the site of skin entry. Intestinal involvement may result in fever, nausea, vomiting, diarrhea, abdominal pain and weight loss. Diagnosis can best be made by examination of duodenal aspirate but can also be done by examination of concentrated stool specimens. Treatment is usually successful with thiabendazole 50 mg/kg/day in 2 doses for 2 days. Disseminated strongyloidiasis may occur in immunocompromised individuals and is recognized as an AIDS-defining illness. Therapy in immunocompromised individuals may need to be continued for at least 7 days, and some may require chronic therapy.

3.5.7 PNEUMOCYSTIS CARINII

Pneumocystis carinii is recognized as a common cause of pulmonary infection. Extrapulmonary infections of Pneumocystis have been recognized especially in patients who have received aerosolized pentamidine rather than systemic therapy for Pneumocystis carinii pneumonia (PCP) prophylaxis. Infection of the liver, spleen, intestine, bone marrow and peritoneal cavity (producing ascites) have all been reported. Diagnosis is made by demonstrating typical organisms on a methenamine-silver stain of clinical specimens. Therapy is similar to that of pneumocystis pneumonia.

3.6 Viral Infections

3.6.1 CYTOMEGALOVIRUS

Cytomegalovirus is a common infection, with greater than 50% of Canadian adults showing serologic evidence of previous exposure to CMV. Homosexual men and intravenous drug users have a seroprevalence of CMV as high as 90%. In immunocompetent patients the infection is latent and rarely causes clinical illness. Reactivation of latent infection occurs as HIV-infected patients become immunocompromised and is usually seen when the CD4 lymphocyte count is below 50×10^6/mL. CMV infection is increasing as an important clinical problem in HIV patients.

The two most common sites for CMV infection in HIV-infected patients are the retina and gastrointestinal tract. The infection can involve any part of the GI tract, where it produces ulcerating lesions. The esophagus and colon are the most common sites of GI involvement. Esophageal involvement usually presents with odynophagia and dysphagia. Endoscopy shows large shallow ulcerations that may be circumferential. Involvement of the colon produces an acute colitis presenting with diarrhea that may be bloody, often with severe abdominal pain. Sigmoidoscopy or colonoscopy shows a colitis with friable edematous mucosa and scattered ulcerations, a picture similar to Crohn's disease. Small intestinal, gastric and hepatic involvement are less common. Since CMV is commonly found in HIV patients, culture of virus from mucosal biopsies is not sufficient to make a diagnosis of CMV infection. The diagnosis is based upon demonstrating the presence of intranuclear inclusion bodies in biopsy specimens. The presence of an accompanying vasculitis with viral inclusions in endothelial cells further supports CMV as the cause of the lesion. Systemic infection can be confirmed by viral cultures of white blood cells from the buffy coat of a centrifuged specimen of blood.

Therapy of symptomatic CMV requires ganciclovir 5 mg/kg IV q12h initially for 14–21 days. Foscarnet 60 mg/kg IV q8h for 14–21 days can be used as an alternative. These treatments usually result in clinical improvement and healing of mucosal lesions. Recurrence is high, however, and many experts recommend chronic suppressive therapy with ganciclovir 6 mg/kg IV daily 5 times per week or foscarnet 90–120 mg IV daily after acute therapy. Chronic therapy appears to be required lifelong. Recently an oral formulation of ganciclovir has been developed and shown to be effective for chronic suppression of CMV retinitis. Its efficacy for suppression of gastrointestinal CMV infections has not yet been established.

3.6.2 HERPES SIMPLEX VIRUS

Herpes simplex virus (HSV) most commonly infects the esophagus to produce multiple esophageal ulcerations. Clinically herpetic esophagitis presents with prominent odynophagia and dysphagia that are indistinguishable from symptoms of CMV esophagitis. Differentiation from other causes of esophagitis in these patients requires endoscopy. The ulcers produced by herpes simplex virus are usually multiple and small. Biopsies will show multinucleated giant cells and Cowdry type A intranuclear inclusion bodies. Viral culture of biopsy material should be positive for HSV.

HSV esophagitis can usually be treated effectively with oral acyclovir 200 mg p.o. 5 times per day. In patients unable to take oral medications because of odynophagia, acyclovir can be given intravenously in a dose of 5 mg/kg q8h. Initial therapy should continue for 10–14 days. Recurrence is common, and many patients require chronic therapy with oral acyclovir. Foscarnet has been used as alternative therapy in those unable to take acyclovir or who fail therapy with acyclovir.

3.6.3 HUMAN IMMUNODEFICIENCY VIRUS

It is not clear whether the HIV itself causes gastrointestinal pathology. Two situations where direct pathologic effect of the HIV in the GI tract is suspected are nonspecific esophageal ulcerations and HIV enteropathy. Esophageal ulcerations are most commonly due to CMV and herpes virus, as discussed above. Ulcerations thought possibly to be directly due to the HIV occur as one of the seroconversion syndromes and as the idiopathic nonspecific esophageal ulcers seen in later stages of HIV infection. Acute infection with the HIV is usually associated with a nonspecific viral illness. As part of this seroconversion syndrome some patients develop severe odynophagia and are found on endoscopy to have multiple superficial esophageal ulcers. Electron microscopy of these ulcers has shown viral particles consistent with retroviruses. The ulcerations and odynophagia typically spontaneously resolve.

Later in the course of HIV infection, esophageal ulcerations may occur which are negative for the usual pathogens. These ulcers are usually deep with undermined edges and may be multiple. Although usually found in the esophagus, they can also occur in the posterior pharynx. Symptomatically they present with severe odynophagia that often limits oral intake. Interestingly they usually respond dramatically to treatment with corticosteroids taken orally or injected intralesionally. The etiology of these lesions is not clear; the dramatic response to steroids and other immune modifiers such as thalidomide implies an immunologic basis to the ulcerations.

HIV enteropathy is a term that has been applied to describe chronic diarrhea, often accompanied by weight loss, where no identifiable pathogen can be found. It is unclear if this enteropathy is due to an unidentified pathogen or to a direct effect of the HIV on the gut. The HIV potentially could affect the gut directly by infecting enterocytes, or indirectly by inducing the local release of cytokines and other inflammatory mediators, which then may affect enterocyte function. Improvement in some patients has occurred with anti-retroviral therapy. Otherwise, treatment is symptomatic only.

3.7 Neoplasms

3.7.1 KAPOSI'S SARCOMA

Kaposi's sarcoma (KS) is the most common neoplasm seen in HIV-infected patients. It has been more common in homosexual or bisexual males than in other risk groups for HIV infection, and its incidence appears to be decreasing within this risk group over the last 10 years. An infective cofactor has been postulated to explain the epidemiology of HIV-related KS, although such a factor has not been definitely identified. KS predominantly involves the skin and oropharynx; gastrointestinal involvement is seen in up to 40% of patients with skin involvement. Rare cases of visceral KS in the absence of skin lesions have been reported.

In most cases, GI involvement with KS is asymptomatic. Mucosal lesions can occur throughout the GI tract and are usually incidentally found at endoscopy, where they appear as raised red to violaceous macules. Large lesions may be nodular and may ulcerate. Symptoms are usually the result of hemorrhage from ulceration or obstruction from bulky lesions. Diarrhea and protein-losing enteropathy have also been reported. The exact presentation will depend upon the location of the lesions in the GI tract. Visceral KS should be suspected in any HIV patient with skin KS who has GI symptoms.

The diagnosis is made by histologic examination of mucosal biopsies. A recently described infection, bacillary angiomatosis, has identical histology to KS; differentiation is made by demonstrating organisms on silver stains. Gastrointestinal involvement with bacillary angiomatosis has also recently been described. HIV-related KS can be treated by local or systemic therapy. Oral lesions are best treated with local radiation or laser excision. Symptomatic visceral involvement requires systemic therapy, usually with combination chemotherapy. Good responses to subcutaneous or intralesional interferon have also recently been reported.

3.7.2 LYMPHOMA

B-cell lymphomas represent the second most common neoplasm occurring in HIV-infected patients. These are usually high-grade lymphomas of the large cell type; however, patients with Burkitt's lymphoma and Hodgkin's disease have also been reported. The gastrointestinal tract represents the second commonest site of involvement after the central nervous system. The lymphomas occurring in HIV infection are commonly extranodal.

Any part of the gastrointestinal tract can be involved, with the presentation and symptoms depending on the particular site. Systemic symptoms of fevers, night sweats and weight loss are commonly associated. The diagnosis is made by histologic examination of material obtained from endoscopy, or ultrasound- or CT-guided biopsy. Treatment requires combination chemotherapy similar to that for other high-grade lymphomas. Tolerance of therapy is generally poor, often as a result of the poor functional status of these patients when they develop lymphoma and the presence of other opportunistic infections. Full remissions can occur in patients who can tolerate combination chemotherapy, but the prognosis is generally poor.

3.7.3 ANAL CARCINOMA

Squamous cell carcinoma of the anal canal is seen with higher frequency in homosexual and bisexual men who practice anoreceptive intercourse. The increased risk is independent of HIV infection and, like cervical carcinoma in women, appears to be related to previous infection with human papilloma virus. Colorectal carcinoma is not seen with higher frequency in this risk group. Anal carcinoma may present with a mass and associated fissure or fistula. Local pain is usually present and there may be bleeding. The differential diagnosis includes infections such as syphilis, lymphogranuloma venereum and condyloma acuminatum, and benign perianal conditions of fissure in ano and anal trauma from intercourse or instrumentation. Definitive diagnosis is made through biopsy of suspicious lesions, especially those that fail to heal after treatment of any secondary infections. Treatment modalities include surgical excision, but many may be treated with combined radiation and chemotherapy, which has effected cures with good preservation of anorectal function.

4. HEPATOBILIARY AND PANCREATIC INVOLVEMENT IN HIV INFECTION

The liver is commonly involved during the course of HIV infection, with hepatomegaly and/or abnormal liver chemistry being seen in approximately 60% of AIDS patients. Involvement of the biliary tree and gallbladder is much less common. Hepatic disease may occur as a result of opportunistic infections (HSV, CMV, MAI, fungi) or neoplasms (KS, lymphoma). In such cases the liver is usually involved as part of more diffuse systemic involvement and is rarely the sole site of infection. Other infections such as hepatitis B and hepatitis C are common as a result of associated risk factors such as intravenous drug use and sexual transmission. Malnutrition, alcohol and hepato-toxicity of medications are other common factors that should be considered in the evaluation of hepatic abnormalities in these patients.

Co-infection of HIV with either hepatitis B or hepatitis C virus is often seen, as a result of common risk factors. The effect of HIV-related immunosuppression on chronic hepatitis B often results in clinical improvement of the chronic hepatitis. Since it is the immune reaction to hepatitis B that causes the hepatic inflammation, biochemical parameters of hepatitis often improve, as does the activity on liver biospy as the HIV-associated immunosuppression progresses. Despite the clinical improvement, hepatitis B viral replication increases. Hepatitis C, on the other hand, is directly hepatotoxic, and advancing immunosuppression is not uncommonly associated with worsening of the hepatitis and progressive liver disease. Treatment with interferon for either hepatitis B or C in this setting is generally associated with a poor response.

Biliary involvement in HIV infection is commonly termed *AIDS cholangiopathy* and results from inflammation of the biliary tree and gallbladder. There can be a spectrum of involvement ranging from acute acalculous cholecystitis to papillary stenosis with bile duct obstruction or more diffuse involvement of the biliary tree producing a picture similar to sclerosing cholangitis. Cholangiopathy is most commonly due to CMV infection of the biliary tree but has also been reported to result from biliary infection with Cryptosporidium or Microsporidium. Acute acalculous cholecystitis presents with RUQ pain, fever and tenderness on examination. Cholecystectomy is usually required. Cholangiopathy may present with less acute RUQ pain, fever and nausea, with cholestatic liver enzyme abnormalities. Diagnosis of cholangiopathy is made by ERCP. Patients with dilated common bile ducts who presumably have papillary stenosis secondary to an acute papillitis have responded symptomatically to endoscopic sphincterotomy. Patients in whom CMV is proven or suspected as the cause may improve with specific treatment for CMV. Rarely Kaposi's sarcoma or lymphoma can involve the gallbladder or biliary tree.

Symptomatic pancreatic involvement in HIV infection is not common, but clinically will usually present as acute pancreatitis. Asymptomatic elevations of serum amylase or lipase are common and are seen in up to 45% of patients. These are often related to medications but may also be due to asymptomatic involvement of the pancreas with opportunistic infection or neoplasm. Acute pancreatitis presents in a similar manner in patients with and without HIV infection. In addition to the commonly recognized causes of pancreatitis, other possibilities need to be considered in HIV patients. Drugs commonly used in HIV patients, including sulfonamides, pentamidine and the reverse transcriptase inhibitor dideoxyinosine (ddI), are common causes of pancreatitis. Pancreatic involvement with opportunistic infection and neoplasm, although usually asymptomatic, may cause pancreatitis. The principles of treatment of acute pancreatitis are the same for HIV-infected patients as for those without HIV infection. Drugs potentially involved should be stopped. Where no obvious etiology is apparent, CT scan of the pancreas is useful to rule out focal lesions that might indicate infections or neoplasms involving the pancreas.

5. NUTRITIONAL CONSIDERATIONS AND THE WASTING SYNDROME

Weight loss is a common problem in HIV infection, especially in the more advanced stages of AIDS. Weight loss of greater than 40% of lean body mass is an independent predictor of mortality. Weight loss of greater than 10% of body weight with no obvious underlying opportunistic infection or neoplasm has been termed *the HIV wasting syndrome* and is an AIDS-defining illness. The cause of weight loss in HIV-infected patients is multifactorial and includes diminished intake, malabsorption and increased metabolic rate. The major cause for weight loss in most patients has been shown to be inadequate caloric intake. Anorexia is a common result of systemic infection and drug side effects. Patients with oropharyngeal and esophageal pathology have discomfort related to eating and will decrease intake. The presence of gastrointestinal involvement is often associated with variable degrees of malabsorption so that the limited calories that are taken in are not assimilated efficiently. Increased basal metabolic rate as well as inefficient use of energy has been demonstrated in some cases. All of these contribute to weight loss.

There is no reliably effective treatment for wasting. Underlying opportunistic infections should be treated if possible. Caloric intake should be optimized; assistance of a dietitian is invaluable in helping patients maximize caloric intake. Intervention with enteral or parenteral nutritional support has not been shown to be generally effective, but may be used successfully in selected cases. Appetite stimulants such as megestrol acetate have been shown to be effective, producing weight gain in patients with anorexia and limited intake. The weight gained appears to be predominantly fat, and whether this translates into an improved survival rate or quality of life has not been established. Metabolic agents such as anabolic steroids and growth hormone have been used with limited success but are not currently in widespread use.

6. CONCLUSIONS

Care of HIV-infected patients with gastrointestinal involvement represents a growing clinical challenge. Differential diagnosis and investigations should be guided by the degree of immunosuppression indicated by the CD4 lympho-cyte count. As curative therapies for most of the GI problems are not avail-able, therapy is usually directed at symptom relief with the goal to improve the quality of life. Functional status and psychosocial issues need to be con-sidered for the successful management of these patients.

10
Inflammatory Bowel Disease
R.N. Fedorak and A.B.R. Thomson

1. CROHN'S DISEASE

Crohn's disease, or regional enteritis, is a chronic inflammatory disorder that can affect the small intestine and/or the large intestine. Inflammation, which may or may not be accompanied by noncaseating granulomas, extends through all layers of the gut wall to involve adjacent mesentery and lymph nodes. The inflammatory process is frequently discontinuous, with normal bowel separating portions of diseased bowel. This disease is characterized by an indolent variable course, by its diverse clinical manifestations, by its perianal and systemic complications, and by its tendency to recur after surgical resection.

1.1 Pathology
The key pathological feature of Crohn's disease is an inflammatory process that extends through all layers of the bowel wall. Microscopic examination reveals (1) hyperplasia of perilymphatic histiocytes, (2) diffuse granulomatous infiltration, (3) discrete noncaseating granulomas in the submucosa and lamina propria, (4) edema and lymphatic dilation of all layers of the gut, and (5) monocytic infiltration within lymph nodules and Peyer's patches on the serosal surface of the bowel.

The mesentery in the vicinity of the diseased bowel is markedly thickened, fatty and edematous. Finger-like projections of thick mesentery characteristically extend over the serosal surface toward the antimesenteric border. The mucosal surface in the diseased segment has a characteristic "cobblestone" appearance, resulting from the combination of deep mucosal ulceration and

Ileitis   **"String Sign"**

FIGURE 1.   Crohn's disease. Barium contrast x-rays showing (a) ulcerations and narrowing characteristic of terminal ileal involvement and (b) the "string sign" as a consequence of stricturing following ulceration.

nodular submucosal thickening. Ulcers are frequently elongated and tend to lie along the long axis of the bowel.

Since the serosa and mesentery are inflamed, a characteristic feature of Crohn's disease is the tendency for involved bowel loops to be firmly matted together by fibrotic bands. This adhesive process is often associated with the fistula formation characteristic of Crohn's disease. Fistulas begin as ulcerations and gradually burrow through the serosa into adjacent organs. Such fistulas communicate between the loops of small bowel themselves, as well as between loops of small bowel and colon, skin, perineum, bladder or vagina, or they may end blindly in indolent abscess cavities located within the peritoneal cavity, mesentery or retroperitoneal structures.

When the lesions of Crohn's disease are discontinuous, the intestine that lies adjacent to or between diseased segments (skip lesions) shows no gross or histological abnormalities.

1.2 Anatomic Distribution

Patients with Crohn's disease can be divided into those with small bowel disease alone (30%), those with both small and large bowel involvement (50%), and those with disease involving only the colon (20%) (Table 1). When Crohn's disease involves the small bowel, 80% of the time the terminal ileum is involved (Figure 1). In only 20% of cases are other areas of small bowel also affected. When the colon is involved in Crohn's disease (Crohn's colitis),

TABLE 1.   Anatomic distribution of Crohn's disease

Major site of involvement	Percentage
Small bowel only	30
Small bowel and colon	50
Colon only	20

TABLE 2.   Epidemiology of inflammatory bowel disease

Factor	Ulcerative colitis	Crohn's disease
Incidence (per 100,000)	2–10	1–6
Prevalence (per 100,00)	35–100	10–100
Racial incidence	High in whites	High in whites
Ethnic incidence	High in Jews	High in Jews
Sex	Slight female preponderance	Slight female preponderance

all segments of the colon can be affected. Although absence of rectal disease is more characteristic of Crohn's disease than of ulcerative colitis, the rectum is involved in half those cases of Crohn's disease in which colonic disease exists.

1.3 Epidemiology
Crohn's disease occurs throughout the world, with a prevalence of 10 to 100 cases per 10^5 people (Table 2). The disorder occurs most frequently among people of European origin, is 3 to 8 times more common among Jews than among non-Jews, and is more common among whites than nonwhites. Although the disorder can begin at any age, its onset most often occurs between 15 and 30 years of age. There appears to be a familial aggregation of patients with Crohn's disease such that 20–30% of patients with Crohn's disease have a family history of inflammatory bowel disease.

1.4 Etiology
The etiological agent responsible for inflammatory bowel disease has not yet been determined. The abnormalities of T cells and/or macrophages and their interaction still remains the most feasible hypothesis (1–4). In synthesizing existing literature, one could propose the following sequence of pathological events leading to the development of inflammatory bowel disease. The gastrointestinal immune system becomes exposed to a mucosal antigen, perhaps even an antigen normally present within the lumen – i.e., a bacterial constitu-

ent of normal flora. However, on this occasion the antigen does not evoke the typical antigen-specific suppressor T-cell activity, mucosal unresponsiveness. Rather, because of an antigen-specific immunoregulatory defect, it evokes helper T-cell activity and sets in play an ongoing immune response. This immune response as an epiphenomenon leads eventually to the development of self-antigens and appearance of autoantibodies. Subsequently, in an attempt to down-regulate the antigen-specific response, antigen-nonspecific suppressor T cells appear. Initially, these antigen-nonspecific suppressor T cells may prevent disease progression; however, they are gradually depleted, leaving the unregulated antigen-specific helper T-cell activity to predominate. This unregulated antigen-specific immune response leads to the production of lymphokines, which stimulate migration of inflammatory and cytolytic cells to the region. Through this process the microscopic and gross morphological changes of inflammatory bowel disease are manifest.

The initiating antigen in the above process has yet to be identified. Mycobacteria have remained a contender as initiating antigen for a number of decades. However, recent studies have found no evidence for Crohn's disease–specific humoral or T-cell reactivity against a variety of mycobacterium species (5). Recent studies demonstrating an increase in intestinal permeability in healthy relatives of patients with Crohn's disease have proposed the hypothesis that Crohn's disease is caused by an epithelial permeability defect that allows exposure to an increased number of mucosal antigens (6). Whether the permeability abnormality is a genetic defect or of environmental origin remains to be determined.

1.5 Clinical Features

The typical patient with Crohn's disease is a young adult whose illness begins with right lower quadrant pain, diarrhea and a low-grade fever. Examination reveals tenderness, guarding and a palpable mass in the right lower quadrant. If the illness has come on acutely and diarrhea is not prominent, these findings, along with an elevated white blood cell count, often lead to a clinical diagnosis of appendicitis with consequent laparotomy and discovery of the Crohn's disease.

More often, however, the clinical picture is insidious. The patient has recurrent episodes of mild diarrhea, abdominal pain, and fever lasting from days to weeks, and then has a spontaneous improvement in symptoms. If disease is confined to a small segment of intestine, this can go on for many years before a correct diagnosis is made.

The abdominal pain of Crohn's disease is localized to the right lower quadrant. When the colon is involved, crampy pain may occur in one or both lower abdominal quadrants. Fever, in the absence of complications, rarely exceeds

TABLE 3.   Mechanisms responsible for malabsorption and malnutrition in Crohn's disease

---

Inadequate dietary intake (most important)
Anorexia
Specific dietary restrictions to avoid diarrhea/pain symptoms

Inflammatory involvement of small bowel
Decreased absorption of nutrients
Acquired disaccharidase deficiency
Protein-losing enteropathy
Iron deficiency due to chronic blood loss

Small bowel bacterial overgrowth due to strictures and fistulas
Malabsorption of cobalamin
Altered bile salt metabolism and fat malabsorption

Intestinal surgery
Loss of absorptive surface area due to resection
Ileal resection causing cobalamin malabsorption, bile salt deficiency, and steatorrhea

Diarrhea
Fluid and electrolyte losses

Combination of above factors

38°C. Diarrhea tends to be moderate in severity, with five to six bowel movements per day when the disease is confined to the ileum. When the disease involves the colon, urgency, incontinence and rectal bleeding may also occur.

If the disease is not diagnosed, gradual deterioration will occur over a period of years; there will be shorter and shorter asymptomatic intervals, along with weight loss and increasing fatigue. A slow and persistent blood loss combined with poor food intake leads to anemia.

Malnutrition and malabsorption, with subsequent weight loss, are common at all stages of Crohn's disease. A variety of factors are responsible. Nevertheless, a voluntary decrease in food intake for fear of exacerbating abdominal symptoms is the primary cause of weight loss (Table 3).

Approximately 10–15% of individuals present without any of the above abdominal symptoms and are seen for the first time with perirectal disease, fever or one of the extraintestinal manifestations (Table 4).

Whatever the presenting clinical features, only 20% of patients will remain completely asymptomatic during the next 10 years. The remainder will have recurrent attacks of abdominal pain, diarrhea, and low-grade fever. If the disease progresses to the state where surgery is required, recurrence is common,

TABLE 4.   Extraintestinal manifestations of inflammatory bowel disease

	Crohn's disease	Ulcerative colitis
Local		
Perianal disease		
Anal fissures, rectovaginal fistulas, rectovesical fistulas	+++	+
Pararectal abscess	+++	+
Rectal prolapse	++	+
Hemorrhage		
Mild – may lead to anemia	+++	+
Massive – may be life-threatening	+	+++
Toxic megacolon	+	+++
Perforation		
Free, with or without toxic megacolon	+	+++
Walled-off	+++	–
Stricture		
Fibrous – permanent	+++	–
Muscularis mucosa hypertrophy – reversible	+	+++
Cancer	+	+++
Systemic		
Skin manifestations		
Erythema nodosum	+++	+
Aphthous ulcers of the mouth	+++	–
Pyoderma gangrenosum	+	+++
Eye lesions		
Conjunctivitis	+++	+
Iritis, uveitis, episcleritis	+++	+
Arthritis		
Peripheral joints – migratory, nondeforming, seronegative	+++	+
Ankylosing spondylitis, sacroiliitis	+	+++
Hepatic disease		
Biliary		
Pericholangitis	+	+
Primary sclerosing cholangitis	+	+++
Bile duct carcinoma	+	+
Gallstones	+++	–
Hepatocellular		
Chronic active hepatitis	+	+
Cirrhosis	–	+
Miscellaneous		
Fatty change (malnutrition)	+	+
Amyloidosis	+	–

(cont'd)

TABLE 4.   Extraintestinal manifestations of inflammatory bowel disease (cont'd)

	Crohn's disease	Ulcerative colitis
Hematologic manifestations		
Megaloblastic anemia	+++	+
Iron deficiency anemia	+++	++
Autoimmune hemolytic anemia	++	+
Thrombocytosis	++	++
Clotting abnormalities (hypercoagulable state)	+	+++
Renal disease		
Nephrolithiasis	+++	–

particularly at the site of anastomosis. Seventy-five percent of patients operated on for small bowel Crohn's disease have recurrences within 5 years and require another operation within 15 years. Additionally, the interval between operations appears to be shorter after the second or third operation than after the initial resection.

1.6 Complications

1.6.1 *SMALL BOWEL OBSTRUCTION*
Small bowel obstruction is the most common reason for surgery when Crohn's disease involves the small intestine. The obstruction results from inflammation and edema in an already strictured segment of bowel. The obstruction is often partial and is transient once the edema and inflammation are treated and allowed to resolve. Progression to complete obstruction is often slow and results from fibrotic stricturing. Complete obstruction may, however, occur suddenly when the small bowel becomes kinked off as a result of an adhesive inflammatory process.

1.6.2 *FISTULAS AND FISSURES*
Perianal and perirectal fistulas and fissures are particularly common in Crohn's disease and may be so severe as to overshadow other intestinal manifestations. Enteroenteric fistulas can develop between loops of bowel and may contribute to nutritional problems if they cause ingested nutrients to bypass areas of small bowel absorptive surface. Additionally, the presence of enteroenteric fistulas may lead to recirculation of intestinal contents and stasis, thus causing bacterial overgrowth within the lumen. Fistulas between loops of bowel and the urinary bladder ultimately lead to chronic urinary tract infec-

tions. Fistulas can also occur between bowel and cutaneous surfaces, bowel and the vagina, or bowel and other internal organs.

1.6.3 *PERFORATION*
Free perforation is unusual in Crohn's disease. When free perforation does occur, it leads to frank peritonitis.

1.6.4 *GASTROINTESTINAL BLOOD LOSS*
Insidious blood loss occurs with small bowel disease and often leads to an iron deficiency anemia. Frank bleeding of bright red rectal blood occurs with colonic disease and with perianal fistulas.

1.6.5 *MALIGNANT NEOPLASMS*
Malignant neoplasms occur both in the involved bowel and in the noninvolved bowel of patients with Crohn's disease three times more frequently than in the general population. Nevertheless, the frequency of malignancy is much lower than that observed in patients with ulcerative colitis.

1.6.6 *EXTRAINTESTINAL MANIFESTATIONS*
Extraintestinal manifestations of Crohn's disease (Table 4) frequently develop alongside colonic involvement and perianal disease. Patients with one extraintestinal manifestation are at increased risk for developing a second.

Arthritis is the most common systemic manifestation and presents as migratory arthritis involving large joints, or as sacroiliitis or ankylosing spondylitis. Spondylitis or sacroiliitis may occur for many years prior to the manifestation of intestinal disease. There is no relationship between the course of spondylitis and sacroiliitis and the course of Crohn's disease. Migratory monoarthritis involves large joints and again runs a course independent of the intestinal disease.

Inflammation of the eye, skin and mucus membranes may also occur during the course of Crohn's disease. Iritis and episcleritis are frequent eye manifestations. Erythema nodosum and, less often, pyoderma gangrenosum are common skin conditions. Aphthous ulcerations of the buccal mucosa, tongue and lips are frequent, often refractory, problems.

Clinically important liver disease is not generally seen with Crohn's disease. Mild abnormalities in liver function studies may be observed in a few patients, and liver biopsy will often show a mild pericholangitis in these cases. Cholelithiasis occurs with a frequency of approximately 30% in patients with ileal disease and/or ileal resection. This high incidence is probably related to a bile salt deficiency that causes the production of a lithogenic bile conducive to cholesterol gallstone formation.

Nephrolithiasis occurs in 30% of patients with Crohn's disease. Oxalate stones and hyperoxaluria are common and are related to steatorrhea. Fat malabsorption increases the amount of dietary oxalate available for absorption in the colon.

1.7 Diagnosis

Diagnosis of Crohn's disease, as of ulcerative colitis, is made through the accumulation of history and physical findings, as well as laboratory, radiologic, endoscopic and histologic findings.

Initially, other causes of bowel inflammation must be excluded (Table 5). In the acute phase of Crohn's disease, viral gastroenteritis, appendicitis, Yersinia enterocolitis and Salmonella gastroenteritis must be excluded. If the Crohn's disease presents as a chronic recurrent illness, then culture of the stools and rectal mucosa for giardiasis, amebiasis, intestinal tuberculosis, nongranulomatous ulcerative jejunoileitis, fungal infections and pseudomembranous enterocolitis must be done. If the inflammatory state is limited to the colon or rectum, ulcerative colitis, ischemic colitis, diverticulitis, and occasionally cancer of the colon may simulate Crohn's disease.

1.7.1 *LABORATORY INVESTIGATIONS*

A complete blood count (CBC) will reveal leukocytosis, an elevated erythrocyte sedimentation rate and thrombocytosis, all of which suggest that an active inflammatory process is present. Indices may be microcytic hypochromic if an iron deficiency anemia exists, macrocytic megaloblastic if a vitamin B_{12} (absorbed in the terminal ileum) or folic acid deficiency exists. If both these states are present then the automated Coulter counter will present a normochromic, normocytic–type anemia that must then be investigated through peripheral smear and measurement of serum iron, total iron binding capacity (TIBC), ferritin, vitamin B_{12} and folic acid levels.

Urinalysis may demonstrate a urinary tract infection if a fistula is present and proteinuria if amyloidosis has developed. The serum albumin is a useful indication of the patient's overall condition. It is low in those patients not eating, those with extensive malabsorption, and those whose disease is causing significant enteric loss of proteins. Serum alkaline phosphatase activity is frequently elevated in patients with Crohn's disease who have no other indication of liver disease. Serum carotene, calcium, phosphorous, Schilling test and stool fat assessment are useful in determining whether or not frank malabsorption is present. Lactose hydrogen breath test and ^{14}C-labeled glycocholate breath test are useful in assessing the degree of lactose intolerance and bacterial overgrowth, respectively. Note that the ^{14}C-labeled glycocholate breath test will also be abnormal in the presence of ileal disease or ileal resection.

TABLE 5.   Differential diagnosis of Crohn's disease (includes
colonic and/or small bowel involvement)

Infectious
   Yersinia species
   Campylobacter species
   Salmonella species
   Amebiasis
   Tuberculosis
   Balantidium coli
   Cytomegalovirus
   Histoplasmosis
   Anisakiasis
Eosinophilic gastroenteritis
Vasculitis
Solitary rectal ulcer syndrome
Colonic cancer
Appendicitis
Appendiceal abscess
Appendiceal mucocele
Meckel's diverticulitis
Pelvic inflammatory disease
Ectopic pregnancy
Ovarian cysts or tumors
Cecal diverticulitis
Carcinoma of the cecum involving the ileum
Carcinoid tumor
Ileal plasmacytoma
Ischemic bowel disease
Intestinal lymphoma
Nongranulomatous ulcerative jejunoileitis
Pseudomembranous enterocolitis
Ulcerative colitis
Radiation enteritis
Small bowel tumors
Systemic vasculitis
Fabry's disease
Zollinger-Ellison syndrome
Benign lymphoid hyperplasia

Endoscopy, flexible sigmoidoscopy, and/or colonoscopy are useful for identifying and performing biopsies on discrete mucosal ulcerations. These ulcers
vary in size and may appear round and punched out, serpiginous or linear.
Often islands of normal mucosa protrude into the colonic lumen as a result of
submucosal inflammation and edema. When prominent islands of mucosa are
separated by linear ulcerations, the intestine assumes a cobblestone appear-

ance. This pattern is characteristically different from that seen in ulcerative colitis, where diffuse ulceration extends without patches of normal mucosa.

The decision to perform colonoscopy should take into account the specific diagnosis and/or therapeutic issues that the procedure may be asked to resolve. These include (1) establishing a diagnosis; (2) activity of disease; (3) extent of involvement; (4) type of disease; and (5) suspicion of cancer.

1.7.2 RADIOLOGIC FINDINGS

The plain x-ray of the abdomen will reveal dilated bowel when a partial obstruction is present. Intra-abdominal masses resulting from matted inflamed loops of bowel or from abscesses can also be seen on the plain film.

An air contrast barium enema will demonstrate involvement of the colon and show narrowing, ulcerations, strictures or fistula formation. As with colonoscopy, a barium enema should be deferred in patients acutely ill with Crohn's colitis, since the examination is not critical for immediate management decisions and the risk of toxic megacolon and perforation is appreciable.

A barium enema may reveal disease of the terminal ileum as a result of reflux of barium past the ileocecal valve. However, determination of the extent of small bowel involvement requires administration of contrast medium orally or via enteroclysis. The small bowel abnormalities seen on x-ray are similar to those observed in the colon and include the characteristic cobblestone appearance, stenosis, and diseased segments separated by small bowel that appears normal (Figure 1).

It is important to note that changes in the appearance of both the large and small bowel on x-ray film correlate poorly with the course of the disease. There is thus no reason to take "routine" evaluative x-rays.

1.7.3 HISTOLOGIC EXAMINATION

Mucosal biopsies obtained from the rectum, colon, terminal ileum or duodenum at the time of colonoscopy or upper endoscopy provide histologic documentation. Granulomatous inflammation of bowel mucosa strongly supports a diagnosis of Crohn's disease (Figure 2).

1.8 Therapy

The management of Crohn's disease varies greatly depending upon the clinical status of the individual patient. No single therapeutic regime is considered routine for patients with Crohn's disease, and treatment must be individualized.

When the patient presents with acute Crohn's disease, the history and physical examination are critical in determining the severity of the disease, in addition to gathering evidence of intestinal obstruction, bowel perforation or

**Transmural
Inflammation**

FIGURE 2.   Crohn's disease. A transmural process.

abscess. The use of steroids or immunosuppressive agents in the presence of gross infection is disastrous. In mild cases, diarrhea and abdominal cramps can be treated effectively with codeine, diphenoxylate (Lomotil®) or loperamide (Imodium®). In moderate or severe cases, the patient should be admitted to hospital, remain n.p.o. and be maintained with intravenous fluids. When symptoms and findings suggest small bowel obstruction, nasogastric suction is usually required until edema and spasm of the bowel subside. If evidence of abscess formation, fever and leukocytosis suggests a systemic infection, broad-spectrum antibiotic coverage should be initiated after appropriate cultures of blood, urine, fistulas or other possible sources of infection have been collected.

1.8.1 *SUPPORTIVE THERAPY*

Symptomatic therapy may be necessary to control diarrhea in cases of chronic stable disease. As indicated above, diphenoxylate, loperamide and codeine are useful agents for controlling diarrhea, but they should be used carefully; they are potentially hazardous and should be promptly withdrawn if the patient's clinical status deteriorates.

Additionally, for patients with Crohn's disease, the diarrhea may be due to unabsorbed deconjugated bile acids that cause a cholerrheic diarrhea. Cholestyramine, an ion-exchange resin, effectively binds the unabsorbed bile salts and controls the diarrhea. Fat malabsorption may be treated with a low-fat diet supplemented with medium-chain triglycerides. Bacterial overgrowth proximal to areas of stenosis causes deconjugation of bile salts, again resulting in diarrhea; it responds well to courses of broad-spectrum antibiotics (e.g., tetracycline). Finally, lactase deficiency may occur secondary to the active inflammation and a trial of lactose-free diet is warranted.

The patient with Crohn's disease also requires continuous emotional support for this chronic, complicated illness; this support is necessary not only during acute attacks, but also during periods of remission. Although many consultants may be required to manage the varying aspects of complicated cases, one physician should be directly and continuously responsible for the overall care of the patient. Psychiatric consultation may occasionally be necessary for specific problems; however, successful management requires that continuous emotional support come from the physician who is directing the overall care of the patient.

1.8.2 NUTRITIONAL THERAPY

Nutritional deficiencies are frequent with Crohn's disease and often result from inadequate food intake by patients who have "learned" that ingestion of food aggravates diarrhea and abdominal pain. In addition, several pathophysiologic mechanisms contribute to nutritional problems in patients with Crohn's disease (Table 3). Nutritional problems may be further aggravated by surgical resection of diseased intestine, which decreases absorptive surface area; this decrease may be sufficient to interfere with an adequate absorption of multiple nutrients. Of particular importance, because of the distal small bowel involvement, is the malabsorption of bile salts and vitamin B_{12}, both of which have receptors located solely in the distal ileum.

Whatever the combination of mechanisms responsible for the impaired absorption and nutritional deficiencies in Crohn's disease, the physician must be attuned to assessing nutritional parameters, including ideal body weight, anthropometrics, serum proteins, and serum vitamin and mineral levels. The consequences of nutritional disturbances are particularly serious in children with Crohn's disease. Delayed growth and sexual maturation can and do occur, and if they are not corrected prior to closure of the epiphysis, permanent shortness of stature will result. Adjunctive nutritional therapy is, as well, required by patients who are malnourished at the time of their Crohn's exacerbation or who are unable to ingest adequate calories because of their disease.

Increasingly, patients with extensive and complicated Crohn's disease are being treated partially or completely with enteral or parenteral nutritional programs as a means of "resting" the gut, allowing fistulas to heal, inducing a positive nitrogen balance, and even causing weight gain. Short-term remission is often achieved through the use of "bowel rest"; however, relapse rates are high within a few months of discontinuing therapy. Recently, Greenberg et al.

TABLE 6.   Drug therapy in inflammatory bowel disease

Corticosteroids
Rectal
   Foam
   Suppositories
   Enemas
Oral

Sulfasalazine
Oral
Enemas

Mesalamine (5-ASA)
Oral
Rectal
Enemas
Suppositories

Metronidazole

Immunosuppressive agents
Azathioprine
6-mercaptopurine
Cyclosporine
Methotrexate

---

have demonstrated that disease remission could be induced provided the patient received an adequate number of calories. Furthermore, it did not matter whether these calories were provided through oral intake, oral intake supplemented with enteral elemental feeding, or total parenteral nutrition.

1.8.3 *DRUG THERAPY*

Although a small percentage of patients with Crohn's disease enjoy prolonged symptom-free intervals when treatment is not required, the vast majority experience long periods of symptomatic active disease or frequent relapses that necessitate treatment of the disease with anti-inflammatory and immunosuppressive agents (Table 6). Evaluation of the efficacy of such agents is extremely difficult, given the fluctuating activity and unpredictable long-term course of Crohn's disease. Recently, randomized double-blind control studies have attempted to answer some of the questions relating to drug therapy.

1.8.3.1 *Corticosteroids*

1.8.3.1.1 *Rectal corticosteroid preparations*   Rectal instillation of steroid-containing preparations is useful when Crohn's disease involves the rectum

TABLE 7.   Comparison of oral 5-ASA products

5-ASA	Average dose for acute therapy	Average dose for maintenance therapy	Approximate cost per month
Predominant colonic delivery			
Salazopyrin®	4 g/d	2 g/d	$ 75.00
Asacol®	4 g/d	2 g/d	$140.00
Dipentum®	2 g/d	1 g/d	$130.00
Salofalk®	4 g/d	2 g/d	$130.00
Mesasal™	4 g/d	2 g/d	$140.00
Small bowel and colonic delivery			
Pentasa®	4 g/d	2 g/d	$150.00

and the sigmoid region. The topical application of steroids allows for rapid healing of the area and restoration of the rectum and sigmoid to their stool reservoir capacity and, therefore, often leads to fewer episodes of diarrhea.

1.8.3.1.2 *Systemic corticosteroid preparations*   Corticosteroids are beneficial in the management of acute exacerbations of small and large intestinal Crohn's disease, in which they induce remission of symptoms and decrease disease activity indices (7). Although steroids continue to be used by many practitioners on a chronic basis in the management of Crohn's disease, there is little evidence to support administration to prevent disease relapse. Steroid therapy for acute disease is best begun at prednisone 40 mg/day (outpatient oral treatment in mild cases or inpatient intravenous therapy in severe cases). As improvement occurs, parenteral therapy may be replaced by oral administration of a dosage that is gradually reduced by 5 mg/week to the minimum level needed to suppress signs of the inflammatory process (20 mg) and then by 2.5 mg/week; the ultimate goal is to end steroid therapy. Unfortunately, this objective cannot always be achieved, and many patients become symptomatic when the dose of prednisone is reduced below 5–10 mg/day. This "steroid dependence" occurs frequently, and the amount necessary for maintenance varies from patient to patient. If possible, patients requiring long-term steroid therapy should be weaned onto an alternate-day regime; alternatively, the immunosuppressive therapy will allow steroid withdrawal or a lowering of the steroid dose.

1.8.3.2 *Mesalamine (5-aminosalicylic acid mesalazine [5-ASA])*
5-ASA products can be broadly divided into those with predominant thera-

peutic effect in the colon and those with therapeutic effect in both the small bowel and the colon (Table 7). In Crohn's colitis, colon-specific mesalamine is equally effective in mild to moderate disease. In Crohn's disease involving the small bowel, the mixed, slow-release and pH-dependent mesalamine (Pentasa®) and the pH-dependent release mesalamine (Mesasal™) appear to be effective in reducing small intestinal inflammation. In addition, both these products have been shown to be effective in reducing the frequency of Crohn's disease relapse. When used for acute treatment the average daily dose of 5-ASA products is 4 g/day (except for Dipentum®, which is 2 g/day). When used for maintenance therapy the average dose is 2 g/day (Dipentum® 1 g/day) (8).

1.8.3.3 *Immunosuppressive agents*
Immunosuppressive agents are reserved for steroid-dependent or steroid-resistant patients. When combined with steroids, azathioprine (150 mg/day), its active metabolite, 6-mercaptopurine (1.5 mg/kg/day), cyclosporine (7.5–15 mg/kg/day), and methotrexate (15–25 mg/day) are useful in cases of both ileal and colonic Crohn's disease. A large number of case reports and open studies have found that immunosuppressive agents will induce remission in steroid-resistant or steroid-dependent patients in approximately 60–70% of cases; nevertheless, the relapse rate is high once the immunosuppressive agent is withdrawn (9–11). Methotrexate and cyclosporine appear to work more quickly than 6-mercaptopurine and azathioprine. While cyclosporine can be effective in inducing disease remission, a recently completed Canadian multi-center trial demonstrated that cyclosporine (7.5 mg/kg/day) was no more effective than placebo in maintaining Crohn's disease in remission. An on-going multicenter trial continues to examine the role of methotrexate in maintenance therapy for Crohn's disease.

1.8.3.4 *Metronidazole*
Metronidazole (250 mg t.i.d.) is as effective as sulfasalazine in acute colonic disease if the patient has not received prior therapy, in patients whose disease does not respond to sulfasalazine, and in the treatment of perianal disease. Side effects include metallic taste, disulfiram-like effects with ingestion of alcohol, paresthesias and peripheral neuropathy. Most side effects are reversible upon withdrawal of the drugs; however, the peripheral neuropathy may persist.

1.8.4 *SURGICAL TREATMENT*
In view of the high rate of recurrence of Crohn's disease following resection of diseased bowel, operative therapy should be reserved for complications of

the disease or for those cases where the disease unequivocally fails to respond to optimal medical management. Complications requiring surgery are (1) chronic obstruction; (2) symptomatic abscess or fistula formation; (3) enterovesical fistulas; (4) free perforation; and (5) retarded physical or sexual development in children with Crohn's disease. Removal of the diseased segment(s) in a young child will normally allow the child to grow and mature normally until the Crohn's disease recurs. Patients should be forewarned that surgery is not curative but is necessary for the treatment of complications. Patients should also be warned about the common recurrence of Crohn's disease after resection of the small bowel or after colonic disease. The recurrence rate is 40% within 5 years, 60% within 10 years and 85% within 15 years.

1.8.5 TREATMENT FOR MAINTENANCE OR REMISSION OF INACTIVE CROHN'S DISEASE
No therapeutic agents have been proven useful for maintaining a remission in Crohn's disease; therefore, once the active disease has been treated and controlled, there is no rationale for continuing medical therapy. Recently, evidence has become available to suggest that mesalamine (Pentasa®, Mesasal™) may be effective in preventing Crohn's disease relapse in a subset of patients.

1.8.6 POSSIBLE NEW THERAPEUTIC APPROACHES
In the past few years, a number of basic research studies have investigated the nature of the inflammatory process involved in inflammatory bowel disease. As a result, it is now known that several mediators, such as prostaglandins, leukotrienes, cytokines and platelet-activating factor, are involved in the inflammation. There is increasing evidence that 5-lipoxygenase products (leukotrienes) play a key role in causing and perpetuating mucosal inflammation, while cyclooxygenase products (prostaglandins) may provide a mucosal protective function (12,13). It has been recently shown that eicosapentaenoic acid, a fatty acid obtainable from marine fish, is metabolized by the lipoxygenase pathway to a less inflammatory leukotriene (LTB_5). Dietary supplementation with 3 g/day of eicosapentaenoic acid for 6 weeks reduced the capacity of neutrophils to produce LTB_4, and in a small open study, inflammatory bowel disease patients showed significant decrease in neutrophil inflammation and improvement in symptoms and histological appearance of rectal mucosa (14). Blocking the synthesis of leukotrienes with selective 5-lipoxygenase inhibitors or blocking the leukotriene activity at the receptor level with leukotriene B_4-receptor antagonists is another new approach to therapy.

Our understanding of the immunological complexities in inflammatory bowel disease is growing. Immune modulators have been proposed as therapeutic agents for treatment of Crohn's disease. Indeed, interleukin-10 (an anti-inflammatory cytokine) when administered intravenously to a small number of patients in a pilot project significantly improved disease activity in patients who had otherwise failed all conventional management. Similarly, antibodies to tumor necrosis factor (TNFα) have also resulted in marked improvement in Crohn's disease in a limited number of patients. It is exciting to speculate that future advances in the management of inflammatory bowel disease will be found in immunomodulatory therapy.

2. ULCERATIVE COLITIS

Ulcerative colitis is an inflammatory disease of unknown etiology affecting the colonic mucosa from the rectum to the cecum. It is a chronic disease characterized by rectal bleeding and diarrhea, and given to remissions and exacerbations.

Ulcerative colitis is not a distinct entity, since most of the histological features of the disease may be seen in other inflammatory states of the colon, such as those caused by bacteria or parasites. The diagnosis of ulcerative colitis, therefore, rests on discovery of a combination of clinical and pathological criteria, investigation of the extent and distribution of lesions, and exclusion of other forms of inflammatory colitis caused by infectious agents (Entamoeba histolytica, Clostridium difficile, Campylobacter, E. coli and Shigella).

2.1 Pathophysiology

Ulcerative colitis is an inflammatory state confined to the mucosa, unlike Crohn's disease, which extends into deeper muscle layers of the serosa. Since the inflammatory process involves only the mucosa, sharp localized abdominal pain, perforation and fistula formation are uncommon in ulcerative colitis; this is in contrast to Crohn's disease, where they frequently appear. Under light microscopy, the colonic tissue displays small microabscesses, called crypt abscesses, which involve the crypts of Lieberkühn. Polymorphonuclear cells accumulate in the crypt abscesses, and frank necrosis of the surrounding crypt epithelium occurs; thus the polymorphonuclear infiltrates extend into the colonic epithelium. These microabscesses in the crypts are not visible to the naked eye; however, several crypt abscesses may coalesce to produce a shallow ulceration visible on the mucosal surface (Figure 3). Occasionally, lateral extension of crypt abscesses may undermine the mucosa on three sides, and the resulting hanging fragment of mucosa will appear endoscopically and radiographically as a "pseudopolyp." Following this mucosal destruction, highly vascular granulation tissue develops in denuded areas, resulting in friability and bleeding. The two most prominent symptoms of ulcerative colitis

crypt
cells
devoid
of mucin

muscularis

crypt
abscess
diffuse
inflammation
throughout
lamina
propria

FIGURE 3.   Cross-section of colonic mucosa showing typical crypt abscess seen in ulcerative colitis.

– diarrhea and rectal bleeding – are related both to the extensive mucosal damage that renders the colon less capable of absorbing electrolytes and water, and to the highly friable vascular granulation tissue, which bleeds readily.

Radiographically, evident foreshortening and narrowing of the colon, loss of haustral margins, and apparent stricture formation will often be seen. These findings, however, are often reversible, since they are due to hypertrophy and spasm of the muscularis mucosa and not to fibrosis.

2.2 Clinical Features

Ulcerative colitis typically occurs in patients between 20 and 50 years of age and may present as an early acute fulminating attack or may follow a rather indolent and often chronic course. Approximately 70% of patients will have complete symptomatic remissions between intermittent attacks. Ten percent of patients will have one initial attack and will experience no subsequent attacks, and 15–20% will be troubled by continuous symptoms that occur without remission.

The initial and most common symptom of ulcerative colitis is rectal bleeding. A blood stain on the toilet tissue or the appearance of bloody mucus on the surface of stools is usually the first symptom noticed. This initial bleeding is often mistaken for bleeding from hemorrhoids. Indeed, this first evidence of blood may follow a bout of constipation, which can sometimes be the presenting complaint. When constipation is the presenting complaint, the colitis is most often associated with disease limited to the rectum, where spasm prevents feces from entering the area involved. Hence, initial constipation or normal bowel habits may be the hallmark of ulcerative proctosigmoiditis.

Diarrhea occurs with more extensive colonic involvement, and blood is usually mixed with the feces. The principal mechanism responsible for diarrhea in ulcerative colitis is exudation with resultant secretion of interstitial fluids and loss of mucosal surface area for absorbing fluid and electrolytes and water. In addition, involvement of the rectum prevents this segment of the colon from acting as a reservoir for fecal contents prior to defecation. This rectal irritability causes frequent bowel evacuation of minute amounts of blood and mucus, an activity that can be termed "pseudodiarrhea."

Since the severity of the disease will affect the therapeutic approach and, indeed, the prognostic implications, it is important for the physician to assess the severity of the disease for every patient. The best indices of severity are clinical signs and symptoms. Large volumes of diarrhea indicate that the colonic mucosa has been involved to the extent that sodium and water absorption are significantly impaired. Frequency, however, is an unreliable indicator of severity because frequent bowel movements can indicate either large-volume diarrhea or rectal irritability. Large quantities of blood in the stools, a fallen hemoglobin concentration, and hypoalbuminemia as a consequence of loss of albumin into the stool are signs of widespread disease. Elevated erythrocyte sedimentation rate, fever, and abdominal pain and tenderness may point to transmural extension of the disease and the development of severe ulcerative colitis.

Ulcerative colitis can be classified according to grade of clinical severity:

1. *Severe.* Diarrhea comprising six or more movements per day, macroscopic blood in the stools, fever, tachycardia greater than 90/min, anemia and an elevated erythrocyte sedimentation rate.
2. *Moderate.* Diarrhea comprising four or fewer movements per day, small amounts of macroscopic blood in stools, no fever, no tachycardia, mild

anemia and a minimally elevated erythrocyte sedimentation rate.
3. *Mild.* Diarrhea comprising fewer than four bowel movements per day without anemia, fever, tachycardia, weight loss or hypoalbuminemia.

2.2.1 *SEVERE ULCERATIVE COLITIS*

Severe ulcerative colitis, the least common form of the disease, occurs in 15% of all patients with ulcerative colitis. This form of the disease may be the initial presentation or may represent a progression from a less severe attack. Diarrhea is profuse and rectal bleeding is constant and severe. Fever is marked and sustained, and appetite and weight are both severely diminished. Abdominal cramps are severe and tenderness may be localized, indicating impending perforation. Leukocytes greater than 10,000, severe anemia, and hypoalbuminemia resulting from low protein intake (anorexia) and increased chronic loss of albumin are hallmarks of this form of the disease.

Medical therapy is often ineffective for this type of patient, and colectomy is often required.

2.2.2 *MODERATE ULCERATIVE COLITIS*

Moderate ulcerative colitis affects 25% of all patients with ulcerative colitis. Diarrhea is the major symptom, and it occurs three to four times per day. Invariably, the diarrhea contains macroscopic amounts of blood. Abdominal pain may occur and may awaken the patient at night; usually the cramps are relieved by defecation. Low-grade fever may exist, and the patient may complain of fatigue, anorexia and some mild weight loss.

Generally, moderate ulcerative colitis responds quickly to appropriate therapy. Immediate mortality in this group is low. However, the long-term prognosis is for repeated attacks of equal or greater severity, and the risk of ultimately developing cancer in the affected colon is appreciable. As well, at any time during the moderate attack of ulcerative colitis, the patient may become severely ill, developing a severe fulminant colitis characterized by high fever, profuse diarrhea, progressive dilation of the colon (toxic megacolon) and rapid deterioration.

2.2.3 *MILD ULCERATIVE COLITIS*

Mild ulcerative colitis is the most common form of the disease, occurring in 60% of patients. In 80% of those affected with mild disease, the ulcerative colitis will be limited to the distal colon (sigmoid and rectum); in the other 20% the whole colon will be involved. The age, sex and familial incidence of ulcerative colitis are the same for mild disease as for severe disease. As well, the number of patients who have only one attack, intermittent attacks, or continuous disease is the same for both mild and severe ulcerative colitis.

In the case of mild disease limited to the rectal sigmoid, most often the disease will remain in this area; however, in 10% of these patients it will eventually involve the entire colon and bring about the simultaneous development of severe diarrhea and bleeding.

Neither colonic bleeding nor diarrhea is severe in mild ulcerative colitis, and the systemic complications of anorexia, weight loss and fatigue are not seen. Occasionally, the patient may suffer from a few days of crampy lower abdominal pain; however, hospitalization is usually not required and mild ulcerative colitis responds rapidly to therapy.

For patients who have mild ulcerative colitis, particularly proctosigmoiditis, the rate of colonic cancer is similar to that of control populations. Thus, colonic cancer occurs in mild cases of ulcerative colitis only one-fifth as often as in the more severe forms of the disease.

2.3 **Diagnosis**
The diagnosis of ulcerative colitis is made on the basis of the clinical symptoms listed above, on physical findings, and on the results of laboratory and endoscopic investigations.

2.3.1 *PHYSICAL EXAMINATION*
Physical examination during mild ulcerative colitis or between attacks may yield completely normal findings. In contrast to Crohn's disease, there are no palpable masses and no specific areas of tenderness, unless serosal involvement, peritoneal irritation or impending perforation (toxic megacolon) exists. Occasionally, the liver is palpable because of fatty infiltration or other hepatic abnormality. Auscultation of the abdomen may reveal increased bowel sounds and audible borborygmi. With toxic megacolon, bowel sounds are quiet or absent.

Rectal examination is usually painful and the anal sphincter is often spastic. The examiner may be able to detect gritty, coarse, granular changes in the rectal mucosa on digital palpation. Pseudopolyps may also be palpated, and a rectal stricture may be detected. In addition, it may be possible to feel a carcinoma. Rectal and perianal complications are far less frequent and destructive than in Crohn's disease and ordinarily consist only of minor fissures.

Examination of the skin and joints may confirm extracolonic complications (uveitis, stomatitis, pyoderma gangrenosum, erythema nodosum, large-joint arthritis, ankylosing spondylitis).

2.3.2 *LABORATORY INVESTIGATIONS*
There is no single laboratory test that will confirm ulcerative colitis. Anemia, leukocytosis and an elevated erythrocyte sedimentation rate often reflect the

TABLE 8.   Endoscopic grading of activity in ulcerative colitis

Activity	Appearance
Quiescent	Distorted or absent mucosal vascular pattern Granularity
Mildly active	Continuous or focal erythema Friability (touch bleeding)
Moderately active	Mucopurulent exudate (mucopus) Single or multiple ulcers (<5 mm); fewer than 10 per 10 cm segment
Severe	Large ulcers (>5 mm); more than 10 per 10 cm segment Spontaneous bleeding

severity of the disease. Iron studies reflect iron deficiency anemia (low serum iron, high TIBC, low ferritin). Electrolyte abnormalities including hypokalemia, metabolic acidosis, hypocalcemia, hypomagnesemia and/or hypoalbuminemia may exist in patients with severe diarrhea. Liver function studies will demonstrate an elevated alkaline phosphatase as a manifestation of sclerosing cholangitis. Blood cultures may be positive in patients with toxic megacolon.

Examination of the stool will reveal abundant red and white blood cells. Stool cultures for Shigella, Campylobacter, Salmonella, Clostridium difficile (culture and toxin), E. coli 0157 and Entamoeba histolytica should be done in all cases to exclude the possibility of infectious colitis.

2.3.3 ENDOSCOPIC FINDINGS

The most useful method of establishing a diagnosis of ulcerative colitis is to assess the integrity of the mucosa directly. Since 97% of people with ulcerative colitis have involvement of the rectum, simple sigmoidoscopy can be used to establish the diagnosis in the majority of cases.

The normal colonic mucosa is a smooth, glistening, pink surface. Seen underneath this smooth surface are the ramifying superficial submucosal blood vessels, which present a prominent vascular pattern. When brushed by a cotton swab, the normal colonic mucosa does not bleed because the mucosa is not friable.

Endoscopic examination of inactive or quiescent ulcerative colitis shows a distorted or absent mucosal vascular pattern with a mild granularity (Table 8). Mildly active disease shows continuous or focal erythema and friability. Moderately active disease displays mucopurulent exudate (mucopus) and ulcers less than 5 mm in diameter and fewer than 10 per 10 cm segment. Severe col-

TABLE 9.   Inflammatory bowel disease: indications for colonoscopy

Differentiating IBD from other diseases and differentiating Crohn's from ulcerative colitis

Establishing the extent of the disease

Screening for malignancy and malignant precursors

Evaluation of abnormalities on radiographs
  Strictures
  Masses

Evaluation of patients not responsive to standard therapy or examination to explain recent flare; searching for complications

Examination prior to surgery
  Detection of intestinal involvement (active IBD) in fistulous disease
  Differentiation of ulcerative colitis from Crohn's colitis

itis demonstrates ulcers larger than 5 mm and more than 10 per 10 cm segment; these ulcers are often accompanied by spontaneous bleeding.

Colonoscopy is rarely necessary in diagnosing a new case of ulcerative colitis. The rectal and distal sigmoid mucosa is almost always involved in cases of ulcerative colitis, and a carefully performed sigmoidoscopy with either a rigid or flexible instrument can usually lead to the correct diagnosis. Colonoscopy should never be performed in the case of acute, moderately severe or severe ulcerative colitis because of the risk of perforation during the procedure itself.

Colonoscopy for ulcerative colitis is, therefore, performed for specific indications only. These are (1) to determine the extent and/or activity of the disease in patients who are considered to be in poor symptomatic control; (2) to perform cancer surveillance or diagnosis; and (3) to determine the type of inflammatory disease, whether ulcerative colitis or Crohn's disease (Table 9).

2.3.4 *RADIOLOGIC FINDINGS*
A plain film of the abdomen should always be obtained, particularly with severe colitis, where the risk of toxic megacolon exists. The plain film may demonstrate foreshortening or loss of haustration; sufficient air in a segment of colon to silhouette the mucosa may reveal irregular mucosa, ulceration and mucosal tags. Patients with toxic megacolon will have mid-transverse colon dilation to a diameter of 6 cm or more.

An air contrast barium enema examination can be used for the same indications as for colonoscopy: to determine disease extent and/or activity, examine for cancer, or differentiate from Crohn's disease. Barium enema examination should thus be performed on all patients with ulcerative colitis, but only at an appropriate time. During the active disease phase, the colonic preparation, and even the barium enema itself, may precipitate a toxic megacolon. It is therefore prudent to delay the barium enema examination until the disease has been brought under medical control.

Radiologic features vary according to the location and state of the disease. There may be a loss of haustration on the left side of the colon (this can be the normal appearance of the colon in elderly patients) (Figure 4). Additionally, the radiolucent filling defects of pseudopolyps may be seen scattered throughout the colon.

Despite significant advances in radiography, comparisons of results from colonoscopy and double contrast barium enema suggest that the extent of the disease is often considerably underestimated with the barium enema. Nevertheless, colonoscopy is best reserved for investigating the disease of patients who have considerable symptoms of colitis yet have minimal changes on sigmoidoscopy and in barium enema results, and for obtaining biopsies of suspicious areas.

2.4 Differential Diagnosis

The disorder from which ulcerative colitis needs to be distinguished is Crohn's disease of the colon. In addition, a host of other diseases may resemble ulcerative colitis. The possibility of these diseases must also be excluded (Table 10).

Methods of distinguishing between ulcerative colitis and Crohn's colitis are illustrated in Table 11. It is important to note that, because of the anatomic distribution of ulcerative colitis, proctosigmoidoscopic examination is abnormal in virtually all cases. By contrast, even when Crohn's disease affects the colon, it often does not involve the rectum. In addition, perianal disease is much more characteristic of Crohn's disease. Although diarrhea and weight loss occur with approximately equal frequency in both diseases, abdominal pain is more evident with Crohn's disease. Extraintestinal manifestations occur in about the same proportion with both diseases.

2.5 Therapy

2.5.1 HOSPITALIZATION

Hospitalization is indicated for the following reasons:

1. Failure of mild disease to improve significantly within four weeks of the start of outpatient treatment. Hospitalization removes the patient from an aggravating environment and provides the physician with the opportunity to initiate more effective and intensive therapeutic measures.

reflux
ileitis

FIGURE 4. "Instant" double-contrast barium enema in total ulcerative colitis. The distal ileum is dilated with a granular surface indicating reflux or "backwash" ileitis.

TABLE 10.   Differential diagnosis of ulcerative colitis

Infectious
  Viral
    Cytomegalovirus
    Herpes

  Bacterial
    Salmonella species
    Shigella species
    Yersinia enterocolitica
    Vibrio parahaemolyticus
    Aeromonas hydrophila
    Neisseria gonorrhoeae
    Chlamydia trachomatis
    Syphilis
    Staphylococcus aureus
    Escherichia coli

  Protozoan
    Amebiasis
    Balantidiasis
    Schistosomiasis

  Fungal
    Histoplasmosis
    Candidiasis

  Other
    Clostridium difficile

Radiation colitis

Crohn's colitis

Medication/drugs
  Enemas
  Laxatives
  Local nonsteroidal anti-inflammatory drugs
  Sulfasalazine
  Penicillamine
  Gold
  Methyldopa

Eosinophilic gastroenteritis

Behçet's syndrome

Colitis in graft-versus-host disease

TABLE 11.   Clinical differentiation of ulcerative colitis from Crohn's colitis

Feature	Ulcerative colitis	Crohn's colitis
Clinical features		
Rectal bleeding	Very common – 90%	Uncommon: may be occult
Diarrhea	Early, frequent, small stools	Less prevalent or absent
Abdominal pain	Predefecatory, urgency	Colicky, postprandial
Fever	Uncommon if uncomplicated	Frequent
Palpable mass	Rare	Frequent, right lower quadrant
Recurrence after resection	Rare	Frequent
Clinical course	Relapses/remissions 65% Chronic/continuous 20–30% Acute/fulminating 5–8%	Usually slowly progressive; fulminant
Endoscopic features		
Proctosigmoidoscopy	Diffuse pinpoint ulcerations, continuous lesions	Discrete aphthoid ulcerations, patchy lesions
Radiologic features		
Rectal involvement	Invariable	Infrequent
Distribution	Continuous	Segmental, discontinuous
Mucosa	Fine ulcerations	"Cobblestones"
Strictures	Rare	Frequent
Fistulas	Rare	Frequent
Histologic features		
Distribution	Mucosal	Transmural
Cellular infiltrate	Polymorphs	Lymphocytes
Glands	Mucin depletion Gland destruction Crypt abscesses	Gland preservation
Special features	None	Granulomas, aphthoid ulcers, histiocyte-lined fissures

2. Severe illness with anorexia, nausea, vomiting, fever and uncontrollable bloody diarrhea (severe ulcerative colitis). Early hospitalization is critical for such patients so that they may be provided with therapy to control the disease and prevent complications, especially toxic megacolon.

3. Development of local or systemic complications including massive hemorrhage, persistent anemia, severe hypoalbuminemia, and/or cancer. Hospitalization at this time provides for assessment of the need for surgical therapy.

2.5.2 *SUPPORTIVE THERAPY*

Supportive therapy consists of medications that improve the patient's general state of health or alleviate symptoms. Chronic losses of potassium, sodium and water must be replaced with oral and/or intravenous fluids, since uncorrected fluid and electrolyte deficits have been implicated in the development of toxic megacolon and renal calculi. Blood loss due to severe disease should be replaced with transfusions. With mild disease, oral iron replacement is indicated. The use of antidiarrheal agents – e.g., diphenoxylate (Lomotil®) or loperamide (Imodium®) – for patients with ulcerative colitis is generally contraindicated. In severe disease where the colonic mucosa is severely damaged, antidiarrheal agents are generally ineffective, since there is a loss of absorbing capacity. Furthermore, they may contribute to the development of toxic megacolon. Similarly, anticholinergics can also precipitate toxic megacolon and thus should not be prescribed for patients with ulcerative colitis.

2.5.3 *NUTRITIONAL THERAPY*

Neither total parenteral nutrition nor enteral nutrition has yet been shown to have any beneficial effect in inducing remission of ulcerative colitis.

2.5.4 *DRUG THERAPY*

2.5.4.1 *Corticosteroids*

Corticosteroids should be used to treat active ulcerative colitis. They have no role in maintenance treatment to prevent relapse. The dosage and routes of administration vary with the severity and location of ulcerative colitis.

2.5.4.1.1 *Rectal corticosteroid preparations*   These are available in enema formulations as hydrocortisone 100 mg in a 60 mL aqueous suspension (Cortenema®) and as budenoside (a first-pass metabolized steroid) 2 mg in 100 mL aqueous suspension (Entocort®), in foam formulation as hydrocortisone acetate 80 mg in a propylene glycol gel (Cortifoam®), and in ointment formulation as hydrocortisone acetate 10 mg or 40 mg in an ointment base (Cortiment®). In general, enema preparations will cover a larger surface area of the colon, while the effect of foam and ointment preparations is generally limited to the rectum. With mild disease, especially that of the distal colon, rectal instillation of steroids will induce or maintain remission for a high percentage of patients. With mild to moderately severe ulcerative proctitis, twice-daily rectal steroids combined with systemic therapy will promote remission and more quickly return the rectum to its normal functional reservoir capacity. Patients should instill the solution while in the left lateral decubitus position and then change their position to right decubitus followed by prone for at least 20 minutes after each position, to allow for maximal topical coverage. Studies indicate that up to one-half of rectally administered steroids is absorbed. Even though systemic absorption does occur, adrenal cortical responsiveness is not adversely affected.

2.5.4.1.2 *Systemic corticosteroid preparations* In active pancolonic disease of mild to moderate severity, prednisone should be started in a dose of 40 mg/day. A single daily dose of prednisone is most convenient; however, such a dose does produce adrenal suppression. No significant difference in healing between groups given single daily doses or divided daily doses of oral steroids has been detected. For patients whose disease responds promptly to oral steroids, withdrawal should be undertaken at 5 mg/week until a dose of 20 mg/day is reached; then the drug should be tapered by 2.5 mg/week to off. In the case of severe ulcerative colitis, the patient requires hospitalization, and intravenous steroids (prednisone 40 mg equivalent/day) should be started. The tapering off protocol is as outlined above.

Once the disease is in remission, further steroid treatment should be avoided until a subsequent exacerbation occurs. Treatment is then reinstituted at a level appropriate to the severity of exacerbation (steroid enemas for mild to moderate exacerbations of proctosigmoiditis, oral or intravenous steroids for moderate to severe pancolonic relapses). If, however, symptoms recur with the attempted withdrawal of steroids, then long-term steroid therapy may be necessary until the patient experiences remission. The use of high doses of steroids to maintain the patient relatively symptom-free is not recommended, however, in view of the potential side effects of steroid therapy. If a patient requires more than 15 mg of oral prednisone daily for many months in order to keep the colitis in control, elective colectomy should be considered as an alternative means of treatment.

Steroids, particularly steroids in the high doses necessary for severe cases, may "mask" a perforation of the colon and lead to peritoneal soiling and death; therefore, careful monitoring of the patient on such high doses is vitally important.

2.5.4.2 *Mesalamine derivatives*
Mesalamine (5-aminosalicylic acid mesalazine, or 5-ASA) has been shown to be the active part of sulfasalazine and is effective in the treatment of active disease and in maintenance therapy to prevent relapse.

2.5.4.2.1 *Mesalamine (5-ASA) rectal preparations* During the past decade mesalamine has been developed in the form of rectal enemas and suppositories. Mesalamine enemas have an overall efficacy of about 80% in patients with active left-sided colitis. Side effects occur in less than 2% of ulcerative colitis patients, many of whom would have had previous allergic reactions to sulfasalazine. In comparison studies, mesalamine enemas are as effective as corticosteroid enemas in the treatment of proctitis and proctosigmoiditis (15). In patients with distal proctitis, mesalamine suppositories (500 mg b.i.d.) are rapidly effective without side effects (16).

2.5.4.2.2 *Mesalamine (5-ASA) oral preparations*   5-ASA is available as sulfasalazine (Salazopyrin®) or as second-generation 5-ASA products that deliver the active ingredient (5-ASA) to the colon without the toxic sulfapyridine moiety (Asacol®, Dipentum®, Mesasal™, Pentasa®, Salofalk®) (Table 7).

Sulfasalazine is metabolized by colonic flora, thus releasing sulfapyridine, an absorbable antibiotic, and 5-aminosalicylic acid (5-ASA), the active ingredient. The sulfapyridine acts only to carry the 5-ASA to the colon and, when released by bacterial metabolism, it is absorbed and is responsible for the dose-related side effects of sulfasalazine. The acetylation rate of sulfapyridine is genetically determined; slow acetylators develop side effects at lower dose levels of sulfasalazine than fast acetylators. The most common dose-related symptoms are anorexia, nausea, dyspepsia and diarrhea. Common hematological complications include impairment of folate absorption (thus supplemental folate therapy is a requirement for all patients on sulfasalazine) and Heinz-body hemolytic anemia. Hypospermia may occur and is reversible through withdrawal of the drug. Hypersensitivity reactions are rare; symptoms include fever, rash, bone marrow suppression, infiltrative lung disease, a lupus-like syndrome, pancreatitis and hepatic toxicity. Sulfasalazine is inferior to corticosteroids in the treatment of acute, moderately severe colitis. For this reason, sulfasalazine is used as an adjunctive to steroid therapy and not as the first line of therapy for acute attacks of ulcerative colitis. Therefore, once steroids have been started and the patient is tolerating oral fluids well, sulfasalazine can be started at a dose of 1 g/day and gradually increased to 4–6 g/day within 7 days. The second-generation site-specific compounds capable of delivering mesalamine to the colon appear to have less systemic toxicity than sulfasalazine. Patients doing well on sulfasalazine are usually not changed to mesalamine product. Nevertheless, new patients presenting with ulcerative colitis are often started on second-generation mesalamine product rather than sulfasalazine.

The two main pharmacological approaches of the second-generation mesalamine compounds adopted are (1) the creation of azo-derivative compounds similar to sulfasalazine but linked with mesalamine through a diazo-bond with another mesalamine molecule (olsalazine, as in Dipentum®); and (2) the incorporation of mesalamine either into pH-dependent delivery capsules such as Asacol® (pH 7.0) or Mesasal™ and Salofalk® (pH 6.0), or into a mixed slow-release pH-dependent polymer (Pentasa®). These second-generation compounds have shown comparable efficacy to sulfasalazine, with generally fewer side effects (17). Comparative studies assessing which compound might favor a higher mesalamine release into the colon and thus would be more suitable for patients with colonic inflammation are yet to be finalized. Comparison of mesalamine product dose and cost is presented in Table 7.

Once remission has been induced by either corticosteroid or mesalamine therapy, the risk of ulcerative colitis relapse can be reduced from 60% to approximately 20% with maintenance mesalamine therapy in approximately one-half the active treatment dose.

2.5.4.3 *Immunosuppressive agents*

In general, the use of immunosuppressive agents (azathioprine, 6-mercaptopurine) has been disappointing in ulcerative colitis. Encouraging preliminary results with methotrexate in severe ulcerative colitis have been published; however, larger trials to confirm these results are yet to be completed (18). High doses of intravenous cyclosporine (10–15 mg/kg/day) have been shown effective in improving severe ulcerative colitis that might otherwise have gone to surgery. However, once the cyclosporine is stopped, the vast majority of these patients relapse and end up requiring surgical therapy (colectomy). In this regard, cyclosporine may be useful in patients who are not psychologically ready for a total colectomy. Since ulcerative colitis is curable with a colectomy, the majority of experts would not use immunosuppressive agents in the treatment of ulcerative colitis over the long term because of their significant side effects.

2.5.4.4 *Metronidazole*

Unlike Crohn's disease, ulcerative colitis does not respond to metronidazole.

2.5.5 *SURGICAL THERAPY*

Twenty to 25% of patients with extensive ulcerative colitis eventually undergo colectomy, usually because their disease has not responded to medical therapy. The decision between surgery and continued medical therapy is often not clear-cut, and in many cases arguments can be made for either course. In ulcerative colitis, colectomy is a "curative" procedure, in contrast to Crohn's disease, in which there is a significant likelihood of recurrence some time after the colectomy. The development of the ileoanal anastomosis, eliminating the need for an ileostomy, has made the thought of colectomy more tolerable for many. In general, patients who require continuous high-dose corticosteroids and/or immunosuppressants to keep their disease under control should be strongly advised to consider colectomy. Those at high risk for colonic carcinoma (pancolitis of greater than 10 to 15 years duration) should also be considering colectomy or alternatively entry into a colonoscopic surveillance program.

2.6 Complications

Ulcerative colitis may be complicated by a variety of associated conditions. These are (1) local complications arising in and around the colon, and (2) systemic complications arising at sites distant from the colon (Table 12).

2.6.1 *MINOR LOCAL COMPLICATIONS*

Minor local complications in ulcerative colitis, unlike those in Crohn's colitis, are infrequent and generally heal with conservative management. Enteroenteric perianal fistulas develop in a very small number of patients with ulcerative colitis. In these instances the physician must be certain that he or she is not dealing with Crohn's colitis, in which enteroenteric fistulas are common.

2.6.2 *MAJOR LOCAL COMPLICATIONS*

2.6.2.1 *Toxic megacolon*

Toxic megacolon is characterized by an acute dilation of all or part of the colon to a diameter greater than 6 cm (measured in the mid-transverse colon) and is associated with severe systemic toxicity. Toxic megacolon occurs in 1–2% of patients with ulcerative colitis. Histological examination reveals extensive deep ulcerations and acute inflammation that involves all muscle layers of the colon and often extends to the serosa. This widespread inflammation accounts for toxic megacolon's systemic toxicity (fever, tachycardia, localized abdominal pain and leukocytosis). The loss of colonic muscular tone results in the dilation of the colon.

Though the association between a barium enema and toxic megacolon has not been experimentally proven, there are many reports of toxic megacolon developing after the patient has undergone a barium enema. Thus, a barium enema should not be performed on patients who are acutely ill with ulcerative colitis.

Clinically, the patient with toxic megacolon presents as severely ill with a fever, tachycardia, dehydration, abdominal pain and distention (Table 13). Examination reveals absent bowel sounds, tympany and rebound tenderness. Leukocytosis (greater than 10,000), anemia and hypoalbuminemia are often present. A plain x-ray of the abdomen will reveal dilation of a colonic segment or of the entire colon. On plain supine x-ray, dilation of the transverse colon

TABLE 12.   Complications of ulcerative colitis

Local complications	Frequency (%)
Minor	
Hemorrhoids	20
Pseudopolyps	15
Anal fissures	12
Anal fistulas	5
Perianal abscess	5
Rectal prolapse	2
Rectovaginal fistulas	2
Major	
Toxic megacolon	2
Colonic perforation	3
Massive colonic hemorrhage	4
Colonic carcinoma	–
Colonic stricture	5

Systemic complications	Frequency (%)
Hepatic	
Biliary	
Pericholangitis	30
Sclerosing cholangitis	1
Bile duct carcinoma	0.5
Hepatocellular	
Fatty infiltration	30
Chronic active hepatitis	5
Cirrhosis	3
Amyloidosis	1
Hematologic	
Anemia	15
Iron deficiency	5
Autoimmune hemolytic anemia	1
Microangiopathic hemolytic anemia	<1
Heinz-body hemolytic anemia (with sulfasalazine therapy)	<1
Thrombocytosis	20
Thromboembolic disease	2
Joint	
Peripheral arthritis, migratory, nondeforming, large-joint, seronegative	20
Ankylosing spondylitis, sacroiliitis	20

(cont'd)

TABLE 12.   Complications of ulcerative colitis (cont'd)

Systemic complications	Frequency (%)
Skin	
Erythema nodosum	3
Pyoderma gangrenosum	4
Ocular	
Episcleritis, uveitis	5
Iritis	5

TABLE 13.   Diagnosis of toxic megacolon

Signs of toxicity (three of the following criteria are required)
Fever >38.6°C
Tachycardia >120 beats per minute
Leukocytosis >10,000/mm^3
Anemia <60% of normal
Hypoalbuminemia <3 g/dL

Associated signs (one of the following criteria is required)
Dehydration
Mental confusion
Hypotension
Electrolyte disturbance

Signs of dilation
Colonic diameter >6 cm or progressive distention with abnormal haustral pattern

is most often seen. This distention of the transverse colon does not indicate severity of disease in this segment of the colon; rather, the distention is determined by the anterior position of the transverse colon. Repositioning the patient to a prone position will redistribute the gas to the more posterior descending colon and will dramatically decrease gaseous tension in the transverse colon.

If toxic megacolon is the presenting symptom of ulcerative colitis, diagnosis may be difficult, since a history of rectal bleeding and diarrhea is sometimes obscured by toxic megacolon. Most often, toxic megacolon complicates chronic intermittent ulcerative colitis and the diagnosis is not difficult. Occasionally, however, a patient seriously ill with ulcerative colitis and the resultant profuse bloody diarrhea will experience a sudden decrease in the frequency of bowel motions upon development of toxic megacolon. This decrease in stool frequency represents diminished colonic evacuation rather than improvement in the patient's status. In this instance, a delay in diagnosis could result in perforation and death.

Treatment of toxic megacolon consists of general supportive measures, including replacement of fluid and electrolyte deficits, correction of hypokalemia, transfusions and nasogastric suction. Intravenous steroids (prednisone equivalent 60–80 mg/day) should be utilized for 48 to 72 hours. If there is insufficient response, surgery should be seriously considered. If the systemic symptoms subside and the abdominal signs improve, high-dose steroids should be continued for 10 to 14 days, after which the dose should be gradually tapered off.

Patients whose disease does not respond to appropriate intensive medical therapy within three days have a risk of colonic perforation of 50%. Mortality in the face of recognized or unrecognized perforation is approximately 85%; thus, surgery should be considered at an early stage rather than at a later.

2.6.2.2 *Cancer of the colon*

Carcinoma of the colon afflicts patients with ulcerative colitis 7 to 30 times more frequently than it does the general population. The risk of colon cancer in ulcerative colitis is related to two factors: (1) duration of the colitis, and (2) extent of colonic involvement. The risk of colon cancer for patients who have had the disease less than 10 years is low, but this risk steadily increases. The cancer risk for patients who have had disease activity for 10 to 20 years is 23 times that of the general population, while a disease duration of more than 20 years is associated with a cancer risk 32 times greater than that of the general population. The extent of colonic involvement in colitis also influences the risk of cancer. The incidence of cancer when ulcerative colitis is limited to the rectum or to the left side of the colon is much lower than when ulcerative colitis involves the entire colon.

The colonic malignancy associated with ulcerative colitis is generally an adenocarcinoma evenly scattered throughout the colon. The adenocarcinoma is often flatter than cancers in the general population and has fewer overhanging margins. It is generally considered extremely aggressive.

Because of this high cumulative risk of cancer, prophylactic diagnostic procedures have been employed in an attempt to detect early malignant changes in the colon of patients with ulcerative colitis. Colonoscopy and biopsy have revealed that colorectal dysplasia is associated with colonic malignancy. However, areas of dysplasia can be missed at the time of biopsy, and the interpretation of dysplasia in the presence of active inflammatory disease is difficult, since regenerative epithelium may exhibit many of the features of dysplasia.

In summary, no test or group of diagnostic tests (not even frequent colono-scopies and biopsies) can absolutely guarantee that the patient with long-term ulcerative colitis is free of focal malignancy.

Patients with ulcerative colitis should have a colonoscopy and multiple biopsies performed after 5 years of disease. If no dysplasia is revealed by mul-tiple colonic biopsies, repeat colonoscopy can be performed every 2 years thereafter. For patients with moderate or severe dysplasia on colonoscopic biopsies, repeat colonoscopy every 6 months to 1 year is recommended. Until more diagnostic tools are available to identify those patients at risk for cancer, colectomy at 10 years to cure the ulcerative colitis and prevent colonic cancer is highly recommended.

2.6.2.3 *Colonic stricture*
Colonic stricture occurs infrequently but may mimic colonic adenocarcinoma clinically and radiologically. If there is any question regarding the diagnosis, surgical removal is advocated.

2.6.2.4 *Massive colonic hemorrhage*
Although rectal bleeding is universal in cases of ulcerative colitis, massive, life-threatening colonic hemorrhage is rare. For most patients, massive colonic hemorrhage can be medically managed with blood transfusions, ste-roids and 5-ASA products. Hemorrhage usually resolves spontaneously.

2.6.3 *SYSTEMIC COMPLICATIONS*

2.6.3.1 *Hepatocellular disease*
Pericholangitis is seen in 30% of patients with ulcerative colitis. It tends to occur more often in patients with pancolitis than in those with ulcerative coli-tis limited to the distal colon. This liver lesion is characterized by periportal inflammatory infiltrates, degenerative changes in bile ductules, and varying degrees of periportal edema and fibrosis. The lesion of pericholangitis is patchy; therefore, sampling error on needle biopsy of the liver often occurs. Clinical manifestations of pericholangitis or its progression to cirrhosis are exceedingly rare, and many patients have only minor abnormalities in serum alkaline phosphatase.

Sclerosing cholangitis develops in less than 1% of patients with ulcerative colitis. In this disorder, the bile duct becomes severely narrowed and resultant recurrent attacks of jaundice, right upper quadrant pain, fever and leukocytosis occur. This lesion must be distinguished from other causes of obstruction of the common bile duct. Sclerosing cholangitis does not respond to any therapy.

Fatty infiltration of the liver is seen in 30% of patients with ulcerative colitis. The etiology of the fat deposition is unknown, but it may be due to malnutrition and protein depletion resulting from diarrhea and protein-losing enteropathy. Liver function studies are normal or only mildly abnormal in patients with fatty infiltration.

2.6.3.2 Hematologic abnormalities

The most common hematologic abnormality in ulcerative colitis is iron deficiency anemia secondary to gastrointestinal blood loss. Most often this can be treated with oral ferrous sulfate (300 mg t.i.d.). However, for some patients, gastrointestinal intolerance of ferrous sulfate will necessitate parenteral iron injections (Imferon®).

Heinz-body hemolytic anemia can be seen in patients receiving sulfasalazine. This type of hemolytic anemia is directly related to the sulfasalazine and resolves when the offending agent is withdrawn. Additionally, autoimmune hemolytic anemia and microangiopathic hemolytic anemia, with or without disseminated intravascular coagulation, can occur.

Secondary thrombocytosis may appear. It is not associated with coagulation defects. However, in addition to thrombocytosis, increased levels of factor V and fibrinogen can be seen, together with reductions in levels of antithrombin III. In rare instances, pulmonary embolism and thrombosis of mesenteric or cranial vessels due to thromboembolic disease can occur. Repeated pulmonary embolisms in spite of adequate anticoagulation therapy or massive colonic hemorrhage during anticoagulation therapy will necessitate a vena cava ligation with colectomy.

2.6.3.3 Joint manifestations

The arthritis of ulcerative colitis may antedate the colonic symptoms. It tends to be migratory and affect the larger joints, is associated with a synovitis and swollen painful joints, and is nondeforming with no involvement of adjacent cartilage or bone. Rheumatoid factors are negative in these patients. Arthritis usually subsides with control of the colitis.

There is a high incidence of ankylosing spondylitis and sacroiliitis in patients with ulcerative colitis. Unlike peripheral arthritis, the ankylosing spondylitis in ulcerative colitis is chronic, progressive, deforming and generalized. It does not respond to corticosteroids and will progress in the face of quiescent colitis. The incidence of sacroiliitis is higher than that of ankylosing spondylitis in patients with ulcerative colitis. However, the sacroiliitis is often asymptomatic and can be identified only through appropriate x-rays of the pelvis.

2.6.3.4 *Skin manifestations*

Erythema nodosum with raised tender erythematous swellings on the extensor surfaces of the legs and arms is less frequent with ulcerative colitis than with Crohn's disease.

Pyoderma gangrenosum complicates severe ulcerative colitis but is rarely seen with mild disease. This skin lesion begins as a small, elevated nodule, which gradually becomes gangrenous, thus resulting in progressive necrosis of the surrounding skin. It tends to ulcerate deeply, involving underlying soft tissue and sometimes bone.

Usually both erythema nodosum and pyoderma gangrenosum will respond to control of the colitis. Occasionally, despite control of the colonic disease, the pyoderma gangrenosum will progress. Persistent severe pyoderma gangrenosum is thus an indication for colectomy.

2.6.3.5 *Ocular manifestations*

Iritis occurs in 5% of patients with ulcerative colitis and presents as blurred vision, eye pain and photophobia. The attack may be followed by atrophy of the iris, anterior and posterior synechiae, and pigment deposits on the lens. Episcleritis and other ocular lesions are only rarely seen with ulcerative colitis.

REFERENCES

1. Mayer L, Eisenhardt D. Lack of induction of suppressor T-cells by intestinal epithelial cells from patients with inflammatory bowel disease. J Clin Invest 1990; 86:1255–1260.
2. Saxon A, Shanahan F, Landers C, Ganz T, Targan S. A distinct subset of antineutrophil cytoplasmic antibodies is associated with inflammatory bowel disease. J Allergy Clin Immunol 1990; 86:202–210.
3. Gitnick G. Etiology of inflammatory bowel disease: Where have we been? Where are we going? Scand J Gastroenterol 1990; 25(Suppl 175):93–96.
4. Das KM, Vecchi M, Sakamaki S. A shared and unique epitope(s) on human colon, skin, and biliary epithelium detected by a monoclonal antibody. Gastroenterology 1990; 98:464–469.
5. Seldenrijk CA, Drexhage HA, Meuwissen SG, Meijer CJ. T-cellular immune reactions (in macrophage inhibition factor assay) against Mycobacterium paratuberculosis, Mycobacterium kansasii, Mycobacterium tuberculosis, Mycobacterium avium in patients with chronic inflammatory bowel disease. Gut 1990; 31:529–535.
6. Katz KD, Hollander D, Vadheim CM, et al. Intestinal permeability in

patients with Crohn's disease and their healthy relatives. Gastroenterology 1989; 97:927–931.

7. Modigliani R, Mary YJ, Simon JF, et al. Clinical, biological, and endoscopic picture of attacks of Crohn's disease: evolution on prednisolone. Gastroenterology 1990; 98:811–818.

8. International Mesalazine Study Group. Coated oral 5-aminosalicylic acid versus placebo in maintaining remission of inactive Crohn's disease. Aliment Pharmacol Ther 1990; 4:55–64.

9. Present DH. 6-Mercaptopurine and other immunosuppressive agents in the treatment of Crohn's disease and ulcerative colitis. Gastroenterol Clin North Am 1989; 18:57–71.

10. Present DH, Meltzer SJ, Krumholz MP, Wolke A, Korelitz BI. 6-Mercaptopurine in the management of inflammatory bowel disease: short- and long-term toxicity. Ann Intern Med 1989; 111:641–649.

11. Brynskov J, Freund L, Rasmussen SN, et al. A placebo-controlled, double-blind, randomized trial of cyclosporine therapy in active chronic Crohn's disease. N Engl J Med 1989; 321:845–850.

12. Fedorak RN, Empey LR, MacArthur C, Jewell LD. Misoprostol provides a colonic mucosal protective effect during acetic acid–induced colitis in rats. Gastroenterology 1990; 98:615–625.

13. Wallace JL, Keenan CM. An orally active inhibitor of leukotriene synthesis accelerates healing in a rat model of colitis. Am J Physiol 1990; 258:G527–534.

14. Salomon P, Kornbluth AA, Janowitz HD. Treatment of ulcerative colitis with fish oil n-3-omega-fatty acid: an open trial. J Clin Gastroenterol 1990; 12:157–161.

15. Campieri M, De Franchis R, Bianchi Porro G, Ranzi T, Brunetti G, Barbara L. Mesalazine (5-aminosalicylic acid) suppositories in the treatment of ulcerative proctitis or distal proctosigmoiditis: a randomized controlled trial. Scand J Gastroenterol 1990; 25:663–668.

16. Campieri M, Gionchetti P, Belluzzi A, et al. Topical treatment with 5-aminosalicylic in distal ulcerative colitis by using a new suppository preparation: a double-blind placebo controlled trial. Int J Colorectal Dis 1990; 5:79–81.

17. Riley SA, Turnberg LA. Sulphasalazine and the aminosalicylates in the treatment of inflammatory bowel disease. Q J Med 1990; 75:551–562.

18. Kozarek RA, Patterson DJ, Gelfand MD, Botoman VA, Ball TJ, Wilske KR. Methotrexate induces clinical and histologic remission in patients with refractory inflammatory bowel disease. Ann Intern Med 1989; 110:353–356.

SUGGESTED READING LIST

Calkins BM. A meta-analysis of the role of smoking in inflammatory bowel disease. Dig Dis Sci 1989; 34:1841–1854.

Delpre G, Avidor I, Steinherz R, Kadish U, Ben-Bassat M. Ultrastructural abnormalities in endoscopically and histologically normal and involved colon in ulcerative colitis. Am J Gastroenterol 1989; 84:1038–1046.

Ekbom A, Helmick C, Zack M, Adami HO. Ulcerative colitis and colorectal cancer: a population-based study. N Engl J Med 1990; 323:1228–1233.

Gyde S. Screening for colorectal cancer in ulcerative colitis: dubious benefits and high cost [Editorial]. Gut 1990; 31:1089–1092.

Hamilton PW, Allen DC, Watt PCH. A combination of cytological and architectural morphometry in assessing regenerative hyperplasia and dysplasia in ulcerative colitis. Histopathology 1990; 16:59–68.

Lashner BA, Kane SV, Hanauer SB. Colon cancer surveillance in chronic ulcerative colitis: historical cohort study. Am J Gastroenterol 1990: 85:1083–1087.

Lennard-Jones JE, Melville DM, Morson BC, Ritchie JK, Williams CB. Precancer and cancer in extensive ulcerative colitis: findings among 401 patients over 22 years. Gut 1990; 31:800–806.

11
The Colon
G.K. Turnbull, S.J. Vanner and M. Burnstein

1. INTRODUCTION

This chapter presents an overview of colonic physiology and diseases affecting the colon. It discusses lower gastrointestinal bleeding, infectious diseases affecting the colon and diseases specifically involving the anus. The main inflammatory bowel diseases have been discussed in Chapter 10. Diarrhea and its causes are examined in Chapter 7, "The Small Intestine." Other infections are presented in Chapter 7 and in Chapter 9, "Gastrointestinal Manifestations of Human Immunodeficiency Virus Infection."

2. PHYSIOLOGY OF THE COLON / S.J. Vanner

2.1 Function
The colon contributes to three important functions in the body: (1) concentration of fecal effluent through water and electrolyte absorption, (2) storage and controlled evacuation of fecal material and (3) digestion and absorption of undigested food. Although the colon is not essential for survival, its functions contribute significantly to the overall well-being of humans. The colon can be functionally divided through the transverse colon into two parts, the right and left colon. The right colon (cecum and ascending colon) plays a major role in water and electrolyte absorption and fermentation of undigested sugars, and the left colon (descending colon, sigmoid colon and rectum) is predominantly involved in storage and evacuation of stool.

2.2 Functional Anatomy
The human colon is a muscular organ measuring approximately 125 cm in length in vivo. Its wall consists of the four basic layers found in other GI hol-

low visceral organs – the mucosa, submucosa, circular muscle and longitudinal muscle – but several important differences exist. The mucosa lacks the villous projections found in the small intestine and presents a relatively smooth surface, but numerous crypts extend from its surface. Cell types lining the surface and the crypts resemble those in the small intestine but are composed of significantly greater numbers of goblet cells. These cells secrete mucus into the lumen, and mucus strands can often be identified in association with stool. This observation is misconstrued by some patients as a response to underlying colonic pathology. The haustral folds, which help define the colon on barium x-ray, are not a static anatomical feature of the colon but rather result from circular muscle contractions that remain constant for several hours at a time. The outer or longitudinal muscle is organized in three bands, called taeniae coli, which run from the cecum to the rectum where they fuse together to form a uniform outer muscular layer. These muscular bands and elongated serosal fat saccules, called appendices epiploicae, aid in the identification of the colon in the peritoneal cavity.

The colon is innervated by the complex interaction of intrinsic (enteric nervous system) and extrinsic (autonomic nervous system) nerves (Figure 1). The cell bodies of neurons in the enteric nervous system are organized into ganglia with interconnecting fiber tracts, which form the submucosal and myenteric plexi. These nerves are organized into local neural reflex circuits, which modulate motility (myenteric), secretion, blood flow and probably immune function (submucosal). Release of excitatory neurotransmitters such as acetylcholine, substance P and serotonin (5-HT) serves to activate local circuits such as those innervating muscle contractions. Their receptor subtypes provide pharmacological targets for the development of drugs designed to alter colonic functions such as motility. The major inhibitory neurotransmitter is nitric oxide. The importance of the enteric nervous system is exemplified by Hirschsprung's disease, where there is a congenital absence of nitric oxide – containing inhibitory neurons over variable lengths of the rectum and colon. This results in an inability of the colon to relax in the affected region. Infants typically present with bowel obstruction or severe constipation. Barium x-rays identify the affected region as a constricted segment because the excitatory effects of the neurotransmitter acetylcholine are unopposed as a result of the absence of inhibitory neurotransmitter.

The autonomic nervous system comprises sensory nerves, whose cell bodies are found in the dorsal root ganglia, and motor nerves, the sympathetic and parasympathetic nerves. Parasympathetic nerves innervating the right colon travel in the vagus nerve, and those innervating the left colon originate from the pelvic sacral nerves. Parasympathetic nerves are predominantly excitato-

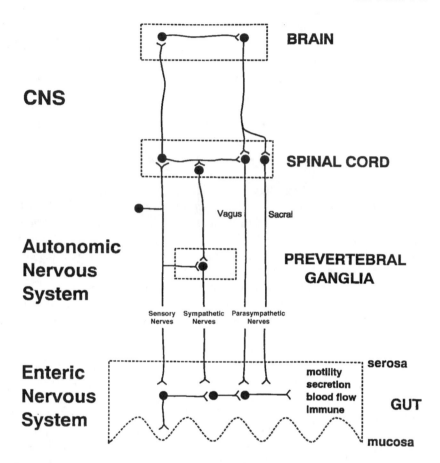

FIGURE 1. Innervation of the colon.

ry, and sympathetic nerves inhibitory. Autonomic nerves modulate the enteric neural circuits within the colon and participate in neural reflexes at the level of the autonomic ganglia, spinal cord and brain. Brain–gut connections are important both for perception of visceral stimuli (sensory) and in modifying colonic function (motor) in response to central stimuli. An example of a central stimulus that can evoke significant changes in colonic activity through this connection is acute stress. This stimulus provokes release of central hormones, such as corticotropin releasing factor. These hormones activate parasympathetic pathways that stimulate motility patterns in the colon and can result in diarrhea.

2.3 Absorption and Secretion

The colon is highly efficient at absorbing water. Under normal physiological conditions, approximately 1.5 L of fluid enters the colon each day, but only about 100–200 mL is excreted in the stool. The maximal absorptive capacity of the colon is up to about 4.5 L per day, so that diarrhea (increased water in stools) will not occur unless the ileocecal flow rate exceeds the absorptive capacity and/or the colonic mucosa itself is secreting. The fundamental feature of colonic electrolyte transport that enables this efficient water absorption is the ability of the colonic mucosa to generate a large osmotic gradient between the lumen and the intercellular space. This osmotic gradient is created by electrogenic sodium transport. This depends upon the energy-dependent Na^+/K^+-ATPase pump on the basolateral membrane, which pumps sodium from inside the cell against a large concentration gradient into the intercellular space (see Figure 5 in Chapter 7, "The Small Intestine"). Luminal sodium in turn enters the apical membrane of the cell through sodium channels, flowing down the concentration gradient created by the pump. In contrast to the small intestine, where sodium in the intercellular space can diffuse back into the lumen and become iso-osmotic, hypertonic solutions are maintained in the intercellular space because the tight junctions are much less permeable to sodium diffusion. The net result is that the hypertonic fluid within the intercellular space draws water passively into the mucosa from the lumen. It also results in highly efficient absorption of sodium. Of the 150 mEq of sodium that enters the colon each day, less than 5 mEq is lost in the stool. The tight junctions are highly permeable to potassium, in contrast to sodium, allowing potassium to move from plasma to the lumen. Potassium pumped into the cell by the Na^+/K^+-ATPase pump can also be secreted into the lumen. Potassium is normally secreted into the lumen unless intraluminal potassium rises above 15 mEq/L. This handling of potassium may account for hypokalemia seen with colonic diarrhea and may play a role in maintaining potassium balance in the late stages of renal failure. Other transport mechanisms, similar to those found in the small intestine (see Chapter 7, Section 5), are also found on colonic enterocytes, which maintain electrical neutrality, intracellular pH and secretion. Nutrient cotransporters, however, are not found in the colon.

The regulation of water and electrolyte transport in the colon also involves the complex interplay between humoral, paracrine and neural regulatory pathways (see Chapter 7). One important difference is the effect of aldosterone, which is absent in the small intestine. This hormone is secreted in response to total body sodium depletion or potassium loading and stimulates sodium absorption and potassium secretion in the colon.

2.4 **Motility of the Colon**

Much less is known about the motility of the colon compared to other regions of the GI tract. The movement of fecal material from cecum to rectum is a slow process, occurring over days. Functionally, the contraction patterns in the right colon (cecum and ascending colon) cause significant mixing, which facilitates the absorption of water, whereas in the left colon (sigmoid and rectum) they slow the movement of formed stool, forming a reservoir until reflexes activate contractions to advance and evacuate stool.

Several fundamental contractile patterns exist within the colon. Ring contractions are due to circular muscle contraction and can be tonic or rhythmic. Tonic contractions are sustained over hours and form the haustral markings evident on barium x-rays; they appear to play a role in mixing. Rhythmic ring contractions can be intermittent or regular. Regular contractions are non-occlusive, occur over a few seconds, and migrate cephalad (right colon) and caudad (left colon). Presumably, they too play a role in mixing. Intermittent ring contractions occur every few hours, occlude the lumen, and migrate caudad. They result in the mass movement of stool, particularly in the sigmoid colon and rectum. Contractions of the longitudinal muscle appear to produce bulging of the colonic wall between the taeniae coli, but the importance of this action remains poorly understood. The origin of these contractions is also poorly understood but appears to depend on slow-wave properties of the smooth muscle (regular rhythmic contractions) in some cases, and predominantly neural factors (intermittent rhythmic contractions) in others. These in turn are modulated by the interaction of paracrine, humoral and other neural pathways.

The nature of the contractile patterns within the colon depends upon the fed state. This is best exemplified during eating when the "gastrocolic reflex" is activated. Food in the duodenum, particularly fatty foods, evokes reflex intermittment rhythmic contractions within the colon and corresponding mass movement of stool. This action, which is mediated by neural and humoral mechanisms, accounts for the observation by many individuals that eating stimulates the urge to defecate.

2.5 **Digestion and Absorption of Undigested Food Products**

Greater numbers of bacteria (more anaerobes than aerobes) are found within the colonic lumen than elsewhere in the GI tract. These bacteria digest a number of undigested food products normally found in the effluent delivered to the colon, such as complex sugars contained in dietary fiber.

Complex sugars are fermented by the bacteria, forming the short-chain fatty acids (SCFAs) butyrate, propionate and acetate. These SCFAs are essential nutrient sources for colonic epithelium, and in addition can provide up to 500 cal/day of overall nutritional needs. They are passively and actively transported into the cell where they become an important energy source for the cell through the β-oxidation pathway. The importance of this role is illustrated by the effects of a "defunctioning" colostomy, which diverts the fecal stream from the distal colon. Examination of this area typically reveals signs of inflammation, termed *diversion colitis*. This inflammation can be successfully treated with the installation of mixtures of short-chain fatty acids into the rectum.

Fermentation of sugars by colonic bacteria is also an important source of colonic gases such as hydrogen, methane and carbon dioxide. These gases, particularly methane, largely account for the tendency of some stools to float in the toilet. Nitrogen gas, which diffuses into the colon from the plasma, is the predominant gas. However, the ingestion of large quantities of undigested complex sugars such as found in beans or the maldigestion of simple sugars such as lactose can result in large increases in production of colonic gas. This can lead to patients' complaints of abdominal bloating and increased flatus.

When bile salts in long-chain fatty acids are malabsorbed in sufficient quantities, their digestion by colonic bacteria generates potent secretagogues. Bile salt malabsorption causing "choleraic diarrhea" typically occurs following terminal ileum resection, usually for management of Crohn's disease. When the resection involves segments greater than 100 cm this problem is further complicated by depletion of the bile salt pool, because bile salt production cannot compensate for the increased fecal loss. In these circumstances diarrhea also results from fat malabsorption. The proposed mechanisms by which multiple metabolites of bile salts and hydroxylated metabolites of long-chain fatty acids act as secretagogues provide an example of how multiple regulatory systems can interact to control colonic function. These mechanisms include disruption of mucosal permeability, stimulation of Cl^- and water secretion by activating enteric secretomotor neurons, enhancement of the paracrine actions of prostaglandins by increasing production, and direct effects on the enterocyte that increase intracelluar calcium.

3. SPECIFIC COLONIC DISEASES / G.K. Turnbull

3.1 Colon Polyps and Cancer

Colon cancer is the second most common cancer (after lung cancer) in men and women combined in Canada. Unlike lung cancer, it has a high survival rate in patients diagnosed before it has spread beyond the confines of the bowel wall. Since it is a very common cancer, has a high survival rate with early curative surgery and is poorly responsive to other forms of cancer ther-

TABLE 1.   Presenting features of colon cancer

Abdominal pain, including symptoms of bowel obstruction
Change in bowel habit
Abdominal complaints of recent onset
Abdominal mass
Iron deficiency anemia
Hypokalemia

TABLE 2.   Colorectal adenocarcinoma staging

Dukes' stage	TNM stage	Tumor invasion	5-year survival
	0	Mucosa	100%
A	I	Submucosa No lymph node or distant metastases	90%
B	II	B1: Circular muscle B2: Longitudinal muscle No lymph node or distant metastases	70–75%

C	III	C1: 1–4 lymph nodes
		  positive
		C2: > 4 lymph nodes
		  positive
			45%

D	IV	Distant metastases (e.g., liver)	20% or less

apy, a high index of suspicion must be maintained in approaching patients with symptoms of colonic dysfunction (Table 1), especially if they are over the age of 40, when the incidence of colon cancer begins to rise. Increased colon cancer risk is also seen in patients with ulcerative colitis, a history of female genital or breast cancer, or a family history of colon cancer or adenoma (including familial polyposis syndromes).

The Dukes' classification is used to stage colon cancer after surgical resection. It is based on the pathological extent and invasion of the primary colonic tumor (adenocarcinoma) at the time of resection (Table 2). Dukes' A stage is adenocarcinoma confined to the mucosa and submucosa; the cure rate for this stage of adenocarcinoma with surgery is about 90%. Dukes' B stage has two subdivisions: B1 for adenocarcinomas that have invaded the muscularis propria, and B2 for tumors that have invaded through to the circular longitudinal muscle although regional lymph nodes are free of cancer. Dukes' C stage is adenocarcinoma that has spread to regional lymph nodes, and Dukes' D stage is adenocarcinoma that is metastatic to distant sites, usually the liver and beyond. Cure rates with stage C and D adenocarcinoma of the colon are very low with surgery; as well, both chemotherapy and radiotherapy have limited success, reinforcing the need to make an early diagnosis. Table 2 also describes the newer TNM colorectal adenocarcinoma staging system, which is similar to the Dukes' A–D staging system. The TNM staging system includes stage 0 when the carcinoma is limited to the mucosa and is called "in situ."

Early recognition is of the utmost importance to try to identify early cancer at a curative stage. Therefore, patients with intermittent symptoms are as important to investigate as patients with persistent symptoms, and the story of occasional blood in the stool in a patient over 40 years of age should not be attributed to local anorectal disease without excluding a more proximal lesion. Many patients may present with no gastrointestinal symptoms, but rather an iron deficiency anemia due to chronic bleeding from the tumor. Patients may not see blood in the stool or note a melena stool, particularly when there is a right-sided colonic lesion. A change in bowel habit, often with constipation alternating with diarrhea, may be the first sign of obstructive symptoms from a colon cancer, and should never be ignored in a patient over 40 years of age with a recent onset of these symptoms. Some patients may present with primarily diarrhea if they have a high output of mucus and fluid from the tumor; in this instance the tumor may be a villous adenoma, and some patients may have hypokalemia due to large amounts of potassium lost with the mucus secretion from the tumor.

Carcinoembryonic antigen (CEA) is a tumor marker that has limited use in diagnosing colon cancer but is often useful in following patients with colon cancer. A high CEA level before surgery often suggests a poor prognosis with probable metastases. CEA that does not fall to normal levels one month after surgery suggests that all the cancer has not been resected. After this, regular monitoring of CEA levels can identify patients with early recurrence. Sometimes a search for metastases will discover a solitary lesion in the liver that may be resected with the use of chemotherapy, which may lead to a cure of the cancer.

3.1.1 POLYP–CARCINOMA SEQUENCE

It is now agreed that the majority of colon cancer patients have a colonic adenocarcinoma arising from an adenomatous polyp. Polyps of 2 cm or greater have about 50% incidence of cancer, compared to 1% in adenomas of 1 cm or less. Adenomatous polyps are a premalignant condition, and their identification and removal before becoming malignant prevents the development of colon cancer. These polyps can arise anywhere in the colon, but (as is the case for colon cancer) they are more frequently seen in the left colon. The majority of polyps are completely asymptomatic, but the occurrence of occult bleeding does increase as they grow. Unfortunately, however, polyps can still be missed, even with occult blood testing of the stool, since the blood loss may be intermittent.

Three histologic types of adenomatous polyps occur: tubular, tubulovillous and villous. The malignant potential is greatest in villous polyps (40%) and lowest in tubular polyps (5%), with an intermediate risk in tubulovillous polyps (22%). The malignant potential may also be described pathologically as the degree of "dysplasia": the more severe the dysplasia, the greater the rate of malignancy. These tubular, tubulovillous and villous polyps can often be completely removed by snare polypectomy at colonoscopy if they are pedunculated on a stalk, but sessile polyps that carpet a wide area of colonic mucosa (often villous polyps) can usually be completely removed only by resection surgery. Since polyps precede cancer and removal of polyps "cures" the cancer, it has been hoped that screening colonoscopy may help reduce the incidence of cancer. Other polyps as well may be present at the initial or index colonoscopy, and polyps and cancer tend to recur. This sets the stage for the rationale for performing follow-up surveillance colonoscopies (colon cancer surveillance program). The best time interval for this surveillance is probably every three years; longer intervals between surveillance colonoscopies may be safe but have yet to be tested. The cost-effectiveness of screening all patients over the age of 40 has not been proven, and until particular subgroups of patients likely to have polyps are identifiable, routine colonoscopy screening is not indicated.

Particular conditions have been associated with an increased risk of colon cancer. The polyposis syndromes of familial polyposis and Gardner's syndrome are manifested by early onset (usually before age 30) of innumerable colonic adenomatous polyps that eventually and invariably lead to colon cancer (usually before age 40). Since the colon has too many polyps to remove by endoscopy-guided polypectomy these patients are referred at an early age for total colectomy to remove the risk of colon cancer. After colectomy these patients still need regular gastroscopic surveillance. Biopsies are taken from the ampulla of Vater to look for adenomas that frequently occur in the proximal duodenum around the ampulla, and also the stomach is examined endoscopically for evidence of adenomas of the stomach. An experimental approach at present is to do tests on blood monocytes looking for mutation of the APC gene, which is the cause of this autosomal dominant disease. There are other families (site-specific colorectal cancer, family cancer syndrome) that have a high risk of colon cancer (autosomal dominant inheritance), with more than two first-degree relatives having had colon cancer. This disease is called hereditary nonpolyposis colorectal cancer (HNPCC). It would be prudent to enter such patients into a colon cancer surveillance program of colonoscopy and/or air contrast barium enema if they have colonic polyps when screened at age 40. Female patients with HNPCC also appear to have an increased risk of endometrial and ovarian cancer.

Also at a high risk for colon cancer are patients with chronic ulcerative colitis for more than 10 years; this risk also appears to be present in patients with Crohn's pancolitis. The patients at highest risk are those who have had total colon involvement and those with left-sided disease, up to and including the hepatic flexure; patients with proctosigmoiditis are at least risk – probably not greater than the general population. Curiously, the risk of cancer does not correlate with the degree of disease activity. Therefore, patients with just one bout of proven subtotal ulcerative colitis would have an increased risk of cancer after 10 years of disease, and the younger the patient at the time of onset of his or her disease, the greater the cumulative risk of cancer will be for that patient. Unlike those who experience the "polyp–carcinoma sequence," patients with colitis do not develop adenomatous polyps before they develop cancer; therefore they require colonoscopy about every one to two years, with endoscopic biopsies of the colon performed to identify dysplasia of the mucosa. Particular attention should be paid to "elevated" or "flat" lesions seen at colonoscopy where the incidence of early colon cancer is high. If there is dysplasia, either "high grade" or "low grade," colectomy should be recommended to the patient.

3.2 Diverticulosis

In Western societies diverticulosis occurs in at least one person in two over the age of 50 years. The frequency increases with age. Diverticulosis or diverticular disease of the colon is due to pseudodiverticula in that the wall of the diverticulum is not full-thickness colonic wall, but rather outpouchings of colonic mucosa through points of weakness in the colonic wall where the blood vessels penetrate the muscularis propria. These diverticula are prone to infection or "diverticulitis" presumably because they trap feces with bacteria. If the infection spreads beyond the confines of the diverticula in the colonic wall, an abscess is formed. Patients present with increasing left lower quadrant pain and fever, often with constipation and lower abdominal obstructive symptoms such as bloating and distention. Some patients with severe obstructive symptoms may actually describe nausea or vomiting. This can occur with

TABLE 3.   Complications of diverticulitis

Abdominal abscess/Liver abscess
Colonic obstruction
Fistulas
   Colovesical
   Colovaginal
   Colocutaneous

---

or without abscess formation. Other causes of these symptoms include Crohn's colitis with stricture formation, colonic cancer and ischemic colitis (see Section 4).

On physical examination the patient often has localized tenderness in the left lower quadrant, and with severe infection and an abscess may have rebound tenderness in the left lower quadrant. A palpable mass is often identifiable where the sigmoid colon (the most common site of diverticulitis) is infected. Treatment consists of intravenous fluids and bowel rest by placing the patient on no oral intake or just a clear liquid diet; intravenous antibiotics are administered. Generally broad-spectrum antibiotics are used to cover both gram-negative enteric bacteria and anaerobic bacteria that are normally found in the colon. CT scan may be helpful in outlining the colon and identifying an abscess, and is preferable to barium enema for diagnosis in patients with acute illness.

Many complications can occur in diverticulitis. These are listed in Table 3. Colonic stricture after resolution of diverticulitis is described further in Section 3.3.

Bleeding occurs in less than 5% of diverticulosis patients; is abrupt in onset, painless, and often massive. A bleeding diverticulum can be from either the left or right colon. The bleeding frequency is approximately equal because of the much higher frequency of left colonic diverticulosis, even though bleeding is more likely to occur in right colonic diverticulosis. It is rare for patients with diverticulosis to have significant bleeding. Over 80% of diverticulosis patients will stop bleeding, but the rest will continue and require investigation and treatment (see Section 5). Segmental colonic resection is reserved for that small group of patients who continue bleeding or have recurrent bleeding. Recent reports recommend that patients under the age of 40 with symptomatic diverticulitis should have surgical resection because this small subgroup is at greater risk of complications.

3.3 Colonic Obstruction

Acute colonic obstruction is a surgical emergency that must be recognized early and dealt with expeditiously in order to avoid the high fatality rate due to colonic perforation. The highest risk patients for colonic perforation are those with an intact ileocecal valve that does not allow air to reflux back into the small bowel from the obstructed colon. The cecum is the most frequent site of perforation, because wall tension is highest in the bowel with the largest diameter (Laplace's law).

Patients with colonic obstruction usually have pain as a prominent symptom, with constipation often preceding the complete obstruction. Patients may initially present with diarrhea as the bowel distal to the obstruction empties, but diarrhea may be persistent, especially with a partial obstruction, because of the increased intestinal secretion proximal to the obstruction. The small intestine is the most common site of intestinal obstruction because of the narrower caliber of the bowel, and similarly the left colon is the most common site for colonic obstruction, especially since the stool is more formed in the left colon and unable to pass through a narrowed lumen.

On physical examination the general state of the patient depends upon the duration of the obstruction. With a recent sudden obstruction the patient will be in extreme pain, will often have distention of the abdomen if the ileocecal valve is intact and may describe initially diarrheal stool as the bowel distal to the obstruction is emptied. Abdominal palpation can often discern a mass lesion at the site of the obstruction. Prompt identification of the site of obstruction is mandatory, with the use of supine and erect abdominal x-rays. An urgent surgical consultation is required if the rectum is empty of air with dilation of more proximal colon, indicating a complete colonic obstruction.

Many patients may present with a more gradual history. If they have had protracted diarrhea up to the point of obstruction, the amount of abdominal pain may be less; they may have abdominal distention, but be less tender on abdominal exam; and they will often show signs of dehydration. Fever and an abdominal mass is particularly common in patients with diverticulitis and a resulting colonic obstruction. A third type of colonic obstruction can be seen that is actually a form of ileus limited to the colon and is sometimes referred to as Ogilvie's syndrome. These patients are most often seen in intensive care units, but the condition can also occur postoperatively (even when no bowel surgery has been performed). As with a "mechanical" bowel obstruction described above, patients with Ogilvie's syndrome may have marked abdominal distention, but frequently they have little abdominal pain and the abdominal x-rays show a picture of dilated colon with impaired movement of air into the distal colon.

Once a diagnosis of colonic obstruction has been made, the site of obstruction should be determined by plain abdominal x-rays and/or with a water-soluble contrast enema (such as iothalamate meglumine) to identify whether

TABLE 4.   Causes of colonic obstruction

Common
Left-sided cancer
Diverticulitis
Ogilvie's syndrome

Others
Hernia
Strictures
  Crohn's
  Postischemic
  Postsurgical

Intussusception
Volvulus
Adhesions

---

urgent surgery is indicated. Urgent colonoscopy is being done increasingly in this setting, especially if a colonic ileus or Ogilvie's syndrome is suggested, since the excess colonic air can be aspirated via the colonoscope and colonic decompression tubes can be placed in the colon to prevent dangerous reaccumulation of air until the ileus resolves.

Some authorities dispute the safety of colonoscopy in Ogilvie's syndrome and recommend prokinetic drugs instead. Unfortunately, drug therapy alone rarely works in severe cases of Ogilvie's syndrome, and if surgery is to be avoided the colon must be decompressed endoscopically. A dual approach of both careful colonoscopic decompression and prokinetic therapy may be best but is untested in clinical trials.

There are many causes of colonic obstruction (Table 4). Colon cancer and diverticulitis are the most common causes. Most colon cancers that obstruct are in the left colon. They cause circumferential disease or "apple-core" lesions (so called because of the irregular mucosal appearance with luminal narrowing seen at x-ray). Diverticulitis commonly occurs in the sigmoid colon, where diverticular disease is most common; the acute abscess formation with swelling of the inflamed diverticulum compresses and obstructs the affected sigmoid colon. Ogilvie's syndrome may initially have been considered to be due to a cancer or diverticulitis, but contrast x-ray or colonoscopy demonstrates a patent lumen and the diagnosis appears to be clear.

Less common causes of colonic obstruction are hernias, in which a loop of colon (usually sigmoid) becomes strangulated and the bowel is acutely obstructed. This is a much more common cause of small bowel obstruction. Strictures in the colon can also be associated with obstruction, especially when they occur in the left colon. These can occur with Crohn's colitis, after a bout of ischemic colitis or at the site of anastomosis following colonic surgery. This latter cause of obstruction should always be visualized endoscopically if possible, since most colonic resections are for cancer and the possibility of a local cancer recurrence can complicate a postsurgical stricture.

Intussusception can occur in the colon, and in adults it almost always occurs at the site of a polyp, which "leads" the intussusception. Typically, this will cause intermittent acute bowel obstruction associated with severe pain and often rectal bleeding from the vascular compromise produced in the intussuscepting bowel. Because of the intermittent nature of the obstruction, a diagnosis may not made be until after repeated attacks. A barium enema should always be considered in this setting, as it identifies the mucosal lesion "leading" the intussusception and can occasionally be used to reduce the intussusception without the need for urgent surgery.

Volvulus of the colon tends to happen in the cecum and/or the sigmoid colon, because the mesentery can be long and redundant in these areas and cause the bowel to rotate upon itself. This can be a surgical emergency, since the affected bowel will strangulate if the volvulus is not relieved quickly. Again, an urgent barium enema may be able to reduce the volvulus, thus allowing a more elective surgical procedure to correct the problem. A sigmoid volvulus will usually be reduced by this approach, and success with colonoscopic decompression of a sigmoid volvulus has been reported. A cecal volvulus may not be easily treatable with either a barium enema or colonoscopic therapy; thus, surgical advice should be sought urgently if cecal volvulus is diagnosed.

Adhesions are often described as a common cause of bowel obstruction, but this is probably true only for small bowel obstruction. Since much of the colon is retroperitoneal or on a limited mesentery, adhesive disease with obstruction of the colon is rare. However, it can occur, particularly in the sigmoid colon if the mesentery is quite long, and particularly after pelvic operations.

3.4 Irritable Bowel Syndrome
Most commonly, patients exhibiting symptoms from the GI tract are suffering from the irritable bowel syndrome. This is a condition that may be a variant of normal function. Causes of irritable bowel are still being evaluated, but the syndrome does sometimes occur after an episode of infectious diarrhea. It appears that patients have no organic disease of the gastrointestinal tract, yet they experience frequent symptoms from the bowel. Large epidemiologic studies would suggest that the condition occurs in at least 15% of the population.

The commonest symptom that brings a patient to a doctor is abdominal pain. Criteria have been developed to identify with more certainty those patients who have the irritable bowel syndrome. A more positive diagnosis can be made, particularly in women, if the abdominal pain is not localized and tends to have been present for at least three months. The pain is associated with bowel movements and relieved after defecation. Abdominal pain is also associated with increased looseness of stool as well as increased frequency. For a "strict" diagnosis of the irritable bowel syndrome, along with the above criteria it is felt that three of the following symptoms should also be present: (1) patients have difficult defecation; (2) patients complain of abdominal bloating or distention; (3) mucus is present in the stool; (4) there is increased stool frequency; (5) there is increased looseness of the stool at the onset of the abdominal pain.

Patients who have difficulty with defecation can have the following complaints. There can be "urgency," with the sudden urge to pass stool and a fear of incontinence if defecation is not performed immediately. Many patients with this symptom will relate that they always identify where the toilet is when they are away from home. The fear of incontinence can often greatly limit a patient's ability to function normally in society. Other patients with difficult defecation may have to strain – defined as having to hold their breath and push when attempting defecation. Straining is defined as "constipation" when a patient must strain 25% or more of the time when trying to defecate. Finally, some patients describe a feeling of incomplete emptying after passing stool. This symptom has to be asked for specifically, as most patients will not spontaneously report it. Nevertheless, the symptom is commonly reported by patients with an irritable bowel.

The presence of mucus in the stool can be alarming to some patients, since they may interpret this to mean they have "colitis." In the past, some doctors used to refer to irritable bowel as "mucus colitis," which is a misnomer since there is no "colitis" or inflammation of the colon in irritable bowel. Mucus is a normal product of the colon, and only if mucus and blood are seen together should other diagnoses such as "colitis" be considered.

The typical stool pattern described by patients with an irritable bowel is the change in stool character and frequency with the onset of abdominal pain. Typically, patients will pass a normally formed stool (sometimes even a constipated stool) first thing in the morning. Then with the attacks of abdominal pain the stools become more frequent and looser, sometimes becoming just liquid diarrheal stools. Once bowel movements cease the pain is relieved, but it can recur again later in the day, often precipitated by eating high-fat foods or other gut stimulants (e.g., coffee).

There have been reports that in men the above criteria (called the Manning Criteria) may not be as helpful as they are in women. It is also important to note that the vast majority of people with an irritable bowel have their symptoms begin in young adult life. One should consider other colonic diseases in patients over the age of 40 who develop these symptoms for the first time without previous episodes suggesting irritable bowel. Sometimes later in life patients can develop irritable bowel after severe infectious diarrhea, but in this population as well, further investigations are warranted to ensure no other cause for the change in bowel function.

The irritable bowel syndrome is a disorder affecting the entire gut, and although many of the symptoms appear to arise from the colon, these patients frequently have symptoms from other parts of the GI tract as well as from other organs. Upper GI symptoms are very common in irritable bowel; these consist of increased frequency of esophageal reflux. As well, nonulcer dyspepsia is associated with irritable bowel. Dyspepsia symptoms in general occur more commonly than lower bowel symptoms, but are obviously due to many other causes, including reflux esophagitis, gastritis, peptic ulcer disease and, less commonly, biliary tract and pancreatic disease. When upper GI symptoms are associated with irritable bowel, other underlying diseases must be considered. Other associated symptoms include frequent headaches and urinary symptoms that are similar to bowel symptoms, in that patients can have urgency and frequency of urination. These symptoms are often worse at times when the bowel symptoms are troublesome. In women, irritable bowel symptoms can often be exacerbated or worsened around the time of menstruation. Studies suggest that bowel symptoms associated with menstruation occur in at least 50% of the normal female population.

When assessing a patient complaining of irritable bowel symptoms, remember that only a small proportion of patients with an irritable bowel present to doctors with these symptoms. Recent studies would suggest that patients who see doctors about their symptoms often have psychological problems, with increased levels of distress and depression as common findings. It is important to inquire about these problems, as successful treatment often consists of dealing with the distress and/or depression that accompanies the irritable bowel symptoms. They may often be the reason that the patient has sought medical attention in the first place.

3.4.1 DIFFERENTIAL DIAGNOSIS

The Manning Criteria provide a more positive diagnosis of irritable bowel: abdominal pain with the association of increased frequency and increased looseness of stool, relief of abdominal pain with defecation, abdominal bloating, mucus in the stool and defecation difficulties such as a sensation of incomplete rectal emptying after defecation. However, lactose intolerance is a common cause of change in bowel habit in young adults, particularly if their racial background is not northern European. Therefore, investigating for lactose intolerance in patients who present with increased frequency and looseness of stool is worthwhile, since the ingestion of lactose-containing foods may be the reason for their symptoms. All patients should have a thorough physical examination, looking for evidence of disease in other organ systems such as the thyroid, which can present with a change in bowel habit. Patients with an irritable bowel will often have pain over the colon, particularly the sigmoid colon, on palpation. The identification of an enlarged liver or spleen or other abdominal masses necessitates further investigations. A barium enema is rarely required in a young healthy adult with new onset of irritable bowel symptoms. However, a patient over the age of 40 presenting with symptoms that may be irritable bowel yet of new onset and without previous complaints would warrant at least a barium enema and a sigmoidoscopic examination. The barium enema should also evaluate the terminal ileum if there is pain on palpation in the right lower quadrant. A complete blood count with platelet count should be done, as an elevated platelet count is often a sensitive finding for underlying inflammation and in the presence of bowel symptoms could mean the presence of early inflammatory bowel disease. Crohn's disease is more likely to present this way than irritable bowel. The persistence of the abdominal pain, even though lessened after bowel movements, would suggest possible underlying inflammation of the gut rather than an irritable bowel. Ulcerative colitis usually presents with rectal bleeding. Rectal bleeding is not a symptom of irritable bowel and its cause must always be investigated. Fever, weight loss and symptoms that wake a patient from sleep, as opposed to early waking in the morning, are all symptoms that should be further investigated.

The presence of nocturnal symptoms, particularly with diarrhea waking the patient at night, is almost never due to an irritable bowel. Occasionally patients with depression who have early morning waking report this symptom, but in general further investigations are indicated.

3.4.2 THERAPY

The therapeutic approach in irritable bowel is as much reassurance as any specific therapies, as most patients do not have any "disease." It is most important to do a thorough history and physical examination to ensure that the complaints are not due to any underlying disease. Once this has been confirmed, explain to the patient how the bowel can produce these symptoms and that there is no cause for concern. Since patients presenting with irritable bowel symptoms frequently have more distress and tend to be more prone to seek medical attention for other minor medical conditions than other patients (so-called illness behavior), these patients may require considerable reassurance to convince them that they do not have serious disease. Part of this reassurance will be provided by screening blood tests such as a complete blood count with platelet count. Sigmoidoscopic examination will rule out most underlying early inflammatory bowel disease and any rectal pathology, particularly in patients complaining of defecation difficulties or a sensation of being unable to empty the rectum adequately. The stool should be analyzed for pathogens if diarrhea is present. Following these initial screening tests emphasis should be placed on the stresses present in the patient's life. Evaluating the level of stress and taking steps to correct it will often be helpful. Many patients, particularly those who have symptoms of constipation, may be helped with a high-fiber diet (see Section 3.6).

Drug treatment for irritable bowel is generally discouraged. There is no single drug that treats all the varied symptoms in irritable bowel, but occasional patients will continue to have intractable symptomatology. In this situation selected medications for specific symptoms may be helpful. Table 5 outlines some drugs that may be useful for specific symptoms. Drug therapy for irritable bowel should always be restricted to short periods during exacerbation of symptoms, and patients should be taken off medications when well. As irritable bowel is a chronic condition and is probably "normal" for these patients, the chronic use of medications often reinforces the notion that they have a "disease." Reassuring the patient that there is no association between irritable bowel symptoms and the development of more serious bowel disease such as colon cancer or inflammatory bowel disease can often alleviate some of the unreasonable yet very real concerns of many patients who present to doctors with these symptoms.

3.5 **Fecal Incontinence**

Understanding fecal incontinence requires knowledge of the normal function of the anorectum. Anatomically, it consists of the internal anal sphincter surrounded by the external anal sphincter and puborectalis muscles. The internal anal sphincter consists of smooth muscle and is a continuation of the circular smooth muscle of the rectum. The external anal sphincter is made up of skeletal muscle and surrounds the internal anal sphincter, whereas the puborectalis (also consisting of skeletal muscle) is a large U-shaped muscle that wraps around the upper anal canal at the anorectal junction above the external anal sphincter and loops anteriorly to attach to the pubic bone. This creates an anatomical sling of muscle that pulls the anorectal junction forward when it tightens, thus closing the upper anal canal and creating the anorectal angle that is vital to the maintenance of fecal continence.

When stool (or gas or liquid) enters the rectum or sigmoid colon, a normal rectoanal inhibitory reflex (RAIR) or rectosphincteric reflex is initiated – that

TABLE 5. Drug therapy in irritable bowel syndrome

Symptom	Drug	Dosage
Abdominal pain	Anticholinergics	
	Hyoscyamine	0.125 mg sl q4h prn
	Dicyclomine	10–20 mg po tid–qid before meals
	Calcium antagonists	
	Pinaverium bromide	50–100 mg po tid before meals
	Antidepressants	
	(e.g.) Amitriptyline	10–25 mg po hs (increase by 10–25 mg increments every 5 to 7 days as tolerated)
	Enteric opioids	
	Trimebutine	100–200 mg po tid before meals
Constipation	High-fiber diet	≥ 30 g daily plus 2 L liquid daily
	Osmotic laxatives	
	Milk of magnesia	15–30 mL po bid–tid
	Prokinetic agent	
	Cisapride	20 mg po bid–qid
	Other agents	
	Misoprostol	200 µg po bid–qid before meals
Diarrhea	Binding agent (resin)	
	Cholestyramine	4 g po once to four times daily
	Antimotility agents	
	Loperamide	2–4 mg po prn to a maximum daily dose of 16 mg
	Diphenoxylate	2.5 mg po qid prn
Abdominal bloating, "gas"	Simethicone	≤ qid prn
	Peppermint oil, enteric coated	1 cap po qid prn
	? motility agents	
	Cisapride	10–20 mg po bid–qid
	Domperidone	10–20 mg po qid

is, the internal anal sphincter relaxes and, if voluntary muscle action occurs, the rectum empties through the anal canal (Figure 2). Fecal continence is maintained by contraction under voluntary control of the striated-muscle sphincters – i.e., the external anal sphincter (EAS) and puborectalis (PR) –

FIGURE 2. Physiology of defecation.

until the rectal pressure rise decreases and the resting tone of the internal anal sphincter is restored. Thus, the "voluntary" sphincters (i.e., the EAS and PR) have the ability to be maximally contracted for approximately one minute, beyond which fecal continence is lost as a result of fatigue in the muscle if the tone of the internal anal sphincter has not recovered.

The patient with fecal incontinence will often describe the problem as "diarrhea" rather than loss of control of bowel function. All patients with a complaint of diarrhea should be asked if they have lost control of stool, as this may indicate where the problem actually lies. Once fecal incontinence has been noted, it is then necessary to identify the frequency of the incontinence, whether both liquid and solid stool have been leaked and whether the individual has an urge to defecate before the leakage occurs. A history of previous anorectal trauma (surgical or otherwise) is important to note, as is the strength of voluntary anal canal tone on digital rectal exam.

Most patients presenting with fecal incontinence have "idiopathic" fecal incontinence, but recent investigations in females with this complaint indicate they have suffered damage to the pudendal nerves during childbirth and, with time, this has led to gradual striated-muscle anal sphincter weakness. Surgical trauma is the next most common cause of fecal incontinence; it should be remembered that surgery (e.g., a vaginal hysterectomy) can put excess stretch on the pelvic floor nerves and muscles, causing injury that may lead to weakness of the anal sphincters. Another common source of fecal incontinence is disruption of the internal anal sphincter, either during a lateral internal sphincterotomy to treat an anal fissure or, more commonly, with the older "Lord's" procedure of forceful three- or four-finger dilation of the anal sphincter under anesthetic, where the extent of damage to the sphincters is not predictable. The finding of perineal descent can be noted on examination of the perineum when the patient is asked to strain and appears to be associated with weakness of the pelvic floor muscles as well as disruption of the normal anatomy. This gives rise to a mechanical disadvantage affecting the sphincter mechanism. Perineal descent may be associated with a rectocele or, in female patients, with a uterine prolapse. Rectal prolapse can also accompany weakness of the pelvic floor muscles and give rise to fecal incontinence.

Therapy of fecal incontinence has improved over the past decade, primarily because of the introduction of biofeedback training. This technique allows the patient to practice tightening of the striated-muscle portion of the anal sphincter, usually with a surface electromyography (EMG) plug electrode held in the anal canal with audio and visual feedback that the patient can see and hear to encourage maximal contraction of these muscles. Attention should also be given to increasing dietary fiber to help reduce the amount of liquid stool. Other drug therapy is limited, but loperamide has been shown to increase the resting tone of the anal sphincters and is a useful adjunct, especially if the stool frequency is increased (loperamide reduces this contributing factor). Cholestyramine may be useful when the patient has diarrhea or loose stool(s) since cholestyramine can make stool more solid (constipating effect). Surgery is sometimes required and is of greatest benefit in those patients who appear to have a mechanical problem such as rectal prolapse or disruption of the sphincter. Surgery to correct perineal descent is often less helpful, since the problem of muscle weakness that gives rise to the descent is not satisfactorily reversed by any of the surgical procedures currently used, and attempts to "suspend" the pelvic floor muscles cannot strengthen these muscles. Patients should refrain from excess straining if they have significant perineal descent, since this will serve only to worsen the pelvic floor muscle weakness.

3.6 Constipation

In the approach to a patient with constipation, it is first necessary to define what the patient means by the term. Many definitions exist, but the best clinical definition is that over 95% of the North American population has a stool frequency from three times a day to three times a week: therefore, patients who have a bowel frequency less than three times a week would be defined as being constipated. Many patients will describe their stool as "constipated," usually meaning that the stool is hard or in pellets (scybalous), while other patients may have a stool frequency that falls within the "normal" range yet feel that their bowels have not completely emptied. This latter symptom is a frequent complaint of the irritable bowel syndrome, and many patients with this disorder will describe a constipated bowel habit. Those constipated patients who have infrequent stool alternating with occasional diarrheal stool have the most common presentation of irritable bowel syndrome. Yet there are a great many patients, almost all female, who have infrequent stool passage, and this group must be considered as separate from the usual irritable bowel syndrome patient for they may be among those rare patients with a secondary cause of constipation.

In Western culture the most frequent cause of constipation is a lack of dietary fiber. The concept of "fiber" has become quite confusing to many patients with the increased emphasis on "oat fiber" for elevated cholesterol treatment. Many foods that patients consider to be high in fiber (e.g., salads, lettuce, tomatoes and celery) are in fact mainly water, and some vegetables may aggravate their symptoms. Fiber is complex carbohydrates that are incompletely digested by the small bowel and are then "digested" by colonic bacteria, liberating fermentation gases and short-chain fatty acids that may provoke and aggravate many of the associated abdominal symptoms (e.g., abdominal pain, "gas" and bloating). It should be emphasized that cereal grain fibers that have more insoluble fiber (as opposed to soluble oat bran fiber) are best to increase stool frequency, but should be added gradually over 8 to 12 weeks to a daily dose of about 30 g. Other fibers in the form of "bulk laxative" preparations containing psyllium, methylcellulose Sterculia or isphagula may be added to wheat bran fiber to accomplish this level of fiber without completely altering a patient's diet. Many patients who are constipated continue to pass dry, hard stool despite an increase in dietary fiber because they do not increase the water content of their diet. Fiber works in the gut by holding onto water and keeping the stool soft; to achieve this effect, the intake of liquids must be increased. For a 30 g/day fiber diet, it is recommended that patients drink eight 8 oz. glasses (i.e., 2 L) of non–caffeine-containing beverages per day.

Secondary causes of constipation must be excluded. The patient with bowel obstruction can present with constipation, and this possibility should always be considered in a patient with the onset of constipation after the age of 40 years (when the incidence of colon cancer rises). A rarer cause of constipation is hypothyroidism; not infrequently, patients with an underactive thyroid will present with a primary symptom of constipation. Hypercalcemia rarely reaches levels that produce constipation but should always be considered, since it can be a life-threatening disorder; constipation in this setting is always resistant to therapy until the hypercalcemia is treated. Proctitis can present with a complaint of infrequent stool passage due to the functional obstruction caused by the inflammation of the rectum; the colon more proximally continues to produce formed stool, which cannot pass easily through the inflamed rectum. Proctitis will usually be associated with excess mucus production, with or without blood in the stool, and proctosigmoidoscopy will always diagnose this entity.

Another cause of constipation is diabetes mellitus, often as a result of impaired motility; dietary factors may also play a role, along with autonomic neuropathy of the enteric nervous system. A small proportion of these diabetic patients with constipation can go on to develop diarrhea, which again has been linked to the autonomic neuropathy seen with long-standing diabetes mellitus.

Inactivity from whatever cause seems to increase the likelihood of a patient's complaining of a constipated bowel habit. This is presumed to be secondary to reduced colonic activity but could be aggravated by a low fiber intake in many of these patients. Severe cardiopulmonary diseases of whatever cause that limit activity can result in constipation. Neurologic disorders that cause the patient to have a reduced ability to ambulate can have constipation as a feature. Some patients with diseases of the nervous system may have impaired awareness of rectal distention to signal a need to defecate, and nerve dysfunction (both peripheral and central) may impair normal colonic propulsion. Finally, the elderly may develop problems with defecation, and although constipation with fecal impaction occurs they may complain of "diarrhea" or "soiling" due to overflow incontinence of stool from the fecal impaction of the rectum inhibiting the normal resting tone of the anal sphincter. Not surprisingly, many of these patients may respond to laxative therapy after the fecal impaction is removed, since this prevents the recurrence of the fecal impaction with overflow incontinence. Some patients can aggravate long-standing constipation with regular laxative abuse, and some theoretical concerns remain that this practice may indeed damage the normal innervation of the colon, rendering it atonic and nonfunctional.

The physical findings are often minimal in the majority of patients with constipation, but specific secondary causes must be looked for. Signs of hypothyroidism may be present; signs of dehydration should be sought, as this may be an early indicator of hypercalcemia. Thorough cardiopulmonary and neurologic examinations are necessary to pick out associated diseases that may be treated, thereby improving the patient's overall health and thus improving bowel function. On abdominal examination, inspection for evidence of distention or hyperperistalsis or masses may point out the source of the impaired stool passage. Localized tenderness of the abdomen must be noted, along with any evidence of liver, spleen or renal enlargement. A complete rectal examination and proctosigmoidoscopy is required in any patient with constipation so that the presence or absence of a fecal impaction, dilation or enlargement of the rectum or the presence of proctitis can be determined.

3.6.1 MEGARECTUM

When the rectum is enlarged, further investigations are required to exclude other causes, particularly Hirschsprung's disease (Section 3.6.2). The majority of patients with constipation and a dilated rectum and/or colon at proctosigmoidoscopy or barium enema have idiopathic or acquired megarectum. A useful guideline for the diagnosis of a "megarectum" is a rectal diameter of greater than 6 cm on a lateral film at the level of the S2 vertebral body. These patients can often present in childhood (many of them presenting with encopresis) and in the elderly with a fecal impaction. The cause of the megarectum is unknown, but if the onset is in childhood it may be the result of chronic stool holding by the child, leading to progressive distention of the rectum and eventual loss of awareness of rectal distention. Once this has occurred the patient can no longer recognize when stool is present in the rectum; the distention of the rectum causes chronic inhibition of the resting tone of the internal anal sphincter. This leads to the loss of control of liquid or semisolid stool that passes by the fecal impaction without the patient being aware of it.

3.6.2 HIRSCHSPRUNG'S DISEASE

The majority of patients with this disorder present soon after birth or in early childhood. This is a lesion, present at birth, where variable lengths of distal colon have no myenteric plexus. The distal colon remains contracted and the normal proximal colon dilates as it fills with stool. Most of these patients present early in life with obstipation and colonic obstruction, and require surgery. However, a few patients have a very short segment of denervated distal colon, so that they can overcome the obstruction and force stool out of the rectum. They usually have lifelong constipation; the normal rectum proximal to the denervated segment dilates over time so that the patient presents with constipation and a "megarectum." These patients rarely have fecal incontinence or fecal "soiling" as seen with idiopathic megarectum, since the internal anal sphincter and denervated distal rectum maintain a high resting tone. This condition can be diagnosed by anorectal manometry in that a normal rectoanal inhibitory reflex cannot be identified (Figure 2). However, a definite diagnosis requires deep rectal biopsy from the denervated segment, which will show absence of the myenteric plexus ganglion cells and hypertrophy of nerve fiber bundles. It should be added that an identical condition can be acquired with Chagas' disease from South America, which attacks the myenteric plexus and other autonomic ganglion cells; patients with this condition can also present with achalasia or intestinal pseudo-obstruction as well as cardiac arrhythmias. These patients will also have an absent rectoanal inhibitory reflex if the disease involves the rectal myenteric plexus.

3.6.3 PELVIC FLOOR DYSSYNERGIA

The majority of patients with constipation have a form of irritable bowel syndrome, but there is a small subgroup of patients who may have a specific disorder in colonic and/or anorectal function that produces constipation. These patients are almost all female, may have delayed colonic transit or present with anorectal dysfunction with impaired awareness to rectal distention (without a megarectum), or may demonstrate a phenomenon of rectal outlet obstruction due to inappropriate contraction of the voluntary anal sphincters during defecation. This has been termed pelvic floor dyssynergia or anismus. These patients can present major therapeutic dilemmas and warrant further investigation in specialized coloproctology units involved in the care of such patients.

3.7 Infections of the Colon

3.7.1 SHIGELLA

This infectious diarrhea is the classic cause of "bacillary dysentery." Typical presentation is with fever, abdominal cramping and watery diarrhea that usually becomes bloody within 24 to 48 hours of onset. The incubation period is from 36 to 48 hours. As the disease progresses the symptoms become typical of colonic dysentery, with small, frequent stools and cramping and tenesmus that may lead to rectal prolapse in some individuals with prolonged straining.

The causative organism is a gram-negative bacterium with only humans as its host. The organism is well adapted to causing disease in humans. As few as 200 organisms are needed to cause infection as compared with other enteric infections requiring 10^6 organisms or more. It can persist in food for weeks and on contaminated body surfaces for several hours. Pathogenesis is through production of a cytotoxin called Shiga toxin or similar toxins that are both cytotoxic and neurotoxic, very similar to the toxin produced by E. coli 0157:H7 species. Shigella is a microinvasive bacterium that enters the host via the M cells in the intestine and then spreads laterally through the colonic mucosa to involve the basolateral membrane of the surrounding cells. It is seen mostly in travelers returning from endemic areas (tropical and subtropical). There is also a higher incidence in male homosexuals who practice oral–anal sex.

Treatment depends on the antibiotic resistance of the infecting strain of bacteria. Shigella species quickly develop antibiotic resistance; patients should be encouraged to complete their course of antibiotics to prevent this. Antibiotics shorten the duration of both symptoms and carriage of the organism. Fluoroquinolones are the antibiotics of choice because of the low incidence of resistance at present, but this may change. Ampicillin and trimethoprim-sulfamethoxazole are also effective against sensitive strains. If infection has been acquired overseas, a confirmed Shigella infection is best treated with a fluoroquinolone twice daily for 5 days, but there are reports of a single large dose eradicating infection. Antimotility agents such as loperamide, diphenoxylate or narcotic analgesics are contraindicated with this infection because of the risk of a toxic colon. In general, antimotility agents should never be used in acute infectious diarrhea when bloody stool is present.

3.7.2 SALMONELLA

Infection with nontyphoidal strains of Salmonella results from ingesting foods contaminated with organisms. These bacteria are endemic to poultry and cattle populations. Large epidemics have resulted from undercooked eggs, and these bacteria are also frequently found in reptiles and amphibians. Salmonella contamination of marijuana can be an important infection source in young adults. The usual incubation period is from 8 to 48 hours after ingestion.

S. typhi, which causes typhoid fever, is found only in humans. It will not be discussed further other than to emphasize that all Salmonella species are related and therefore can cause systemic illness of similar severity, especially in patients who are immunocompromised and those at the extremes of age (i.e., those under 2 and the frail elderly).

Salmonella is an invasive bacterium that can cause septicemia after first multiplying in the mesenteric lymph nodes. Resistance to infection is first a result of the presence of gastric acid and then of the integrity of the intestinal flora and of motility. Increased infection is associated with the use of purgatives, antimotility agents and broad-spectrum antibiotics along with acid-suppression therapy. Bowel surgery will also increase the chance of symptomatic infection. Diseases that predispose to infection as a result of impaired host defenses include sickle cell disease, systemic lupus erythematosus (SLE) and AIDS.

Treatment is usually symptomatic. Antibiotics should be used only if the patient is showing signs of bacteremia; antibiotics often increase the development of a chronic carrier state. The antibiotics of choice are ampicillin and trimethoprim-sulfamethoxazole, but recently the fluoroquinolones and the third-generation cephalosporins (especially ceftriaxone with its high biliary excretion) have been shown to be very effective in patients who need antibiotic therapy. Treatment with antibiotics should normally be considered only for patients under the age of 2 years and elderly patients with vascular disease, as well as patients with metal implants in bones, lymphoproliferative disease, sickle cell disease or AIDS. The site of chronic infection is usually the biliary tract. Disease of the biliary tree, especially cholelithiasis, requires surgery to correct the disease followed by a two-week course of therapy, which often leads to resolution of the chronic carrier state.

3.7.3 *CLOSTRIDIUM DIFFICILE*
This spore-forming anaerobic gram-positive bacterium is the commonest cause of infectious diarrhea in hospitalized patients. The organism is not invasive, but with reduction of the normal colonic bacterial flora it multiplies and produces two toxins, known as toxins A and B. Toxin A causes colitis. Toxin B is a cytotoxin that is often used as a diagnostic test for this infection.

Most commonly, infection is preceded by antibiotic therapy. Outbreaks in hospital frequently occur among the sickest patients, some not receiving antibiotics beforehand. Penicillins, cephalosporins and clindamycin are more likely to be associated with C. difficile infection, but all antibiotics, including metronidazole and vancomycin, have been associated with it. Other risk factors include agents that affect gut motility such as enemas and anti-diarrheal medications, and intensive chemotherapy. Patients with severe illnesses and advanced age are also more prone to manifest disease symptoms.

Diarrhea is the commonest symptom of presentation and is usually non-bloody, but with prolonged diarrhea some blood can result from local anorectal irritation. The typical appearance at endoscopy of the colon and rectum is of "pseudomembranes" or whitish plaques on the surface of the colonic mucosa with intervening areas of mucosa that appear almost normal. For this reason, infection is often called "pseudomembranous colitis" (PMC). Unfortunately, these characteristic changes may not be present in the rectum, so diagnosis is usually confirmed by the presence of cytotoxin in the stool placed on tissue culture. The clinician must be alert to the possibility of this infection in susceptible patients since in some patients, neither culture of C. difficile nor the presence of the cytotoxin in the stool is positive. A careful inventory of any antibiotic therapy in the last three months is crucial in considering this cause for diarrhea, as many patients will have taken the offending antibiotic several days to weeks before symptoms begin.

Metronidazole (Flagyl®) treatment is preferred to vancomycin because both antibiotics show similar efficacy in treating this infection and metronidazole is about one-tenth the cost of vancomycin. Treatment is for 7 to 10 days, usually in a dose of 250 mg p.o. q.i.d. in the studies that have been reported. The vancomycin dosage is 125 mg p.o. q.i.d. but is effective only via the oral route, whereas metronidazole is also effective intravenously in the occasional patient with postoperative ileus. With both regimens there is a high relapse rate of infection, of up to 20%. The best method to prevent relapse is unknown, but relapsing symptoms may respond to retreatment of the infection with either metronidazole or vancomycin.

3.7.4 ENTAMOEBA HISTOLYTICA (AMEBIASIS)

Entamoeba histolytica, the parasite that causes amebiasis infection, appears to be the only ameba that causes disease in humans. Other amebas are often found in the colon as normal commensals. E. histolytica is a cyst-forming parasite, but the cysts do not cause disease. The cysts are ingested and are protected by gastric acid; then the trophozoite develops in the colon from the ingested cyst. The cysts spread disease to others, and frequently unaffected carriers spread disease by excreting cysts. The trophozoites, which invade the colonic mucosa, cause disease, but trophozoites passed in the stool of symptomatic individuals cannot survive outside the body and rarely transmit infection. The disease is most prevalent in areas of the tropics where sanitation is poor.

The colon is the usual site of initial disease. Invasion of the mucosa by trophozoites is due to the production of an "amebapore" molecule that causes the lining colonocytes to lyze; the lyzed colonocytes are then ingested by the amebas, leading to ulceration of the colon and dissemination throughout the body. The amebas infect the colon and rarely the ileum, but the cecum is usually involved. E. histolytica is an invasive pathogen and can spread hematogenously to other organs, especially the liver.

Diagnosis is usually made by identification of E. histolytica on microscopic analysis of stool, but can also be made on identification of the ameba on histological diagnosis of colonic biopsies. There is a decreased yield on stool analysis after barium studies and if antibiotics or mineral oil is used prior to collection. At endoscopy the ulcers of the rectum and colon may appear characteristic with undermined edges, and sometimes the intervening mucosa looks normal in contrast to acute bacillary dysentery (see Section 3.7.1) and ulcerative colitis. Diagnosis can also be made by indirect hemagglutination and ELISA tests on serum to detect infection, but if the patient is a carrier with only cyst excretion these tests are often negative. Chronic infection of the cecum leads to a "coned" appearance on x-ray. Other colonic complications include perforation, ameboma (a granulomatous tissue reaction in the colon;

the mass effect can lead to obstruction or be mistaken for colonic malignancy), pericolic abscess and fistulas. The liver is the commonest extraintestinal organ infected, but E. histolytica can also spread to the brain, lungs, pericardium and eyes. There is an increased risk of disseminated disease and abscess formation if the patient is on steroids, is pregnant or is immunocompromised.

Treatment is usually metronidazole 400–750 mg t.i.d. × 5–10 days for acute colitis. If the patient has chronic colonic disease with chronic shedding of cysts, diloxanide 500 mg t.i.d. × 10 days is the drug of choice. If this cannot be obtained, then iodoquinol 650 mg t.i.d. × 20 days can be used, but this is the maximal dose because it can cause optic neuritis. Patients with amebic liver abscess should first be treated with metronidazole for 10 days and then be given 10 days of diloxanide. All patients should be reassessed two to three months after treatment to ensure clearance of the parasite and that there is no chronic carrier state with cyst excretion.

3.7.5 BALANTIDIUM COLI

A very large, ciliated protozoan that uncommonly causes an illness similar to amebic dysentery, B. coli is usually easy to identify in stool samples owing to its large size. It is acquired in tropical or subtropical countries from exposure to pigs, which frequently carry this organism without signs of illness. Treatment is with tetracycline 500 mg q.i.d. for 10 days. B. coli is also sensitive to ampicillin and metronidazole.

3.7.6 BLASTOCYSTIS HOMINIS

A yeast frequently found in asymptomatic individuals, recently B. hominis has been suggested as a cause of unexplained diarrhea in some patients found to have large numbers of this protozoan in the stool. Treatment appears to be with either metronidazole 750 mg t.i.d. × 10 days or iodoquinol 650 mg t.i.d. × 20 days. Iodoquinol may be more successful, but the best treatment has not been identified to date.

3.8 Intestinal Nematode Infections

3.8.1 ROUNDWORM (ASCARIS LUMBRICOIDES)

Roundworm or ascaris, one of the more common nematodes found in humans, is most often found in the tropics. Usually eggs are ingested from contaminated foods or dirty hands. The eggs hatch in the intestine and spread by the blood to the liver and then to the lungs. An eosinophilic pneumonitis can develop and then the larvae migrate through the alveoli, up to the trachea and through the larynx where they are swallowed. They develop into adult worms in the small intestine. The adults can cause intestinal obstruction symptoms if large numbers are present, and can cause biliary symptoms if they migrate into the common bile duct.

3.8.2 HOOKWORM (ANCYLOSTOMA DUODENALE; NECATOR AMERICANUS)

Hookworm can infiltrate skin from contaminated earth and is prone to be found in areas with fecal contamination of the soil. A pruritic rash develops at the site of entry into the body. The filarial larvae then travel to the lungs, migrate through the alveoli and then up through the larynx where they are swallowed. After being swallowed, they cause nausea, diarrhea, vomiting, abdominal pain and flatulence. Many patients present with iron deficiency from a daily blood loss of 0.1–0.4 mL with each worm.

3.8.3 WHIPWORM (TRICHURIS TRICHIURA)

Whipworm can also cause iron deficiency if large numbers infect the GI tract. It primarily invades the colon. Bloody diarrhea develops with larger infestations. It is easily diagnosed by stool analysis looking for the typical eggs, but is increasingly diagnosed at colonoscopy during investigation of the bloody diarrhea, where the worms are easily seen if present.

3.8.4 PINWORM (ENTEROBIUS VERMICULARIS)

Pinworm is probably the commonest nematode worldwide. It usually causes pruritus ani, often worse at night when the worms migrate onto the perianal skin and lay their eggs. Pinworm is probably the most common nematode encountered in Canada, especially in children. Diagnosis is by identification of the eggs from the perianal skin, usually collected in the early morning before defecation.

3.8.5 STRONGYLOIDES STERCORALIS (STRONGYLOIDIASIS)

Strongyloides stercoralis is widely found in the tropics. It is the only nematode that can multiply and reproduce its entire life cycle within the human host, thus causing persistent reinfection over many years after the original infection. Larvae can penetrate intact skin or the eggs can be ingested. Filariform larvae that penetrate the skin travel hematogenously to the lungs and then, as with the other worms, travel into the airways and are swallowed. In the intestine the larvae become adult worms. When the eggs are ingested, they become filariform larvae in the intestine; then the larvae invade the blood vessels, thus reinfecting the host.

Symptoms of strongyloidiasis vary and may include abdominal pain, diarrhea, nausea and vomiting. With mostly intestinal involvement diarrhea can develop; especially in children, a syndrome similar to celiac disease with protein-losing enteropathy can develop. The majority of adult infections are asymptomatic or are only intermittently symptomatic. Recurrent urticaria can develop where the worms infiltrate the skin, particularly the perianal skin and gluteal areas.

Diagnosis can be confirmed by stool analysis but can be negative in up to 25% of cases, even after repeated stool analysis. The larvae look similar to hookworm. An ELISA test is useful for diagnosis, but there may be overlap with the presence of Filaria species. Eosinophilia is often present, even in asymptomatic individuals.

Thiabendazole is usually used to treat, 25 mg/kg twice daily to a maximum of 3 g daily for two days, or five days for disseminated disease. Albendazole or ivermectin may be used if the patient is unable to tolerate thiabendazole, but these drugs appear to be less effective against S. stercoralis. With the hyperinfection syndrome, when large numbers of the worms are present (often in association with immune suppression, as with steroid therapy), antibiotics are often needed to treat the septicemia that results if the intestinal damage allows secondary bacterial invasion.

3.9 Microscopic Colitis

A rare condition has been recognized increasingly in which the patient presents with usually painless diarrhea. Investigations often find signs of inflammation, but the colon appears normal on both radioscopic and colonoscopic examination. This condition is sometimes called "lymphocytic colitis" and may also be part of a spectrum of colitis conditions that include "collagenous colitis." The natural history of these diseases is unclear at present, and no infective agent has been found. These disorders can be diagnosed only by colonoscopic biopsy. The colonic mucosa appears normal, yet on histological examination there is an increase in the inflammatory infiltrate of the lamina propria. In collagenous colitis the basement membrane of the colonic mucosa is thickened by a band of collagen. In most patients the disease appears to follow a benign course, but about half of patients continue to have significant diarrhea for more than two years. The disease is controlled by antimotility agents such as loperamide or by use of 5-aminosalicylic acid–based therapies directed at the colon (see Chapter 10, "Inflammatory Bowel Disease"), which often help to lessen the diarrhea. Glucocorticoids also control the diarrhea, but in view of the benign course of this illness in most patients, steroid therapy should be used only in severely symptomatic patients who cannot be controlled by other therapy.

3.10 Eosinophilic Colitis

Eosinophilic gastroenteritis is an uncommon inflammatory condition that affects primarily the upper GI tract and small intestine (see Chapters 5, 6 and 7). However, there have been recent reports of an apparently separate condition called "eosinophilic colitis" in which patients with connective tissue disease present with diarrhea of uncertain cause with negative stool investigations. These patients have all been diagnosed at colonoscopy by biopsy of essentially normal-looking mucosa, yet with increased eosinophils in the lamina propria. All patients respond to steroids, but it would appear that not all patients resolve over time and some may need prolonged steroid therapy.

4. THE ANAL CANAL / M. Burnstein

4.1 Functional Anatomy of the Anal Canal and Anorectal Spaces

4.1.1 *THE ANAL CANAL*
The anal canal begins where the terminal portion of the large bowel passes through the pelvic floor muscles, and it ends at the anal verge. It measures roughly 4 cm in length. The wall of the anal canal is formed by a continuation of the circular muscle of the rectal wall; the smooth muscle is thickened in this area to form the internal anal sphincter. This smooth-muscle sphincter is wrapped by skeletal muscle, the external anal sphincter. The top of the external anal sphincter is formed by the U-shaped puborectalis muscle, which loops around the anus, arising and inserting on the pubis. This is felt posteriorly and laterally as the anorectal ring on digital examination. The longitudinal muscle coat of the rectum descends in the plane between the sphincters as the conjoined longitudinal muscle, and it sends fibers across the lower part of the external anal sphincter to insert on the skin (corrugator cutis ani, responsible for the anocutaneous reflex or "anal wink"). These fibers also traverse the internal anal sphincter to insert on the submucosa ("mucosal suspensory ligament").

In approximately the mid-anus there is a rolling line of demarcation called the dentate line. Above the line is columnar epithelium; below it is squamous epithelium without appendages (the anoderm). The demarcation does not really occur at a line, but at a transitional zone of 0.5–1 cm in length.

As the rectum narrows into the anal canal, the mucosa develops 6 to 14 longitudinal folds, Morgagni's columns. Between the distal ends of the columns are small crypts. Anal glands open into the crypts. There are 4 to 10 glands, and they are lined by stratified columnar epithelium. About half of these tubular glands end in the intersphincteric plane.

Blood is supplied to the anus via the inferior rectal artery, a branch of the internal pudendal artery. The inferior rectal artery crosses the ischiorectal fossa. The superior rectal vein drains the upper part of the anal canal via the inferior mesenteric vein to the portal vein. The middle and inferior rectal veins drain the upper and lower anal canal into the systemic circulation via the internal iliac and internal pudendal veins, respectively.

Lymphatic drainage above the dentate line is via the superior rectal lymphatics (accompanying the superior rectal vessels) to the inferior mesenteric nodes, and laterally along the middle and inferior rectal vessels to the internal iliac nodes. Lymphatic drainage from the anal canal below the dentate line may be in a cephalad or lateral direction, but is primarily to the inguinal nodes.

Motor innervation of the external anal sphincter is via the inferior rectal branch of the pudendal nerve and the perineal branch of the fourth sacral nerve. The internal anal sphincter has sympathetic (motor) and parasympathetic (inhibitory) innervation. Parasympathetic supply is from the nervi erigentes (S2, S3, S4). Sympathetic innervation is from the first three lumbar segments via the preaortic plexus. Fibers from the preaortic plexus ultimately join the nervi erigentes to form the pelvic plexuses. Sensation below the dentate line (and for up to 1.5 cm above the dentate line) is carried by the inferior rectal nerve. Above the level of the inferior rectal nerve sensory distribution, there are only dull perceptions, mediated by parasympathetic fibers.

4.1.2 ANORECTAL SPACES

Around the anorectum are a number of potential spaces filled with fat or connective tissue. These may become the sites of abscess formation. The perianal space is at the anal verge, and is continuous with the intersphincteric space. The pyramid-shaped ischiorectal (ischioanal) fossa is medially bounded by the external anal sphincter and the levator ani muscles. The lateral wall is the obturator internus muscle and fascia. The inferior boundary is the skin of the perineum, and the apex is the origin of the levator ani from the obturator fascia. Posteriorly is the gluteus maximus muscle, and anteriorly the transverse perinei muscles. On the obturator fascia is Alcock's canal, containing the internal pudendal vessels and pudendal nerve. The fossa is filled with fat and also contains the inferior rectal nerve and vessels, and the fourth sacral nerve. The two ischiorectal spaces communicate with one another behind the anal canal.

4.2 Evaluation of Anorectal Complaints

This section will review the symptoms associated with anorectal pathology and the techniques of anorectal examination.

4.2.1 HISTORY

As in most of medicine, taking a careful history is the most productive step in leading to a diagnosis. In the evaluation of the patient with anorectal complaints, there is a limited number of questions to be asked:

4.2.1.1 *Pain*

There are three common lesions that cause anorectal pain: fissure in ano, anal abscess and thrombosed external hemorrhoid. If the pain is sharp and occurs during, and for a short time following, bowel movements, a fissure is likely. Continuous pain associated with a perianal swelling probably stems from thrombosis of perianal vessels, especially when there is an antecedent history of straining, either at stool or with physical exertion. An anal abscess will also produce a continuous, often throbbing pain, which may be aggravated by the patient's coughing or sneezing. Anorectal abscesses are generally associated with local signs of inflammation. The absence of an inflammatory mass in the setting of severe local pain and tenderness is typical of an intersphincteric abscess; the degree of tenderness usually prevents adequate examination, and evaluation under anesthesia is necessary to confirm the diagnosis and to drain the pus.

Anal pain of any etiology may be aggravated by bowel movements. Tenesmus, an uncomfortable desire to defecate, is frequently associated with inflammatory conditions of the anorectum. Although anal neoplasms rarely produce pain, invasion of the sphincter mechanism may also result in tenesmus. Tenesmus with urgency of evacuation suggests proctitis.

Transient, deep-seated pain that is unrelated to defecation may be due to levator spasm ("proctalgia fugax").

Anorectal pain is so frequently, and erroneously, attributed to hemorrhoids, that this point bears special mention: pain is *not* a symptom of uncomplicated hemorrhoids. If a perianal vein of the inferior rectal plexus undergoes thrombosis, or ruptures, an acutely painful and tender subcutaneous lump will appear. This is the "thrombosed external hemorrhoid." Internal hemorrhoids may prolapse and become strangulated to produce an acute problem of anorectal pain, tenderness, and mucous, bloody discharge. Gangrene and secondary infection may ensue.

4.2.1.2 *Bleeding*

The nature of the rectal bleeding will help determine the underlying cause. However, the clinician must remember that the historical features of the bleeding cannot be relied upon to define the problem with certainty. Bright red blood on the toilet paper or on the outside of the stool, or dripping into the bowl, suggests a local anal source, such as a fissure or internal hemorrhoids. Blood that is mixed in with the stool, or that is dark and clotted, suggests sources proximal to the anus. Melena is always due to more proximal pathology.

The associated symptoms are very helpful. A history of local anal bleeding, as described above, associated with painful defecation, suggests a fissure. The same bleeding pattern without pain suggests internal hemorrhoids; this may be associated with some degree of hemorrhoidal prolapse. Bleeding and diarrhea may occur with inflammatory bowel disease. When bleeding is associated with a painful lump and is not exclusively related to defecation, a thrombosed external hemorrhoid is likely. Bleeding associated with a mucopurulent discharge and tenesmus may be seen with proctitis, or possibly with a rectal neoplasm.

Bleeding per rectum is an important symptom of colorectal cancer, and although this is not the most common cause of hematochezia, it is the most serious and must always be considered. This does not mean that every patient who passes blood must have contrast radiography of the colon or total colonoscopy. If the bleeding has an obvious anal source, it may be prudent not to proceed with a total colon examination, especially in a patient at low risk for colorectal neoplasms (i.e., age under 50 years; no history of Crohn's or ulcerative colitis; no family history of colon cancer; and no personal history of colorectal neoplasms). However, if bleeding persists after treatment of the anal pathology, more ominous lesions have to be excluded.

4.2.1.3 *Prolapse*

In evaluating protrusion from the anal opening, there are several relevant questions: Is the prolapse spontaneous or exclusively with defecation? Spontaneous prolapse is less characteristic of internal hemorrhoids than of hypertrophied anal papillae or complete rectal prolapse. Does the prolapsing tissue reduce spontaneously (as may be the case with second-degree internal hemorrhoids) or does it require manual reduction (as with third-degree internal hemorrhoids or complete rectal prolapse)? The patient may be able to describe the size of the prolapsing tissue, and this may suggest the diagnosis.

Complete rectal prolapse (procidentia) must be distinguished from mucosal prolapse or prolapsing internal hemorrhoids. Procidentia occurs mainly in women (female:male = 6:1), with a peak incidence in the seventh decade. Procidentia is often associated with fecal incontinence. In later stages, protrusion occurs even with slight exertion such as coughing or sneezing. The extruded rectum becomes excoriated, leading to tenesmus, mucus discharge and bleeding. (Examination of the patient with procidentia usually reveals poor anal tone, and with the tissue in a prolapsed state, the mucosal folds are seen to be concentric, whereas with prolapsed hemorrhoids there are radial folds.)

Rarely, a large polypoid tumor of the rectum may prolapse through the anal canal.

4.2.1.4 *Perianal mass*

A painful perianal lump may be an abscess or a thrombosed external hemorrhoid. Knowing whether there has been a discharge of blood or pus may be helpful. An intermittent mass suggests a prolapsing lesion.

External or "skin" tags are very common deformities of the anal margin. They may be the result of previous or active fissure disease, or the sequelae of a thrombosed external hemorrhoid. Condylomata acuminata – or venereal warts – are caused by a sexually transmitted virus. The perianal skin is frequently affected, and the condition occurs with greatest frequency in gay men.

The differential diagnosis also includes benign and malignant neoplasms.

4.2.1.5 *Pruritus*

Itching is a common associated feature of many anorectal conditions, especially during the healing phase or if there is a discharge. But pruritus ani may also be an isolated symptom or the patient's primary complaint. As a chief complaint, pruritus may be caused by infections (e.g., pinworms, condylomata, Candida) or skin conditions (e.g., contact dermatitis, psoriasis). More commonly, no specific underlying pathology is identified, and the problem is idiopathic.

Idiopathic pruritus ani is more common in men, and is typically worse at night. When chronic, the characteristic changes of hypertrophy and lichenification, nodularity, scarring and fissuring of the skin become apparent.

4.2.1.6 *Discharge*

Although mucus is a normal product of the colorectal mucosa, it is not normally seen in the stool. Increased mucus may be the result of proctocolitis or a colorectal neoplasm, especially a villous adenoma of the rectum. Both inflammatory and neoplastic conditions may present with mucus and blood. Phosphate enemas are irritating and often elicit copious mucus production. Patients with the irritable bowel syndrome may complain of mucous stools.

Mucus staining of the underclothes may be associated with prolapsing tissue. When the staining has a fecal component, or when there is associated inability to control gas or to discriminate gas from solids within the rectum, a disturbance of the continence mechanism exists. A history of "accidents," or the need to wear pads during the day or night, will help indicate the magnitude of the problem. The discharge may arise from an obvious external lesion – e.g., blood from a thrombosed external hemorrhoid, or pus from an abscess, from the external opening of a fistula, from a pilonidal process or from perianal hidradenitis suppurativa.

Other issues that will prove helpful in coming to a diagnosis of anorectal pathology include bowel habits, associated medical conditions and medications, sexual practices, travel history and family history.

4.2.2 *EXAMINATION*

The patient about to undergo examination of the anorectum may not only be embarrassed, but also afraid of impending pain and discomfort. Explanation of the examinations to be performed, and reassurance, will lessen the patient's anxiety and contribute greatly to patient cooperation.

The four steps in anorectal evaluation are inspection, palpation, anoscopy and proctosigmoidoscopy.

4.2.2.1 *Positioning*

The patient is placed either in the left lateral position or (preferably) in the prone-jackknife position. The prone-jackknife position requires a special table that tilts the head down and raises the anorectal region, with the buttocks tending to fall apart. This provides the best and easiest access for the examiner, although patient comfort may be slightly less.

The left lateral (Sims') position has the advantages of patient comfort and of being suitable for any examining table, bed or stretcher. The patient's buttocks are allowed to protrude over the edge of the table, with hips flexed and knees slightly extended. The examiner may sit or stand.

The patient is unable to see "what's going on back there," and it is important to continually explain what you are doing and what can be expected.

4.2.2.2 *Inspection*

Looking at the anal area may reveal obvious external pathology. The resting anal aperture should be observed: a patulous opening may be seen with procidentia, sphincter injury or neurologic abnormality. Straining and squeezing by the patient may provide information about anorectal function.

Gentle spreading of the buttocks may elicit pain in a patient who has an anal fissure. Asking the patient to strain down may provide information: internal hemorrhoids may protrude or procidentia may be seen. However, if procidentia is suspected, it should be sought with the patient squatting or sitting at the toilet.

4.2.2.3 *Palpation*

A disposable plastic glove and water-soluble lubricant are required. The patient is told that a finger will be gently placed into the rectum. While one hand separates the buttocks, the index finger is placed on the anal verge, and with the patient bearing down, thereby relaxing the anus, the digit is advanced into the anal canal.

A methodical approach is best. Palpation anteriorly checks the prostate in males, and the cervix in females. The finger then sweeps backward and forward to palpate the rest of the circumference of the anorectum. This may be the only part of the examination that identifies submucosal lesions, which may easily go undetected by endoscopy. Resting tone and ability to squeeze should also be assessed. The location of tenderness or a palpable abnormality should be precisely recorded.

4.2.2.4 *Anoscopy*
The anoscope is the optimal instrument for examining lesions of the anal canal. It is not a substitute for proctosigmoidoscopy, and the proctosigmoidoscope does not provide as satisfactory a view of the canal as does the anoscope. Many anoscopes are available; the best instrument is end-viewing, with an attached fiberoptic light source.

4.2.2.5 *Proctosigmoidoscopy*
The rigid 25 cm sigmoidoscope (or proctoscope) is the best instrument for examining the rectum. A barium enema, because of the balloon-tipped catheter used in administering the contrast material, does not adequately evaluate the rectal ampulla and is never a sufficient workup of a lower GI complaint.

A variety of rigid sigmoidoscopes are available: disposable or reusable, in a range of diameters (1.1 cm, 1.9 cm, 2.7 cm) and with proximal or distal lighting. The 1.9 cm instrument provides good visibility with minimal patient discomfort. The instrument includes a 25 cm tube, a magnifying lens, a light source, and a bulb attachment for air insufflation. Long swabs may be helpful in maintaining visibility, but suction is best.

A single Fleet® enema provides excellent preparation of the distal bowel and should be used just before the examination. The Fleet® enema may produce transient mucosal changes, and if inflammatory bowel disease is suspected, it should be avoided.

The digital examination has set the stage for instrumentation by permitting the sphincter to relax. With the tip well lubricated, the sigmoidoscope is inserted and passed quickly up the rectum. As always, the patient is informed of what is being done, and is reassured that the sensation of impending evacuation is caused by the instrument, and that the bowels are not about to move.

Air insufflation should be kept to a minimum, as it may cause discomfort, but it is of value both on entry and on withdrawal in demonstrating the mucosa and lumen and in assessing rectal compliance and the presence of normal sensation of rectal distention. Advancement should occur only with the lumen clearly in sight. When the lumen is "lost," withdraw and redirect to regain it.

As the rectosigmoid is reached (approximately 15 cm along), the patient should be warned of possible cramping discomfort that will disappear as the scope is removed. Frequently, even with experience, the rectosigmoid angle cannot be negotiated, and the examination should be terminated. Most importantly, the patient should not be hurt or caused significant discomfort. The scope should be withdrawn making large circular motions, carefully inspecting the circumference of the bowel wall, flattening the mucosal folds and valves of Houston. The posterior rectal wall in the sacral hollow must be specifically sought out, or it will be missed.

In most large studies, the average depth of insertion is 18–20 cm; the full length of the instrument is inserted in less than half the patients.

Perforation of the normal rectum by the sigmoidoscope is extremely rare (1 in 50,000 or less). However, advancing the instrument or insufflating air may be hazardous in settings such as inflammatory bowel disease, radiation proctitis, diverticulitis and cancer. Of course, biopsy and electrocoagulation have to be performed with care and with knowledge of the technique and equipment.

The incidence and significance of bacteremia following anorectal manipulations is controversial, and has been reported in 0–25% of proctoscopies. Prophylactic antibiotics should be considered in patients with prosthetic heart valves.

4.3 Specific Anorectal Problems
This section will briefly review some of the more common anorectal problems.

4.3.1 *HEMORRHOIDS*

4.3.1.1 *Background*
The upper anal canal has three sites of thickened submucosa containing arterioles, venules and arteriovenous communications. These three vascular "cushions" are in the left lateral, right anterior and right posterior positions. Minor cushions may lie between the three main ones. The cushions are held in the upper anal canal by muscular fibers from the conjoined longitudinal muscle of the intersphincteric plane.

Hemorrhoids exist when the anal cushions prolapse after disruption of their suspensory mechanism, or when there is dilation of the veins and arteriovenous anastomoses within the cushions. Various theories can be put forward for the development of internal hemorrhoidal disease: raised intra-abdominal pressure, pressure on the hemorrhoidal veins by an enlarging uterus, poor venous drainage secondary to an overactive internal anal sphincter, straining at stool with a resultant downward displacement of the cushions, etc.

Skin tags are projections of skin at the anal verge. They may be the result of previous thrombosed external hemorrhoids, fissure in ano, or inflammatory bowel disease.

External hemorrhoids are dilated veins of the inferior hemorrhoidal (rectal) plexus. This plexus lies just below the dentate line and is covered by squamous epithelium.

Internal hemorrhoids are the symptomatic, enlarged submucosal vascular cushions of the anal canal. The cushions are located above the dentate line and are covered by columnar and transitional epithelium. The patient's history allows internal hemorrhoids to be subdivided. First-degree hemorrhoids produce painless bleeding but do not protrude from the anal canal; at anoscopy, they are seen to bulge into the lumen. Second-degree hemorrhoids protrude with bowel movements, but reduce themselves spontaneously. Third-degree hemorrhoids prolapse outside the anal canal, either spontaneously or with bowel movements, but require digital reduction. Fourth-degree hemorrhoids are always prolapsed, and cannot be reduced.

4.3.1.2 Diagnosis and treatment

4.3.1.2.1 *Thrombosed external hemorrhoids* As a rule, external hemorrhoids are asymptomatic until the complication of thrombosis (intravascular clot) or rupture (perianal hematoma) supervenes. In either case, the presentation is severe pain with a perianal lump, often after straining. The natural history is one of continued pain for 4 to 5 days, then slow resolution over 10 to 14 days. The treatment depends on the severity of the pain and the timing of presentation. A patient who presents within 24 to 48 hours and with severe pain is best dealt with operatively. Under local anesthesia, the involved perianal vessel and clot are excised. The wound may be left open or may be closed. Simple evacuation of the thrombus is less effective. A patient presenting later, after 3 to 4 days, is advised to take frequent warm baths, a bulk laxative, a surface-active wetting agent, and oral analgesics. This regimen is also prescribed post-excision.

4.3.1.2.2 *Internal hemorrhoids* Painless, bright red rectal bleeding (usually with or following bowel movements) is the most common symptom of this condition. Blood appears on the toilet paper or on the outside of the stool, or drips into the bowl. It is very rare for the volume of blood lost from internal hemorrhoids to be sufficient to explain iron deficiency anemia; further workup is always indicated.

Prolapse with defecation or other straining activities is also a common symptom of internal hemorrhoids. Chronic prolapse is associated with mucus discharge, fecal staining of the underclothes and pruritus.

Anal sphincter spasm may result in thrombosis and strangulation of prolapsed hemorrhoids. This presents as an acute problem of a painful, discharging, edematous mass of hemorrhoids.

Inspection will identify the later stages of the disease, especially when the patient is asked to bear down. Digital examination can rule out other pathology, as well as assess the sphincters. A palpable abnormality suggests some other process. Anoscopy provides a diagnosis in first- and second-degree disease. With the anoscope in place, the patient is once again asked to strain, and the degree of prolapse observed. Proctosigmoidoscopy should always be performed to exclude other diseases, particularly rectal neoplasms and inflammatory bowel disease.

If the symptoms are at all atypical, or the physical findings leave any doubt about the source of blood, a colon-clearing examination (either colonoscopy or barium enema) should be performed.

In patients over the age of 50, it is reasonable to take the opportunity to screen (or to practice "case-finding") for colorectal cancer by performing sigmoidoscopy with the 60 cm flexible instrument. If risk factors for colorectal neoplasia are present, then colonoscopy or barium enema should certainly be performed.

Occasional bleeding, especially if it is related to hard stools or straining, should be managed by improving bowel habits using high-fiber diet and bulk agents (e.g., psyllium). If bleeding persists or is frequent, intervention is indicated, and in most cases should take the form of rubber-band ligation. Prolapsing hemorrhoids that reduce spontaneously, or can be easily reduced, are also nicely treated by rubber-band ligation. If prolapsing tissue is not easily reduced, or if there is a significant external component, surgical hemorrhoidectomy offers the best cure. Similarly, prolapsed, thrombosed internal hemorrhoids should be surgically excised.

4.3.1.2.3 *Rubber-band ligation* In this technique, strangulating rubber bands are placed at the cephalad aspect of the internal hemorrhoids. The absence of somatic pain fibers above the dentate line renders this a relatively painless procedure, as long as the rings are properly positioned. The banded tissue infarcts and sloughs over the next week, resulting in reduction of hemorrhoidal tissue, as well as fixation of the residual hemorrhoid in the upper anal canal. It is a simple office procedure requiring an anoscope and ligator. In general, only one or two areas are banded at a time, so that several treatments are often required. Long-term success is expected in approximately

75% of patients with second-degree hemorrhoids. Pain, bleeding and infection are rare complications.

4.3.1.2.4 *Hemorrhoidectomy*   Since the popularization of rubber-band ligation, excisional hemorrhoidectomy has been much less frequently performed. The important principles of all excisional procedures are removal of all external and internal hemorrhoids, protection of the internal anal sphincter from injury, and maintenance of the anoderm, so as to avoid anal stenosis.

4.3.2 FISSURE IN ANO

This is a linear crack in the lining of the anal canal, extending from the dentate line to the anal verge. It is seen equally in men and women, and at all ages, but is a common entity in young adults. It is encountered mainly in the posterior midline, but also occasionally in the anterior midline. If a fissure persists, secondary changes occur. These include the "sentinel pile" at the distal end of the fissure and the "hypertrophied anal papilla" at the proximal end. They are due to edema and low-grade infection.

4.3.2.1 *Pathogenesis*

Fissure in ano is probably the result of trauma during the passage of hard stool, but not all patients with fissure in ano give a history of "constipation." While most fissures will readily heal with an appropriate change in bowel habits, some will persist. This may be due to continued trauma or to spasm of the internal anal sphincter.

There is an association between fissures and inflammatory bowel disease, particularly Crohn's disease, and this should be kept in mind.

4.3.2.2 *Diagnosis*

Pain with defecation is the chief complaint. The pain may persist for minutes to hours. Bright red blood is often seen on the toilet paper and on the stool. The patient with an edematous, tender skin tag (sentinel pile) may complain of a painful hemorrhoid. The patient may be constipated in response to painful defecation.

With gentle separation of the buttocks, most fissures will be visible. The sentinel pile of a chronic fissure may be the initial finding. With acute fissures, digital and anoscopic examination are usually not possible because of local tenderness. However, these examinations should be performed later to rule out other pathology. With chronic fissures, anoscopy reveals the defect in the anoderm, with exposed muscle fibers of the internal anal sphincter at the fissure base. The hypertrophied anal papilla may be seen.

Fissures off the midline should raise the possibility of other diseases.

Crohn's disease may be associated with atypical-looking fissures that are off the midline and have atypical symptoms. Anal and rectal carcinoma should be palpably different from fissures, but if any doubt exists, a biopsy should be done. A syphilitic chancre may occasionally look like an idiopathic fissure.

4.3.2.3 *Treatment*
The mainstay of therapy for acute fissures is to achieve daily soft bowel movements. This will prevent further tearing and relieve the anal spasm, allowing most acute fissures to heal within one to two weeks. Warm tub baths are soothing and cleansing, and may also reduce spasm. A high-fiber diet supplemented with bulk agents and surface-active wetting agents will accomplish the desired effect.

If the history is longer than a few weeks and the physical findings suggest chronicity (i.e., exposed sphincter fibers, hypertrophied papilla, sentinel pile and palpable induration), this conservative therapy may not help. If symptoms warrant, such a fissure should be treated operatively, generally by lateral internal sphincterotomy. This relieves the internal anal sphincter spasm and allows the fissure to heal in over 90% of cases. Minor disturbances of continence, especially for flatus, may complicate a sphincterotomy in 5–10% of patients.

4.3.3 *FISTULA-ABSCESS DISEASE*
Anorectal abscess and fistula are the acute and chronic phases, respectively, of the same disease. The disease begins as an infection in the anal glands and initially presents as an abscess. When the abscess is surgically drained, or drains spontaneously, a communication (i.e., a fistula) exists between the gland of origin and the perianal skin.

The infection begins in the intersphincteric plane, where many of the anal glands terminate. The infectious process may remain in this plane as an intersphincteric abscess, or, more commonly, it may track downward in the intersphincteric plane to present as a perianal abscess. Similarly, infection may penetrate the external sphincter to enter the ischiorectal fossa. Many complex variations are seen, determined by the direction of spread and sometimes by inappropriate intervention. The infection may track circumferentially from one side of the anal canal to the other to cause a "horseshoe" abscess. Perianal and ischiorectal abscesses account for at least three-quarters of anorectal abscesses.

The classical signs of inflammation are generally present, although with an intersphincteric abscess there may be nothing to see. In the case of intersphincteric abscess, the patient will be too tender for adequate examination, and examination under anesthesia will be necessary.

Management of the abscess consists of incision and drainage, and this can usually be accomplished under local anesthesia. To ensure adequate drainage, a cruciate or elliptical incision is made. For the one-half to two-thirds of patients who go on to develop a fistula in ano, a fistulotomy, or laying-open, with curettage of the track is required. The wound heals secondarily. Non-healing or recurrence of the fistula usually indicates a failure to destroy the gland of origin. In performing fistulotomy, the utmost attention must be paid to the anatomic relationship between the fistula track and the sphincter mechanism. Excessive division of muscle contained within the fistula can lead to partial or complete fecal incontinence.

4.3.4 *PILONIDAL DISEASE*
This is an acquired condition in which body hair is drilled into the skin of the natal cleft by the back-and-forth motion of the buttocks. This produces a primary midline opening or track, from which abscesses and secondary tracks and openings may form.

The disease is mainly seen in young, hirsute males. It commonly presents as an acute abscess, but may also present as a chronic "sinus," usually with multiple openings.

The abscess stage is treated by incision and drainage, usually under local anesthesia. After the abscess has healed, some of these patients will require definitive surgery to deal with the primary and secondary tracks. The preferred treatment consists of opening the anterior wall of the tracks and suturing the edge of the track to the skin edge. This technique is called "marsupialization."

4.4 Sexually Transmitted Diseases of the Anorectum
There is an increasing incidence of venereal infections of the anorectal region, mainly accounted for by sexual practices among gay men. Many of these diseases may mimic nonvenereal conditions of the anorectum, and multiple venereal infections may coexist.

While immunocompetent gay men are subject to infection with the usual venereal pathogens, AIDS patients may additionally suffer from opportunistic infections of the gut.

The common anorectal venereal infections seen in North America are discussed here.

Condylomata acuminata, or venereal warts, are seen in the perianal region and anal canal, as well as the vulva, vagina and penis. They are most often seen in male homosexuals. The causative agent is believed to be a papilloma virus with an incubation period of one to six months. Symptoms are generally minor – itching, and occasionally bleeding. Perianal warts are frequently accompanied by warts within the anal canal, and these must be looked for at anoscopy.

Many treatments exist. None has a better than 70% chance of eradicating the disease by a single application. For perianal and anal canal warts, electro-coagulation or laser destruction is preferred. For extensive persistent disease, immunotherapy with an autologous vaccine has been very successful.

Squamous cancer has been seen to arise in condylomata acuminata.

Neisseria gonorrhoeae may produce proctitis. The incubation period of *gonococcal proctitis* is five to seven days. Gonococcal proctitis is most often asymptomatic; symptoms may include mucopurulent discharge and tenesmus. Proctoscopy reveals a thick, purulent discharge on a background of mild, non-ulcerative inflammation of the distal rectum. Gram's stain is unreliable, but culture of the pus confirms the diagnosis. Serologic testing for syphilis should be carried out. Treatment for homosexual men is ceftriaxone, 250 mg IM once.

Syphilis can affect the anal region. The incubation period ranges from 9 to 90 days. The primary lesion is a chancre, and because it is painful, it may be mistaken for a fissure. However, chancres are off the midline, are often multi-ple, and have an atypical appearance. Bilateral inguinal lymphadenopathy may be present. The chancre regresses over 6 weeks. Treponema pallidum is demonstrated from the primary lesion by darkfield microscopy. Serologic testing will be positive within a few weeks of the appearance of the chancre. If untreated, the secondary stage of syphilis may involve the anal area 6 to 8 weeks after healing of the chancre. This takes the form of a rash or of condylomata lata – flat, wart-like lesions teeming with Treponema palli-dum. Treatment of primary and secondary syphilis is with benzathine peni-cillin G, 2.4 million units IM once. Sexual contacts should be treated prophy-lactically.

Herpes simplex 2 may infect the anorectum. The incubation period is 4 to 21 days. Constitutional symptoms are followed by severe anorectal pain. Small vesicles and aphthous ulcers are seen perianally and in the anal canal and lower rectum. Examination may reveal tender inguinal lymphadenopathy. Viral cultures of the vesicular fluid will be positive and rectal biopsy has a characteristic appearance. Spontaneous resolution occurs over several weeks. Recurrences are frequent but less severe. Immunosuppressed patients may develop a severe, destructive process. Treatment is with tub baths and analge-sics. Topical acyclovir q8h × 5 days shortens the symptomatic period and the duration of viral shedding. Intravenous acyclovir is used when there is procti-tis in addition to anal and perianal disease. In the AIDS patient, acyclovir is used intravenously in the acute phase, followed by oral acyclovir for 6 months.

Chlamydia proctitis with non-LGV (lymphogranuloma venereum) serotypes is almost identical to gonococcal proctitis. However, the LGV serotypes are invasive and produce a severe proctocolitis with pain, tenesmus, discharge and diarrhea. Chlamydia is isolated from the rectum. Treatment is with tetracycline.

5. LOWER GASTROINTESTINAL BLEEDING / S.J. Vanner

Lower GI bleeding often presents as a medical emergency. Like other medical emergencies, optimum patient care requires careful assessment and resuscitation. The history and physical findings provide important clues to the etiology and are critical for determining the severity and location of the bleeding site.

Lower GI bleeding can be classified arbitrarily as major or minor. Patients presenting with the passage of significant amounts of bright red blood per rectum and hemodynamic compromise have major GI blood loss and are at risk of life-threatening hypovolemia. Be wary of the patient who may have stabilized temporarily or received intravenous fluids prior to a full clinical assessment. Historical clues to a major bleed include the occurrence of syncope or presyncope prior to seeking medical care. The vital signs, with particular attention paid to postural changes, are crucial to assessing severity. *The passage of bright red blood per rectum almost always orginates from the colon. However, it is important to remember that brisk bleeding from a site in the upper GI tract may masquerade as a major lower GI bleed.* In contrast to the patient with major lower GI bleeding is the patient who describes the passage of bright red blood per rectum as blood on the tissue paper or on the outside of formed stool in the absence of other symptoms. Such patients, whose general physical examination is normal, usually have a minor lower GI bleed. Most often this is due to local perianal pathology.

5.1 Determining the Site of Bleeding (Upper or Lower GI Tract)

In the clinical setting of a major lower GI bleed with the passage of bright red blood per rectum and hemodynamic compromise, there are a number of important clues that may raise the suspicion of an upper GI source. These include a past history or symptoms of peptic ulcer disease, NSAID use, prior abdominal aneurysm repair, alcohol abuse and coexisting liver disease. Unfortunately, the lack of upper GI symptoms does not exclude peptic ulcer disease, as a number of duodenal ulcers present as major GI bleeds without a previous typical ulcer history. On physical examination, the finding of hypovolemic shock, particularly in a young person, should trigger immediate consideration of a proximal source of bleeding. Features of chronic liver disease and portal hypertension suggest varices as a possible cause. Most major upper GI bleeding, even in a young person, is accompanied by a transient rise in the BUN (blood urea nitrogen), whereas this is not typical in a lower GI bleed unless there is renal comorbidity.

When an upper GI source is considered, several actions are necessary. A nasogastric tube returning bloody gastric aspirate positively identifies a proximal source of bleeding, but a negative aspirate may not. A negative aspirate will exclude significant bleeding from the esophagus or stomach but may fail to identify bleeding from the duodenum. Even aspirates with bile staining and no blood may fail to identify 5–10% of bleeding duodenal ulcers. When an upper GI source cannot be excluded with confidence, urgent upper endoscopy is required.

Another potentially confusing scenario involves the patient presenting with melena. Melena results from the digestion of blood as it travels through the GI tract, and almost always originates from the upper GI tract. However, occasionally transit of blood from a bleeding right colon is sufficiently slow that stool can appear as melena or melena mixed with dark red blood.

Positive fecal occult blood tests are another clue to lower gastrointestinal bleeding. Many results prove to be false positives; testing should be done with patients on a controlled diet (no red meat, vitamin C or aspirin) to minimize this possibility. Occult positive stools can result from bleeding sites in either the upper or lower GI tract.

5.2 Major Lower GI Bleeding

Angiodysplasia and diverticular bleeding are the two most common causes of major lower GI bleeding, accounting for up to 60–70% of cases.

Angiodysplastic lesions result from dilation and tortuosity of submucosal veins associated with small arteriovenous communication with submucosal arterioles. These lesions are typically multiple, less than 5 mm in diameter, and are most commonly found in the right colon and cecum. The pathogenesis of these lesions is unknown but they occur most commonly in elderly patients and differ from congenital vascular lesions. Diverticula are located predominantly in the left colon, but angiographic studies have shown that those in the right colon bleed more frequently. The pathophysiology underlying diverticular bleeding is also uncertain but is thought to result from rupture of arteries that penetrate the dome of the diverticulum.

A number of other possible but less common causes exist (Table 6), but many of these more typically present with minor lower GI bleeding and a clinical picture dominated by other features such as diarrhea. Angiodysplasia, unlike diverticular bleeding, can also present with minor chronic GI bleeding, and may even present as chronic anemia secondary to microscopic blood loss.

TABLE 6.   Causes of major lower GI bleed

Very common
Diverticular disease
Angiodysplasia

Less common
Ischemia
Neoplasia
Inflammatory bowel disease
Hemobilia
Perianal disease
Aortoenteric fistula
Solitary rectal ulcer

In contrast to angiodysplasia and diverticular bleeding, which are relatively painless, bleeding secondary to colonic ischemia is typically preceded by minutes to hours of significant abdominal pain. Abdominal x-rays may demonstrate thumb-printing, but this finding is neither specific nor sensitive.

Most major lower GI bleeding will stop without intervention and can be investigated electively, but up to 25% will continue to bleed and require immediate investigation and treatment (Figure 3). After resuscitation, the next priority is to identify the site of bleeding. Radionuclide scanning using technetium-labeled red blood cells is least invasive and readily available in most centers, but interpretation is fraught with false negative and positive results. Although angiography is less available and more invasive, it is more accurate and has the advantage of therapeutic intervention with embolization of the arteriole feeding the bleeding lesion. Colonoscopy can also be attempted to identify the bleeding lesion, and if angiodysplasia is evident it can be treated with electrocautery. However, unless the rate of bleeding is relatively slow, ongoing bleeding usually obscures the lumen, making it difficult to identify the responsible lesion and technically difficult to advance the colonoscope to the site of bleeding. In some cases, continuing bleeding (requiring transfusions of 6–10 units of blood) requires either urgent angiography with embolization or surgical resection with a subtotal colectomy.

5.3 Minor Lower GI Bleeding

Minor bleeding from the lower GI tract is a common complaint and requires a careful approach (Figure 3) to differentiate minor pathology such as hemorrhoids and fissures from serious problems such as colonic tumors. Patients may notice blood only on the outside of formed stool or on the tissue paper, suggesting that the blood originates from the anal canal or the rectosigmoid

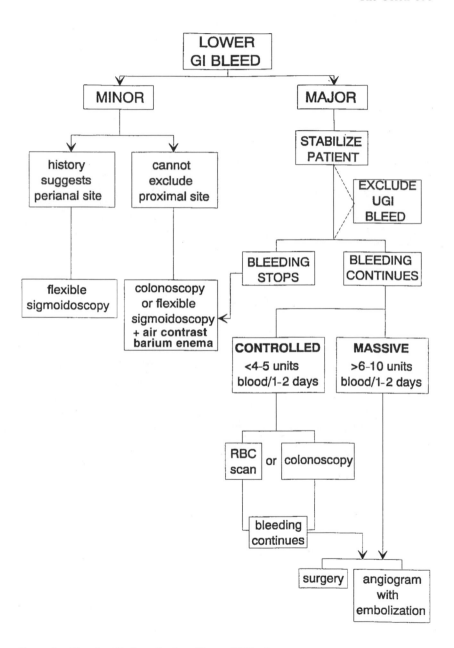

FIGURE 3.   Flowchart for investigation of lower GI bleed.

TABLE 7.   Causes of minor lower GI bleed

Very common
Hemorrhoids
Fissures
Other perianal disease
Proctitis

Less common
Neoplasia
Inflammatory bowel disease
Infectious colitis
Radiation colitis
Angiodysplasia
Ischemia
Rectal ulcer

region. Alternatively, some patients notice that the blood is mixed in the stool, suggesting that bleeding is more proximal within the colon.

Hemorrhoids are the commonest cause of minor bleeding (Table 7), but even when the history is very suggestive, proctoscopic or sigmoidoscopic assessment should be carried out to ensure that a rectal lesion such as proctitis or a tumor is not mimicking this presentation. Patients with ulcerative proctitis often have frequent bowel movements but pass only bright red blood and mucus on many occasions. Radiation proctitis can present shortly after radiotherapy treatment but is often delayed by many months or years. This condition results from chronic inflammation within the blood vessels, called endarteritis obliterans, and this indolent process underlies the delayed presentation.

SUGGESTED READING LIST

Konvolinka CW. Acute diverticulitis under age forty. Am J Surg 1994; 167:562–565.
Cash R. Inappropriate treatment for dysentery. Br Med J 1996; 313:181–182.
Reinus JF, Brandt LJ. Vascular ectasias and diverticulosis. Gastroenterol Clin North Am 1994; 23:1–20.
Jensen DM, Machicado GA. Diagnosis and treatment of severe hematochezia. Gastroenterology 1988; 95:1569–1574.
Griffiths JK, Gorbach SL. Other bacterial diarrhoeas. Clin Gastroenterol 1993; 7:263–305.
Farthing MJG. Intestinal parasites. Clin Gastroenterol 1993; 7:333–364.
Benson JT (ed.). Female pelvic floor disorders. New York: WW Norton, 1992.
Phillips SF, Pemberton JH, Shorter RG (eds.). The large intestine: physiology, pathophysiology and disease. New York: Raven Press, 1991.

Sleisenger MH, Fordtran JS (eds.). Gastrointestinal disease: pathophysiology, diagnosis, management. 5th ed. Philadelphia: WB Saunders, 1993.

Rubin RH, O'Hanley P. Infections due to gram-negative bacilli. In: Scientific American medicine. New York: Scientific American, 1995.

Mayer RJ. Gastrointestinal Cancer. In: Scientific American medicine. New York: Scientific American, 1996.

Quinolones in acute non-travellers' diarrhoea [Editorial]. Lancet 1991; 335:282.

OBJECTIVES

The student should be able to discuss the following with regard to colonic and anorectal function and disease.

Physiology
1. The role of the colon in the intestinal transport of fluid and electrolytes.
2. The mechanism of defecation.
3. The different motility patterns in the right and left colon and how they determine colonic function.
4. The coordination of colonic motility with eating and the innervation of the colon and its relationship with the central nervous system.
5. The role of the colon in digestion.

Carcinoma of the Colon
1. The epidemiology of colonic carcinoma and the predisposing causes to colon cancer.
2. The use of CEA in diagnosis and follow-up of patients with colon cancer.
3. The Dukes' classification of carcinoma of the colon and the percentage survival after five years for each group in the classification.
4. The role of diet in the etiology of colon cancer.
5. The role of chemotherapy and radiation therapy in carcinoma of the colon.
6. Classification of colonic polyps and how to determine their malignant potential.
7. How polyposis syndrome differs from other conditions associated with polyps.

Diverticular Disease
1. The pathophysiology of diverticular disease.
2. The complications and management of diverticular disease.

Colonic Obstruction
1. The symptoms and signs of colonic obstruction.

2. The causes of colonic obstruction in adults and children.
3. The diagnostic approach to a patient with presumed large bowel obstruction.
4. The x-ray findings of partial large bowel obstruction.

Irritable Bowel Syndrome
1. The Manning criteria and how to make a positive diagnosis of an irritable bowel.
2. The symptoms that are not associated with an irritable bowel.
3. When a patient with an irritable bowel should have further investigations to confirm the diagnosis and the appropriate screening tests to rule out other diseases.
4. The factors that influence patients with an irritable bowel seeking medical attention.
5. The treatment of irritable bowel and the approach to differential diagnosis.

Fecal Incontinence
1. The pathophysiology of fecal incontinence.
2. The mechanism by which the anal sphincter maintains continence.
3. The investigation and management of fecal incontinence.

Constipation
1. The etiological classification of constipation.
2. The investigation and differential diagnosis of constipation.
3. The management of constipation.
4. The identification of "laxative abuse."
5. The causes of solitary rectal ulceration.

Colonic Ischemia
1. The colonic blood supply and the areas of the colon at greatest risk for ischemia.
2. The symptoms and signs of colonic ischemia.
3. The diagnosis and management of ischemia.

Infectious Diarrhea
1. The common causes of dysentery in the tropics.
2. The treatment of common bacterial infections of the colon and choice of the most appropriate antibiotic.
3. The infectious causes of persistent diarrhea.

4. The nematode infections that cause diarrhea and the presentation of nematode intestinal infections.

Perianal Disease

1. The proper techniques of examining the perineum and doing a complete rectal examination (students should be able to demonstrate these techniques).
2. The symptoms of hemorrhoids and their management.
3. The difference between internal and external hemorrhoids.
4. The symptoms and management of fissure in ano.

12
The Pancreas
F. Habal

1. ANATOMY AND PHYSIOLOGY

The pancreas is an endocrine and exocrine organ located retroperitoneally in the upper abdomen overlying the spine. The head and uncinate process lie within the curve of the duodenum, while the body and tail extend to the gastric border of the spleen. The pancreas is supplied by the gastroduodenal arteries and by branches of the splenic artery. The splenic vein and artery run superiorly and posteriorly; the mesenteric vein lies in the angle between the head and body of the gland. At this point the superior mesenteric vein and splenic vein join to form the portal vein (Figure 1).

The islets of Langerhans, clumps of cells scattered throughout the gland, produce the *endocrine* secretion of the pancreas. Their hormones, secreted directly into capillaries, include insulin, which is produced by the beta cells, and glucagon, pancreatic peptide, somatostatin and other hormones secreted by nonbeta cells.

The *exocrine* portion of the pancreas accounts for about 80% of the total glandular volume. It consists of at least two functional units: *acinar cells*, which secrete primarily digestive enzymes; and *centroacinar* or *ductal cells*, which secrete fluids and electrolytes (Figure 2). Pancreatic secretion is regulated by several peptides that are released from the gastrointestinal tract. Some of these peptides, such as secretin and cholecystokinin (CCK), stimulate pancreatic secretions, whereas somatostatin and pancreatic polypeptide inhibit their release. The pancreas secretes about 20 digestive enzymes and cofactors. Some enzymes are activated in the duodenum by enterokinases and calcium (Figure 3). These enzymes account for most of the intraluminal digestion of

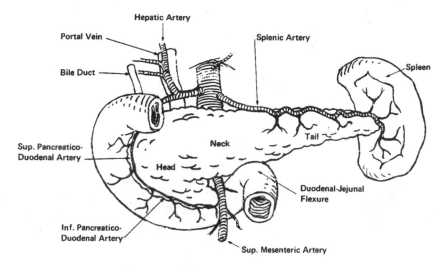

FIGURE 1.   Relationships and blood supply of pancreas.

dietary proteins, triglycerides and carbohydrates. They are also important in the cleavage of certain vitamins (such as A and B_{12}) from carrier molecules, thereby allowing them to be absorbed efficiently. Because pancreatic enzymes are secreted in great excess, maldigestion and serious nutritional deficiencies occur only when over 90% of the gland has been destroyed.

2. PANCREATIC SECRETION

2.1 Bicarbonate Secretion

The pancreas secretes an isosmotic juice at a daily rate of 1,500–3,000 mL. It has a pH ranging between 8.0 and 8.5 and contains enzymes for fat, carbohydrate and protein digestion, water and electrolytes. The total concentration of the major anions Cl^- and HCO_3^- approaches 150 mEq/L (Figure 4). At maximum output, as would be observed following a meal, HCO_3^- concentration reaches 150 mEq/L, whereas Cl^- concentration is less than 50 mEq/L. This ratio is reversed at low flow rates. The high pH of the postprandial juice neutralizes acidic gastric chyme and raises duodenal contents to an optimal pH for enzymatic digestion. Pancreatic juice also contains Ca^{++} and traces of Mg^{++}, $HPO_4^=$ and $SO_4^=$, although the role of these electrolytes is not known.

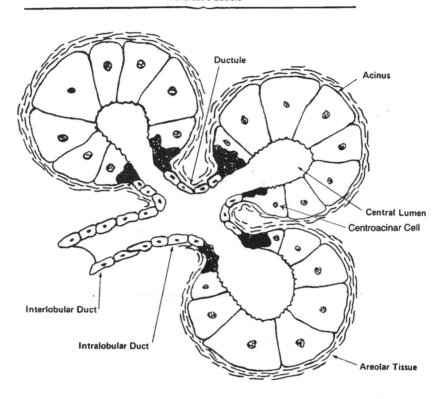

FIGURE 2.   Schematic representation of acinar structure of exocrine pancreas.

2.2 Enzyme Secretion

Four classes of enzymes are secreted by the pancreas; these are proteolytic, lipolytic, carbohydrate-hydrolyzing and nucleolytic enzymes.

Two of the proteolytic enzymes, trypsin and chymotrypsin, are secreted as zymogens. Both trypsinogen and chymotrypsinogen are activated by enterokinases that are secreted by the mucosa of the proximal intestine. Once trypsinogen is activated into trypsin, it in turn activates further zymogens. Trypsin and chymotrypsin are endopeptidases and constitute the largest component; they act by cleaving the peptide bonds of dietary protein, producing oligopeptides and amino acids. Other enzymes include carboxypeptidases A and B, and elastase.

Lipolytic enzymes are secreted in active form. Lipase is the major compo-

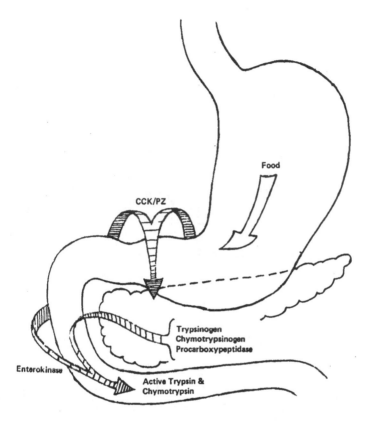

FIGURE 3. Role of cholecystokinin/pancreozymin and of enterokinase activation in pancreatic secretion.

nent. This enzyme hydrolyzes triglycerides to diglycerides, monoglycerides and fatty acids. Lipase acts as the oil–water interface of fat droplets. Its action is thus facilitated when the fat droplets are emulsified by bile salts and fatty acids. Bile salts also form molecular aggregates, micelles, to solubilize the products of lipolysis in the aqueous duodenal juice, removing them from the oil–water interface and so enhancing lipase activity. Colipase, a small-molecular-weight cofactor, is secreted by the pancreas. It combines with lipase to prevent the latter from being inhibited and removed from the oil–water interface by bile salts. Colipase also lowers the pH optimum of lipase from 8.5 to 6.5, which is the normal pH in the proximal intestine.

Amylase hydrolyzes starch to form maltose, maltotrioses and dextrins.

FIGURE 4. Secretion by centroacinar cells and by cells of the extralobular ducts of the pancreas. Chloride concentrations (right) were determined on fluid collected by micropuncture, and the bicarbonate concentrations were inferred from the fact that the fluid is isotonic. These data are for the cat pancreas, but other species seem to be similar.
SOURCE: Adapted from Lightwood R, Reber HA. Micropuncture study of pancreatic secretion in the cat. Gastroenterology 1977; 72:61.

The fourth class of enzymes comprises nucleolytic enzymes, which hydrolyze the phosphodiester bonds that unite nucleotides in nucleic acid.

2.3 Regulation of Pancreatic Secretion

There are two patterns of pancreatic secretion. The first pattern is *basal secretion*, which is punctuated every 1 to 2 hours by bursts of increased bicarbonate and enzyme secretion that last 10 to 15 minutes. The second pattern is the *postprandial stage*, which results from a complex interaction of neural and hormonal mechanisms. It is divided into three phases. The cephalic phase occurs in response to the sight or taste of food and is probably mediated by the vagus nerve. The stimulation of cholinergic nerve fibers results in the production of enzymes and bicarbonate. The gastric phase occurs partially in response to distention of the stomach, which may stimulate gastrin release, probably by vagal reflexes. The released gastrin and neural reflexes stimulate acid secretion by the gastric parietal cells and pancreatic enzyme secretion. The intestinal phase, which is the most important, is initiated in response to acid entering the duodenum. When the pH of duodenal contents falls to 4.5 or below, secretin is released from the intestine; secretin in turn stimulates the pancreatic ducts to secrete bicarbonate. The presence of fatty acids, oligopeptides and amino acids results in the release of cholecystokinin (CCK), which stimulates the secretion of pancreatic enzymes. It appears that CCK and secretin each augments the action of the other on the secretion of both bicarbonate and enzyme.

The ultimate result of these interactions is food digestion and then absorption. Although secretin and cholecystokinin induce pancreatic secretion, other hormones – such as pancreatic polypeptide (PP) and peptide YY – inhibit basal and stimulated pancreatic secretion. Produced by the intestinal mucosa, they appear to act as a feedback mechanism to inhibit pancreatic production of further enzymes and electrolytes.

Stimulation of the vagus nerve induces bicarbonate secretion by the pancreas. This activity is thought to be in part mediated by vasoactive intestinal peptide (VIP). VIP hormone is present in vagal nerve endings and throughout the entire gastrointestinal tract. Its physiological role has not been established.

3. PANCREATIC FUNCTIONS

3.1 Secretory Studies
It is easy to diagnose pancreatic insufficiency in the presence of the clinical triad of pancreatic calcification, diabetes and steatorrhea. Most pancreatic diseases, however, remain clinically silent until approximately 90% of the gland is destroyed. Lipase secretion appears to decrease earlier than trypsin secretion; hence, steatorrhea appears earlier than azotorrhea in patients suffering from pancreatic disease. Earlier recognition of pancreatic dysfunction may improve the management of the patient's disease and his or her quality of life.

Pancreatic function tests may be divided into two main groups: direct (duodenal intubation) and indirect (Table 1).

3.2 Direct Tube Tests
Tube tests require an oroduodenal tube that aspirates pancreatic secretion

TABLE 1.   Exocrine pancreatic function

Direct invasive intubation tests
CCK/secretin stimulation
Lundh meal
ERCP and pancreatic aspiration

Indirect noninvasive tests
Stool fats and nitrogen
Stool trypsin and chymotrypsin
Breath tests
Oral function tests (bentiromide test and pancreolauryl test)

Blood determination
Trypsinogen
Lipase
Pancreatic amylase

from the duodenum near the papilla of Vater so that the response to stimulating factors can be measured. The stimulants used are secretin, cholecystokinin and the Lundh test meal. The accuracy of these tests can be compromised by ineffective tube placement and lack of success in aspiration. This is partly compensated for by using measures of concentration of enzymes and bicarbonate. The collection period varies from 45 to 120 minutes.

The stimulation of the pancreas can be accomplished directly by infusing secretin alone or in combination with cholecystokinin. The combination allows the assessment not only of bicarbonate secretion (with secretin) but also of enzyme secretion, mainly trypsin.

A more physiological stimulation test of the pancreas by a meal is called the Lundh test. It assesses the response of the pancreas to endogenous secretin and pancreozymin (or CCK) released in response to a test meal of protein, fat and carbohydrates. The concentration of trypsin and the volume of secretion are measured in samples obtained in the duodenal aspirate. The Lundh meal is virtually always abnormal in pancreatic insufficiency. Unfortunately there is a borderline zone of abnormal values that are uninterpretable. In addition, many other factors influence the results of a Lundh meal, including small bowel mucosal disease, rate of gastric emptying, and surgical interruption of gastroduodenal anatomy. Although this is a more physiological test, its sensitivity and specificity are lower (70–80%) than those of direct hormonal stimulation.

Cannulation of the pancreatic duct during endoscopic retrograde cholangiopancreatography (ERCP) has been combined with direct stimulation of the pancreas. This technique allows the measurement of pure pancreatic juice uncontaminated by biliary or intestinal secretions, but this method is possibly no more sensitive than other tests in the diagnosis of pancreatic disease.

3.3 Indirect Pancreatic Function (Tubeless) Tests

The intubation tests tend to be unpleasant for patients; they are also time-consuming and expensive and are performed mostly in specialized centers. Indirect tests of pancreatic function detect the result of pancreatic disease. The standard indirect test is the 72-hour fecal fat determination. The patient is placed on a 100 g/day fat diet and the stool is collected daily for three days. Individuals with normal pancreatic functions excrete less than 7% of the total amount of fat ingested, whereas those with pancreatic insufficiency excrete more than 20%. Although steatorrhea occurs in mucosal malabsorption, it is not as great as that encountered with pancreatic insufficiency. Measurements of stool nitrogen and stool chymotrypsin have not proved superior to fecal fat determinations. The major drawbacks to stool fat estimations are the lack of specificity and the inconvenience of collecting and analyzing the specimens. Attempts to screen for steatorrhea with less offensive tests (such as urine oxalate levels, ^{14}C-triolein/^{3}H-oleic acid assimilation test tripalmitate or palmitic acid breath tests) are promising but not generally accepted. After a rice-flour challenge, breath hydrogen is negligible in normal individuals but is dramatically increased in those with pancreatic insufficiency, in whom it is in turn reduced when the challenge rice flour is given with pancreatic enzymes.

There are two oral function tests available for assessing pancreatic functions: the bentiromide test and the pancreolauryl test.

The bentiromide test is useful in distinguishing patients with pancreatic steatorrhea from those with normal fat absorption. Bentiromide, a synthetic compound attached to para-aminobenzoic acid (PABA), is hydrolyzed by pancreatic chymotrypsin in the duodenum. This yields a low-molecular-weight substance, para-aminobenzoic acid, which is absorbed in the proximal small bowel and is partially conjugated in the liver. Metabolic byproducts of PABA are excreted in the urine. The excretion of less than 50% of the ingested dose in six hours indicates pancreatic exocrine insufficiency. Thus, the urine output of PABA should reflect duodenal chymotrypsin activity. Falsely abnormal results occur in patients with intestinal mucosal, liver or renal disease as a result of abnormalities of absorption, conjugation or excretion of PABA. A two-stage test has therefore been proposed in which PABA excretion following bentiromide is compared with the urine recovery of an equivalent dose of free PABA given on a subsequent occasion. PABA may also be measured in plasma instead of urine, and the plasma test may be more reliable in identifying patients with pancreatic insufficiency. The greatest use of this test may be in excluding pancreatic disease as a cause of diarrhea, steatorrhea, or weight loss.

The pancreolauryl test, using fluorescein dilaurate, has been extensively evaluated in Europe. It can detect only severe pancreatic insufficiency. This test is rarely used.

Chronic pancreatitis may give rise to an abnormal Schilling test, but rarely causes B_{12} deficiency. Vitamin B_{12} is released from food by gastric hydrochloric acid. This B_{12} is bound to an R factor that is present in the saliva and the gastric juices. In the upper intestine, pancreatic enzymes release the R factor from B_{12}, which is then bound to intrinsic factor; the complex is subsequently absorbed in the terminal ileum. The Schilling test is relatively simple, but unfortunately it is not predictably abnormal except in instances of obvious pancreatic insufficiency.

3.4 Miscellaneous Tests

Differentiating pancreatic carcinoma from chronic pancreatitis can at times be difficult; many tests have been described to aid diagnosis, but none are of proven value. Assay of carcinoembryonic antigen (CEA) in serum or from pure pancreatic juice obtained during ERCP has not proved to be a useful discriminator. The pancreatic oncofetal antigen has proved to be of uncertain significance. Serum galactosyl II transferase activity has recently been shown to be a reasonably specific indicator of pancreatic carcinoma in some patients. A sophisticated assay, it is unlikely to be suited to widespread use.

Trypsinogen, a proteolytic proenzyme, is exclusively produced in the pancreas. This enzyme can be detected by radioimmunoassay. It is elevated during an attack of pancreatitis and in renal failure, and is decreased in severe pancreatic insufficiency, cystic fibrosis and insulin-dependent diabetes without exocrine insufficiency. The levels of trypsinogen in cystic fibrosis decrease with age if the pancreas is involved. Low levels are found in about 60% of patients with pancreatic insufficiency. Patients with pancreatic insufficiency who have ongoing inflammation may have normal or raised levels. This fact, in addition to low levels in non–insulin-dependent diabetes, casts some doubt on the usefulness of this test in diagnosing pancreatic insufficiency. It may be useful in patients with steatorrhea that is due to nonpancreatic causes.

3.5 Tests Suggestive of Active Disease

When faced with a patient with hyperamylasemia, it is necessary to exclude disease involving many organs other than just the pancreas (Table 2).

Amylase is produced and released from a variety of tissues, including the salivary glands, intestine and genitourinary tract. Normal serum contains three

TABLE 2. Conditions associated with hyperamylasemia

Pancreatic amylase
(Pancreatic pancreatitis/carcinoma/trauma, including surgical
    and post-ERCP complications of pancreatitis)
Intra-abdominal
Drugs
Diabetic ketoacidosis

Salivary amylase
Malignant neoplasms
Pulmonary diseases/pneumonia/tuberculosis/carcinoma
Diabetic ketoacidosis/ruptured ectopic pregnancy/ovarian cyst

Mixed or unknown
Renal insufficiency
Thermal burns
Macroamylasemia

---

types of isoamylases as identified by isoelectric focusing. The pancreatic gland secretes one amylase at an isoelectric point of 7.0 that constitutes 33% of the total serum amylase. The parotid secretes several isoamylases with isoelectric points of about 6.4 and 6.0. Electrophoresis on polyacrylamide gel can separate five isoamylases on the basis of electrode mobility. Amylases originating in the fallopian tubes, tears, mucus and sweat have the same mobility as salivary amylase. All amylases have similar molecular weight and amino acid composition, but vary in terms of their glycosylation or deamination.

Amylase is filtered through the glomerular membrane and is reabsorbed in the proximal tubule. In healthy individuals, the amylase clearance parallels creatinine clearance. During acute pancreatitis, there is an increase in amylase clearance as opposed to creatinine clearance. Although this ratio was once thought to be specific to acute pancreatitis, other conditions that produce hyperamylasemia (such as diabetic ketoacidosis, burns, renal failure and perforated duodenal ulcer) may demonstrate a similar elevation. Occasionally, the serum amylase may be markedly increased in the absence of pancreatic or salivary diseases, whereas the urinary amylase is normal. In this instance, one must suspect either renal disease or macroamylasemia. In the latter condition normal serum amylase is bound by an IgA globulin, forming a complex that is too large to be filtered by the glomerulus. Affected individuals have an elevated serum amylase and a low to normal urinary excretion rate.

Frequently physicians are faced with a patient who has no overt salivary gland disease but has hyperamylasemia and no specific abdominal findings.

As a rule, the level of amylase in pancreatitis usually is elevated to greater than 3 times the upper limit of normal and returns to normal within 2 to 10 days. If the amylase continues to be elevated in the absence of pancreatic complications, other causes (such as malignancy and macroamylasemia) should be investigated.

A rapid rise and fall in serum amylase in a patient with abdominal pain suggests the passage of a stone through the ampulla of Vater. When the serum amylase remains elevated for several days, the gallstone disease is usually complicated by pancreatitis.

Marked hyperamylasemia has been observed in patients with metastatic disease with ovarian cysts and tumors, and ruptured ectopic pregnancy. Isoamylase analysis reveals that the amylase has the same electrophoretic mobility as salivary-type isoenzyme. Macroamylase consists mostly of salivary amylase complexed with globulins, being therefore too large to be filtered at the glomerulus. Therefore these individuals have elevated serum amylase and low urinary amylase, with a low amylase-to-creatinine clearance ratio.

While the amylase levels in serum and urine are usually used as a measure of acute pancreatitis, measurements of lipase may be more specific and sensitive than total serum amylase. The assay of lipase is as accurate as the pancreatic isoamylase assay, and is likely to replace the amylase assay. Measuring both offers no advantage. Amylase and lipase measurements are readily available clinically, whereas radioimmunoassays are still being developed for other pancreatic enzymes (such as trypsin, chymotrypsin and elastase). Their role in the diagnosis of pancreatic disease needs to be established.

4. PANCREATITIS

4.1 Etiology and Pathogenesis

Inflammatory disease of the pancreas is a common problem in North America, with gallstones and alcohol being the major causes (Table 3). Pancreatitis tends to present with abdominal pain, which may improve with no sequelae or may run a more severe course that can lead to death. When the pancreas is continuously injured, such as with alcohol, a chronic condition results in obstruction and fibrosis of the gland, which leads to pancreatic insufficiency and chronic pain. Even one attack of pancreatitis from alcohol use can lead to some residual pancreatic damage.

Pancreatitis results from an autodigestive process. Pancreatic digestive enzymes, vasoactive materials and other toxic materials extravasate out of the pancreas into the surrounding areas, leading to a widespread chemical irritation resulting in simple edema to severe hemorrhage and necrosis. Serious

TABLE 3.   Causes of acute pancreatitis

Alcoholism

Gallstones

Postoperative (post–coronary bypass)

Traumatic
  Abdominal trauma
  Iatrogenic intraoperative, post-ERCP, diagnostic and therapeutic

Penetrating duodenal ulcer

Metabolic
  Hyperlipoproteinemia, especially types I, IV and V
  Hypercalcemia
  Renal failure
  Acute fatty liver of pregnancy

Viral infections
  Mumps
  HIV (AIDS)
  Varicella
  Viral hepatitis
  CMV
  Epstein-Barr virus

Parasitic infections
  Ascariasis

Drug-associated
  Diuretics (e.g., thiazides, furosemide)
  Tetracycline
  Sulfonamides
  Estrogens
  Azathioprine and mercaptopurine
  Pentamidine
  Valproic acid
  Salicylates
  Steroids

(cont'd)

complications include hypovolemia and hypotension. Trypsin and chymotrypsin are the initiating enzymes; their release can in turn result in the release and activation of other proenzymes (including proelastase, procollagenase and phospholipases). Trypsin damages endothelial cells and mast cells, resulting in the release of histamine. This major inflammatory mediator enhances vascular permeability, leading to edema, hemorrhage and the activation of the kallikrein system, which in turn results in the production of vasoactive peptides or kinins. The latter are thought to cause pain and further

TABLE 3.   Causes of acute pancreatitis (cont'd)

Toxins
  Ethyl alcohol
  Methyl alcohol
  Scorpion venom
  Organophosphorous insecticides
  Amanita (toxin in some mushrooms)
Miscellaneous
  Hereditary
  Regional enteritis
  Connective tissue disorders with vasculitis
  Systemic lupus erythematosus (SLE)
  Polyarteritis
  Thrombotic thrombocytopenic purpura (TTP)
  Duodenal diverticulum

Undetermined

---

aggravate the inflammatory response. The other released enzymes destroy the supporting matrix of the gland and the plasma membrane of the acinar cell, precipitating further release of digestive enzymes, which in turn leads to further damage. Lysolecithin, which is released by the action of phospholipase on lecithin (a phospholipid found in bile), has also been implicated in pancreatic damage, because of its cytotoxic and hemolytic properties. When the pancreas is inflamed but remains viable, the condition is termed *interstitial pancreatitis*; this may occur in up to 80% of cases. In the remaining cases, there is significant pancreatic necrosis resulting from disruption of the microcirculation, destruction of the pancreatic parenchyma and peripancreatic necrosis. Although these enzymes result in pancreatic damage, the triggering mechanism is not well known. In the case of gallstones, the major theories include (1) reflux of bile into the pancreatic duct; (2) reflux of duodenal content into the pancreatic duct; and (3) distal obstruction of the pancreatic duct, with continued pancreatic secretion leading to increased ductal pressure and resulting in pancreatitis.

Although alcohol has been implicated as a major cause of acute pancreatitis, there is no evidence that an occasional bout of excessive alcohol intake can lead to an acute attack. It is suggested that chronic ingestion may lead to chronic damage and sensitization, which may result in acute pain even with small amounts of alcohol. Alcohol can cause direct damage to acinar cells in a manner similar to that in which it damages liver cells.

Hyperlipoproteinemia types I, IV and V are associated with the majority of lipid-associated cases of pancreatitis. The incidence of pancreatitis varies

TABLE 4. Poor prognostic indicators in acute pancreatitis (Ranson's criteria, 1978, modified by Hollander et al., 1983)

First 24 hours
Age > 55
Leucocytosis > 16,000
Hyperglycemia, serum glucose > 200 mg/dL
LDH > 350 units/L

After 24 hours
Decrease in hematocrit by > 10%
Hypocalcemia (< 2.0 mmol/L)
Hypoxemia pO_2 < 60 mm Hg
Hypovolemia
Base deficit > 4.0 mmol/L
Amylase > 1,000

from 15–40% of patients. Hyperlipidemia has been suggested to be the cause of pancreatitis; however, recent evidence suggests that mild to moderate elevation of serum triglyceride levels is likely to be an epiphenomenon of the pancreatitis rather than the primary etiology. Hypercalcemia and hyperparathyroidism may also induce pancreatitis. Although the incidence of pancreatitis in patients with hyperparathyroidism was at one time shown to vary from 7–19%, recent findings suggest this variation to be closer to 1.5%. This discrepancy can be accounted for by the difference in the degree or duration of the hyperparathyroidism and by the earlier treatment of hypercalcemia. Other causes of pancreatitis are shown in Table 3.

4.2 Acute Pancreatitis

4.2.1 *CLINICAL MANIFESTATIONS*
The clinical spectrum of acute pancreatitis ranges from mild, self-limiting disease to fulminant lethal disease. Up to 80% of patients will have an uneventful recovery; the remainder will have serious complications with a high mortality rate. Objective measurements such as Ranson's criteria (Table 4) show a good correlation with the risk of major complications and death. The overall mortality rate of acute pancreatitis ranges from 7–20%. The mortality rate correlates well with complications such as shock and hemorrhage.

4.2.2 *SYMPTOMS*
Pain from acute pancreatitis is a knife-like, steady, sharp pain that starts suddenly and reaches its zenith rapidly. It is commonly localized to the epigastric

area and may radiate directly to the back. It improves on leaning forward and is frequently associated with nausea or vomiting. Depending on the location of the inflammation, the pain may be referred to either the left upper quadrant or the right upper quadrant. When the pancreatitis is severe, it may result in shock and may lead to death. Frequently the pain is dyspeptic in quality and aggravated by food. This is due partially to the fact that eating stimulates secretion. Classically the pain lasts between three and four days. When the pancreatitis is severe, it may result in peripheral circulatory failure; under these conditions, the mortality rate approaches 60%.

Recurrent nausea and vomiting may be due to a reflex mechanism secondary to pain and occurs in over 90% of the cases. Other causes include pseudo-obstruction secondary to ileus and distention or obstruction secondary to a pancreatic mass or pseudocyst. Since the common bile duct traverses the pancreatic head before entering the duodenum, jaundice may occur, often transiently.

4.2.3 SIGNS
Depending on the severity of pancreatitis, the patient may appear in distress or be in shock. Jaundice may be caused by edema of the head of the pancreas or by an obstructing stone. Tachycardia could be secondary to pain, volume depletion or the inflammatory process. Low-grade fever could be secondary to the inflammation in the pancreas or result from such complications as abscess formation.

Abdominal examination may reveal epigastric and abdominal tenderness with guarding or rigidity. Bluish discoloration of the flanks (Grey Turner's sign) or of the periumbilical area (Cullen's sign) indicates that blood from hemorrhagic pancreatitis has entered the fascial planes. The signs are not specific and may occur in any condition that causes retroperitoneal hemorrhage. Tender red and painful nodules that mimic erythema nodosum may appear over the extremities. These are often due to circulating lipases.

4.2.4 COMPLICATIONS
Since the signs and symptoms of acute pancreatitis may mimic those of surgically correctable intra-abdominal disorders, the diagnosis of acute pancreatitis is often one of exclusion. Other diseases to be considered are a perforated peptic ulcer, mesenteric thrombosis, intestinal obstruction, dissecting aneurysm, peritonitis, acute cholecystitis and appendicitis. The diagnostic process is complicated by the fact that hyperamylasemia can occur in disorders other than pancreatic inflammation (such as ectopic pregnancy, parotiditis, carcinoma of the lung, posterior penetrating ulcer, ruptured aortic aneurysm and opiate administration). Although amylase values greater than

1,000 units have been said to occur principally in conditions requiring surgery (e.g., biliary tract disease), this distinction is not absolute.

Local involvement of pancreatitis includes phlegmon (18%), pancreatic abscess (3%), pancreatic pseudocyst (10%) and thrombosis of the central portal system. Phlegmon is an area of edema, inflammation and necrosis without a definite structure (unlike an abscess). A phlegmon results from acute intrapancreatic inflammation with fat necrosis and pancreatic parenchymal and peripancreatic necrosis. This arises from the ischemic insult caused by decreased tissue perfusion and release of the digestive enzymes. When this damage is not cleared, further inflammation ensues, declaring itself by increased pain, fever and tenderness. In severe cases a secondary infection ensues, a process termed *infected necrosis of the pancreas*, which occurs within the first one to two weeks of the illness and carries a high mortality. This diagnosis can be made by computerized tomography (CT) and percutaneous aspiration of the area with subsequent bacterial staining and appropriate cultures. In 3% of acute pancreatitis an abscess develops, usually several weeks into the illness. An abscess is a well-defined collection of pus occurring after the acute inflammation has subsided.

A pseudocyst develops as a result of pancreatic necrosis and the escape of activated pancreatic secretions through pancreatic ducts. It contains blood and debris. This fluid coalesces and becomes encapsulated by an inflammatory reaction and fibrosis. These patients usually have pain and hyperamylasemia, but may be asymptomatic. They may present with an abdominal mass, causing compressive symptoms.

Systemic complications of acute pancreatitis are numerous (Table 5) and correlate well with the severity of the inflammatory process. They may be manifested by shock (circulatory collapse secondary to sequestration of retroperitoneal fluid or hemorrhage), respiratory and renal failure and profound metabolic disturbances.

Although acute pancreatitis may run a mild self-limiting course, severe pancreatitis occurs in up to 25% of acute attacks, with a mortality approaching 10%. The majority of deaths occur within the first week of hospital admission and are caused by local and systemic complications, including sepsis and respiratory failure. Most clinical studies in adults cite pancreatic infection as the most common cause of death, accounting for 70–80% of deaths.

4.2.5 DIAGNOSTIC EVALUATION

The diagnosis of acute pancreatitis is based on a combination of clinical findings and the use of laboratory and radiographic techniques. Elevation of serum amylase in acute pancreatitis is short-lived. Amylase is rapidly cleared by the renal tubules and may return to normal within 24 hours from the time

TABLE 5.   Systemic complications of pancreatitis

Metabolic
 Hypocalcemia, hyperglycemia, hypertriglyceridemia, acidosis

Respiratory
 Hypoxemia, atelectasis, effusion, pneumonitis
 Acute respiratory distress syndrome (ARDS)

Renal
 Renal artery or vein thrombosis
 Renal failure

Circulatory
 Arrhythmias
 Hypovolemia and shock; myocardial infarct
 Pericardial effusion, vascular thrombosis

Gastrointestinal
 Ileus
 Gastrointestinal hemorrhage from stress ulceration; gastric
   varices (secondary to splenic vein thrombosis)
 Gastrointestinal obstruction

Hepatobiliary
 Jaundice
 Portal vein thrombosis

Neurologic
 Psychosis or encephalopathy (confusion, delusion and coma)
 Cerebral emboli
 Blindness (angiopathic retinopathy with hemorrhage)

Hematologic
 Anemia
 DIC (disseminated intravascular coagulopathy)
 Leucocytosis

Dermatologic
 Painful subcutaneous fat necrosis

of onset. Although amylase-to-creatinine clearance was used in the past to diagnose pancreatitis, it is now rarely used. Lipase levels appear to be a more sensitive and specific method of diagnosing acute pancreatitis and may remain elevated for several days following the onset of pain. Immunologic assays for trypsinogen or immunolipase are experimental and do not add any more information than the serum lipase.

4.2.6 RADIOLOGIC EVALUATION
A plain film of the abdomen is very helpful. It may reveal calcification of the pancreas (indicative of a chronic process) or it may reveal gallstones (if calci-

fied). The presence of free air suggests perforation, whereas the presence of thumb-printing in the intestinal wall may indicate a mesenteric ischemic process. A localizing ileus of the stomach, duodenum or proximal jejunum (all of which are adjacent to the pancreas) is highly suggestive of pancreatic inflammation. Similarly, when the transverse colon is also involved, air filling the transverse colon but not the descending colon (colon "cut-off" sign) may be seen. The chest x-ray can show atelectasis or an effusion, more often involving the left lower lobe.

Although clinical, biochemical and simple radiographic evaluation suffice for the diagnosis of pancreatitis, ultrasonographic and computerized tomography imaging are essential. These confirm the diagnosis, provide an early assessment regarding the course of the disease and detect complications such as phlegmon, pseudocyst and abscess formation. A pseudocyst or an abscess may also be drained percutaneously under CT or ultrasound guidance.

The most common ultrasonographic and CT finding in patients with acute pancreatitis is diffuse glandular enlargement. Ultrasonographically there is a decrease in echogenicity of the organ; on CT scan there is decreased attenuation from edema of the tissues. Frequently intravenous contrast is given, and this may demonstrate a uniform enhancement in the pancreatic parenchyma. A normal examination does not rule out the presence of acute disease. In up to 30% of uncomplicated cases of acute pancreatitis CT scan may be normal; these patients usually have a mild form of pancreatitis. When a stone or an obstruction of the distal common bile duct is present, the common bile duct and the intrahepatic biliary tree may be dilated.

Endoscopic retrograde cholangiopancreatography (ERCP) involves cannulating the ampulla of Vater and then injecting contrast material into the pancreatic duct and the biliary tree. This procedure is usually contraindicated during the acute phase, except when the pancreatitis is caused by an impacted common bile duct stone. Under those conditions, a sphincterotomy and stone removal may be performed. If performed as early as 24 hours following admission, this procedure may result in significant improvement in morbidity and mortality.

4.2.7 TREATMENT

The aims of therapy of acute pancreatitis are (1) hemodynamic stabilization, (2) alleviation of pain, (3) stopping the progression of the damage, and (4) treatment of local and systemic complications. As yet there are no specific medical therapies capable of reducing or reversing the pancreatic inflammation. Hence therapeutic interventions are aimed at the complications of the disease.

Once the diagnosis is established with certainty, the patient's intravascular volume is replenished, and electrolytes, calcium, magnesium and blood sugar are closely monitored. Depending on the severity of the attack, an indwelling urinary catheter and close monitoring of urinary output may be necessary. Analgesics such as meperidine should be administered regularly during the first several days of the attack. This may alleviate the pain, decrease the patient's apprehension and improve respiration, thus preventing pulmonary complications such as atelectasis. The risk of narcotic addiction is minimal during the first days; most patients settle within 72 hours. The patient is kept off oral feeding; nasogastric suctioning is maintained if the disease is severe and complicated by vomiting and ileus. Mild cases with minimal symptoms may be managed without suctioning. The rationale behind nasogastric suctioning is to place the pancreas at rest by removing the acidic gastric juices. This suppresses secretin release and decreases pancreatic stimulation. The validity of this postulate has not been substantiated. Similarly, the use of acid-suppressive medications such as cimetidine has failed to show benefit in the treatment of acute pancreatitis. The use of enzyme inhibitors such as soybean trypsin inhibitor to prevent further damage is controversial, as is the use of prostaglandins and corticosteroids.

The routine administration of antibiotics does not improve the course of mild to moderate disease. However, when the development of pancreatic abscess is suspected from an increase in fever and abdominal pain, antibiotic therapy should be instituted using an aminoglycocide and cephalosporin.

Respiratory insufficiency may occur in up to 40% of the cases, usually in patients with severe or recurrent pancreatitis. In such patients, arterial oxygen saturation should be monitored and corrected. Fluid overload should be avoided. Intubation and ventilation may be required.

Peritoneal lavage has been advocated in patients with severe disease, such as those with marked hypovolemia or hypotension or those who continue to deteriorate despite appropriate medical therapy. Although this technique reduces the circulatory and renal complications, it does not seem to alter the local complications.

Intravenous hyperalimentation has been advocated in patients who continue to have pain and whose symptoms are aggravated postprandially. If during a trial of six weeks or longer, complications develop (such as an abscess or an enlargement of phlegmon), a surgical debridement may be warranted, albeit as a last resort.

4.3 Chronic Pancreatitis

Chronic pancreatitis is defined as a continued inflammation characterized by irreversible morphologic changes. These changes include fibrosis, ductal abnormality, calcification and cellular atrophy. Alcohol is the major etiologic factor, accounting for about 75% of the cases. Repeated attacks of gallstone-related pancreatitis rarely if ever result in chronic pancreatitis. Other causes include diabetes, protein-calorie malnutrition, hereditary pancreatitis, cystic fibrosis and idiopathic causes.

Alcohol presumably causes pancreatic injury by the intraductal formation of protein plugs secondary to increased protein concentration and precipitation, with or without calcification. These plugs lead to obstruction and secondary pancreatic damage caused by autodigestion. In developed countries chronic pancreatitis occurs after a long history (6 to 17 years) of alcohol ingestion of 150 to 170 g per day. Alcoholic pancreatitis is known to occur with much less consumption of alcohol, as low as 50 g per day. The mean age of a patient with new onset of disease is around 32 years, with a male predominance. Despite heavy drinking only a small number of alcoholics develop chronic pancreatitis, suggesting other factors that potentiate the injurious side effects of alcohol, including high-protein diet with either very high or very low fat content.

4.3.1 CLINICAL MANIFESTATIONS

Chronic pancreatitis is characterized by irreversible injury to the pancreas and clinically by intractable abdominal pain and loss of exocrine and endocrine pancreatic function. The pain is localized to the upper abdomen, with radiation to subcostal regions and to the back. The pain is aggravated by meals and improves with fasting.

When more than 90% of exocrine pancreatic function is lost, maldigestion and malabsorption ensue. This is manifested by steatorrhea (fat malabsorption) associated with diarrhea and bloating, azotorrhea (protein malabsorption) and progressive weight loss. These patients frequently present with loss of adipose tissue, judged by hanging skin folds, and more objectively by demonstrating that the skin fold at the mid-triceps is less than 8 mm in males and less than 12 mm in females. In addition, patients manifest muscle wasting and edema, indicating protein deficiency. Latent fat-soluble vitamin deficiency (vitamins A, D, E and K) in addition to deficiencies of magnesium, calcium and essential fatty acids may occur and are closely related to dysfunction of fat digestion. Endocrine insufficiency presenting as diabetes mellitus may present at the same time as exocrine insufficiency or a few years later.

4.3.2 COMPLICATIONS

4.3.2.1 Pancreatic pseudocyst

Pancreatic pseudocyst is localized fluid collection occurring within a pancreatic mass or in the peripancreatic spaces following acute or chronic pancreatitis. The pseudocyst is usually surrounded by a non-epithelial-lined fibrous wall of granulation tissues. Its frequency varies from 10–50% of patients experiencing severe pancreatitis. When a pseudocyst is present for less than six weeks, it is considered acute; after that it becomes chronic. The pseudocyst may be asymptomatic or may present as an acute exacerbation of pancreatitis, with abdominal pain, nausea, vomiting and weight loss. These pseudocysts may obstruct intra-abdominal viscera, cause pancreatic ascites, rupture into viscera or the abdominal cavity, hemorrhage or become infected. Spontaneous resolution occurs in 20% of the cases within the first six weeks of the pseudocyst's development. Chronic pseudocysts or pseudocysts greater than 5 cm rarely improve. Asymptomatic patients with persistent psuedocysts should be observed and intervention may be considered if symptoms appear. Successful percutaneous catheter drainage may be accomplished by CT- or ultrasound-guided drainage techniques. The catheter may be required for up to six weeks and is frequently associated with infections. Surgical drainage is sometimes necessary for failed percutaneous drainage or for complicated pseudocysts. If the pseudocyst is in the head of the pancreas, drainage can be done via ERCP.

4.3.2.2 *Pancreatic ascites*
Pancreatic ascites results from the leakage of pancreatic juices into the peritoneal cavity through a fistula or ruptured pseudocyst. It presents with gradually increasing massive ascites, high levels of amylase, abdominal pain and weight loss. Painful areas of subcutaneous fat necrosis result from the high levels of circulating pancreatic lipase.

4.3.2.3 *Common bile duct stricture*
Common bile duct compression is another manifestation of chronic pancreatitis, but it rarely results in significant obstruction. As the distal common bile duct traverses the head of the pancreas, it may be narrowed secondary to inflammation, with edema or fibrosis of the gland.

Although pancreatic carcinoma was formerly thought to be increased in chronic pancreatitis, the incidence is now believed to be the same as in the general population. Pancreatic carcinoma may present as pancreatitis.

4.3.3 *DIAGNOSTIC AND RADIOGRAPHIC EVALUATION*
The diagnosis of chronic pancreatitis is straightforward in patients with advanced pancreatic disease, especially in the presence of radiologic evidence, such as calcification seen exclusively in the ductal system on plain radiographic abdominal films, by ultrasonography or on computerized tomography. This radiologic evidence may be seen in up to 30% of patients with

FIGURE 5. Pancreatic foil pseudocyst. Transverse sonogram showing a cystic septated well-defined mass in the pancreatic tail. It is touching and compressing the line of the splenic vein.

chronic pancreatitis. Although ultrasonography may demonstrate pancreatic enlargement, ductal dilation or pseudocysts (Figure 5), these findings may be better seen on computerized tomography (Figure 6). Abnormalities of the ducts associated with chronic pancreatitis can also be demonstrated by endoscopic retrograde pancreatography. In mild to moderate disease these findings may be subtle and even normal. In more severe disease there is narrowing and dilation of the ducts, stenosis and filling of side ductules. Examination may reveal a tortuous main duct containing stones or protein plugs, or obstruction of the common bile duct (Figure 7). These changes may not be closely relat-

FIGURE 6. Computerized tomography of a pancreatic pseudocyst in the tail of the pancreas.

ed to the degree of pancreatic insufficiency; hence the need for pancreatic function studies.

The only tests that appear to accurately measure pancreatic function in chronic pancreatitis are the direct tube tests that measure the response of the pancreas to various stimuli. The commonest manifestation is a decreased bicarbonate concentration (<50 mEq/L) and decreased volume of secretion.

4.3.4 TREATMENT

The ultimate goals of treatment in chronic pancreatitis are to alleviate pain, maintain adequate nutritional status, and reduce symptoms associated with steatorrhea such as abdominal pain, bloating and diarrhea.

The mechanism of pain in chronic pancreatitis is not known. Abstinence from alcohol may decrease the frequency and severity of painful attacks in patients with alcoholic pancreatitis. Large meals with foods rich in fat should be avoided. Analgesics should be given prior to meals, since the pain is maximal postprandially. The continuous use of narcotics often leads to drug addic-

FIGURE 7. ERCP of a patient with chronic pancreatitis demonstrating dilation of the duct (PD) with filling of side branches in the tail. This is complicated by pancreatic pseudocyst.

tion, which makes the management of pain more difficult. Large doses of pancreatic extracts may reduce the frequency and severity of the pain in patients with no demonstrable duct obstruction. These enzymes appear to suppress pancreatic exocrine output, thus putting the pancreas at rest and resulting in pain relief. Pancreatic replacement is given with meals and at bedtime. Patients who respond to this therapeutic regimen tend to be middle-aged women with idiopathic pancreatitis who suffer from mild or moderate disease. These patients tend to have a bicarbonate output greater than 55 mEq/L and normal fat absorption. Patients with more severe disease, whose peak bicarbonate output is less than 50 mEq/L, tend not to respond to this regimen.

Patients with intractable pain who fail to respond to medical therapy may benefit from surgical intervention. When there is a dilated pancreatic duct with obstructive areas, longitudinal pancreatojejunostomy (modified Pustow operation) may induce immediate pain relief. When the duct is small, partial surgical resection of the pancreas may control the pain in a certain percentage of patients. Although pain alleviation with surgery may be achieved in certain patients, its long-term benefit is limited since pain recurs in the majority of

TABLE 6.   Causes of failure of pancreatic replacement

Incorrect diagnosis (nonpancreatic causes of steatorrhea, such as sprue, bacterial overgrowth)
Poor compliance
Incorrect timing of the medications (should be given with meals)
Variability in the enzyme content of the pancreatic replacement or loss of potency of the enzyme (inadequate amount of enzymes)
Inactivation of the enzymes by gastric juices or by sunlight

patients. An alternative to surgical drainage may be achieved by endoscopic insertion of an an endoprosthesis (stent) into the pancreatic duct. Although this approach is promising, its long-term benefit has not been proven.

Octreotide, a long-acting somatostatin analogue, appears to decrease the pain of chronic pancreatitis. Its action is mediated by suppressing pancreatic secretion, hence resting the pancreas. The role of octreotide remains uncertain.

Administration of high-potency, enteric-coated pancreatic enzymes remains the main therapy for the treatment of steatorrhea in the majority of patients with idiopathic and alcoholic pancreatitis. This will improve fat digestion, increase absorption and allow weight gain, although it will not correct the steatorrhea completely. Azotorrhea is more easily reversed than steatorrhea, since trypsin is more resistant to acid inactivation than lipases. It seems that the most important barrier preventing correction of steatorrhea is the destruction of enzymes in the stomach, which prevents the delivery of enough active enzyme into the duodenum.

Replacement pancreatic enzymes are made from hog pancreas and contain a mixture of proteases, lipase and amylase, along with a variety of enzymes normally present in pancreatic secretions. Different preparations vary in the amount of lipase activity and the method of enzyme delivery (e.g., tablets, capsules or enteric-coated microspheres). Treatment with these enzymes is lifelong. Pancreatic enzymes are inactivated by pH 4 or below; hence, enteric-coated preparations such as Pancrease™ or Cotazym® may be appropriate. In patients who do not respond well, the use of histamine H_2-receptor antagonists (cimetidine, ranitidine or famotidine) or antacids with meals may overcome the detrimental effect of acid on the enzymes. The causes of failure to respond to pancreatic enzyme supplementation are shown in Table 6.

Hypersensitivity to pancreatic enzymes has been reported in patients who have hypersensitivity to pork proteins. Hyperuricosuria may occur in patients receiving high doses of pancreatic extracts, although recent reports have ques-

TABLE 7. Commonest sites of metastases from pancreatic carcinoma

Local nodes
Liver
Peritoneum
Adrenal glands
Lung
Kidneys
Spleen
Bone

tioned this relationship. There appears to be a relationship between urinary urate concentration and the severity of pancreatitis. It appears that oral pancreatic enzymes may bind to folic acid, thereby impairing its absorption, but the clinical significance of this is not clear. Fat-soluble vitamins (e.g., vitamins A and E) are poorly absorbed when steatorrhea exceeds 20 g of fat loss per day. Vitamin D and calcium malabsorption leads to osteopenia and tetany. Vitamin K is also malabsorbed, but bleeding is rare. Malabsorption of vitamin B_{12} occurs in up to 40% of patients with chronic pancreatitis, although vitamin B_{12} deficiency is rare. This malabsorption is thought to be due to the failure of R factor to cleave from the vitamin B_{12} intrinsic factor complex, resulting in failure to absorb vitamin B_{12}.

5. CARCINOMA OF THE PANCREAS

The incidence of cancer of the pancreas has increased steadily over the past 25 years. In males it is the fourth commonest cancer causing death, exceeded only by cancers of the lung, colon and rectum, and prostate. In females it is the fifth commonest cause of death, with only cancers of the breast, colorectum, lung, and ovary/uterus being more frequent. The incidence is higher in males, with a sex ratio of two males to each female; peak incidence occurs in the fifth through seventh decade.

The overall five-year survival rate is less than 3%, and most patients who develop carcinoma of the pancreas die within six months of diagnosis. The poor prognosis in this condition is secondary to the inability to diagnose the carcinoma at an early stage. When symptoms present, the tumor is far advanced and often has metastasized to regional lymph nodes and to adjacent and distant organs, as shown in Table 7.

Ductal cell adenocarcinoma accounts for 90% of pancreatic tumors. Approximately 5% of pancreatic carcinomas are of islet cell origin; the rest consist of cystadenocarcinoma, giant cell carcinoma and epidermoid carcinoma. The head of the pancreas is the commonest site of involvement, accounting for 70% of the cases, whereas the body and tail account for 20% and 10% of the cases, respectively.

Several etiological agents have been invoked in the pathogenesis of pancreatic carcinoma, although most of the studies have not yielded consistent results. Epidemiologically, long-term cigarette smoking is a well-established risk factor. The mechanism causing carcinoma is not proven and has been explained on the basis of the presence of a carcinogen in tobacco smoke. High-fat or high-protein diets tend to stimulate CCK release from the duodenum, which in turn can cause pancreatic hypertrophy and may predispose to carcinoma, although the evidence is not convincing. Diabetics are at twice the risk of developing carcinoma of pancreas as the general population. The mechanism of this is not known. There is no evidence to suggest that alcoholic chronic pancreatitis predisposes to carcinoma. A recent study has shown a four- to five-fold increase in pancreatic carcinoma in individuals exposed to DDT (dichlorodiphenyltrichloroethane).

Some epidemiological studies have suggested an increased rate of pancreatic carcinoma in patients who drank chlorinated water; this remains to be proven. Genetic defects have also been invoked, such as oncogenes and 53 p tumor suppressor mutation, in addition to some evidence suggesting an increase in epidermal growth factor receptor activity.

5.1 Clinical Manifestations

The major symptoms of pancreatic carcinoma include pain, jaundice and weight loss.

Rapid and progressive weight loss is probably the commonest symptom of carcinoma of the pancreas, and is not related to the location or the extent of the tumor.

Most (up to 90%) of the patients suffer from pain during the course of the disease. The pain frequently is a dull aching or boring. Located in the epigastrium, it radiates to the back and increases in severity at night. Depending on the site of the tumor, the pain may radiate to the right or left upper quadrant. Unrelenting pain results from retroperitoneal extension, with invasion of the neural plexuses around the celiac axis.

Jaundice may be the presenting symptom in up to 30% of the patients, and the incidence increases as the disease progresses. It may be associated with pain and pruritus. Jaundice is more common when the head of the pancreas is involved, but obstruction or jaundice can occur secondary to spread to the liver or to lymph nodes around the bile duct. Other nonspecific symptoms include bloating, nausea and vomiting, weakness and fatigue, and diarrhea.

5.2 Signs

The commonest finding in carcinoma of the head of the pancreas is jaundice, with abdominal tenderness and an enlarged liver. Less common signs include a palpable gallbladder, an abdominal mass and edema. Thrombophlebitis occurs in less than 10% of the patients.

The development of diabetes in a middle-aged man or elderly patient with no family history of diabetes should suggest pancreatic carcinoma, especially when this is associated with abdominal pain or weight loss.

5.3 Diagnostic Evaluation

Laboratory tests are often normal or nonspecific. Serum alkaline phosphatase and bilirubin are evaluated when the bile duct is obstructed or there are hepatic metastases. Serum amylase may be moderately elevated but also may be normal. Pancreatic secretory studies are not often helpful, since findings overlap with chronic pancreatitis.

Several tumor markers have been detected in the sera of patients with pancreatic carcinoma. These include pancreatic oncofetal antigen (POA), α-fetoprotein (AFP), carcinoembryonic antigen (CEA), and pancreatic cancer associated antigen. Certain serum tumor markers such as CA 19-9 and CA 242 have been useful in following the progression of pancreatic cancer but not in its diagnosis. These tests are nonspecific and not sensitive enough for screening purposes. Cytologic specimens can be obtained by percutaneous needle aspiration under ultrasound or CT guidance and by aspiration of duodenal or pancreatic juices at ERCP. Positive cytology may guide further management; on the other hand, negative cytology does not rule out the disease.

Ultrasonography is the procedure of choice for detecting pancreatic cancer. Its usefulness is dependent on the examiner's expertise (Figure 8). Examination may be less than optimal in the presence of increased bowel gas. The sensitivity of this test in pancreatic cancer is reported to be 76–94%, with a specificity of 96%. Once a lesion is detected, a guided biopsy may be helpful in establishing the diagnosis. When obstructive jaundice is present, ultrasound may reveal the presence of hepatic lesions or obstruction of the biliary tree. This procedure is simple and involves no radiation exposure.

Computerized tomography (CT) is more accurate and gives more information than ultrasonography (Figure 9). However, it is also more expensive and involves low radiation exposure; also, small centers may not have the equipment. With this technique, bowel gas does not interfere with the visualization of the pancreas. There is better identification of any retroperitoneal invasion. A guided biopsy of the lesion is also possible. However, small early lesions (especially in the head of the pancreas) may be missed on CT scan; hence, its usefulness in early diagnosis is not clear.

FIGURE 8.   Pancreatic head carcinoma. Transverse sonogram shows the confluence of splenic vein and portal vein. The pancreatic body and tail are normal. The head is enlarged and bulbous with an abnormal texture, appearing hypoechoic on the image.

When there is a clinical suspicion of a pancreatic lesion and the ultrasound or CT scan is normal, an ERCP is helpful. It has the advantage of combining gastroduodenoscopy, cholangiography and pancreatography. The papilla may also be examined and cytologic sampling may be obtained. When obstruction is present, therapeutic drainage via stents may be attempted. Angiography is no longer used for diagnosing pancreatic carcinoma, but is still useful to evaluate patients who have known carcinoma for resectability, outlining vascular anatomy. Newer diagnostic tools such as endoscopic ultrasound may further improve selection of patients who might benefit from curative surgery. Magnetic resonance imaging has no apparent advantage over CT.

5.4 Treatment

At the time of presentation, 75%–80% of patients have an unresectable tumor. Pancreatectomy or pancreatoduodenal resection for localized disease is the only treatment that carries a potential for cure. Despite this intervention, the disease carries a poor long-term prognosis, with a survival rate of 3% at five

FIGURE 9. Computerized tomography showing a cancer in the head and body of the pancreas. The tumor is overlapping the superior mesenteric artery posteriorly.

years. Factors that lead to a poor prognosis in pancreatic carcinomas include the presence of tumor in the lymph nodes, vascular invasion, tumor size greater than 2.5 cm and histologically poorly differentiated tumour. Complications can occur in up to 20% of patients following pancreaticoduodenectomy. These include delayed gastric emptying, pancreaticojejunal leak, intra-abdominal sepsis, biliary anastomotic leak, gastrointestinal bleeding and other intra-abdominal hemorrhage. Factors favoring longer survival include jaundice at presentation, a small tumor mass, early tumor stage and a well-differentiated tumor. Palliative operations for unresectable tumor offer some relief, such as alleviating biliary or duodenal obstruction. Operative intervention is frequently associated with high morbidity and mortality; hence, nonsurgical intervention may be preferable. Biliary obstruction can be relieved by percutaneous drainage or by endoscopic stenting of the bile duct. Unfortunately these stents tend to occlude and may require frequent changes.

Adjuvant chemotherapy has not been demonstrated to be beneficial in long-term survival. Irradiation therapy has been advocated in treating larger tumors; it may offer local control and pain management, although its benefit in long-term survival has not been proven.

6. PANCREATIC ISLET CELL TUMORS

Pancreatic islet cell tumors are divided into two types: (1) an endocrine type that elaborates excessive gastrointestinal tract hormones, causing specific clinical syndromes, and (2) a nonfunctioning type that is characterized by symptoms related to the size, location and invasion of the tumor mass. Pancreatic islet cell tumors have a better prognosis than those associated with ductal cell adenocarcinoma. They may be diagnosed by the classic clinical manifestation, by the detection of hormones in the serum and by dynamic CT scan with intravenous and oral contrasts.

Several pancreatic islet cell tumors have been identified. These tumors tend to elaborate a variety of biologically active peptides, resulting in a variety of clinical presentations. These peptides include glucagon, insulin, gastrin, vasoactive intestinal peptide (VIP), somatostatin and pancreatic polypeptide (PP).

Insulinoma is the most common neoplasm of the endocrine pancreas. The insulinoma syndrome is associated with Whipple's triad, which includes symptoms of (1) fasting hypoglycemia (confusion, seizures, personality changes, in addition to palpitation, tremulousness and diaphoresis), with (2) a low serum glucose level, and (3) a relief of symptoms by the administration of glucose. The diagnosis can be made by the demonstration of high serum insulin and low blood sugar, and an elevation in the insulin-to-glucose ratio (IG). The tumor may be localized by dynamic CT scan. Treatment includes surgery to remove the tumor if it is well localized or amenable to surgery, and a combination chemotherapy including streptozocine, doxorubicin and 5-fluorouracil.

Glucagon-secreting tumors (*glucagonomas*) arise from the alpha cells of the pancreas. Patients commonly present with mild diabetes, dermatitis, delayed gastric emptying, stomatitis, ileus and constipation. The dermatitis is manifested by a skin rash termed necrolytic migratory erythema, commonly appearing over the lower extremities. The diagnosis is established by the demonstration of elevated plasma glucagon levels that increase, paradoxically, with challenge by intravenous tolbutamide. Glucagonoma tends to present with large tumors and can be demonstrated by dynamic CT scan.

Gastrin-secreting tumors (*gastrinomas*; Zollinger-Ellison syndrome) arise from nonbeta islet cells. They are frequently malignant and tend to be multiple. They commonly present with recurrent severe peptic ulceration accompanied by marked gastric acid hypersecretion and occasionally diarrhea. The diagnosis is established by the demonstration of marked fasting hypergastrinemia and marked gastric acid hypersecretion. In patients who have borderline increases in gastrin, provocative testing with secretin is indicated. Following secretin stimulation, gastrin levels increase in patients with gastrinoma, whereas in patients with common duodenal ulcer, gastrin levels may show a minimal increase, a decrease or no change. High levels of gastrin may be present in a condition known as G-cell hyperplasia. This can be distinguished from gastrinoma by the sharp rise of gastrin levels (> 200%) in response to meals. Patients with gastrinoma show minimal or no rise in gastrin levels.

Vasoactive intestinal peptide–secreting tumors (*VIPoma*; Werner-Morrison syndrome) produce the pancreatic cholera syndrome, which is characterized by severe diarrhea, hypokalemia and hypochlorhydria or achlorhydria. Fluid secretion may exceed 3–5 L, with a loss of 200–300 mEq of potassium daily. Although the diagnosis is established by the demonstration of high levels of VIP, other substances, such as prostaglandins and secretin-like substances, may contribute to this syndrome.

Somatostatin-producing tumors (*somatostatinomas*) are the least common of pancreatic islet cell tumors, so by the time of diagnosis they tend to be malignant and have usually metastasized. They commonly present with mild diabetes mellitus, gallstones with a dilated gallbladder, anemia, hypochlorhydria and malabsorption. The diagnosis is established by the demonstration of high serum levels of somatostatin.

Pancreatic polypeptide–producing tumors have not been shown to produce any clinically defined syndrome.

6.1 Treatment
Pancreatic endocrine tumors are ideally treated by resection. Unfortunately, despite all our available techniques, up to 40% of these tumors tend to escape localization. These tumors tend to be single or multiple and may be located in any portion of the pancreas or ectopically in the duodenum or any other part of the gastrointestinal tract. It appears that endoscopic ultrasonography may play an important role in tumor localization, but this technique is operator dependent and is not widely used.

Recently, octreotide scintigraphy has shown promise in detecting endocrine islet cell tumors, which appear to have somatostatin receptors. Radiolabeled somatostatin analogues bind to these receptors and can be demonstrated by a gamma camera scintigraphy. This test offers some hope in differentiating endocrine from ductal cell tumors. It may assist the surgeon in delineating and removing the tumor and possibly the metastatic lesions.

7. PANCREAS DIVISUM

Pancreas divisum is the most common variant of human pancreas, occurring in nearly 10% of the population. This anomaly results from the failure of fusion of the dorsal and ventral pancreatic ducts, which usually occurs in the

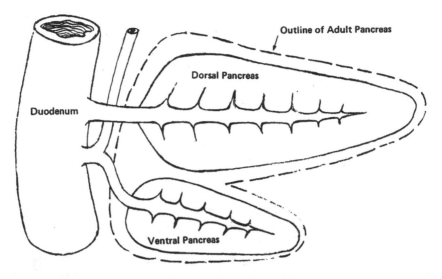

FIGURE 10.   Pancreas at approximately 7 weeks fetal life.

second month of fetal life. This results in the drainage of the main pancreatic duct (including the superior-anterior aspect of the head, the body and the tail) into the dorsal duct via the accessory papilla. The ventral duct, which drains the posterior-inferior aspect, joins the common bile duct and empties into the major papilla (Figure 10). The diagnosis of this condition is made by ERCP.

Most patients having this anomaly are symptom-free, although some reports have suggested a high incidence of abdominal pain and pancreatitis. It has been suggested that the relative stenosis of the accessory papillary orifice, the major outflow tract for pancreatic secretions, is the cause of problems.

Endoscopic sphincterotomy or transduodenal sphincteroplasty has been advocated as the operation of choice in these individuals. The results obtained with this intervention have been controversial. Some studies have reported a success rate of 90% in patients with pancreas divisum pancreatitis after two years, whereas other reports did not support such findings. From the available literature, surgical intervention in pancreas divisum is as controversial as its causative relationship in abdominal pain and pancreatitis.

8. CYSTIC FIBROSIS IN THE ADULT

Cystic fibrosis (CF) is no longer solely a pediatric disease. CF is the most common potentially lethal genetic disease affecting Caucasians. Its incidence shows regional variations, but overall incidence in Caucasians is approximately 1 per 2,500 live births; it is inherited as an autosomal recessive trait. CF is also the most common cause of chronic lung disease and pancreatic insufficiency in patients under the age of 20.

Over the past decade the fundamental biochemical defect in CF has been identified. The gene has been cloned and up to 300 alleles have been discovered. The gene product is a protein called the cystic fibrosis transmembrane conductance regulator. This regulator, the main chloride transport system, is defective in individuals with CF. The regulator is synthesized within the epithelial cell, then transported to the apical cell membrane of the epithelial duct cells of the proximal pancreatic duct. Its main function is to act as a chloride channel activated through cAMP-mediated phosphorylation, thus allowing secretion of chloride ions into the pancreatic duct or to the outside of the body. In addition to cystic fibrosis transmembrane conductance regulator, these cells contain "Cl^-/HCO_3^- exchangers," which are responsible for bicarbonate secretion and are dependent on luminal chloride, which is supplied by cAMP-activated chloride channels. Thus, in CF, altered chloride secretion results in decreased bicarbonate production and ultimately failure to adequately hydrate and alkalinize the concentrated protein secretions of the acinar cells. This proteinaceous material becomes inspissated, resulting in ductal obstruction and ultimately acinar cell destruction, fibrosis and malabsorption. The decrease in bicarbonate secretion also results in failure to neutralize duodenal acid, thus leading to further malabsorption by decreasing lipase activity and altering the bioavailability of enteric-coated enzyme supplement.

The "classic" picture of a chronically malnourished child with a progressive lung disease and pancreatic dysfunction culminating in early death is an oversimplification. CF should now be regarded as a syndrome with a heterogeneous assortment of presentations involving variable degrees of organ dysfunction and damage. Pulmonary disease and its complications still dominate the clinical picture in most patients, and are the primary determinants of overall morbidity and mortality. However, as many as 20% of CF patients are not diagnosed until after the age of 15 because they have atypical presentations (e.g., recurrent sinusitis, nasal polyps, chronic bronchitis, recurrent abdominal pain, loose, foul-smelling stools, cirrhosis and infertility).

The advent of vigorous physiotherapy, more effective antibiotics, improved pancreatic extracts and continuing care in specialized CF clinics has resulted in a median survival of at least 18 years. Indeed, in many CF centers, half the patients survive 26 years, and up to 90% of patients may live more than 18 years after the diagnosis has been made. With such increased survival, gastrointestinal complications are becoming increasingly common.

TABLE 8. Nonpulmonary complications in adult CF patients

Steatorrhea, diarrhea
Impaired nutritional status
Meconium ileus equivalent, intussusception
Gallbladder disease
Multilobular biliary cirrhosis
Glucose intolerance, diabetes mellitus
Pancreatic exocrine dysfunction
Psychological problems

Abnormalities have been identified in glycoproteins, mucus secretions, circulating proteases and cell transport mechanisms. Liver and biliary tract disease may occur in individuals with CF. The incidence of biliary cirrhosis reaches 14% during the second decade of life in these who have pancreatic insufficiency. In these individuals subclinical hepatic involvement, manifested as biochemical or ultrasound abnormalities of the liver, are common. High losses of sodium and chloride through sweating during periods of heat in the summer months can lead to sodium depletion, dehydration, cardiovascular collapse and death. The abnormally thick mucus produced obstructs ductules and tubules, and results in distal organ damage, which leads to chronic obstructive lung disease, pancreatic insufficiency, hepatic fibrosis and intestinal obstruction. The mucosal and submucosal glands of the small intestine are dilated, with acidophilic concretions. Steatorrhea and enteral protein loss result from exocrine pancreatic failure, low duodenal pH and perhaps also impaired absorption of fatty acids. These patients require supplementation with fat-soluble vitamins A, D, E and K.

Abdominal pain is common in CF patients. It may be related to steatorrhea, constipation, meconium ileus equivalent, intussusception, cholelithiasis, duodenal ulcer or pancreatitis. In contrast to infants and children, adults are less affected by malabsorption, although close questioning may reveal that they experience cramps, flatulence and frequent, greasy, foul-smelling, bulky stools.

8.1 Complications

There are a number of nonpulmonary complications of CF in adults (Table 8). Most CF patients have height and weight levels that are less than the mean for their age and sex. Although during adulthood nutritional status declines progressively with advancing age, not all patients are malnourished at the time of diagnosis or in early adulthood. In early adulthood, some 10% of patients are above the 90th percentile, while others are even overweight.

There is no correlation between the patient's nutritional status and the severity of the steatorrhea or gastrointestinal symptoms, or age at diagnosis. The height and weight attained seem to correlate only with the severity of the pulmonary disease; those individuals with the least pancreatic insufficiency tend to have better preservation of pulmonary function.

Pancreatic insufficiency markedly overshadows the other complications of CF. In spite of the clinical impression of a voracious appetite, overall energy intake in the CF patient is usually inadequate. Maldigestion and malabsorption, along with the increased energy requirements associated with pulmonary disease, further compound the energy problem.

CF patients also show biochemical evidence of essential fatty acid deficiency. Improvement may be achieved with oral linoleic acid monoglyceride or with total parenteral nutrition. Essential fatty acid deficiency is associated with impaired intracellular oxygenation, decreased membrane fluidity and impaired transport mechanisms. It has not yet been established, however, what benefit will be derived by treating and preventing essential fatty acid deficiency.

In addition to the problems of essential fatty acid and energy deficiency, there is a third major problem in the nutrition of the CF patient: deficiency of fat-soluble vitamins. Even with a standard supplementation of vitamin A 4,000 IU/day, vitamin A levels, retinol binding protein levels and serum carotene may remain low. Approximately 25% of patients have evidence of vitamin D deficiency.

The management of pancreatic insufficiency in adults with cystic fibrosis is similar to the management of pancreatic insufficiency due to other conditions. About half of the adults with CF show some degree of glucose intolerance. Diabetes mellitus is easy to control with insulin; because glucagon levels are decreased, ketoacidosis is extremely uncommon. The presumed pathogenesis of the pancreatic islet cell dysfunction is fibrosis-induced islet cell disarray and strangulation.

Meconium ileus is seen in approximately 10% of neonates with CF and is primarily related to the secretion of abnormal mucinous (glycoprotein) material by the intestinal glands. Children, adolescents and adults have a counterpart, termed *meconium ileus equivalent*, that is characterized by recurrent episodes of intestinal obstruction. Typically, there is colicky abdominal pain, a palpable, indentable right lower quadrant mass and evidence of mechanical obstruction. Constipation is considered a milder form of this disorder, and must be differentiated from intussusception, which occurs in a small number of CF patients. There is usually a history of precipitating cause, such as immobilization, use of antidiarrheal agents, dietary indiscretions, or reduction or abrupt discontinuation of oral enzyme therapy.

The diagnosis of meconium ileus equivalent is suggested by the presentation. Plain abdominal radiographs may show an empty colon with bubbly granular material proximally, and ileal distention with air fluid levels. It is necessary to confirm the diagnosis by early Gastrografin® enema studies because of the high mortality of this condition and the need to rule out intussusception. Nasogastric suction and correction of electrolyte imbalance result in resolution of the obstruction in 80% of cases. Decompressive surgery may be necessary if medical management fails.

Pancreatitis is relatively uncommon in CF patients, but tends to occur in those patients (some 15%) whose pancreatic function is initially normal. The pathophysiology of the pancreatitis is presumably related to precipitation of abnormal secretions in the tubules, with subsequent damage. Biliary tract disease and alcohol are other possible causes of pancreatitis in these patients.

An increase in the incidence of duodenal ulcer might be expected in CF patients because of the loss of pancreatic bicarbonate buffer, but in fact duodenal ulcer is uncommon.

Patients with untreated pancreatic insufficiency commonly have profound malabsorption of bile acids in the terminal ileum and fecal losses of bile acids. This interrupts the normal enterohepatic circulation of bile acids. The etiology of bile acid wastage is unknown, but it probably relates to the presence of steatorrhea, with bile acid binding to undigested fat, fiber and other intraluminal contents. As a result of the excessive fecal bile acid loss, there is a decrease in the total bile acid pool; the bile becomes saturated with cholesterol. Up to 60% of adolescents and adults with CF have gallbladder abnormalities (e.g., cholelithiasis, nonvisualization, microgallbladder, and marginal filling defects or septation). There is a high incidence of both gallbladder abnormalities and abdominal pain in these patients, but there is not necessarily a cause–effect relationship between the cholelithiasis or gallbladder abnormalities and the clinical symptoms. The hazards of surgery must be weighed against the hazards of nonoperative intervention. The structure and function of the gallbladder may be evaluated by ultrasonography and oral cholecystography.

Treatment of pancreatic insufficiency with oral enzymes will decrease bile acid loss, thus correcting the lithogenic nature of the bile. However, the abnormal glycine:taurine ratio and the preponderance of cholic and chenodeoxycholic acid persist despite enzyme replacement. Ursodeoxycholic acid therapy remains experimental.

With increased age and survival, liver disease is becoming increasingly prevalent in CF patients. The most common hepatic lesion in CF is steatosis, secondary to decreased circulating lipoprotein levels and decreased hepatic triglyceride clearance. Other hepatic lesions seen include nonspecific portal changes, excessive biliary ductal mucus, mild ductal proliferation and focal biliary cirrhosis. A small number of these patients will develop multilobular biliary cirrhosis, the progression remaining clinically silent until portal hypertension supervenes with classical presentation of ascites, hyper-splenism or variceal bleeding. Hepatic decompensation and portal-systemic encephalopathy are extremely uncommon because of the relative hepatic parenchymal integrity and the overall focal nature of the pathology. The only clinical clue is the development of a hard, knobby liver, while liver biochemical tests remain relatively normal. The results of therapeutic portacaval anastomoses are encouraging, with no development of portal-systemic encephalopathy.

8.2 Diagnosis

Classical CF in infants and children is easy to diagnose. However, diagnosis of CF is more difficult in adults and in mild or atypical cases. The cornerstone of diagnosis is the quantitative pilocarpine iontophoresis sweat chloride test. This should be performed on two separate occasions, using a sample of 100 mg of sweat or more. Chloride levels that are continually above 60 mEq/L are virtually diagnostic. Such levels are not found with other chronic pulmonary or gastrointestinal tract diseases. Sweat chlorides may, however, occasionally reach 60 mEq/L or more in a variety of other disorders, including untreated adrenal insufficiency, hereditary nephrogenic diabetes insipidus, hypothyroidism and a variety of genetic mucopolysaccharide disorders.

Sweat chloride testing should be performed in infants and children with chronic pulmonary disease, meconium ileus, steatorrhea, rectal prolapse, failure to thrive, heat prostration or pansinusitis, and in siblings of affected individuals. In addition, children, adolescents and young adults should be screened if they have any type of chronic liver disease, long-standing gastrointestinal complaints, childhood or cryptogenic cirrhosis, aspermia or malabsorption.

8.3 Treatment

Pancreatic enzyme replacement is the mainstay of treatment in patients with CF who suffer from pancreatic insufficiency. Enteric-coated enzymes ideally should be used, since they are not inactivated by gastric acids. Ultimately these enzymes could be used in combination with an H_2 blocker. At least 30,000 USP units of lipase should be administered and taken together with food.

Hyperuricosuria may occur in these patients secondary to the large purine content in the enzyme preparation. This complication can be controlled by decreasing the dose of the enzymes.

OBJECTIVES

Pancreatitis
1. Classify pancreatitis on the basis of the severity of injury to the organ.
2. List four etiologies of pancreatitis.
3. Discuss at least five potential early complications of acute pancreatitis.
4. Discuss four potential adverse outcomes of chronic pancreatitis.
5. Describe the clinical presentation of a patient with acute pancreatitis.
6. Outline the appropriate diagnostic approach for a patient with acute pancreatitis, emphasizing the timing, interpretation and reliability of various studies.
7. Discuss the management of acute pancreatitis, including the specific medical management of the initial phase and indications for surgical intervention.
8. Discuss the criteria used to predict the prognosis for acute pancreatitis.

Pancreatic Pseudocysts
1. Discuss the mechanism of pseudocyst formation with respect to the role of the pancreatic duct.
2. List and discuss five symptoms and physical signs of pseudocysts.
3. Given a patient with a pancreatic mass suspected to be a pseudocyst, discuss the indications for and sequence of diagnostic methods, including laboratory, radiological and invasive studies.
4. Discuss the natural history of an untreated pancreatic pseudocyst.
5. Describe the medical and surgical treatment of a pancreatic pseudocyst.

Carcinoma of the Pancreas
1. List four pancreatic neoplasms; describe the pathology of each with reference to cell type and function.
2. Describe the symptoms and physical signs of pancreatic cancer on the basis of the location of the tumor in the pancreas.
3. Outline the diagnostic approach for pancreatic masses, including laboratory, radiological and invasive methods.
4. List the laboratory tests that would be expected to be abnormal in a patient with a large cancer of the head of the pancreas.
5. Describe the surgical treatment for pancreatic neoplasms.
6. On the basis of pathology and cell type, discuss the long-term prognosis for pancreatic cancers.

Skills
1. Demonstrate the ability to perform a complete abdominal examination of a patient with an upper abdominal mass.
2. Given a patient with suspected pancreatitis, interpret a plain abdominal x-ray and identify pertinent positive and negative findings.
3. Given a patient with obstructive jaundice and a mass in the head of the pancreas, accurately interpret the transhepatic cholangiogram.

13

The Biliary System

E.A. Shaffer

1. GALLSTONE DISEASE

Gallstones (cholelithiasis) are the most common cause of biliary tract disease in adults, afflicting 20–30 million persons in North America. Approximately one-fifth of men and one-third of women will eventually develop cholelithiasis. In Canada, calculous disease of the biliary tract is also a major health hazard, accounting for about 130,000 admissions to hospital and 80,000 cholecystectomies annually. Cholecystectomy is the second most common operation in Canada and the United States, where it is performed six to seven times as often as in the United Kingdom or France. Although the frequency of gallstone disease does vary between countries and regions, it is high in both Western Europe and North America (Table 1). The recent advent of laparoscopic cholecystectomy has further increased the use of surgery. Such variance suggests overuse of our health-care system, particularly as few (20%) ever become symptomatic.

1.1 Classification of Gallbladder and Bile Duct Stones
Two major types of gallstones exist (Table 2).

1. *Cholesterol stones* are hard, crystalline stones that contain more than 50% cholesterol plus varying amounts of protein and calcium salts. They predominate (>85%) in the Western world.
2. *Pigment stones* consist of several insoluble calcium salts that are not normal constituents of bile.

Pigment stones can be further divided into (a) black pigment stones, which consist of a linear polymer of bilirubin, large amounts of calcium salts such as

TABLE 1. Frequency of gallstone disease in different countries

Very common (30–70%)	Common (10–30%)	Intermediate (<10%)	Rare (≈0%)
American Indians	United States (whites)	United States (blacks)	East Africa
Sweden	Canada (whites)	Japan	Canada (Inuit)
Chile	Russia	Southeast Asia	Indonesia
Czechoslovakia	United Kingdom	Northern India	West Africa
United States (Hispanics)	Australia	Greece	Southern India
	Italy	Portugal	
	Germany		

TABLE 2. Classification of gallstones

| | Cholesterol | Pigment | |
		Black	Brown
Composition	Cholesterol	Pigment polymer Calcium salts (phosphates, carbonates)	Calcium bilirubinate Calcium soaps (palmitate, stearate)
Consistency	Crystalline	Hard	Soft, greasy
Location	Gallbladder +/– common duct	Gallbladder Bile ducts	Common duct
Radiodensity	Lucent (85%)	Opaque (50%)	Lucent (100%)
Clinical associations	Metabolic	Hemolysis Cirrhosis	Infection Inflammation Infestation

phosphates and carbonates (making 50% of these radiopaque) and only trace amounts of cholesterol; and (b) brown pigment stones, which are predominantly calcium bilirubinate (an amorphous polymer) and calcium salts of fatty acids – hence their earthy friability.

1.2 Basis for Gallstone Formation

1.2.1 CHOLESTEROL STONES
Cholesterol gallstones form in three stages (Figure 1).

1.2.1.1 Chemical stage
Bile secreted by the liver becomes supersaturated with cholesterol. Such abnormal bile contains an excess of cholesterol relative to the solubilizing

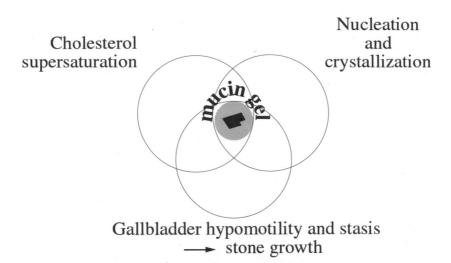

Cholesterol
supersaturation

Nucleation
and
crystallization

Gallbladder hypomotility and stasis
→ stone growth

FIGURE 1. Key events in cholesterol gallstone formation, expressed as a Venn diagram. Excess cholesterol secretion causes bile to become supersaturated. This results in the production of pronucleating proteins (including mucins), which precipitate cholesterol microcrystals (shown as a notched rhomboid). Excessive bile cholesterol also becomes incorporated into the sarcolemma of smooth muscle cells, lessening gallbladder contractility. The resultant stasis traps the microcrystals of cholesterol in a mucin gel, allowing them to agglomerate, attract other insoluble components of bile (such as bile pigment and calcium), become biliary sludge and grow into overt gallstones.

agents, bile salts and the phospholipid, lecithin. This stage may develop as early as puberty and is often associated with obesity. The liver, perhaps as a result of genetic programming, produces supersaturated bile by a decreased secretion of bile salts, an increased secretion of cholesterol, or both. Obesity is associated with excess cholesterol production. With ileal disease or loss, bile salt malabsorption breaks the enterohepatic circulation, decreasing its hepatic return and thus decreasing secretion. Reduced bile flux through the liver produces lithogenic bile with excess cholesterol.

1.2.1.2 *Physical stage*
The excess cholesterol precipitates out of solution as solid microcrystals. A nucleating factor (e.g., mucin) secreted in bile hastens this relatively rapid precipitation. Conversely, there may be a deficiency of antinucleating factors.

1.2.1.3 *Gallstone growth*
The cholesterol microcrystals precipitate from bile, are retained, aggregate

and grow into macroscopic stones. Retention occurs in the gallbladder because the epithelium in stone-formers secretes excess mucus (consisting of mucin, a glycoprotein). This mucus gel forms a colloidal shell that entraps cholesterol microcrystals, preventing them from being ejected from the gallbladder. Mucin also creates a scaffold for the addition of more crystals. A defect in the contractile function of the gallbladder smooth muscle results in failure to properly evacuate the solid material.

"Biliary sludge" consists of calcium bilirubinate, cholesterol microcrystals and mucin. On ultrasound, biliary sludge is echogenic material that layers but does not cast an acoustic shadow (unlike gallstones). Sludge develops in association with conditions causing gallbladder stasis, such as pregnancy or total parenteral nutrition. Though frequently asymptomatic and prone to disappear, sludge in the gallbladder can produce biliary-type pain and progress to overt gallstones or precipitate pancreatitis.

1.2.2 PIGMENT STONES

In North America, black pigment stones constitute about 15% of gallstones found at surgery (cholecystectomy). They are frequently associated with hemolysis or alcoholic cirrhosis (Table 3). The basis for their formation is excessive bilirubin excretion in bile. Brown pigment stones are associated with stagnation and infection (often from a stricture) or infestation (e.g., liver flukes) of the biliary tract. Such conditions predispose to chronic cholangitis and eventually cholangiocarcinoma. Infection and inflammation increase β-glucuronidase, an enzyme that deconjugates bilirubin; the resultant free bilirubin then polymerizes and complexes with calcium, forming calcium bilirubinate in the bile duct system.

1.3 Natural History of Gallstone Disease

Gallstones grow at about 1–2 mm per year over a 5- to 20-year period before symptoms develop. They frequently are clinically "silent," being incidentally detected on routine ultrasound performed for another purpose. Most patients (80%) with gallstones never develop symptoms. Problems, if they do occur, usually arise in the form of biliary pain during the first 5 to 10 years. Complications are from stones obstructing

1. the cystic duct, leading to cholecystitis: this begins as a chemical inflammation and later may become complicated by bacterial invasion; or
2. the common duct, causing biliary obstruction (cholestasis), sometimes accompanied by bacterial infection in the ductal system (cholangitis) (Figure 2).

TABLE 3.   Risk factors for gallstone formation

Factor	Pigment stone	Cholesterol stone
Demography		
Race	Asian	American Indian
Female sex	?	++
Age	+	++
Familial	Hemoglobinopathies	++
Diet	+	Obesity (high calorie)
		Weight reduction
		High animal fats
		Low fiber
Gallbladder stasis	+	++
	Total parenteral nutrition	Reduced meal frequency
		Vagotomy
		Pregnancy
Female sex hormones		
Parity/fertility	—	Early menarche
Oral contraceptives	—	+
Estrogens	—	+
Associated disease	Cirrhosis	Cystic fibrosis
	Hemolytic anemia	Ileal disease or loss
	Biliary infections	Diabetes mellitus
Drugs	Clofibrate	

++ = definite; + = probable; ? = questionable; — = unknown

1.4 Clinical Features

Biliary colic pain ensues when an obstructing stone causes sudden distention of the gallbladder and/or the biliary tract. "Colic" is a poor term, as biliary pain typically does not increase and decrease spasmodically. Rather, abdominal pain onsets suddenly, quickly becomes severe, remains steady for 1 to 3 hours and then gradually disappears over 30 to 90 minutes, leaving a vague ache. Its duration may be less than an hour, but is not as brief as 15 to 30 minutes. Although biliary-type pain can follow a fatty or spicy meal, such "fatty food intolerance" is not specific for biliary tract disease. Its location usually is the epigastrium or right upper quadrant. Mediated by splanchnic nerves, biliary pain may radiate like angina to the back, right scapula or shoulder tip, down the arm or into the neck. The pain may also be confined to the back. Analgesics are usually required for relief. Episodes of pain occur irregularly,

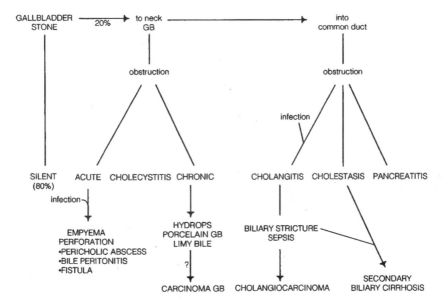

FIGURE 2. Potential complications of cholelithiasis. Migration of the stone in the gallbladder to impact in the neck of the gallbladder or the bile duct can cause obstruction and result in complications. Cystic duct obstruction results in cholecystitis. Chronic calculous cholecystitis may be associated with carcinoma of the gallbladder, but causality is unproven. Common duct obstruction leads to cholangitis, cholestatic jaundice and/or pancreatitis. Chronic cholestasis results in malabsorption. Stricture formation and recurrent cholangitis on occasion can lead to secondary biliary cirrhosis. Chronic duct obstruction and injury may lead to cholangiocarcinoma.

being separated by pain-free periods lasting from days to years. The severity of pain also varies. Being a visceral pain, biliary colic is not aggravated by movement but is deep-seated. The patient is usually restless and may exhibit vasomotor features such as sweating and pallor. Nausea and vomiting often accompany a severe attack. Fever and rigors are absent unless infection supervenes.

Findings consist of right upper quadrant or epigastric tenderness, perhaps with some guarding. During an attack or often soon after one, the pain disappears. There are no peritoneal signs. Often the examination is completely normal.

Laboratory tests are usually normal. In 10–20% of cases, there may be a slight elevation of serum bilirubin, alkaline phosphatase, aminotransferases (AST and ALT) or γ-glutamyl transpeptidase (GGT).

Between attacks the patient feels well. Liver biochemistry is normal. Over long periods the activity of the disease remains fairly constant. If having fre-

TABLE 4. Comparison of biliary colic to acute cholecystitis

	Biliary colic	Acute cholecystitis
Pain	Constant	Constant
Duration	Hours	Hours to days
Vomiting	Yes	Yes
Onset	Rapid	Variable
Jaundice	No	Later (20%)
Tenderness	RUQ	RUQ
Fever	No	Yes
Leukocytosis	Minimal	Marked
Resolution	Spontaneous	Spontaneous ($\approx$66%)

quent episodes of biliary pain, the patient will probably continue to experience this pattern.

Pain lasting more than 6 to 12 hours, especially if accompanied by persistent vomiting or fever, suggests another process such as cholecystitis or pancreatitis (Table 4). Conversely, abdominal pain and bloating relieved by defecation suggests the irritable bowel syndrome.

1.5 Diagnosis
Diagnosis of the gallstones (but not symptomatic disease) is radiological. Plain abdominal x-ray will identify the 10–15% with a high calcium content as radiopaque densities in the right upper quadrant. Ultrasonography is the most sensitive and specific method for detecting gallstones (appearing as echogenic objects that cast an acoustic shadow) or a thickened gallbladder wall (indicating inflammation). In suspected cases of acute cholecystitis, cholescintigraphy will assist the diagnosis by failing to visualize the gallbladder because of a stone obstructing the cystic duct.

1.6 Management

1.6.1 MEDICAL THERAPY

1.6.1.1 Expectant
Management should be expectant in asymptomatic adults with gallstones, as most will never develop problems. In minimally symptomatic patients without major complications or those unfit for or unwilling to undergo surgery, medical therapy offers techniques for dissolving, fragmenting or extracting stones.

1.6.1.2 *Dissolution*

1.6.1.2.1 *Bile acids*   Administered orally, bile acids can dissolve cholesterol gallstones. Two bile acids, chenodeoxycholic acid and ursodeoxycholic acid, work to reduce cholesterol saturation of bile. The stones must be radiolucent and hence presumably composed of cholesterol, and the gallbladder must function (i.e., fill and empty through a patent cystic duct) for the unsaturated bile to bathe the stones. Gallbladder function can be assessed by visualization on either oral cholecystography or cholescintigraphy, or by change in gall-bladder size on fatty meal ultrasonography. The reported success rate varies from 13–80% over one to two years. Gallstone size largely determines the success rate. Stones must be less than 1.5 cm in diameter. Small stones with a relatively great surface area have the best result. Ideal cases have tiny (<0.5 cm) gallstones that float on oral cholecystography (floating indicates a low calcium content); here, dissolution has a success rate greater than 80%. Large stones in obese individuals have less favorable results. Chenodeoxycholic acid (15 mg/kg/day), though cheaper, has significant side effects in terms of dose-related diarrhea and liver damage. Ursodeoxycholic acid (8–10 mg/kg/day) is therefore the drug of choice. It also reduces the frequency of episodes of biliary colic. Combination therapy with both agents at lower doses appears to be equally effective and safe. Ursodeoxycholic acid therapy can result in calcification of gallstones, negating dissolution; combination therapy avoids this. About 15–20% of patients are candidates for ursodeoxycholic acid therapy. Even after successful dissolution, 50% will experience gallstone recurrence, although most are asymptomatic. Prevention of gallstone formation is possible in those at high risk, such as obese people undergoing rapid weight loss either after gastric bypass surgery or while on a very restrictive caloric diet.

1.6.1.2.2 *Shock-wave lithotripsy*   The surface area of gallstones is so critical to successful dissolution that stone fragmentation has been undertaken with shock-wave lithotripsy. This is then followed by bile acid therapy to dissolve the residual fragments. Ultrasonic fragmentation has a low complication rate: 1% develop pancreatitis, 40% experience biliary pain. The cystic duct must be patent (i.e., the gallbladder must function as demonstrated by oral cholecys-tography or cholescintigraphy). Within a year, 60–80% will go on to success-ful clearance of debris from the gallbladder using oral bile acids to dissolve the remnants. Best results (up to 95% success) occur with a single gallstone 2 cm in diameter. Again, only about 20% of patients overall are eligible. Gall-stones can recur, although the rate is low at 15%.

1.6.2 *CHOLECYSTECTOMY*

1.6.2.1 *Open cholecystectomy*
The term "open" connotes the need for an incision to open the abdominal cavity for direct visualization and operation. In contrast, the laparoscopic technique uses endoscopy and tiny incisions. Cholecystectomy is the "gold standard" for treating gallstone disease. The operation is relatively safe, with mortality less than 0.5% when electively performed for biliary colic. Mortality reaches 3% for emergency surgery in acute cholecystitis or for common duct procedures, and is higher in the elderly.

1.6.2.2 *Laparoscopic cholecystectomy*
This technique views the abdominal contents through a laparoscope (with the peritoneal cavity insufflated with gas) and uses instruments inserted through three trocars in the abdominal wall to perform surgical manipulation. In 5% of cases the procedure must be converted to an open cholecystectomy because of technical problems. There is overwhelming enthusiasm for this procedure because it leaves the patient with less postoperative pain and with tiny scars, and it allows for an early discharge from hospital (about two days) and return to work. Selected cases can even be done on an outpatient basis. The disadvantage is a somewhat higher complication rate, particularly from common duct injury and retained common duct stones, plus the potential for overuse. Laparoscopic cholecystectomy is now the standard for elective surgery and for most cases of acute cholecystitis.

Surgery is indicated in those with significant symptoms (e.g., repeated visits to the emergency room for narcotic relief) or with complications. Prophylactic cholecystectomy is not warranted except for rare cases suspected of developing/harboring carcinoma of the gallbladder (e.g., very large stones >3 cm or a calcified gallbladder wall). It generally should not be done on asymptomatic people with gallstones.

2. CHOLECYSTITIS

2.1 Chronic Calculous Cholecystitis
Chronic inflammation of the gallbladder is the most common pathologic process in this organ. Some degree of chronic inflammation inevitably accompanies gallstones, but the stones will have developed first. Even transient obstruction of the cystic duct can produce biliary colic. Yet there is little correlation between the severity and frequency of such biliary episodes and the pathology found in the gallbladder. There may be only modest round cell

infiltration with marked symptoms. Conversely, symptoms may be minimal while gallbladder scarring is marked. Prolonged obstruction can lead to acute cholecystitis (Figure 2). Chronic inflammation may follow acute cholecystitis or evolve insidiously. The inflammatory process is chemical in origin.

2.1.1 CLINICAL FEATURES
The clinical features are those of either biliary colic or a previous episode of acute cholecystitis that has resolved, leaving the gallbladder chronically inflamed. The pain characteristically is a constant dull ache in the right hypochondrium and epigastrium, and sometimes also in the right shoulder or back. Nausea is frequent. There may be local tenderness in the right upper quadrant of the abdomen. Flatulence, fatty food intolerance and dyspepsia occur, but are equally frequent in patients without gallstone disease. Fever or leukocytosis suggests acute cholecystitis or another entity.

2.1.2 DIAGNOSIS
Diagnosis largely depends upon detecting gallstones by plain film of the abdomen (10–15% are calcified), ultrasound or oral cholecystogram. The latter two are more than 95% accurate. If the gallbladder is fibrotic and shrunken, visualization may be difficult. This is considered a positive finding, given the accuracy of these tests. Merely identifying calculi in the gallbladder confirms biliary tract disease but does not necessarily mean that gallstones were responsible for the symptoms. Nuclear medicine scanning helps. Cholescintigraphy normally demonstrates filling of a healthy gallbladder. Nonvisualization (with radioactivity present in the common duct and duodenum) in suspected cases of acute cholecystitis is diagnostic. The test is much less sensitive for chronic cholecystitis, in which the gallbladder commonly fills. If no filling occurs, then biliary tract disease is likely. Failure of the gallbladder to fill can occur with use of narcotics or after a prolonged fast.

2.1.3 MANAGEMENT
Once symptoms begin, they are likely to recur. Medical management depends upon gallstone size, gallbladder function and any co-morbid conditions (e.g., age, obesity, diabetes). Cholecystectomy provides definitive treatment, removing the stones and the gallbladder.

2.2 Acute Cholecystitis
Here the gallbladder becomes acutely inflamed. In most, a stone obstructs the cystic duct, resulting in a vicious cycle of increased secretion of fluid, causing distention, mucosal damage and the release of chemical mediators of the

inflammatory process. Inflammatory damage results from agents such as lyso-lecithin, derived from the hydrolysis of lecithin by phospholipase, and pros-taglandins whose synthesis increases. Any role that bile salts and regurgitated pancreatic enzymes may have is unclear. Bacterial infection is a late complication.

Obstruction of the cystic duct results in the gallbladder becoming distended with bile, an inflammatory exudate or even pus. The gallbladder wall can go on to necrosis and perforation. If resolution occurs, the mucosal surface heals and the wall becomes scarred, but the gallbladder may not function (i.e., fill with contrast agent) on oral cholecystography.

2.2.1 CLINICAL FEATURES

Acute cholecystitis onsets like biliary colic (Table 4). The abdominal pain rises to a plateau and remains constant. Its location is usually the right upper quadrant or epigastrium, sometimes radiating to the back or the right shoulder. There may be a previous history of biliary pain. Pain in acute cholecystitis, unlike biliary colic, persists for more than 6 to 12 hours. As the gallbladder becomes inflamed, the visceral pain is replaced by parietal pain that is aggravated by movement. Anorexia and vomiting are common. Fever is usually low-grade. If rigors occur, suspect bacterial invasion.

Abdominal examination characteristically shows tenderness in the right upper quadrant. During palpation of the right upper quadrant, a deep breath during the inspiratory effort worsens the pain; inspiration suddenly ceases (Murphy's sign). Severe cases exhibit peritoneal signs: guarding and local rebound tenderness. A reflex paralytic ileus may be present. Patients appear unwell and are reluctant to move with such parietal pain. An enlarged gallbladder is sometimes palpable, particularly with the first attack.

2.2.2 DIAGNOSIS

Jaundice with mild hyperbilirubinemia and elevated liver enzymes occurs in about 20% of cases, even in the absence of common duct stones. The higher the bilirubin level, the more likely is a common duct stone. High levels of aminotransferase and of amylase or lipase suggest a common duct stone. Leukocytosis is common. If the patient is febrile, blood cultures may be positive. Cholangitis suggests a common duct stone.

Diagnosis is best confirmed by ultrasound, which detects the stone(s) and a thickened gallbladder wall. In doing the procedure, the physician may elicit tenderness ultrasonographically when pressing over the gallbladder (the ultrasonographic Murphy's sign). A plain film may reveal calcification of the stone(s). Cholescintigraphy typically fails to visualize the gallbladder at one hour, a feature highly accurate for acute cholecystitis. Conversely, a normal scan filling the gallbladder virtually eliminates acute cholecystitis, but cannot detect gallstones. Late visualization (after one hour) sometimes occurs in chronic cholecystitis.

2.2.3 MANAGEMENT
Treatment is surgical and is performed in hospital. General measures include rehydration, observation, analgesia and antibiotics. In mild cases of acute cholecystitis that resolve, cholecystectomy can be delayed for up to six weeks. Because of the risk of recurrent cholecystitis, surgery should be performed early, once the patient has been stabilized during the current admission.

2.2.4 COMPLICATIONS
Acute cholecystitis normally resolves spontaneously, usually within three days. Inflammation may progress to necrosis, empyema or perforation in about one-third of cases. These complications will be heralded by (1) a continuation of the pain, along with tachycardia, fever, peritoneal signs and leukocytosis; (2) features of a secondary infection, such as empyema or cholangitis; or (3) a suspected perforation. Urgent surgery then becomes mandatory.

Empyema is suppurative cholecystitis with an intraluminal abscess (i.e., an inflamed gallbladder containing pus). It develops from continued obstruction of the cystic duct leading to secondary infection. The abdominal findings of acute cholecystitis are accompanied by systemic features of bacteremia, with a hectic fever and rigors. Treatment consists of antibiotics and surgery.

Perforation of the gallbladder occurs when unresolved inflammation leads to necrosis, often in the fundus, a part of the gallbladder that is relatively avascular. Gallstones also may erode through a gangrenous wall. If localized, the perforation spawns an abscess, clinically evident as a palpable, tender mass in the right upper quadrant. Free perforation with bile peritonitis is uncommon, fortunately, as the mortality reaches 30%. With perforation the gallbladder, if enlarged, suddenly disappears. The pain and temperature may also transiently resolve, only to be replaced by acute peritonitis. Both localized and free perforations demand surgical drainage of the abscess. Rupture into adjacent viscera (e.g., the small intestine) creates an internal biliary fistula. Large stones can produce a mechanical small intestine obstruction (*gallstone ileus*). Obstruction usually occurs at the terminal ileum, rarely at the duodenal bulb or the duodenojejunal junction. This is a rather common cause of distal small bowel obstruction in the elderly. Radiologic diagnosis comes from finding air in the biliary system, a small bowel obstruction and perhaps a calcified gallstone ectopically located. Urgent surgery with appropriate antibiotic coverage is imperative.

Hydrops of the gallbladder occurs when the inflammation subsides but the cystic duct remains obstructed. The lumen becomes distended with clear mucoid fluid. The hydropic gallbladder is evident as a right upper quadrant mass that is not tender. Treatment is cholecystectomy.

Limy bile occurs when prolonged gallbladder obstruction causes loss of the pigment material from bile and the residual calcium salts precipitate. The hydropic, obstructed gallbladder secretes calcium into the lumen. Calcium can also accumulate in the wall of the gallbladder, producing a *porcelain gallbladder*. The mural calcifications are easily identified on plain films of the abdomen. Although presumably there has been at least one episode of acute cholecystitis in the past, most patients with a porcelain gallbladder are asymptomatic. One-quarter will develop carcinoma of the gallbladder, making prophylactic cholecystectomy necessary.

2.3 Choledocholithiasis (Common Duct Stones)

Stones in the common duct are classified according to their site of origin: *primary stones* are formed in the bile ducts; *secondary stones* originate in the gallbladder and then migrate into the common duct. In North America, virtually all cholesterol stones and most pigment stones are considered secondary when the gallbladder is intact. Thus, more than 85% of patients with common duct stones also have stones in the gallbladder. Conversely, about 10% of patients undergoing cholecystectomy for chronic cholecystitis also have common duct stones. *Residual stones* are those missed at the time of cholecystectomy; *recurrent stones* develop in the ductal system more than three years after surgery. The composition of stones also varies with their site of origin. Stones are predominantly (approximately 80%) cholesterol when situated in the gallbladder and in the common duct. After cholecystectomy, the proportion of ductal stones that are pigment rises with time: most recurrent ones (more than three years after surgery) are pigment stones. These brown stones result from stasis (e.g., a postoperative stricture) and infection. Bacteria and inflamed tissues release β-glucuronidase, an enzyme that deconjugates bilirubin. The result is calcium bilirubinate, which polymerizes and precipitates along with calcium soaps. Biofilm, a glycoprotein produced by bacteria as its glycocalyx, then agglomerates this pigment material, leading to brown stones.

2.3.1 *CLINICAL FEATURES*

Common duct stones may be asymptomatic, but usually cause biliary colic, obstructive jaundice, cholangitis or pancreatitis (Figure 2). Biliary colic results from sudden obstruction of the common duct, which increases biliary pressure. The abdominal pain is steady, located in the right upper quadrant or epigastrium, and often bores through to the back.

Acute cholangitis results when duct obstruction leads to infection. Obstruction and ductal damage permit bacteria to regurgitate across the ductal epithelium into the hepatic venous blood, causing a bacteremia with chills and a spiking fever. The raised intrabiliary pressure also initiates abdominal pain. The classical "Charcot's triad" consists of jaundice, upper abdominal pain and a hectic fever. Jaundice results from the mechanical obstruction of the ducts plus a component of intrahepatic cholestasis due to sepsis (endotoxin, for example, impairs hepatic bile formation). Pain and fever are common, though jaundice is often less apparent on presentation. Most patients are toxic. There is abdominal tenderness and a large, tender liver (often containing liver abscesses). Hypotension, confusion and a septic picture predominate in critical cases.

2.3.2 DIAGNOSIS

Leukocytosis and abnormal liver biochemistry are common. Urine may be positive for bilirubin. Blood cultures reveal the causal microorganisms, which are usually enteric (e.g., E. coli or Klebsiella) in origin. Ultrasound will show dilated ducts and, in advanced cases, liver abscesses. Cholangiography (by endoscopy from below or via percutaneous transhepatic catheterization from above) is necessary to locate the site and cause of obstruction.

2.3.3 MANAGEMENT

The presence of cholangitis necessitates urgent decompression of the biliary system. In the past, laparotomy was the only recourse. Now, endoscopic surgery (using the ERCP procedure – endoscopic retrograde cholangiopancreatography) is routinely performed under antibiotic coverage (for enteric gram-negative organisms, enterococci and anaerobes). ERCP also allows sphincterotomy followed by extraction of the stone and, if needed, placement of a stent through a stricture. Large common duct stones may need fragmentation, either by mechanical means using a basket for crushing, or by energy delivered as shock or laser waves. This allows cholecystectomy to be done electively. Another option is open cholecystectomy with common duct exploration, removing the gallbladder and all stones.

Pancreatitis can result from gallstones impacting at the ampulla of Vater. Acute biliary pancreatitis does not differ clinically from other forms of acute pancreatitis. Biliary pancreatitis tends to be more commonly associated with jaundice and higher serum levels of bilirubin, alkaline phosphatase and aminotransferase than alcohol-induced pancreatitis, but there is significant overlap. Ultrasound should detect any gallstones and the inflamed pancreas. In patients unfit for surgery, early ERCP with papillotomy may be done, but its role as the definitive procedure is unproven. Most will come to elective cholecystectomy to prevent recurrent pancreatitis. Unlike alcoholic pancreatitis, gallstone-related disease does not progress to chronic pancreatitis.

3. NONCALCULOUS GALLBLADDER DISEASE

3.1 Congenital Anomalies

Congenital abnormalities of the gallbladder and biliary system result from embryonic maldevelopment and are most interesting for the surgeon attempting to identify biliary anatomy at cholecystectomy. Agenesis of the gallbladder is rare. Curiously, it is associated with common duct stones.

3.2 Acalculous Cholecystitis

3.2.1 *ACUTE ACALCULOUS CHOLECYSTITIS*

Inflammation of the gallbladder can occur in the absence of gallstones. Though uncommon in adults, acute acalculous cholecystitis may appear associated with AIDS, pregnancy, trauma, burns, sepsis or following major surgery. In young children, acute cholecystitis frequently occurs without gallstones and follows a febrile illness, although no definite infectious agent is identified. Biliary stagnation sometimes accompanied by sludge appears to be a factor. Impaired blood flow to the gallbladder, coagulation factors and prostaglandin may also have roles. Cytomegalovirus or Cryptosporidia can cause gangrenous cholecystitis in AIDS.

Clinical presentation is identical to that of acute cholecystitis, with pain, fever and abdominal tenderness in the right upper quadrant. These features are often obscured by the patient's underlying critical condition. Diagnosis is then revealed at laparotomy, but sometimes can be determined preoperatively by nonvisualization of the gallbladder on cholescintigraphy (although nonvisualization is less sensitive here because of the prolonged fast many are on) or by ultrasonographic evidence of a thickened gallbladder wall. Perforation, gangrene and empyema are all too frequent complications. The best treatment is prompt cholecystectomy. Prevention is possible in some patients on complete TPN (no oral intake) following major surgery, trauma or burns. Daily injections of cholecystokinin (CCK) can prevent sludge formation and its complication, cholecystitis.

3.2.2 *CHRONIC ACALCULOUS CHOLECYSTITIS*

Recurrent biliary-type pain in the absence of gallstones has been associated with rather modest inflammation. The basis is presumed to be a motility disorder, impaired gallbladder evacuation; hence the alternative term "biliary dyskinesia." Relief can follow cholecystectomy. Difficulties arise in attempting to make this diagnosis: the symptoms are often not clear-cut (sometimes having features of the irritable bowel syndrome or nonulcer dyspepsia), and there are no gallstones to detect. Abnormal gallbladder evacuation in response to CCK may be evident on cholescintigraphy. Sensitivity and specificity of these tests remain unclear. CCK infusion alone can reproduce the biliary pain, but the value of this provocative test is uncertain. The entity remains poorly defined. In some, the origin of the problem is dysfunction of the sphincter of Oddi. In many, it may represent one facet of the irritable bowel syndrome.

3.3 Cholecystoses

Cholesterolosis consists of deposits of cholesterol esters and triglycerides within the gallbladder wall. These submucosal deposits produce a fine yellow reticular pattern on a red background of mildly inflamed mucosa, providing an appearance like a strawberry: hence the term "strawberry gallbladder." Some of the cholesterol deposits protrude like polyps and can be detected on ultrasound. There is no well-defined symptom complex linked to this entity. Although frequently an incidental finding at post mortem, it is sometimes associated with vague dyspeptic complaints, the irritable bowel syndrome or recurrent right upper quadrant abdominal pain. The importance of CCK provocative tests to reproduce the pain or demonstrate reduced gallbladder emptying on quantitative cholescintigraphy in response to CCK is unclear.

Adenomyosis is characterized by hyperplasia of the gallbladder mucosa and by deep clefts. The meaning of any biliary-type symptoms is moot.

3.4 Postcholecystectomy Syndrome

Cholecystectomy relieves the symptoms of most, but definitely not all, patients with biliary calculi. The occasional patient will experience diarrhea following cholecystectomy, perhaps the result of unmasking a malabsorption of bile acids, which leads to a cholerrheic (bile acid–induced) diarrhea. Symptoms persist or recur in 5–50%, depending upon selection bias. Most often the original complaint was not true biliary pain, but rather reflux esophagitis, peptic ulcer disease or the irritable bowel syndrome. There may be recurrent biliary tract problems such as a biliary stricture, retained common duct stone or even pancreatic disease. In suspected cases, ERCP is indicated. Occasionally, narrowing (papillary stenosis) or increased tone in the sphincter of Oddi (sphincter dysfunction) will produce recurrent biliary-type pain, often with abnormal liver biochemistry tests or increased serum amylase. Nuclear medicine scanning (cholescintigraphy) and sphincter of Oddi pressure measurements (manometry) provide diagnostic clues. Endoscopic sphincterotomy relieves pain in selected patients.

3.5 Neoplasms of the Gallbladder

Carcinoma of the gallbladder is fortunately uncommon, as its prognosis is extremely poor. Adenocarcinoma is generally cured only when incidentally discovered at cholecystectomy for cholelithiasis. Gallstones are present in most (75%) cases, probably as innocent bystanders rather than as causal agents (Figure 2). Any risk is too low to advocate prophylactic cholecystectomy in the many people with asymptomatic gallstones. A porcelain gallbladder with calcifications in the wall predisposes to adenocarcinoma and calls for cholecystectomy. Large gallstones (>3 cm) are also a risk factor for carcinoma.

The clinical features of gallbladder carcinoma consist of pain, a hard mass in the right epigastrium, jaundice, pruritus and weight loss. Ultrasound and CT scan help define the mass and metastases. Prognosis is grim, as it is common for the cancer to spread. The five-year survival is less than 5%. Therapy is palliative; most are not resectable unless removed incidentally at the time of cholecystectomy.

Benign tumors of the gallbladder are uncommon. Adenomas are asymptomatic, being detected on ultrasound or found incidentally at surgery. Small masses in the wall of the gallbladder, however, are relatively common findings on ultrasound; when multiple they usually represent cholesterol polyps or adherent gallstones. Polypoidal masses warrant a repeat ultrasound in six months. If these are larger than 1 cm, surgery is necessary to exclude a carcinoma.

4. DISEASES OF THE BILE DUCTS

4.1 Congenital

Caroli's disease (congenital intrahepatic biliary dilation) is a rare condition in which saccular, dilated segments of the intrahepatic bile ducts lead to stone formation, recurrent cholangitis and hepatic abscesses with sepsis. Episodes of abdominal pain, fever and jaundice may onset at any age, most commonly in childhood or young adult life.

Cholangiography reveals the irregularly dilated segments of the intrahepatic bile ducts that connect with the main ducts. The common duct is normal. Endoscopy (or surgery) can remove some stones but does little for the process that affects small bile ducts in the liver. If involvement is unilateral, partial hepatectomy can be curative. Otherwise, management is conservative, using antibiotics for infectious complications of the duct system. These recurrent episodes of cholangitis sometimes progress to secondary biliary cirrhosis, portal hypertension and eventually cholangiocarcinoma. Partial hepatectomy of an affected segment sometimes is feasible. Liver transplantation may become necessary in other cases.

Congenital hepatic fibrosis frequently accompanies Caroli's disease (perhaps reflecting a developmental defect of the small interlobular ducts). It clinically presents as portal hypertension with esophageal varices in children. Liver biopsy is diagnostic, revealing broad bands of fibrous tissue entrapping bile ducts but no cirrhosis (i.e., no regeneration). Liver transplantation may be necessary in complicated cases.

Choledochal cyst is a congenital dilation of a portion of the common bile duct, which may form a diverticulum in the intraduodenal segment. This congenital cystic anomaly can be associated with Caroli's disease: both represent a spectrum of defective budding and cannulation from the primitive foregut. Presentation may be as cholestasis in infants, or intermittent jaundice, pain and fever (cholangitis) later in young adults. Complications include chronic obstruction leading to biliary cirrhosis and the development of ductal carcinoma. Diagnosis is provided by ultrasound or CT scan and verified by endoscopic cholangiography. Surgery involves excising the cyst and re-establishing biliary drainage with a biliary-enteric anastomosis.

Alagille's syndrome is a marked reduction in intrahepatic (actually interlobular) bile ducts. Although it is believed to be congenital, being inherited in an autosomal dominant pattern, presentation may be as a neonatal jaundice or as cholestasis in older children. There are associated triangular facies, cardiovascular anomalies (e.g., pulmonary artery stenosis) and vertebral body abnormalities. Outcome is variable, depending upon the attendant anomalies and the severity of the liver disease.

Biliary atresia is a common cause of neonatal cholestatic jaundice. Although congenital (appearing at birth), it is not inherited. Complete absence of the extrahepatic bile ducts reflects either an arrest in remodeling of the ductal plate in utero or, more probably, an inflammatory destruction of the formed bile ducts during the postpartum period. The latter process is evident by an inflammatory infiltrate in the portal tracts and, in some, features of neonatal hepatitis, perhaps initiated by a viral infection. Large duct obstruction then leads to small duct injury within the liver and hence secondary biliary cirrhosis. Severe cholestasis develops in the neonatal period. The stools are pale and the urine is dark and devoid of urobilinogen. Cholestatic features predominate, with the development of steatorrhea, skin xanthoma, bone disease and failure to thrive. Surgery is usually necessary to confirm the diagnosis and attempt some form of biliary drainage. In some, existence of a patent hepatic duct or dilated hilar ducts potentially allows correction of the obstruction by anastomosis to the small intestine (e.g., a Roux-en-Y choledochojejunostomy). Much more common is an absence of patent ducts; dense fibrous tissue encases the perihilar area and precludes conventional surgery. Such obliteration of the proximal extrahepatic biliary system requires the Kasai procedure. A conduit for biliary drainage is fashioned by resecting the fibrous remnant of the biliary tree and anastomosing the porta hepatis to a Roux-en-Y loop of jejunum. With either surgery, most children eventually develop chronic cholangitis, hepatic fibrosis/cirrhosis and portal hypertension. When the child is larger, hepatic transplantation dramatically improves the prognosis.

4.2 Inflammatory

4.2.1 *CHOLANGITIS*
Cholangitis is any inflammatory process involving the bile ducts, but common usage implies a bacterial infection, usually above an obstructive site. The presence of bacteria in the biliary tree plus increased pressure within the system results in severe clinical features of cholangitis (*suppurative cholangitis*). Any condition producing bile duct obstruction is liable to cause bacterial infection of bile. Most commonly, this takes the form of a common duct stone (Section 2.3), a benign biliary stricture (trauma from biliary surgery, ischemia following liver transplantation or sclerosing cholangitis), stasis in a congenital biliary cyst (Section 4.1), a parasite residing in the ducts (Clonorchis sinensis, Opisthorchis viverrini or Fasciola hepatica), an occluded biliary stent or extrinsic compression from a diseased papilla or pancreas. A less likely cause of infection is neoplastic obstruction. The difference relates to the high-grade, fixed obstruction of neoplasms versus the intermittent blockage with a stone or an inflammatory stricture. Such intermittent blockage allows retrograde ascent of bacteria; the stone may act as a nidus for infection. The bacteria are commonly thought to ascend the biliary tree (hence the term "ascending cholangitis"), but may enter from above via the portal vein or from periductular lymphatics.

In acute bacterial cholangitis, particularly if severe, the classical Charcot's triad of intermittent fever and chills, jaundice and abdominal pain may be followed by septic shock. Most cases are less severe and life-threatening; jaundice may be absent. Mild cases may respond to antibiotics and conservative measures. Investigation and decompression of the biliary system are mandatory in all patients, whether by ERCP, percutaneous transhepatic cholangiography or surgery.

4.2.2 *SCLEROSING CHOLANGITIS*
Primary sclerosing cholangitis is a chronic cholestatic syndrome of unknown etiology characterized by progressive inflammation of the intra- and extrahepatic bile ducts. The entity may appear either alone or in association with inflammatory bowel disease, particularly ulcerative colitis. Primary sclerosing cholangitis may precede inflammatory bowel disease and runs a separate course, not being cured by colectomy. The patchy scarring (sclerosis) leads to

fibrotic narrowing and eventually obliteration of the bile ducts. Like other organs, the biliary tract exhibits a limited number of responses to injury: here it responds with diffuse strictures and segmental dilations. Periductal inflammation and fibrosis in the portal areas, termed "pericholangitis," probably represents the intrahepatic extension of this process. The basis may be an infectious agent, an enterohepatic toxin or an immunological attack on the biliary epithelium.

Diffuse stricturing also occurs in *secondary sclerosing cholangitis*, which may complicate a biliary obstruction from a common duct stone, biliary stricture or cholangiocarcinoma, or some AIDS-related infections.

The presentation in primary sclerosing cholangitis is insidious in most cases, with fatigue, pruritus or just an elevated alkaline phosphatase level. In others, acute cholangitis develops with obstructive jaundice, pruritus, abdominal pain and fever. Biliary stagnation leads to pigment stones. Eventually, secondary biliary cirrhosis supervenes with portal hypertension, pronounced cholestasis and progressive liver failure. Antimitochondrial antibody is negative. ERCP provides the diagnosis, showing thickened bile ducts with narrowed, beaded lumens.

Therapeutic trials of corticosteroids and immunosuppressive agents (for the presumed immunologically mediated inflammatory process), penicillamine (to mobilize copper, because this potentially toxic material accumulates in cholestasis) and proctocolectomy in patients with inflammatory bowel disease have all failed. As some patients may be asymptomatic for a decade, only careful observation is warranted early on. Recurrent bacterial cholangitis requires antibiotics. Predominantly large-duct strictures respond to endoscopic or transhepatic dilation and stent placement. Evaluation of ursodeoxycholic acid (which helps the pruritus but may not change the disease process), cyclosporine, methotrexate and colchicine awaits good clinical trials. Some 10–15% of patients develop cholangiocarcinoma, creating a diagnostic challenge. Primary sclerosing cholangitis is a frequent indication for liver transplantation that has a good outcome.

4.3 Neoplasia (Including Cholangiocarcinoma)
Benign tumors (adenomas, papillomas, cystadenomas) are rare causes of mechanical biliary obstruction.

Adenocarcinoma, the most common malignancy, is uncommon in the Western world. Predisposing factors are chronic parasitic infestations of the biliary tract (e.g., a liver fluke, such as Clonorchis sinensis or Opisthorchis viverrini), congenital ectatic lesions (Caroli's disease, choledochal cyst) and primary sclerosing cholangitis.

Jaundice and pruritus are common, but the presentation is varied. Cholestasis and weight loss eventually develop. There may be a deep-seated, vague pain localized in the right upper quadrant of the abdomen, in contrast to the severe pain of biliary colic and the septic picture of cholangitis. Indeed, cholangitis is not a feature if no biliary manipulations have been performed, such as an ERCP-placed stent. Hepatomegaly is frequent. A distended, nontender gallbladder may occasionally be palpated, feeling like a small rubber ball, if the common duct is obstructed below the entry of the cystic duct ("Courvoisier's sign"). Obstruction produces dilation of the biliary tree that can be readily detected on ultrasound or CT scan. Cholangiography, usually by ERCP, should reveal the diagnosis. This slow-growing tumor presents late. The terminal event is usually hepatocellular failure. Palliation using biliary stents placed across strictures sometimes helps. Occasionally, a distal common duct lesion is amenable to curative surgery. Transplantation does not provide a good outcome.

OBJECTIVES

1. Recognize the normal anatomy of the biliary tree.
2. Discuss the mechanisms for the stimulation of bile secretion and the hormonal mediators of this response.
3. Describe the physicochemical characteristics of normal bile, its production and the physiologic mechanism of bile salt reabsorption.

Acute and Chronic Gallbladder Disease, Carcinomas of the Biliary Tract

1. Identify the common types of gallstones and describe the pathophysiology involved in their formation.
2. Recognize the mechanisms by which risk factors predispose to gallstone formation.
3. List the tests commonly used in the diagnosis of calculous biliary tract disease. Describe the indications for, limitations of and potential complications of each.
4. Describe the probable natural history of a young patient with asymptomatic gallstones.
5. Know the complications that can occur from biliary calculi and describe the history, physical examination and laboratory findings for each.
6. Outline the management of a patient with acute cholecystitis.
7. Describe the symptoms and signs of choledocholithiasis; construct the management of this problem.
8. Outline a diagnostic and management plan for a patient with acute right upper quadrant pain.

9. Describe the diagnostic evaluation and management of a patient with fever, chills and jaundice.
10. Describe the following:
    a. Murphy's sign
    b. Courvoisier's sign
    c. Gallstone ileus
11. Contrast carcinomas of the gallbladder, bile duct and ampulla of Vater with regard to presenting features and survival.

Diagnostic Studies in Biliary Tract Disease
1. Contrast the liver enzyme abnormalities in cholestasis and viral hepatitis.
2. Identify the most common bacteria found in cholecystitis and cholangitis.
3. Describe the indications for and risks of oral cholecystogram, transhepatic cholangiogram and ERCP.
4. Accurately interpret an abnormal ultrasonogram of the gallbladder, oral cholecystogram, transhepatic cholangiogram and ERCP.

Skills
1. Given a patient with acute cholecystitis, demonstrate the right upper quadrant physical findings that indicate this diagnosis.

14
The Liver

L.J. Worobetz (ed.), R.J. Hilsden, E.A. Shaffer,
J.B. Simon, P. Paré, V.G. Bain, M. Ma, F. Wong,
L. Blendis, P. Adams, J. Heathcote, S.S. Lee,
L.B. Lilly, A.W. Hemming and G.A. Levy

1. LIVER STRUCTURE AND FUNCTION / R.J. Hilsden and E.A. Shaffer

1.1 Liver Morphology

The liver is the largest and most metabolically complex organ in humans. Anatomically, it consists of two main lobes, right and left, separated by the round and falciform ligaments, plus two smaller lobes, the caudate lobe located on the posterior surface and the quadrate lobe on the inferior surface. The liver is functionally divided into eight segments based on the distribution of the portal and hepatic veins. Each segment receives a pedicle of the portal vein and is an independent functional unit. The caudate lobe (segment 1) differs from other segments in that it receives blood from both the right and left branches of the portal vein and drains directly into the inferior vena cava.

At a microscopic level, the liver consists of myriads of individual functional units, traditionally called lobules. Each lobule is bounded by four to five portal triads (supplied from the portal vein and hepatic artery) and has a central terminal hepatic venule (central vein). A more physiologically sound concept is the unit termed the acinus. At the center is the portal triad, while the terminal hepatic venules are at the periphery. The acinus is divided into three zones based upon the distance from the feeding vessels (Figure 1).

The liver receives a dual blood supply. The portal vein drains the splanchnic circulation and provides 75% of the total blood flow (1,500 mL/min). The hepatic artery provides the remaining 25%. Small branches of each blood vessel (the terminal portal venule and the terminal hepatic arteriole) enter the acinus at the portal triad (zone 1). Blood then flows through sinusoids between plates of hepatocytes toward the terminal hepatic venule (zone 3), where blood from several adjacent acini merges. The sinusoidal lining is fenestrated;

FIGURE 1. Normal liver. This liver biopsy shows the orderly arrangement of the liver cell plates, central veins (arrowheads) and portal tracts (P). A hepatic lobule is outlined. (Retic. stain, original magnification × 370)

this porosity allows nutrients to gain access to the intervening space of Disse and from it to the hepatocyte. The terminal hepatic venules coalesce to form the hepatic vein, which carries all efferent blood to the inferior vena cava. A rich supply of lymphatic vessels also drains the liver.

Hepatocytes make up the bulk of the organ. They are arranged in plates that radiate out from each portal triad toward adjacent central veins. Those hepatocytes surrounding the portal tract form an interface between the connective tissues of the portal tract and the hepatic parenchyma, termed the limiting plate.

The bile canaliculus is formed by grooves on the contact surface of adjacent liver cells. Bile forms in these canaliculi and progressively flows into ductules, interlobular bile ducts and then larger hepatic ducts. Outside the porta hepatis, the hepatic duct joins the cystic duct from the gallbladder to form the common bile duct, which drains into the duodenum.

Sinusoidal lining cells comprise at least four distinct populations: endothelial cells, Kupffer's cells, perisinusoidal fat-storing cells and pit cells. Endothelial cells differ from the vascular endothelium elsewhere in the body in that they lack a basement membrane and contain numerous fenestrae that permit hepatocytes to have ready access to nutrients and macromolecules in plasma. Endothelial cells are also responsible for endocytosis of molecules and particles, and play a role in lipoprotein metabolism.

Spindle-shaped Kupffer's cells are tissue macrophages. They form an important part of the body's reticuloendothelial system. Their major functions include phagocytosis of foreign particles, removal of endotoxins and other noxious substances, and modulation of the immune response through the release of mediators and cytotoxic agents.

Perisinusoidal fat-storing cells (Ito cells) store vitamin A. They transform into fibroblasts in response to hepatic injury, contributing to hepatic fibrosis.

Pit cells, the least common sinusoidal lining cells, are large, granular lymphocytes, which function as natural killer cells.

The extracellular matrix of the liver includes its reticulin framework and several molecular forms of collagen, laminin, fibronectin and other extracellular glycoproteins.

1.2 Hepatobiliary Function

1.2.1 *METABOLISM*
The liver plays a central role in carbohydrate, protein and fat metabolism. It stabilizes glucose level by taking up and storing glucose as glycogen (glycogenesis), breaking this down to glucose (glycogenolysis) when needed, and forming glucose from noncarbohydrate sources such as amino acids (gluconeogenesis). Hypoglycemia occurs only late in the course of severe liver disease because the liver has a large functional reserve; glucose homeostasis can be maintained with only 20% of the liver functioning. The liver synthesizes the majority of proteins that circulate in the plasma, including albumin and most of the globulins other than gamma globulins. Albumin provides most of the oncotic pressure of plasma and is a carrier for drugs and endogenous hydrophobic compounds such as unconjugated bilirubin. Globulins include the coagulation factors: fibrinogen, prothrombin (factor II), and factors V, VII, IX and X. Factors II, VII, IX and X are vitamin K–dependent. Availability of vitamin K, a fat-soluble vitamin, requires adequate bile salts for the vitamin's absorption. These factors decrease with fat malabsorption (as with prolonged cholestasis) and with the reduced synthetic function of hepatocellular disease. (In hepatocellular diseases, deficiency of these coagulation factors is not corrected by parenteral vitamin K administration.) The liver is also the site of most amino acid interconversions and catabolism. Amino acids are catabolized to urea. During this process ammonia, a product of nitrogen metabolism and a possible neurotoxin, is utilized and therefore detoxified. Fatty acids are

taken up by the liver and esterified to triglycerides. The liver packages triglycerides with cholesterol, phospholipids and an apoprotein into a lipoprotein. The lipoprotein enters blood for utilization or storage in adipocytes. Most cholesterol synthesis takes place in the liver. Bile salts are the major product of cholesterol catabolism.

1.2.2 DRUG DISPOSITION
The liver's rich enzyme system allows the metabolism of many drugs, including alcohol. The liver detoxifies noxious substances arriving from the splanchnic circulation, preventing them from entering the systemic circulation. This particularly makes the liver susceptible to drug-induced injury. The liver converts some lipophilic compounds into more water-soluble agents, which are then easily excreted in the urine or bile. Others are metabolized to less active agents.

1.2.3 BILE FORMATION
Bile provides the main excretory pathway for toxic metabolites, cholesterol and lipid waste products. Bile is also necessary for the efficient digestion and absorption of dietary fats. Bile salts are synthesized exclusively in the liver from cholesterol and are the driving force behind bile formation. After excretion by the liver, bile is stored in the gallbladder during periods of fasting.

Cholecystokinin (CCK), released from the small intestine during digestion by fatty acids and amino acids, stimulates gallbladder evacuation. When the bile reaches the duodenum it aids in fat absorption by acting as a biologic detergent. Bile salts are reabsorbed predominantly in the ileum and return to the liver via the portal vein to be taken up and secreted once again. This is the enterohepatic circulation (intestine-to-liver).

2. APPROACH TO THE PATIENT WITH LIVER DISEASE / J.B. Simon

Because of the liver's complexity, liver disease is often reflected by abnormalities of different hepatic "systems" – i.e., hepatocytes (hepatocellular dysfunction), the biliary excretory apparatus (cholestasis) and the vascular system (portal hypertension). In addition, the liver often is involved in systemic disease by virtue of its rich metabolic and reticuloendothelial activity and its large blood supply.

Patterns of disproportionate involvement often provide an important clue to the underlying disorder. For example, viral hepatitis characteristically produces predominant hepatocellular dysfunction; primary biliary cirrhosis, predominant cholestasis; cryptogenic cirrhosis, predominant portal hypertension;

TABLE 1.   Major clinical manifestations of liver disease (asterisk implies chronicity)

Systemic
  Anorexia, malaise, fatigue
  Fever
  *General deterioration, weight loss, "cirrhotic habitus"
  Cholestasis: pruritus, *xanthelasma/xanthomas, *malabsorption problems

Jaundice

Hepatomegaly ± pain

Portal hypertension

Fluid derangements
  *Ascites ± edema
  Electrolyte disturbances
  Functional renal failure ("hepatorenal syndrome")

Hepatic encephalopathy (portal-systemic encephalopathy)

*Cutaneous and endocrine changes
  Spider nevi, palmar erythema, Dupuytren's contractures
  Gynecomastia, testicular atrophy, impotence
  Amenorrhea
  Parotid enlargement

Coagulopathy
  Hypoprothrombinemia
  Thrombocytopenia
  Dysfibrinogenemia

Circulatory changes
  Hyperdynamic circulation
  *Arterial desaturation, clubbing

---

and alcoholic liver disease, variably predominant dysfunction of any of these three systems. The clinician can usually take advantage of these general patterns to help establish a diagnosis, though overlap and exceptions are frequent.

2.1 Clinical Features of Liver Disease

Table 1 lists the most important clinical manifestations of liver disease. Most can be seen in both acute and chronic hepatic disorders; features marked by an asterisk usually denote chronicity. This distinction can be of diagnostic value at the bedside. For example, a clinical diagnosis of acute hepatitis should be reconsidered if physical examination reveals spider nevi and palmar erythema.

2.1.1 *SYSTEMIC FEATURES*

Nondescript anorexia, malaise and fatigue are common manifestations of both acute and chronic liver disease. An abrupt onset often reflects acute viral or drug-induced hepatitis, whereas insidious development typifies alcoholic liver disease, chronic active hepatitis and other chronic disorders.

Fever is another nonspecific feature of some liver conditions, especially the prodromal phase of acute viral hepatitis, severe alcoholic hepatitis and (sometimes) malignancy. However, frank rigors and chills are rare in these conditions, and instead strongly suggest acute cholangitis, usually secondary to common duct stone.

Patients with advanced chronic liver disease, especially alcoholic cirrhosis, often develop deterioration of general health, weight loss and a characteristic "cirrhotic habitus" in which wasted extremities and shoulder girdle contrast with a bloated belly from ascites.

Generalized pruritus is a hallmark of cholestatic disorders, especially if chronic. When cholestasis is prolonged – for example, in primary biliary cirrhosis – this may be accompanied by cutaneous lipid deposits (xanthelasma, xanthomas) and by features of malabsorption.

2.1.2 *JAUNDICE*

This cardinal feature of liver disease indicates hyperbilirubinemia. Bilirubin arises primarily from the physiologic breakdown of senescent red blood cells, with a minor contribution from other heme sources. It is not water-soluble and is therefore transported in plasma loosely attached to albumin. This form of the pigment is called *unconjugated* or *indirect-reacting bilirubin*. The molecule is then taken up by hepatocytes and conjugated in microsomes with glucuronic acid to form bilirubin diglucuronide; the reaction is catalyzed by the enzyme glucuronyl transferase. Other minor conjugates are also formed; their clinical significance is unknown.

Transformed bilirubin is then secreted into the bile canaliculus along with the other constituents of bile. A small amount normally enters the blood as *conjugated* or *direct-reacting bilirubin*. In contrast to unconjugated bilirubin, this form of the pigment is water-soluble and is therefore excreted into urine, though a portion becomes tightly bound to circulating albumin (the so-called albumin-bound fraction of conjugated bilirubin).

After reaching the gut through the biliary tree, bilirubin is transformed by intestinal bacteria into pigmented breakdown products collectively called urobilinogen; these impart the normal brown color to stool. With impairment of biliary secretion (cholestasis) the stools are therefore often pale, but this is a relatively crude and unreliable diagnostic feature. Some urobilinogen is absorbed from the intestine and recycled through the liver (the enterohepatic circulation), with a portion escaping into the urine.

Various derangements in the above metabolic steps can result in jaundice. An increased bilirubin load from hemolysis may overwhelm the liver's conjugating capacity, resulting in unconjugated hyperbilirubinemia. This is invariably mild, however, unless there is also concomitant hepatic dysfunction. Isolated unconjugated hyperbilirubinemia also occurs in some specific defects of bilirubin metabolism, though these are rare except for Gilbert's syndrome (see Section 3 below).

In the vast majority of cases, jaundice is due to either hepatocellular disease or biliary obstruction. Both produce multiple defects in the pathway of bilirubin metabolism, including impaired hepatocellular uptake and transport, defective conjugation, decreased canalicular secretion, and "leakage" of conjugated bilirubin into the circulation. The resultant hyperbilirubinemia is a mixture of unconjugated and conjugated pigment; usually the latter predominates, but the exact proportion varies widely and has no specific diagnostic value.

Clinically, mild jaundice can usually be detected when serum bilirubin is about twice the upper limit of normal, and is best diagnosed by inspecting the patient's sclerae in natural daylight. More advanced cases are often apparent at a glance. Patients with severe long-standing jaundice sometimes have a generalized muddy-yellow appearance.

2.1.3 HEPATOMEGALY WITH OR WITHOUT PAIN
A readily palpable liver is not necessarily enlarged, for it may merely be low-lying – as, for example, in emphysema. Thus the upper border should be percussed when the edge is palpable.

The "quality" or feel of the liver is at least as important diagnostically as its size. For example, the liver usually retains its rubbery, relatively sharp edge when enlargement is due to fatty infiltration, acute hepatitis or passive congestion, whereas chronic fibrosis typically produces a blunt, indurated edge. Individual cirrhotic nodules are rarely detectable clinically. Palpable lumpiness instead favors malignant infiltration. It is important to remember that major liver disease – including a high proportion of cirrhosis – may not be associated with hepatomegaly.

Abdominal pain is common in biliary or pancreatic disease that might secondarily affect the liver – for example, common duct stone or pancreatic carcinoma – but pain is relatively uncommon in primary hepatic disorders. True hepatic pain is usually due to distention of the liver capsule, typically felt as a deep-seated right upper quadrant ache. This is often accompanied by hepatic tenderness on physical examination, best elicited by compression of the rib cage or fist percussion over the liver. The commonest causes are acute hepatitis, passive congestion from cardiac failure, and malignancy. Pain from malignancy is sometimes pleuritic in character and may be accompanied by a hepatic friction rub or bruit on auscultation. Some individuals claim some discomfort when the liver edge is palpated; this has no special significance and should not be interpreted as hepatic tenderness.

2.1.4 *CUTANEOUS AND ENDOCRINE CHANGES*

These findings as listed in Table 1 are important clues to chronic liver disease. Their pathogenesis is still poorly understood, but altered metabolism of sex hormones by the diseased liver appears important. The abnormalities may be seen in any chronic hepatic disorder, but are especially prevalent in alcoholic liver disease; this probably relates in part to a direct toxic effect of ethanol on gonadal function.

2.1.5 *COAGULATION DISTURBANCES*

The liver synthesizes most clotting factors, including vitamin K–dependent factors II, VII, IX and X. Severe hepatocellular dysfunction is therefore often accompanied by an enhanced bruising and bleeding tendency and by abnormal coagulation studies, particularly an increased INR/prothrombin time. Malabsorption of the fat-soluble vitamin K in prolonged cholestasis can also produce an abnormal INR/prothrombin time.

Thrombocytopenia is common in patients with cirrhosis, primarily as a result of portal hypertension with hypersplenism, but usually the platelet counts are not low enough to induce clinical bleeding. In patients with alcoholic liver disease, thrombocytopenia may also be due to direct marrow suppression by alcohol and/or nutritional folate deficiency.

Dysfibrinogenemia also sometimes contributes to coagulopathy in cases of severe hepatic dysfunction.

2.1.6 *CIRCULATORY CHANGES*

A hyperdynamic circulation and relatively low blood pressure are sometimes seen in patients with severe liver disease, especially fulminant hepatitis and advanced cirrhosis. The mechanism may relate to the accumulation of vasoactive agents normally cleared by the liver, which reduce tone. Occasional patients with cirrhosis develop intrapulmonary A–V shunting, with resultant arterial desaturation and (rarely) clubbing (hepatopulmonary syndrome).

A number of topics will be discussed in later sections, including portal hypertension (Section 11), fluid derangements (Sections 12 and 14) and hepatic encephalopathy (Section 13).

2.2 Laboratory, Radiologic and Histologic Evaluations

No single test can assess overall hepatic function, as the liver is a complex organ with interdependent metabolic, excretory and defense functions. Thus a number of laboratory tests are usually combined to detect hepatobiliary abnormalities and to assess their severity, follow the course of the disease, and help establish an etiology. Diagnosis is often based on patterns of abnormality that help distinguish hepatocellular dysfunction from excretory impairment (cholestasis), though overlap is great. In only a minority of cases does a specific laboratory test establish the diagnosis.

Radiologic imaging techniques and liver biopsy often provide essential diagnostic information, but their use should be tailored to the specific clinical circumstances.

2.2.1 *SERUM BIOCHEMICAL TESTS*

2.2.1.1 *Bilirubin*

This is a relatively insensitive indicator of liver disease, but it provides a clue to the overall assessment of hepatic function. The degree of bilirubin elevation often correlates poorly with clinical severity, but serial values are useful for following the course of the illness. Direct/indirect (conjugated/unconjugated) fractionation is *not* of diagnostic value in most cases of jaundice, and cannot distinguish hepatocellular disease from biliary obstruction. Measuring the presence of unconjugated hyperbilirubinemia is useful only in cases of mild, isolated bilirubin elevation to corroborate hemolysis or Gilbert's syndrome.

Urine bilirubin has little diagnostic value except in early hepatitis, when bilirubinuria precedes clinical jaundice, and in isolated unconjugated hyperbilirubinemia, when bilirubinuria is absent despite jaundice. (Unconjugated bilirubin is not cleared into urine.) Otherwise bilirubinuria is commonly present in hepatobiliary jaundice of any cause.

2.2.1.2 *Aminotransferases (transaminases)*

These liver enzymes include alanine aminotransferase (ALT), found primarily in liver cytosol, and aspartate aminotransferase (AST), also found in several other tissues, most notably skeletal and cardiac muscle. Both are exquisitely sensitive indicators of hepatocellular injury and provide the best guide to hepatocellular necrosis/inflammation.

The magnitude of elevation covers a very wide range. Levels <100 IU are common and nonspecific, and often have no clinical significance; levels of 100–300 IU are seen in numerous mild/moderate inflammatory processes. In acute viral or drug hepatitis aminotransferase levels are typically in the

500–1,500 IU range, but in alcoholic hepatitis they are usually <300 IU, even if the disease is severe. Values >3,000 IU usually are seen only in acute toxic necrosis or severe hypoxia ("shock liver," "ischemic hepatitis"); in both disorders levels typically plummet within two to three days, whereas values fall more slowly in viral hepatitis. Aminotransferase levels are variable in biliary obstruction but usually remain <200 IU, except with acute passage of common duct stone, characterized by a sudden rise to hepatitic levels and a rapid fall over the next one to two days.

The AST to ALT ratio is usually <1 in most circumstances, but is typically >1.5 in alcoholic liver disease; though not absolute, this is diagnostically helpful for alcoholic injury. Alcohol consumption lessens the ALT rise as a result of deficiency of a coenzyme needed for ALT synthesis.

2.2.1.3 *Alkaline phosphatase (ALP)*

The level of this bile canalicular enzyme is disproportionately increased in impaired bile excretion, and therefore an elevated level of ALP is a hallmark of cholestasis. An elevation in its level is due to enhanced synthesis rather than hepatocytic leakage; thus, the level usually rises slowly over days or weeks rather than abruptly. A disproportionately elevated ALP may be seen in infiltrative disorders, especially malignancy.

ALP isoenzymes also are present in bone and placenta. If the source of an isolated increase in ALP is not clinically clear, a concomitant elevation of γ-glutamyl transpeptidase (GGT) indicates a hepatobiliary origin. A form of ALP specific to the liver is 5′-nucleotidase (5′NT).

2.2.1.4 *Gamma-glutamyl transpeptidase (GGT)*

Levels of GGT usually parallel ALP, but this microsomal enzyme is also easily inducible – for example, by ethanol and numerous drugs. Thus, GGT is often disproportionately elevated in alcoholic liver disease, although this is too nonspecific for diagnostic reliability.

2.2.1.5 *Proteins*

2.2.1.5.1 *Albumin* Synthesized by the liver, albumin is the major contributor to oncotic pressure in the serum. Decreased levels usually develop only in severe hepatic dysfunction – most often in advanced cirrhosis – and therefore imply a relatively poor prognosis. Albumin usually remains normal in acute hepatitis; falling values in this setting imply an unusually severe course.

2.2.1.5.2 *Globulins* Nonspecific diffuse elevation is common in chronic liver disease, and of no consequence. Sometimes there is disproportionate elevation

of IgG in autoimmune hepatitis, of IgM in primary biliary cirrhosis, and of IgA in alcoholic liver disease.

2.2.1.6 *International Normalized Ratio (INR) and prothrombin time*

The INR/prothrombin time is a valuable index of the liver's ability to synthesize vitamin K–dependent clotting factors – a true "function" test. Increasing INR/PT implies relatively severe dysfunction, analogous to low serum albumin, and is especially worrisome in acute hepatitis. An abnormal value may be found in chronic cholestasis due to vitamin K malabsorption rather than impaired hepatic synthesis of clotting factors. Improvement after parenteral administration of vitamin K therefore favors a diagnosis of cholestasis over hepatocellular failure, but there are too many exceptions for diagnostic reliability.

2.2.1.7 *Lipids*

Complex lipoprotein derangements are common in liver disease, though usually not routinely studied. Cholesterol is often low in acute or chronic liver failure, whereas hypercholesterolemia is associated with prolonged cholestasis. Striking triglyceride elevations occasionally occur in alcoholic liver disease ("alcoholic lipemia").

2.2.2 *SERUM IMMUNOLOGIC TESTS*

2.2.2.1 *Hepatitis serology*

Serology is crucial for the specific diagnosis of hepatitis A, B, C and D. See Section 4 for details.

2.2.2.2 *Antimitochondrial antibody*

This is actually a complex series of antibodies directed against dehydrogenase components of mitochondrial membranes of various tissues. Nevertheless, it serves as a valuable marker for primary biliary cirrhosis, as it is present in >90% of cases. Antimitochondrial antibody is uncommon in other disorders, though there is some overlap with autoimmune hepatitis.

2.2.2.3 *Antinuclear factor and antismooth muscle antibody*

Such nonspecific immune markers are seen relatively commonly in autoimmune hepatitis; they are infrequent in other hepatic diseases.

2.2.2.4 *Alpha-fetoprotein*

This normal hepatic fetal protein disappears soon after birth. Detection therefore reflects hepatic dedifferentiation. Levels >250 ng/mL serve as a relatively specific marker for hepatocellular carcinoma, though they are also seen occasionally in other tumors. Values <100 ng/mL are nonspecifically seen in hepatic regeneration – e.g., recovering from hepatitis.

2.2.3 IMAGING PROCEDURES

In general, radiologic imaging is essential for the accurate diagnosis of biliary disease, important for focal liver disease (e.g., tumor), but overused and of relatively little value for diffuse hepatocellular disease (e.g., hepatitis, cirrhosis).

2.2.3.1 Ultrasonography (US)

Ultrasound is now the most widely used imaging procedure. Highly reliable for diagnosis of gallstones (>95% sensitivity), it has replaced oral cholecystography. US is less accurate in detecting common bile duct stones (<40% sensitivity), but reliably establishes the presence of a dilated biliary tree, which implies mechanical obstruction. It is therefore the primary initial tool to distinguish intrahepatic from extrahepatic cholestasis. It also detects focal hepatic lesions (e.g., tumor, cysts), sometimes with characteristic diagnostic features. It is less useful in detecting diffuse hepatocellular disease, as features are usually nonspecific. Abdominal ultrasound can be useful in the detection of fatty liver (steatosis), which results in a diffuse increase in echogenicity.

Ultrasonography can also provide important ancillary information relevant to hepatobiliary disease – e.g., splenomegaly or pancreatic mass. Doppler US is valuable in establishing the patency of hepatic vessels, especially the portal vein.

2.2.3.2 Computerized tomography (CT)

An expensive alternative to US, CT sometimes provides additional hepatic information. Generally less valuable than US for biliary disease, CT has proven more valuable for assessing the pancreas.

2.2.3.3 Direct biliary visualization

2.2.3.3.1 Endoscopic retrograde cholangiopancreatography (ERCP) Upper endoscopy allows direct cannulation of the common bile duct and/or pancreatic duct; the injection of contrast agent yields excellent definition of ductal anatomy. ERCP permits definitive visualization of the biliary tree for common duct stone, sclerosing cholangitis and other conditions. It also allows therapeutic intervention – e.g., removal of common duct stones via endoscopic papillotomy or stenting a stricture.

2.2.3.3.2 Percutaneous transhepatic cholangiography (PTC) In PTC, direct contrast visualization of the biliary tree is obtained via percutaneous needle

puncture of liver. This is done less often than ERCP, but is especially useful if there is high biliary obstruction – e.g., a tumor at the bifurcation of the hepatic ducts. It also permits therapeutic intervention such as stent insertion to bypass a ductal malignancy.

ERCP and PTC require considerable technical expertise and have significant risks. They should not be undertaken lightly, but are highly valuable in selected cholestatic situations and often obviate laparotomy.

2.2.3.4 *Radionuclide scanning*
A liver–spleen scan using 99mTc-sulfur colloid can reveal space-occupying lesions and diffuse parenchymal disease, but such scans are much less sensitive than US or CT; therefore, their use has rapidly waned. A 99mTc-labeled RBC scan can visualize suspected vascular lesions, especially hemangiomas. Cholescintigraphy using 99mTc-iminodiacetic acid derivatives (termed HIDA scan) can reveal cystic duct obstruction, especially in acute cholecystitis. The HIDA scan also assesses biliary excretion/patency and anatomy, but results often are less than ideal or misleading. Occasionally 67Ga-citrate scans are used to help detect liver abscess or tumor.

2.2.3.5 *Nuclear magnetic resonance imaging (NMR)*
NMR is an expensive but valuable imaging technique, not yet widely available. It can detect some lesions poorly seen by US or CT and sometimes can better clarify the nature of focal defects. NMR can also show the biliary tree, though in less detail than ERCP, and in selected instances of biliary obstruction may serve as a noninvasive alternative to ERCP.

2.2.4 *LIVER BIOPSY*
Percutaneous liver biopsy provides important diagnostic information at relatively low risk, but is needed in only a minority of cases of hepatic dysfunction. A small core of liver tissue is obtained at the bedside by needle aspiration under local anesthesia. This usually provides a surprisingly reliable reflection of the underlying disorder, though sampling error can occur in focal disease and some cases of cirrhosis.

The major indications are shown in Table 2. Transient right upper quadrant pain is not uncommon after biopsy, but significant hemorrhage, bile peritonitis or other major complications are rare if cases are properly selected.

Relative contraindications include a clinical bleeding tendency, INR > 1.5 or prothrombin time more than three seconds greater than control, severe thrombocytopenia, marked ascites, and high-grade biliary tract obstruction. A transjugular approach can be used with relative safety in cases of coagulopathy or severe ascites.

TABLE 2.   Indications for liver biopsy

Unexplained liver enzyme abnormalities
Hepatosplenomegaly of unknown cause
Diagnosis and staging of alcoholic liver disease
Cirrhosis – diagnosis and etiology
Chronic hepatitis
Unexplained intrahepatic cholestasis
Acute necrosis, if cause unclear
Suspected infiltrative disorder, especially malignancy
Unexplained systemic illness – fever of unknown origin, suspected granulomatous disease, etc.

Fine-needle aspiration of specific hepatic lesions can be obtained under US or CT guidance. This provides a cytologic sample, but is usually inadequate for full histologic assessment. Ultrasound guidance can be used to obtain a "core biopsy" from the liver.

2.3 Clinical Approach

When faced with a patient with known or suspected liver disease, the physician should attempt to answer several central questions: (1) Is the disorder acute or chronic? (2) Is it primarily a hepatocellular problem (e.g., hepatitis), a disorder of hepatobiliary secretion (cholestasis) or a vascular problem (e.g., portal hypertension)? (3) If hepatocellular, is alcohol, a virus or a drug responsible? If cholestatic, is it an intrahepatic problem or due to mechanical biliary obstruction? If vascular, is it due to cirrhosis or to a less common cause? (4) Is this actually a systemic disorder involving the liver rather than a primary hepatic problem? (5) Are there complications that require specific treatment? These and other pertinent questions are approached by bedside clinical judgment coupled with ancillary tests.

Broadly speaking, the most important diagnostic tool is a complete history and physical examination. Laboratory tests, imaging techniques and liver biopsy are valuable and sometimes essential for diagnosis, but in most cases clinical acumen provides the most important diagnostic information. Moreover, clinical judgment determines what additional studies should be undertaken and how to interpret the results. *Diagnostic errors most often arise from an inadequate history and physical examination with undue reliance on ancillary tests.*

The clinical assessment should emphasize aspects discussed above in Section 2.1. Inquire about ethanol, drugs (prescribed, over-the-counter and illicit) and epidemiologic factors relevant to viral hepatitis, especially in cases of suspected hepatocellular injury. In addition, pursuit of systemic illness is often necessary. A positive family history may also be obtained from patients with certain metabolic diseases found in children such as Wilson's disease, α_1-antitrypsin deficiency and autoimmune liver disease. If a cholestatic disorder is suspected, clues to a possible extrahepatic cause should also be sought – e.g., biliary or pancreatic pain, rigors and chills or weight loss. The physical examination may provide valuable information on the size and nature of the liver, presence or absence of signs of chronic liver injury, and complications such as portal hypertension, fluid retention or encephalopathy (see Section 2.1).

The extent and nature of laboratory investigations are guided by the initial clinical evaluation. Broadly speaking, a minimal initial study will include CBC plus bilirubin, AST and/or ALT, and ALP. These few simple tests usually clarify whether the problem is primarily a hepatocellular injury (disproportionate aminotransferase elevations) or an excretory problem (predominant ALP elevation). If the former is clinically apparent but the etiology is not, viral hepatitis markers may help, especially if the disorder is acute. If a cholestatic problem seems most likely, early US (or CT) should help distinguish intrahepatic from extrahepatic causation. If US indicates extrahepatic obstruction, direct biliary visualization by ERCP (or PTC) should be considered, whereas liver biopsy may be warranted if the process appears intrahepatic.

As yet there is no reliable biochemical marker of liver fibrosis. Thus laboratory indicators of hepatic dysfunction are often normal or only mildly deranged in cases of inactive cirrhosis; this is a common circumstance. It is well to remember that alcoholic liver disease is the commonest cause of chronic hepatocellular injury, even in patients who initially deny heavy ingestion.

With appropriate evaluation, a diagnosis can readily be established in the large majority of patients with hepatobiliary dysfunction. In many circumstances, however, especially if the hepatic abnormalities are minor, the wisest approach is simply to follow the patient's progress with periodic clinical and laboratory assessments.

3. CONGENITAL HYPERBILIRUBINEMIA / P. Paré

The importance of recognizing congenital hyperbilirubinemia lies mainly in distinguishing it from other, more serious hepatobiliary disease: congenital conjugated hyperbilirubinemia or hepatobiliary diseases. Except for Crigler-Najjar syndrome, congenital hyperbilirubinemia does not impair either the quality of life or the life expectancy of affected subjects. By definition, patients with familial hyperbilirubinemia have normal standard liver tests, and the liver histology is also normal (except for the pigment accumulation in Dubin-Johnson syndrome). With the exception of Gilbert's syndrome, these syndromes are uncommon and are divided into two groups on the basis of the type of the serum hyperbilirubinemia.

3.1 Unconjugated Hyperbilirubinemia

3.1.1 GILBERT'S SYNDROME

Gilbert's syndrome is the most common congenital hyperbilirubinemia syndrome, occurring in about 5% of Caucasians. It is probably transmitted through an autosomal dominant mode. Its pathogenesis is related to a partial deficiency in hepatic UDPglucuronyl transferase, the enzyme responsible for the glucuronidation of bilirubin. In addition, some patients have reduced bilirubin uptake by the hepatocytes, as observed with diagnostic substances (BSP, indocyanine green) and drugs (tolbutamide). The syndrome is usually detected in adolescents and young adults, most commonly in male persons; the possibility that testosterone inhibits whereas estrogen and progesterone augment the action of UDPglucuronyl transferase may provide the explanation. Complaints leading to the diagnosis are various (fatigue, nausea, vague abdominal discomfort) and unrelated to the condition. Scleral icterus may be present and fluctuating, but the physical examination is otherwise normal. Liver tests and hemogram (to exclude hemolysis) are normal except for unconjugated serum bilirubin, which is elevated between 20 and 100 μmol/L and conjugated bilirubin, which is often unrecordably low. Diagnostic tests are available but usually not necessary: fasting for two days or intravenous administration of nicotinic acid significantly increases serum unconjugated bilirubin, while phenobarbital significantly decreases it. No treatment is warranted and prognosis is excellent.

3.1.2 CRIGLER-NAJJAR SYNDROME

This syndrome may present in two types. Type I is a very rare and serious disease characterized by unconjugated hyperbilirubinemia often greater than 400–500 μmol/L. It is due to an absolute deficiency of UDPglucuronyl transferase. Jaundice occurs almost immediately after birth and may lead to kernicterus with consequent neurologic damage and mental retardation. Kernicterus involves damage to the basal ganglia and cerebral cortex because unconjugated bilirubin is able to penetrate the immature blood–brain barrier of infants. The syndrome is inherited in an autosomal recessive fashion, often with a family history of consanguinity. Phenobarbital treatment is ineffective in inducing UDPglucuronyl transferase activity; an early death occurs. The treatment of choice appears to be hepatic transplantation.

Crigler-Najjar syndrome type II is a much more benign condition in which the unconjugated hyperbilirubinemia usually does not exceed 400 μmol/L. Kernicterus rarely develops in these patients (except with prolonged fasting, in which bilirubin can rise). Hepatic UDPglucuronyl transferase activity is very low or undetectable, but phenobarbital therapy lowers serum bilirubin levels. (Phenobarbital presumably induces even the low levels of this enzyme.) Prognosis is very good despite a lifelong persistent unconjugated hyperbilirubinemia.

3.2 Conjugated Hyperbilirubinemia

Two conditions characterized by congenital conjugated hyperbilirubinemia without cholestasis have been described. Both syndromes are inherited as autosomal recessive traits. Both are uncommon disorders believed to result from specific defects in the hepatobiliary excretion of bilirubin. These conditions are benign, and their accurate diagnosis provides reassurance to the patient. Plasma bilirubin levels are usually in the range of 35–85 μmol/L, although occasionally levels may be as high as 400 μmol/L. Plasma bilirubin may further increase in both conditions during intercurrent infection, pregnancy or use of oral contraceptives. Pruritus is absent and serum bile acid levels are normal, as are routine biochemical liver tests, except for serum bilirubin concentration. Bilirubinuria is usually present. No treatment is necessary.

Some distinctive features allow differential diagnosis between the two syndromes.

3.2.1 *DUBIN-JOHNSON SYNDROME*

Patients with the Dubin-Johnson syndrome have a black liver, which results from the accumulation of a melanin-like pigment in lysosomes. Visualization of the gallbladder during oral cholecystography is usually delayed or absent. Urinary excretion of total coproporphyrin is normal, whereas the proportion of isomer I is higher than in normal controls (>80%). Finally, the BSP plasma retention test is normal in its initial phase, but there is a secondary rise in plasma BSP concentration at 90 minutes due to reflux of BSP from the hepatocyte to the plasma.

3.2.2 *ROTOR'S SYNDROME*

In patients with Rotor's syndrome, the appearance and histology of the liver are normal. Oral cholecystography usually visualizes the gallbladder. Total coproporphyrin excretion is greater than normal, as in other hepatobiliary disorders, and isomer I makes a smaller proportion (<80%) than in Dubin-Johnson patients. The plasma disappearance of injected BSP is delayed, with no secondary rise.

TABLE 3.   Causes of acute hepatitis

Viruses
   Hepatitis A
   Hepatitis B
   Hepatitis C
   Hepatitis D
   Hepatitis E
   Herpes simplex
   Cytomegalovirus
   Epstein-Barr
   Adenoviruses
Drugs
Toxins
Alcohol
Ischemia
Wilson's disease
Other

---

4. ACUTE VIRAL HEPATITIS / V.G. Bain and M. Ma

The term *hepatitis* refers to any inflammatory process of the liver. The most common etiology of acute hepatitis is viral infection (Table 3). In North America, hepatitis A, hepatitis B and hepatitis C are the commonest causes of viral hepatitis. Viral hepatitis occurs less commonly with infections such as Epstein-Barr virus, cytomegalovirus, adenovirus, herpes simplex and Coxsackie virus. In these cases, the clinical picture is usually dominated not by the hepatitis but by other features of the viral illness.

The clinical course of acute hepatitis varies from mild symptoms requiring no treatment to fulminant liver failure requiring liver transplantation. In the last decade, the treatment of acute viral hepatitis has not progressed as rapidly as our understanding of these hepatitis viruses' epidemiology and molecular biology. The mainstay of treatment is still supportive care, because the inflammation is self-limited in most cases. Postexposure prophylaxis is possible for some of the hepatitis viruses.

4.1 The Hepatitis Viruses and Their Epidemiology

4.1.1 *HEPATITIS A VIRUS (HAV)*
Previously termed "infectious hepatitis," hepatitis A virus (HAV) is an RNA virus that belongs to the enterovirus family. It is present in the stool of patients during the prodrome or pre-icteric phase until about two weeks after the onset of jaundice. Both IgM and IgG antibodies to the virus (anti-HAV) can be

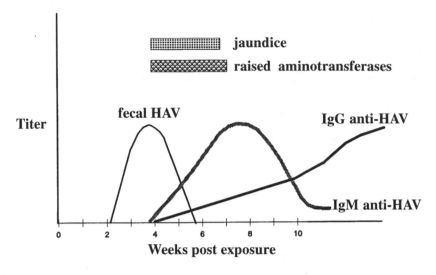

FIGURE 2. Typical clinical and serologic features of acute hepatitis A infection.

detected, with the most helpful sign being the demonstration of an elevated IgM antibody, indicating recent infection (Figure 2).

HAV infection infection is common. The anti-HAV IgG can be detected in 30–40% of the population in developed countries and 90% of the population in developing countries. HAV is usually transmitted by the fecal–oral route. Thus, food or water contamination may lead to epidemic outbreaks. Several outbreaks have been associated with ingestion of raw clams and oysters from polluted water. Person-to-person spread results in sporadic cases. Parenteral transmission is also possible, especially in intravenous drug users, but is much less common.

Infection can occur at any age but is most common in younger age groups. Infection can present as a gastrointestinal illness and therefore diagnosis can be missed. In countries with good water supplies and sanitation, more symptomatic hepatitis A is seen in older age groups, since fewer adults are exposed to hepatitis A as children. The incubation period is about one month, and rarely is longer than 40 days. The mortality rate – usually from fulminant hepatitis – is very low (0.1%). There is no evidence for a chronic carrier state or the development of chronic liver disease.

4.1.2 HEPATITIS B VIRUS (HBV)

In 1965, an antibody in a hemophiliac patient was found to react with an antigen in the serum from an Australian aborigine; this antigen was subsequently

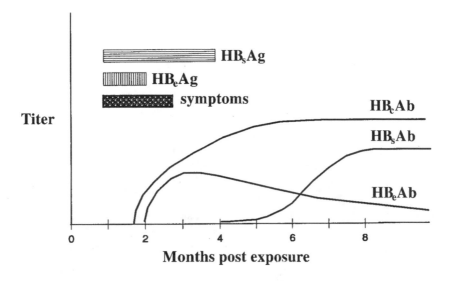

FIGURE 3. Typical clinical and serologic features of acute hepatitis B infection.

found in patients with viral hepatitis. This antigen was termed the Australian antigen and is now known to be the surface coat of the hepatitis B virion, now called the hepatitis B surface antigen (HB_sAg).

HBV is a unique DNA virus that replicates through reverse transcription of its mRNA. It behaves more like a retrovirus than a DNA virus. HBV consists of a 28 nm central core containing the genome (a single molecule of partially double-stranded DNA) and a specific DNA polymerase with a surrounding core protein shell. The core is commonly found in the nuclei of infected hepatocytes, with the outer HB_sAg coat being acquired from the cytoplasm of the hepatocyte. The core antigen is antigenically distinct from the HB_sAg. This allows separate detection of core antibody (anti-HB_c) and surface antibody (anti-HB_s). A further viral antigen, termed HB_eAg, can be detected in the serum, together with DNA polymerase. HB_eAg is a subunit of HB_cAg. HB_eAg positivity implies viral replication and is an indicator of high infectivity. Mutants that do not produce HB_eAg exist; these "pre-core mutants" can cause severe hepatitis.

The typical course of HBV infection, appearance of the viral antigens and host immune response are shown in Figure 3. The significance of HBV markers and their importance in interpretation is summarized in Table 4.

In North America, HBV infection occurs primarily in adolescents and adults. High-risk groups for HBV infection are summarized in Table 5. The

TABLE 4.   Interpretation of hepatitis B markers

Marker	Interpretation
HB$_s$Ag	Active HBV infection; may be acute or chronic
HB$_s$Ab	Immune to HBV; may be natural immunity or following vaccination
HB$_c$Ab-IgM	Acute HBV infection (newer and more sensitive assays may also be positive during reactivation of chronic infections)
HB$_e$Ag	High infectivity, active viral replication
HB$_e$Ab	Low or no infectivity; need only be measured in chronic HBV
HBV-DNA	Direct measure of infectivity or replicative state; becoming increasingly available

TABLE 5.   Risk factors associated with reported cases of acute HBV in the U.S.

Risk factors	%
Heterosexual activity	48
IV drug use	11
Homosexual activity	7
Health-care employment	2
Household contact	1
Transfusion, dialysis	1
Unknown	30

SOURCE: Data from Centers for Disease Control and Prevention, 1992.

transmission may be sexual, vertical or parenteral (most commonly through inoculation by contaminated needles in intravenous drug users). Hepatitis B infection from transfusion has been almost completely eliminated by routine screening by the use of volunteer blood donors. Vertical transmission is common in developing countries, passing from a mother who is a chronic hepatitis B carrier to a fetus or newborn; the infection is acquired at the time of birth or shortly thereafter. This vertical transmission of HBV results in the vast majority of chronic carriers worldwide.

4.1.3 HEPATITIS C VIRUS (HCV)
Hepatitis C virus is a recently discovered single-stranded RNA virus of less

than 80 nm in diameter that has been classified as a member of the flavivirus family. The virus itself has not been isolated or visualized, although the majority of its genome has been cloned and sequenced. It is worldwide in distribution. The prevalence of HCV infection in the general population is approximately 1%. However, prevalence is highly variable among different risk groups. Hemophilia patients have a prevalence rate as high as 90%, whereas health-care workers have a prevalence rate of 1%.

The principal mode of HCV transmission is parenteral exposure, but a significant percentage of patients do not have identifiable risk factors. Parenteral exposure accounts for at least 90% of cases of post-transfusion hepatitis (previously labeled as non-A non-B hepatitis), but these cases make up only 10% of the total hepatitis C cases. Intravenous drug use is the main cause of hepatitis C infection, but interestingly, the exposure may predate clinical hepatitis by decades. HCV also accounts for 12–25% of cases of sporadic hepatitis.

The incubation period is 5 to 10 weeks (mean 7 weeks), with the acute phase being clinically mild and the majority of cases being anicteric. The elevated aminotransferase pattern may be monophasic or multiphasic with the latter suggesting chronicity, which develops in over 75% of cases. Histologically, it is not possible to distinguish between progressive and nonprogressive forms of hepatitis C, and liver biopsy is not suggested.

Serologic testing for this virus has developed rapidly following its discovery in 1989. The third-generation ELISA (enzyme-linked immunosorbent assay) and RIBA (recombinant immunoblot assay) identify antibodies to the nonstructural as well as structural epitopes of the virus. The ELISA test is very sensitive but not specific, and therefore all positives must be confirmed with the highly specific RIBA or another confirmatory test. From Red Cross blood donor data, about 50% of individuals who have normal liver enzymes and are anti-HCV positive by ELISA will be negative on subsequent RIBA testing. Hypergammaglobulinemia is a common reason for a false-positive ELISA test. An additional problem with the ELISA test for anti-HCV is that the antibody cannot be detected in the circulation for approximately three months following the onset of acute hepatitis C, as opposed to six to eight weeks for RIBA testing. Moreover, only 60–70% of patients with acute HCV infection will ever develop anti-HCV ELISA positivity.

Studies detecting HCV-RNA using the highly sensitive polymerase chain reaction have shown that 80% of antibody-positive individuals have viremia and are potentially infectious. In contrast to hepatitis B, sexual and vertical transmission is uncommon. HCV infection from contaminated needles in health-care workers occurs in less than 5%.

4.1.4 *HEPATITIS D VIRUS (HDV)*

HDV is a defective RNA virus that requires the presence of hepatitis B surface antigen for its expression. HDV utilizes the HB_sAg protein as its external coat to attach to and enter hepatocytes. It is found worldwide, but Italy, Eastern Europe, the Middle East, the South Pacific, South America and Africa have the highest incidence. In North America, less than 1% of HB_sAg-positive patients have evidence of HDV infection, whereas in parts of Italy 14–50% of HB_sAg-positive patients are co-infected with HDV. In the United States and Canada, HDV infection is found almost exclusively among intravenous drug abusers and their sexual partners.

Hepatitis D infection may originate as a co-infection with hepatitis B or as a superinfection in a patient who is already a chronic HBV carrier. Co-infection produces a more severe acute hepatitis than that caused by hepatitis B alone, but it is usually self-limited. Superinfection often results in more severe chronic hepatitis than hepatitis B alone. The delta virus circulates in association with the delta antigen, but until more sensitive assays are developed, this antigen can be detected only during the early phases of infection. The serologic marker for acute and chronic hepatitis D infection is the antibody to delta antigen (anti-HDV).

4.1.5 *HEPATITIS E VIRUS (HEV)*

Hepatitis E (epidemic hepatitis) appears to be due to a single-stranded RNA virus of 27–34 nm in size. It shares many similarities with hepatitis A. Although HEV was previously included in the group labeled non-A non-B hepatitis, it has now been classified as an enteric virus transmitted by contaminated water supplies or by the fecal–oral route. Cases of HEV infection may be part of an epidemic or may be isolated, sporadic cases. HEV is the leading cause of acute viral hepatitis in young to middle-aged adults in many developing countries. It is associated with a high mortality rate (approaching 20%) in infected pregnant women in the third trimester. It is seen only rarely in North America and almost exclusively in travelers returning from endemic regions. The incubation period is 10–50 days. There are no distinctive clinical features, with secondary cases being rare. Chronicity of infection does not develop. Testing for anti-HEV is available at reference laboratories.

4.1.6 *HEPATITIS F VIRUS (HFV)*

An as yet unidentified virus is believed to be associated with some cases of fulminant hepatitis that are negative for all other viral serology. Most such cases are fatal without a liver transplant.

4.1.7 *HEPATITIS G VIRUS (HGV)*
In 1995, a new virus that causes hepatitis was cloned. It is known as the GB agent, so named after the initials of a surgeon who contracted this infection. It is similar to flaviviruses and shares 25% homology with hepatitis C. It persists as a mild chronic hepatitis. Very little is known about this new virus or group of viruses.

4.1.8 *OTHER CAUSES OF ACUTE HEPATITIS*
A paramyxo-like virus has been identified in a small number of patients with severe acute liver disease who usually died of liver failure or underwent liver transplantation. The presumptive diagnosis is made by liver biopsy where multinucleated giant cells are present. Paramyxo-like virus particles can also be seen on electron microscopy of the specimen. The epidemiology, presumed infectious agent, response to treatment and forms of prevention have yet to be defined.

4.2 Pathology
Acute viral hepatitis causes inflammation of the liver involving primarily the parenchyma. There is evidence of hepatocellular degeneration (ballooning, acidophilic bodies, spotty necrosis), inflammation (lobular and portal mononuclear infiltrate) and hepatocyte regeneration (Figure 4). More severe cases demonstrate bridging necrosis between central veins and portal tracts (Figures 5 and 6). Because there is usually preservation of the reticular framework, the liver completely restores itself with hepatocyte regeneration. Liver biopsy is not generally helpful in distinguishing between the different types of acute hepatitis, as the histology is quite similar.

4.3 Clinical Features
Most viral hepatitis infections are asymptomatic, especially in younger individuals. When symptomatic, initial symptoms are those of any viral infection, beginning with malaise, nausea, vomiting, fatigue and a low-grade fever. More characteristic are severe anorexia, an aversion to smoking, and the passing of dark urine. Right upper quadrant discomfort is common in acute hepatitis, but severe abdominal pain is not a feature. After several days, jaundice appears, often preceded by dark urine and light-colored stool. The convalescent stage is usually 7 to 10 days, with the total illness lasting 2 to 6 weeks. Physical findings are usually minimal, aside from jaundice and a tender, enlarged liver.

4.4 Diagnosis
Acute viral hepatitis can be suspected by the presence of viral prodrome

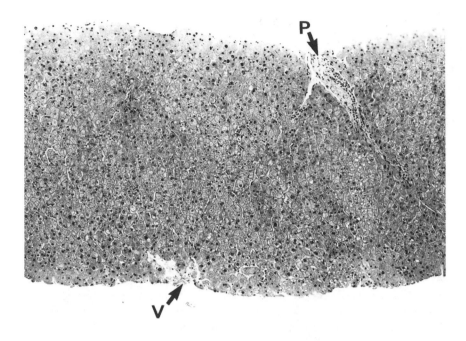

FIGURE 4.   Mild hepatitis. There is some increase in inflammatory cells but no obvious hepato-cellular necrosis. P, portal tract; V, central vein. (H & E, original magnification × 92.5)

symptoms, which often precede the more classical symptoms (including jaundice, dark urine and pruritus). Of diagnostic importance are a history of exposure to jaundiced persons, recent intravenous drug use or transfusions, sexual orientation and sex practices, travel history, drug or toxin exposure (including herbs) and the absence of significant abdominal pain.

If viral hepatitis is suspected clinically, laboratory evaluation will help confirm the presence of acute liver injury, may define the etiology and may help monitor the course and prognosis of hepatitis. Characteristically, the serum aminotransferase level is significantly elevated, often to levels >1,000 IU/L (normal is 10–40 IU/L), with the alkaline phosphatase only mildly to moderately elevated. The serum bilirubin is mainly conjugated and reflects the severity of the hepatitis. The INR/prothrombin time defines the extent of liver injury in the acute stage, with an increasing INR/PT implying a poor prognosis and the need for referral to a regional liver center. Initial serologic testing should include only HAV-IgM and HB$_s$Ag. Anti-HCV should be done at the onset only if specific risk factors are present (especially intravenous drug use) or subsequently if the HAV and HBV serology is negative.

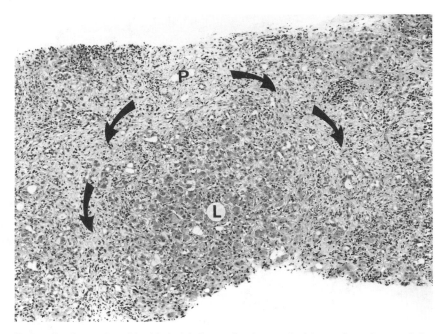

FIGURE 5. Severe hepatitis. Marked inflammation has resulted in confluent hepatocellular necrosis, termed bridging necrosis (curved arrows), along the portal tracts (P) that surround a residual hepatic lobule (L). (HPS, original magnification × 92.5)

The differential diagnosis should include other viral infections (such as infectious mononucleosis or cytomegalovirus infection), drug-induced liver disease, autoimmune hepatitis and Wilson's disease. Biliary tract disease (including cholecystitis and cholangitis) is distinguished by the presence of fever and significant abdominal pain. If doubt exists as to the diagnosis of hepatitis, abdominal ultrasound to investigate extrahepatic biliary obstruction and even liver biopsy may be necessary. In general, however, liver biopsy is rarely required in patients with acute hepatitis.

4.5 Complications

Most patients with viral hepatitis recover completely. The most important complication is the development of chronicity, which may follow hepatitis B, C, D and G. Most other complications are fortunately rare.

4.5.1 FULMINANT HEPATITIS

This is defined as the development of acute liver cell injury proceeding to liver failure and hepatic encephalopathy within eight weeks in a patient without any known previous liver disease. Clinically, the patient deteriorates with

FIGURE 6. Severe hepatitis. High power shows numerous inflammatory cells within the sinusoids as well as foci of hepatocellular necrosis (arrows). Reactive changes, including binucleation and prominent nucleoli, are seen in the viable hepatocytes. (Gomori, original magnification × 370)

development of deep jaundice, confusion and drowsiness. The encephalopathy can progress into deep coma. Because of massive liver necrosis, there is deficiency of clotting factors, and hence the INR/PT is always increased. At this stage, mortality is greater than 50% unless a liver transplant can be performed. Death may occur from infection, hypoglycemia, increased intracranial pressure with cerebral edema, or renal failure. Massive hepatic necrosis with architectural collapse is seen histologically (Figures 7 and 8). Despite this, if regeneration occurs, histologic recovery is the rule.

4.5.2 CHOLESTASIS
Occasionally acute viral hepatitis exhibits a cholestatic phase, in which the patient becomes intensely pruritic and jaundiced, and the enzyme pattern changes with a fall in the aminotransferase but with an increased alkaline phosphatase value. Biliary tract disease and drug toxicity should be ruled out. Resolution within a few weeks is the usual course. This occurs most commonly in hepatitis A.

FIGURE 7.   Submassive necrosis. Extensive hepatocellular necrosis in seen, leaving large areas of connective tissue around the central vein (V) and widening of the portal tracts (P), which have become confluent. Residual bile ducts (arrowheads) are seen in the portal tracts. (HPS, original magnification × 370)

4.5.3 RELAPSING (BIPHASIC) HEPATITIS
Clinically, these patients are improving, only to have a recurrence of the signs and symptoms of their hepatitis. Resolution is almost always complete. This pattern is most characteristic of hepatitis A. In some cases of hepatitis B, the second phase is due to acute hepatitis D. Hepatitis C is characterized by continued and wide fluctuations in liver aminotransferase values, but a biphasic clinical course is uncommon.

4.5.4 IMMUNE COMPLEX DISEASE
In hepatitis B, about 5–10% of cases initially develop a serum-sickness–like syndrome (characterized by skin rash, angioedema and arthritis), which is due to circulating immune complexes of viral particles and antibody with complement activation. Other immunologic manifestations include pericarditis, aplastic anemia or neurologic abnormalities such as Guillain-Barré syndrome. Chronic hepatitis B may have persisting circulating immune complex disease that leads to such diseases as membranous glomerulonephritis with nephrotic

FIGURE 8.   Submassive necrosis. High power shows viable hepatocytes on the left, an island of degenerating cells centrally (arrowheads) and residual bile ducts (arrows) in the widened portal tract. (HPS, original magnification × 185)

syndrome or polyarteritis nodosa. Chronic hepatitis C can cause cryoglobulinemia secondary to viral protein and antibody interaction.

4.5.5 *CHRONIC HEPATITIS*
Chronic hepatitis represents continued disease activity beyond six months. This complicates acute hepatitis B infrequently in adults but occurs in acute hepatitis C in over 75% of cases. It does not occur in hepatitis A or E. Chronic hepatitis can be suspected if there are persistent symptoms or persistent elevation of serum aminotransferase levels after six months.

4.6 **Treatment**
Most cases of acute viral hepatitis resolve spontaneously and require no specific treatment. Strict bed rest is not necessary. The patient may undertake any activity that does not exacerbate symptoms. Diet can be liberal, encouraging a high calorie intake but excluding alcohol. Fatty foods are poorly tolerated and are best avoided. Hospitalization is not necessary. All drugs, especially

tranquilizers and sedatives, should be avoided. Corticosteroids do not alter the degree of hepatitis or rate of healing and should be avoided to allow a normal immunologic response, which then can eliminate the virus. Indeed, their use in acute viral hepatitis may increase the risk of a chronic carrier state. Alpha-interferon may be useful in acute hepatitis C, but this approach remains investigational.

Return to work and activity should be guided by the patient's symptoms. Patient education will help alleviate anxiety. Specialist referral is not usually required. Prophylaxis and prevention of secondary spread is perhaps the most important aspect of treatment.

4.7 Prophylaxis

The control of hepatitis A is dependent on good sanitation and hygiene, because the virus is excreted in the stool early in the course of the infection. An attack of hepatitis A confers lifelong immunity. An effective vaccine has been developed for use by high-risk individuals such as those traveling to endemic areas or in institutions. Serum immunoglobulin (ISG) is also available. This should be provided to all household contacts, and is optimally given within one week of exposure at a dose of 0.02 mL/kg IM. Casual school or work contacts are not usually treated prophylactically unless an epidemic is identified.

A specific globulin preparation and a vaccine are available for HBV. Hepatitis B immunoglobulin (HBIG) should be given when there has been a clear-cut exposure such as inadvertent "needlestick" or sexual contact. It also should be given, along with hepatitis B vaccine, within 24 to 48 hours to the neonates of mothers with acute or chronic hepatitis B. Hepatitis B vaccine, originally manufactured from pooled donor sera, is now synthesized from recombinant DNA. Side effects are minimal with both forms. Vaccination targeted against high-risk groups such as homosexuals, health-care workers, IV drug users, family contacts of chronic carriers, chronic transfusion recipients and dialysis patients has surprisingly failed to affect the incidence of hepatitis B. Universal vaccination is therefore advocated and has been initiated in some provinces. Vaccination for hepatitis B is also protective against hepatitis D.

There is no vaccine or specific immunoglobulin available for hepatitis C. Pooled gamma globulin may reduce post-transfusion hepatitis C and thus it has been given empirically following high-risk exposures such as needlestick or transfusion from a known case of hepatitis C.

4.8 Summary

Table 6 summarizes the important features of the different types of viral

TABLE 6.   Overview of viral hepatitis

	Virus type	Transmission	Incubation (days)	Serologic diagnosis	Chronicity
HAV	RNA	Fecal–oral	20–35	HAV-IgM	No
HBV	DNA	Percutaneous, venereal	60–110	HB$_s$Ag	Adults <5% Preschoolers 25% Neonates >90%
HCV	RNA	Percutaneous	35–75	anti-HCV	>75%
HDV	RNA	Percutaneous, venereal(?)	60–110	anti-HDV	Usual in superinfection; rare in co-infection
HEV	RNA	Fecal–oral	10–50	anti-HEV	No
HFV	?	?	?	?	No
HGV	RNA	Percutaneous	?	(Research only; HGV-RNA)	Yes

hepatitis. Acute viral hepatitis is a self-limited disease and requires supportive care only. For the few patients who develop fulminant liver failure, liver transplantation may be required. Chronic infection can develop in patients with HBV, HCV, HDV and HGV infection.

5. CHRONIC HEPATITIS / V.G. Bain and M. Ma

The term *chronic hepatitis* means active, ongoing inflammation of the liver persisting for more than six months that is detectable by biochemical and histologic means. It does not imply an etiology. The biochemical hallmark of chronic hepatitis is an increased serum aminotransferase (AST and ALT) with minimal elevation of alkaline phosphatase. When the inflammation is severe and/or prolonged, hepatic dysfunction may become apparent with an increase in serum bilirubin and INR/prothrombin time, and a decrease in serum albumin. Typically, biochemical tests are used to identify and follow patients with chronic hepatitis, while liver biopsies serve to more precisely define the nature of the chronic hepatitis and provide useful information regarding the extent of damage and prognosis.

Histologically, chronic hepatitis is characterized by infiltration of the portal tracts by inflammatory cells. These cells are predominantly mononuclear cells including lymphocytes, monocytes and plasma cells. Chronic hepatitis is designated as mild when the infiltrate is confined to the portal triad (Fig-

FIGURE 9. Mild chronic hepatitis. This portal tract contains a chronic inflammatory infiltrate that is confined to the portal triad and does not extend past the limiting plate (arrowheads). V, vein; A, artery; B, bile duct. (Masson, original magnification × 185)

ure 9). It is designated as moderately severe chronic hepatitis (Figure 10) when the infiltrate extends into the parenchyma (piecemeal necrosis) and when it extends to adjacent portal triads (bridging). The inflammatory process can also "bridge" from the portal tract to the central vein. Severe chronic hepatitis is associated with multilobular or confluent necrosis and is much more likely to progress to cirrhosis. The amount of fibrosis is staged separately. These newer terms, *mild, moderate* and *severe chronic hepatitis*, replace the older terminology including *chronic persistent hepatitis* and *chronic active hepatitis*, which are still frequently mentioned in older textbooks.

By far, the commonest cause of chronic hepatitis is viral infections of the liver. Other causes include autoimmune hepatitis, drug-induced hepatitis, Wilson's disease, α_1-antitrypsin deficiency and steatohepatitis. Primary biliary cirrhosis and primary sclerosing cholangitis may occasionally mimic chronic hepatitis, but are not usually classified as such. An approach to help determine the etiology of chronic hepatitis is summarized in Table 7.

FIGURE 10.   Moderately severe chronic hepatitis. Inflammatory cells are shown infiltrating and destroying the periportal hepatocytes (arrow) and disrupting the limiting plate (piecemeal necrosis) (arrowheads). (HPS, original magnification × 185)

5.1 Chronic Viral Hepatitis

5.1.1 GENERAL CONSIDERATIONS

Of the known viral infections of the liver, HBV, HCV, HDV and HGV can cause chronic liver disease; HBV and HCV make up the vast majority of these cases. A careful history is most helpful in determining the cause of chronic hepatitis (Table 7). In most cases, selected laboratory tests will provide the confirmation of diagnosis. Sometimes liver biopsy is required to identify the cause of chronic hepatitis. The liver biopsy will also provide important information about the extent of damage and current activity.

5.1.2 HEPATITIS B VIRUS

5.1.2.1 Evolution to chronic liver disease

A number of factors determine whether an individual will clear an acute HBV infection or progress to a chronic carrier state. Of these, the age at infection is

TABLE 7.   Role of history in diagnosis of chronic hepatitis

Etiology	Key points in the history	Useful lab tests
Hepatitis B	Sexual history (homosexuality, use of prostitute services, promiscuity), family history, country of origin, IV drug use	HB_sAg – if positive, measure HB_eAg, HB_eAb and HBV-DNA (if available)
Hepatitis C	Blood transfusions (pre-1990), IV drug use (even once), tattoos, ear or body piercing, sexual promiscuity, HCV-positive partner, incarceration	anti-HCV
Autoimmune hepatitis	Usually young or middle-aged females, often chronic symptoms – especially fatigue (but may present acutely), other autoimmune disease (e.g., thyroid)	Quantitative immuno-globulins Antinuclear antibodies Smooth-muscle antibody
Drug-induced hepatitis	Careful history of all drugs and herbs: common offenders include isoniazid, nitrofurantoin, NSAIDs, sulfa drugs	None
Wilson's disease	Family history, neurologic or psychiatric symptoms in children or young adults	Serum ceruloplasmin 24-hr urinary copper
α_1-antitrypsin deficiency	Family history of liver or lung disease (emphysema)	α_1-antitrypsin levels and Pi typing
Nonalcoholic steatohepatitis (NASH)	Obesity – especially recent weight gain, diabetes mellitus, corticosteroids, intestinal by-pass surgery	Glucose Hgb Al$_c$ Abdominal ultrasound

most important, with carrier rates of greater than 90% occurring in vertically infected newborns as compared to less than 5% in adults. The immunologic status of the host is also important, with immunocompromised individuals (e.g., HIV, renal failure, post-transplant) being more likely to become chronic carriers. The severity of the acute disease has also been correlated with outcome. In general, the milder the acute illness the more likely that progression to chronic liver disease will occur. Presumably, individuals with mild acute disease are those with a suboptimal immunologic response to the virus, whereas patients with more severe acute disease are manifesting a prompt and effective immunologic attack on hepatocytes harboring HBV.

5.1.2.2 Presentation

The majority of patients with chronic type B hepatitis are asymptomatic or have mild fatigue only. The patients might give a history of risk-taking behavior or a family history of hepatitis B infection. Liver enzyme abnormalities discovered incidentally frequently alert the physician to the possibility of underlying viral infection. Screening of family and sexual contacts of known cases will often discover additional cases.

5.1.2.3 Diagnosis

By the strictest definition, a patient is not a chronic HBV carrier until the HB_sAg test is found to be positive for six months, but the diagnosis is often suspected much earlier.

It is important not to be confused by other viral markers of previous hepatitis B exposure (Table 4). Antibodies to HB_sAg (anti-HB_s) indicate immunity against HBV and may be acquired either after vaccination or after clearance of HBV infection. On the other hand, the presence of HB_eAg and HBV-DNA indicates active HBV replication. The level of HBV-DNA correlates with the amount of virus present in the circulation. When HBV-DNA is strongly positive, there is a high viral load, which indicates a high degree of infectivity (all physiologic fluids are potentially infectious). A negative HBV-DNA indicates very low or absent infectivity. Unfortunately, serum HBV-DNA testing is not widely available. If HB_eAg is negative there is usually lower infectivity. Positive antibodies to the core antigen (anti-HB_c) indicate exposure to the virus only and are therefore of very limited use in patient assessment. The presence of IgM and anti-HB_c suggests recent HBV exposure. In chronic HBV infection the anti-HB_c is is positive but the IgM anti-HB_c is negative because exposure took place more than six months previously. The exception is in patients with reactivation of chronic hepatitis B who may also be IgM anti-HB_c positive, which reduces the usefulness of this test in the diagnosis of acute HBV infection.

5.1.2.4 Natural history

The natural history of chronic HBV infection has been well defined. The first six months of the illness represent the acute hepatitis phase of the infection. This acute phase is not often seen in chronically infected patients who have contracted the virus at birth or in early childhood. Chronic hepatitis has three phases, termed the replicative, inflammatory and inactive phases (Figure 11).

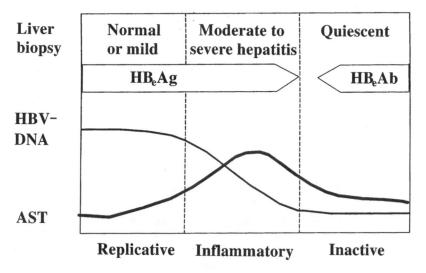

FIGURE 11.   Phases of chronic hepatitis B.

During the replicative phase, HB$_e$Ag is positive as is HBV-DNA, indicating high levels of viral replication. Despite this, the aminotransferases are normal or near normal and the liver biopsy is relatively inactive. For unknown reasons, patients may then enter the inflammatory phase in which their immune system now recognizes those hepatocytes harboring virus and begins to attack them. Accordingly, the aminotransferase becomes elevated and the biopsy shows chronic hepatitis, often of a severe degree The level of viral replication as measured by the HBV-DNA will decline. If the patient has successfully cleared viral replication, he or she will enter an inactive phase characterized by normalization of the aminotransferases and relative inactivity on the liver biopsy. HB$_e$Ag will be cleared and anti-HB$_e$ will form (seroconversion).

It is the severity and duration of the inflammatory phase that determine whether a patient will develop cirrhosis. This progression of chronic hepatitis to cirrhosis occurs in 20–30% of all chronic hepatitis B patients. Even patients who successfully enter the inactive phase are still at risk of hepatocellular carcinoma (relative risk greater than 100 vs the general population). Those with cirrhosis are at highest risk. Screening for hepatocellular carcinoma has been recommended in chronic carriers by performing a serum α-fetoprotein and an abdominal ultrasound each 6 to 12 months; more recently, however, the efficacy and cost benefit of this approach have been questioned. The problem is that even cases discovered by screening are often beyond cure by resection or liver transplantation.

5.1.2.5 *Treatment*

There are few therapeutic options for the treatment of patients with chronic hepatitis B, although different agents have been tried. Of these agents, only interferon-α has been licensed for use. In most studies, 30-40% of chronic hepatitis B patients successfully respond to interferon treatment with a loss of serologic markers of viral replication (HB_eAg and HBV-DNA). A minority of responders will also lose all evidence of infection (clear HB_sAg) during treatment, but up to 50% will become HB_sAg negative during the first five years of follow-up. The relapse rate following discontinuation of therapy is less than 15%.

Since the majority of patients do not respond to interferon, an important question is, which patients warrant a trial of therapy? Those most likely to respond include patients who acquired their infection during adulthood, females, patients with elevated ALT and low HBV-DNA levels, those with active hepatic inflammation on biopsy, patients who are HIV antibody negative and those who are anti-HDV negative. Stated another way, patients in the inflammatory phase (Figure 11) are most likely to benefit from interferon.

A number of new medications are being tested for efficacy against HBV. Lamivudine is a new nucleoside analogue with very potent antiviral effect against HBV. Its role in treatment of chronic hepatitis B is currently being defined in clinical trials; but it may find a use in combination with interferon.

5.1.2.6 *Prevention*

Active immunization is important to prevent transmission of HBV infection from a chronic carrier to sexual and family contacts. The safety of the vaccine is well established. It should be given to all high-risk groups as a minimum, but ultimately the goal is universal vaccination. As universal vaccination becomes a reality, prophylaxis with hyperimmune hepatitis B globulins for HBV contacts will become unnecessary.

5.1.3 *HEPATITIS C VIRUS*

Chronic hepatitis C virus has become the commonest type of chronic viral hepatitis in most areas. The identified cases may represent only the tip of the iceberg, with most cases still undiagnosed. Many cases are identified after investigation of raised liver enzymes in asymptomatic individuals or by the Red Cross during screening of blood donors. Other patients present to physicians with fatigue, malaise and abnormal liver enzymes.

5.1.3.1 Epidemiology

Although HCV infection can be transmitted by the same routes as HBV infection, the majority of cases are related to intravenous drug abuse (60–70%). Ten percent of patients with chronic HCV infection will have had a previous blood transfusion. In the remaining patients, one cannot identify a possible source of infection. Nonparenteral transmission through sexual or intimate contact and maternal–infant exposure can occur with HCV infection, but much less often than with HBV infection.

5.1.3.2 Natural history

The natural history of HCV infection has been better defined with the availability of anti-HCV serologic testing. Widespread application of this test has revealed that more than 75% of patients with acute HCV infection will remain chronically infected. Of the patients with chronic hepatitis, 20% either have or will go on to develop cirrhosis by 20 years. Thereafter, an additional 1% per year develop cirrhosis. Of much concern is the fact that recent data document a strong association between chronic HCV infection and hepatocellular carcinoma. The exact relative risk has yet to be determined but appears to be as high as or higher than that with HBV. Other disorders that have been described in association with chronic HCV infection include cryoglobulinemia, porphyria cutanea tarda and membranoproliferative glomerulonephritis.

5.1.3.3 Treatment

Interferon-α is the only therapy available for chronic HCV infection. Numerous studies have identified a 40–50% response rate (normalization of ALT abnormalities). However, at least 50% of these responders will relapse, with the majority of relapses occurring within three months following discontinuation of therapy. Therefore, only about 10–20% of treated patients enjoy a sustained response (presumed cure). The most recent clinical trials have utilized 12 to 24 months of therapy instead of the standard 6 months. Sustained response rates in excess of 30% have been published; however, longer therapy is associated with increased cost and more side effects. There are no strict guidelines for who should receive interferon treatment for chronic HCV infection. Factors that predict a favorable response to interferon include recent infection, minimally elevated ALT, absence of cirrhosis, low titer of virus in serum and certain hepatitis C genotypes (genetic variants).

A vaccine for HCV has not been developed, but is an active area of research. There are currently insufficient data to advocate the use of immune serum globulin for the prevention of HCV infection. Condoms should be used during the acute phase of the illness and indefinitely for patients who are immunocompromised. Couples in whom one is chronically infected with hepatitis C must make their own decision in regard to condom use after being advised of the risks; the risk of spread to regular sexual partners is 2–5%. Vertical transmission from a normal mother to her newborn is rare; however, the risk of HCV vertical transmission is much higher if the mother is co-infected by HIV.

5.1.4 *HEPATITIS D VIRUS*
Chronic hepatitis D usually results from HDV superinfection of an HBV carrier. Less commonly, acute HBV/HDV co-infection leads to chronic infection. Either way, chronic hepatitis D is usually aggressive and severe with rapid progression to cirrhosis.

The diagnosis is made by testing for anti-HDV in the serum of HBV carriers with risk factors for HDV infection. HDV antigen and HDV-RNA in serum or liver can also be measured, but only in a limited number of laboratories. In North America this virus is most often transmitted by intravenous drug abuse. In Mediterranean countries nonparenteral transmission may also occur. Treatment with interferon for HDV infection has been disappointing. Because of the dependency of HDV on HBV, prevention of HBV infection with vaccine can decrease HDV infection also.

5.2 Drug-Induced Chronic Hepatitis
Many drugs can cause chronic hepatitis. Whether to discontinue an implicated drug depends to some extent on whether the drug is merely causing persistent enzyme abnormalities or hepatic dysfunction with severe histologic abnormalities. In severe cases, fibrosis, cirrhosis and death from liver failure or complications of portal hypertension can result. Examples of drugs that are capable of causing chronic hepatitis that may progress to liver failure and portal hypertension are oxyphenisatin, isoniazid, nitrofurantoin, alpha methyldopa and dantrolene. On the other hand, if a drug is essential to the health of the patient and there are no unrelated agents that can be substituted, it is reasonable to continue therapy under close clinical supervision providing the enzyme abnormalities are mild and not associated with symptoms or functional derangements (i.e., serum bilirubin, albumin and INR/PT remain normal). Liver biopsy may be helpful in defining the severity of liver injury.

5.3 Autoimmune Hepatitis
Autoimmune hepatitis is an immunologically mediated disorder of the liver that often affects young females with a personal or family history of autoimmune disease. The etiology is unknown. The onset may be insidious or acute. The hepatic presentation can be that of sudden hepatic failure, chronic hepati-

TABLE 8.   Differentiating viral and alcoholic hepatitis

	Viral hepatitis	*Alcoholic hepatitis*
History	Risk factors	Significant alcoholic intake
Physical examination	Mild hepatomegaly, extrahepatic stigmata not prominent	Moderate to marked hepatomegaly, florid stigmata
Laboratory examination	AST variable ALT > AST	AST <300 AST > ALT (often 2:1 or more)
Liver biopsy	Mononuclear cells Portal tract centered Ground glass cells (HBV) Special stains (HBV)	Polymorphs Pericentral, diffuse Mallory's hyaline Fat

tis or inactive cirrhosis. The most common complaints include fatigue, amenorrhea, complaints associated with an accompanying rheumatological disorder such as arthritis, or those associated with thyroid disease. Physical findings include jaundice (in severe cases), spider nevi, palmar erythema and hepatosplenomegaly. Laboratory investigations reveal hypergammaglobulinemia with pronounced elevation of IgG levels, reduced serum albumin, positive antinuclear factor and smooth-muscle antibody. A proposed subclassification includes type 1 and type 2 autoimmune hepatitis, with the latter demonstrating antibodies to liver/kidney microsome (anti-LKM 1 hepatitis). Liver biopsy is essential to establish the diagnosis and severity of the underlying disease as well as to exclude other liver disease. Cirrhosis is present in over 50% of autoimmune hepatitis on initial biopsy.

Treatment is initiated with high-dose corticosteroids (prednisone 40–60 mg/day) for 4–6 weeks. The dose is then tapered to a maintenance level (e.g., 5–10 mg/day) just sufficient to keep the liver enzymes within normal values. Often azathioprine is used for its steroid-sparing effect. Following discontinuation of treatment, most patients will relapse, requiring reinitiation of therapy. Untreated autoimmune hepatitis progresses rapidly to cirrhosis (three to five years). Although corticosteroids may not prevent cirrhosis, they are clearly lifesaving in this otherwise fatal condition. With careful titration of their medication, most patients remain in stable condition for years. In the remaining minority, liver transplantation is highly successful.

5.4 Alcoholic Hepatitis

This condition is usually readily diagnosed on clinical grounds (see Section 6). These features are contrasted with those of viral hepatitis in Table 8.

5.5 Fatty Liver

Nonalcoholic hepatosteatonecrosis (fatty liver) is a common disorder, usually asymptomatic, found most commonly in patients who are obese, diabetic and, occasionally, hyperlipidemic. Mild right upper quadrant pain may be present with aminotransferase levels typically <3–4 times normal. The diagnosis can be established by ultrasound (or CT) examination of the liver or by liver biopsy showing macrovesicular fat. The treatment is that of the underlying condition, including weight loss and therapy of diabetes and hyperlipidemia. Most cases of fatty liver are not associated with inflammation and hepatocellular necrosis. However, 10–20% have nonalcoholoic steatohepatitis and have the potential to progress on to fibrosis and cirrhosis.

6. ALCOHOLIC LIVER DISEASE / F. Wong and L. Blendis

Liver disease is the fourth commonest cause of death in adults between the ages of 20 and 70 years in Canada. Alcohol is still the commonest cause of chronic liver disease in this country. Not all those who abuse alcohol develop liver damage: the incidence of cirrhosis among alcoholics is approximately 10–30%. The mechanism for the predisposition of certain people to develop cirrhosis is still unknown. The amount of alcohol ingested has been shown in epidemiological studies to be the most important factor in determining the development of cirrhosis. Males drinking in excess of 80 g and females in excess of 40 g of alcohol per day for 10 years are at a high risk of developing cirrhosis. The alcohol content rather than the type of beverage is important, and binge drinking is less injurious to the liver than continued daily drinking.

Women are more susceptible to liver damage than men. They are likely to develop cirrhosis at an earlier age, present at a later stage and have more severe liver disease with more complications. Genetics may play a role in the development of alcoholic liver disease, although no single genetic marker has been identified. Patterns of alcohol drinking behavior are inherited. Alcohol is metabolized to acetaldehyde by alcohol dehydrogenase and then to acetate by acetaldehyde dehydrogenase. Genetic pleomorphism of the enzyme systems that metabolize alcohol, leading to different rates of alcohol elimination, also contributes to the individual's susceptibility to alcohol damage. Alcoholics with decreased acetaldehyde dehydrogenase activity develop alcoholic liver disease at a lower cumulative intake than others. Malnutrition may play a permissive role in producing alcohol hepatotoxicity. However, there is a threshold of alcohol toxicity beyond which no dietary supplements can offer protection.

The spectrum of liver disease covers the relatively benign steatosis to the potentially fatal alcoholic hepatitis and cirrhosis.

6.1 Alcoholic Fatty Liver

Fatty liver is the most frequent hepatic abnormality found in alcoholics. It is a toxic manifestation of ethanol ingestion, appearing within three to seven days of excess alcohol intake. Metabolic changes associated with ethanol ingestion result in increased triglyceride synthesis, decreased lipid oxidation and impaired secretion by the liver. This results in the accumulation of triglycerides in the hepatocytes, mainly in the terminal hepatic venular zone. In more severe cases, the fatty change may be diffuse. The fat tends to accumulate as macrovesicular (large droplets), rather than microvesicular (small droplets), which represents mitochondrial damage. Fatty liver may occur alone or be part of the picture of alcoholic hepatitis or cirrhosis.

Clinically, the patient is usually asymptomatic, and the examination reveals a firm, smooth, enlarged liver. Occasionally the fatty liver may be so severe that the patient is anorexic and nauseated, and has right upper quadrant pain or discomfort. This usually follows a prolonged heavy alcoholic binge. Liver function tests including bilirubin, albumin and INR are usually normal, although the γ-glutamyl transpeptidase (GGT) is invariably elevated while the aminotransferases and alkaline phosphatase may be slightly increased. A fatty liver is usually detected by ultrasound. Liver biopsy is required to make a definitive diagnosis. When fatty liver is not associated with alcoholic hepatitis, its prognosis is excellent. Complete abstinence from alcohol and a nutritious diet will lead to disappearance of the fat over four to six weeks.

6.2 Alcoholic Hepatitis

Alcoholic hepatitis may occur separately or in combination with cirrhosis. There are all grades of severity. It is a condition characterized by liver cell necrosis and inflammatory reaction. Histologically, hepatocytes are swollen as a result of an increase in intracellular water secondary to increase in cytosolic proteins. Steatosis, often of the macrovesicular type, is present. Alcoholic hyaline (Mallory's) bodies are purplish red intracytoplasmic inclusions consisting of clumped organelles and intermediate microfilaments. Polymorphs are seen surrounding Mallory-containing cells and also within damaged hepatocytes. Collagen deposition is usually present. It is maximal in the zone 3 and extends in a perisinusoidal pattern to enclose hepatocytes, giving it a "chicken wiring" effect. Changes in the portal triad are inconspicuous. Marked portal inflammation suggests an associated viral hepatitis such as hepatitis C, whereas fibrosis suggests complicating chronic hepatitis. When the acute inflammation settles, a varying degree of fibrosis is seen, which may eventually lead to cirrhosis.

Clinically, mild cases of alcoholic hepatitis are recognized on liver biopsy only in patients who present with a history of alcohol abuse and abnormal liver enzymes. In the moderately severe case, the patient is usually malnourished and presents with a two- to three-week prodrome of fatigue, anorexia, nausea and weight loss. Clinical signs include a fever of <40°C, jaundice and tender hepatomegaly. In the most severe case, which usually follows a period of heavy drinking without eating, the patient is gravely ill with fever, marked jaundice, ascites, and evidence of a hyperdynamic circulation such as systemic hypotension and tachycardia. Florid palmar erythema and spider nevi are present, with or without gynecomastia. Hepatic decompensation can be precipitated by vomiting, diarrhea or intercurrent infection leading to encephalopathy. Hypoglycemia occurs often and can precipitate coma. Gastrointestinal bleeding is common, usually from a local gastric or duodenal lesion, resulting from the combination of a bleeding tendency and portal hypertension. Signs of malnutrition and vitamin deficiencies are common. Intake of moderate doses of acetaminophen in an alcoholic may precipitate florid alcoholic hepatitis.

Laboratory abnormalities include elevations of the aminotransferases, bilirubin, alkaline phosphatase and GGT. The aminotransferase levels rarely exceed 300 IU/L, except in association with acetaminophen ingestion; the AST/ALT ratio is usually >2. Hyperbilirubinemia can be quite marked, with levels reaching 300 to 500 μmol/L, and is a reflection of the severity of the illness. The increase in GGT is proportionally greater than that of alkaline phosphatase. There is also leukocytosis of up to 20–25 × 10⁹/L and increased INR/prothrombin time, which does not respond to vitamin K. The serum albumin falls. Serum IgA is markedly increased, with IgG and IgM raised to a lesser extent.

Patients with acute alcoholic hepatitis often deteriorate during the first few weeks in hospital, with a mortality rate of 20–50%. Bad prognostic indicators include spontaneous encephalopathy, markedly increased INR/PT unresponsive to vitamin K and severe hyperbilirubinemia of greater than 350 μmol/L. The condition may take one to six months to resolve, even with complete abstinence. Alcoholic hepatitis progresses to cirrhosis in 25–30% of clinical episodes.

6.3 Alcoholic Cirrhosis
Established cirrhosis is usually a disease of middle age after the patient has had many years of drinking. Although there may be a history of alcoholic hepatitis, cirrhosis can develop in apparently well-nourished, asymptomatic patients. Occasionally the patient may present with end-stage liver disease with malnutrition, ascites, encephalopathy and a bleeding tendency. A history of alcohol abuse usually points to the etiology. Clinically, the patient is wast-

ed. There may be bilateral parotid enlargement and Dupuytren's contracture in alcohol abuse. The patient may have palmar erythema and multiple spider nevi of chronic liver disease. Males develop gynecomastia and small testes. Hepatomegaly is often present, affecting predominantly the left lobe as a result of marked hypertrophy. There may be signs of portal hypertension, which include splenomegaly, ascites and distended abdominal wall veins. At the late stage, the liver may become shrunken and impalpable. There may be signs of alcohol damage in other organ systems, such as peripheral neuropathy and memory loss from cerebral atrophy. Alcoholic cirrhosis is also associated with renal problems, including IgA nephropathy, renal tubular acidosis and the development of hepatorenal syndrome. There is an association between hepatitis B and C and alcoholic cirrhosis.

Histologically, the cirrhosis is micronodular. The degree of steatosis is variable and alcoholic hepatitis may or may not be present. Pericellular fibrosis around hepatocytes is widespread. Portal fibrosis contributes to the development of portal hypertension. There may be increased parenchymal iron deposition. When parenchymal iron deposition is marked, genetic hemochromatosis has to be excluded. With continued cell necrosis and regeneration, the cirrhosis may progress to a macronodular pattern.

Biochemical abnormalities include a low serum albumin, and elevated bilirubin and aminotransferases. AST and ALT levels rarely exceed 300 IU/L and the AST/ALT ratio usually exceeds 2. GGT is disproportionately raised with recent alcohol ingestion and is a widely used screening test for alcohol abuse. With severe disease, the INR/PT may be increased. Portal hypertension results in hypersplenism leading to thrombocytopenia, anemia and leukopenia. Other nonspecific serum changes in acute and chronic alcoholics include elevations in uric acid, lactate and triglyceride, and reductions in glucose and magnesium.

The prognosis of alcoholic cirrhosis depends on whether the patient can abstain from alcohol; this in turn is related to family support, financial resources and socioeconomic state. Patients who abstain have a five-year survival rate of 60–70%, which falls to 40% in those who continue to drink. Women have a shorter survival rate than men. Bad prognostic indicators include a low serum albumin, increased INR/PT, low hemoglobin, encephalopathy, persistent jaundice and azotemia. Zone 3 fibrosis and perivenular sclerosis are also unfavorable features. Complete abstinence may not improve prognosis when portal hypertension is severe. Hepatocellular carcinoma occurs in 10% of stable cirrhotics. This usually develops after a period of abstinence when macronodular cirrhosis is present. It is usually fatal in six months.

6.4 Management

Early recognition of alcoholism is important. Physicians should have a high index of suspicion when a patient presents with anorexia, nausea, diarrhea, right upper quadrant tenderness and an elevated GGT. The most important therapeutic measure is total abstinence from alcohol. Support groups and regular follow-up can reinforce the need for abstinence. Withdrawal symptoms should be treated with chlordiazepoxide or diazepam. A nutritious, well-balanced diet with vitamin supplements should be instituted.

Alcoholic fatty liver responds to alcohol withdrawal and a nutritious diet. Patients with severe alcoholic hepatitis should be admitted to hospital and complications of liver failure treated appropriately. These patients usually have significant metabolic abnormalities that have to be corrected. Hyperglycemia is a common manifestation of chronic liver disease because of insulin resistance, whereas hypoglycemia is a manifestation of (especially fulminant) hepatic failure because of failure of gluconeogenesis and depletion of glycogen stores. Hypomagnesemia and hypokalemia are common as a result of reduced dietary intake and increased urinary excretion. Metabolic acidosis may be present, which may relate to the failure to convert lactic acid to pyruvate as well as possible underlying ketoacidosis. Specific treatments for alcoholic hepatitis include the use of corticosteroids. A recent meta-analysis of 11 controlled trials showed a significant benefit of steroids for patients with severe alcoholic hepatitis complicated by encephalopathy. Propylthiouracil has been used to dampen the hepatic hypermetabolic state in alcoholic hepatitis, and may reduce the two-year mortality rate. Testosterone and anabolic androgenic steroids have been tried with conflicting results. Intravenous amino acid supplements have been given to the severely protein malnourished with varying degrees of success. Oral supplementation is the preferred route if the patient can tolerate a diet.

Cirrhosis is an irreversible process, and therapy is directed at the complications of liver failure and portal hypertension, although colchicine has been used as an antifibrotic agent without much success. Portacaval shunts will reduce the risk of bleeding from esophageal varices, but the establishment of a shunt is associated with a 30% incidence of hepatic encephalopathy (see Section 11). Hepatic transplantation is a treatment option for patients with end-stage alcoholic cirrhosis, although the ethical issues surrounding the use of such a scarce resource for a self-inflicted disease still need to be settled. However, liver transplantation is a reasonable option in patients with alcoholic liver disease providing there is prolonged abstinence (at least six months), good social supports and no evidence of severe damage to other organs due to alcoholism. In the centers that transplant in cases of alcoholic cirrhosis, the results are comparable to those in patients with other forms of cirrhosis.

7. DRUG-INDUCED LIVER DISEASE / J.B. Simon

Drugs are an important and common cause of hepatic injury. This is not surprising, as the liver is the predominant site of drug clearance, biotransformation and excretion. Abnormalities cover a wide spectrum from minor nonspecific derangements to fulminant hepatic necrosis. The two most common, however, are acute inflammation and cholestasis, which can closely mimic viral hepatitis and biliary obstruction, respectively. Various other acute and chronic disease patterns also occur (as noted below). Thus drug-induced liver disease is complex, has protean manifestations, and can simulate a wide variety of other hepatic disorders.

The pathogenesis varies with the offending agent, and in most cases is poorly understood. Sometimes the drug or one of its metabolites exerts a direct toxic effect on liver membranes. This type of injury is predictable and dose-related, but is relatively infrequent. Much more commonly, the injury occurs unpredictably in only a tiny fraction of individuals receiving the drug and is independent of dosage. In some such instances genetic predisposition or idiosyncratic metabolism of the drug may be responsible. Immune hypersensitivity is often invoked, but only a minority of cases have concomitant evidence of an allergic reaction such as a rash, arthralgias or eosinophilia. Many instances of putative hypersensitivity may actually be due to toxic intermediate drug metabolites in rarely susceptible individuals. In most situations the reasons for individual susceptibility are unknown, and the precise pathogenesis of the hepatic injury is equally obscure.

Diagnosis requires first and foremost a careful history of drug ingestion, including over-the-counter and illicit agents as well as prescribed medications. A temporal association is also important in cases of acute dysfunction: injury typically develops within days or a few weeks of starting the drug. Other reactions involve chronic insidious injury and therefore require prolonged drug exposure – e.g., methotrexate fibrosis and oral contraceptive–induced adenomas. Liver biopsy sometimes provides an important clue to certain drug injuries, but more commonly the histologic pattern is nonspecific and/or mimics other primary liver disorders. Thus in many cases the diagnosis of drug injury remains uncertain or unproven even after appropriate patient assessment.

The prognosis is variable. Acute damage usually resolves when the offending agent is withdrawn, but cases of severe acute necrosis can be fatal or result in postnecrotic scarring. In cases of chronic injury, further hepatocellular damage and inflammation will generally cease when the drug is stopped, but any concomitant fibrosis will be irreversible.

No physician can know the innumerable drugs capable of producing liver

TABLE 9.   Drug-induced liver disease

Type and example	Pathogenesis
Acute hepatocellular injury	
Toxic necrosis (e.g., CCl$_4$, acetaminophen)	Membrane damage, some via toxic metabolite; dose-related, predictable
Hepatitis-like (e.g., isoniazid, methyldopa)	Idiosyncrasy; ? immune, ? metabolic; unpredictable, not dose-related
Cholestasis	
Inflammatory (e.g., chlorpromazine)	Unknown; unpredictable; periportal inflammation and cholestasis
Pure (e.g., oral contraceptives)	Exaggeration of normal hormonal effect on bile transport; ? genetic idiosyncrasy; pure cholestasis, no inflammation
Miscellaneous acute/subacute	Variable, usually unknown
Chronic liver disease	
Chronic hepatitis (e.g., isoniazid, methyldopa)	Idiosyncrasy; ? immune, ? metabolic
Chronic cholestasis (e.g., chlorpromazine)	Unknown; rare
Fibrosis/cirrhosis (e.g., methotrexate)	Dose-related, insidious toxic metabolic damage
Tumor: adenomas (oral contraceptives)	Unknown

injury. Rather, it is best to maintain a constant awareness of the possibility, to understand the general types of damage, and to learn the most common agents responsible for each. Table 9 gives an arbitrary classification and examples of drug-induced hepatic injury. A few of the more important examples are briefly discussed below.

7.1 Acute Hepatocellular Injury
This takes at least two distinct forms, both characterized clinically and bio-chemically by features of acute liver cell destruction.

7.1.1 TOXIC NECROSIS
This involves direct membrane damage by the parent drug or a toxic metabolite. It is therefore dose-related and a predictable occurrence in anyone ingesting a sufficient quantity of the drug. Sometimes the histologic injury is characteristic – e.g., zonal necrosis and fat in carbon tetrachloride toxicity.

Acetaminophen is the most important example. This widely used analgesic is largely excreted as harmless conjugates, but a portion is transformed by hepatic microsomes to toxic intermediate metabolites. Normally these are safely eliminated by conjugation with hepatic glutathione, but a large enough dose of acetaminophen will deplete the available glutathione stores. Once this occurs, cell necrosis results from binding of the toxic intermediates to liver macromolecules. The threshold injurious dose of acetaminophen is usually about 10–15 g acutely; this is far beyond the normal dosage and is generally ingested only in suicide attempts. Alcoholics are susceptible at much lower dosage, however, as a result of heightened microsomal transformation coupled with nutritional depletion of glutathione. Acetaminophen should be suspected in an alcoholic with extremely high AST/ALT levels, as values rarely exceed 300 μmol/L in uncomplicated alcoholic hepatitis. Another clue to acetaminophen toxicity is a disproportionately elevated INR.

Acetaminophen hepatotoxicity typically becomes apparent only 36 to 48 hours after ingestion; by then it is too late to modify the process. Fortunately, injury is successfully aborted by early therapy with N-acetylcysteine, which repletes hepatic glutathione levels. This should be given within 10 to 16 hours of acetaminophen ingestion to be effective, though some benefit may be achieved even at 24 to 36 hours. To guide therapy, nomograms are available relating the probability of liver injury to blood acetaminophen levels and to the amount of time since ingestion.

7.1.2 ACUTE HEPATITIS

This pattern of injury closely mimics acute viral hepatitis clinically, biochemically and histologically. Unlike toxic necrosis, it occurs unpredictably, is not dose-related and affects only rare individuals exposed to the drug. Reasons for the idiosyncratic susceptibility are obscure. Numerous agents can produce this injury pattern; methyldopa, isoniazid and halothane are classic examples, the latter usually producing damage only after repeated exposure to the anesthetic. Acute isoniazid hepatitis occasionally develops only after several months of drug therapy. This is an exception to the general rule of a temporal relationship, and the association may therefore be overlooked.

7.2 Cholestasis

This type of reaction also takes at least two distinct forms.

7.2.1 INFLAMMATORY TYPE

Chlorpromazine, other phenothiazines and many other drugs can produce an acute periportal necro-inflammatory reaction. This is characterized clinically and biochemically by a predominant cholestatic disorder with variable fea-

TABLE 10.   Hepatobiliary reactions to oral contraceptives

Cholestasis

Tumors
  Adenomas
  Focal nodular hyperplasia?
  Hepatocellular carcinoma (rare)

Vascular
  Budd-Chiari syndrome ($\uparrow$ clotting tendency)
  Peliosis hepatis (subclinical)

Gallstones ($\uparrow$ lithogenicity of bile)

"Unmasking" of other cholestatic disorders

---

tures of concomitant inflammation. Differentiation from extrahepatic biliary obstruction is usually required.

7.2.2 PURE TYPE

Certain steroid hormonal drugs, most notably oral contraceptives and methyltestosterone, can produce relatively pure impairment of bile flow with little or no associated hepatocellular injury (bland cholestasis). This appears to be due to an idiosyncratic exaggeration of the physiologic effect of sex hormones on bile canalicular transport, and may have a genetic component. The patient typically develops insidiously progressive pruritus, dark urine, and jaundice without associated systemic symptoms. Laboratory tests show high ALP with normal or minimally elevated AST/ALT levels. The liver biopsy is usually unremarkable aside from histologic cholestasis. Women who develop this reaction to oral contraceptives are predisposed to cholestasis of pregnancy, which appears to be similar or identical in pathogenesis (see Section 17).

Oral contraceptives are also associated with other, less common hepatobiliary effects. These are listed in Table 10.

7.3 Miscellaneous Acute and Subacute Reactions

Many hepatic drug reactions involve a variable mixture of hepatocellular and excretory impairments that do not neatly fit any of the above categories. Laboratory and histologic features are variable and nonspecific. Occasionally granulomatous inflammation occurs (e.g., with sulfonamides), often with acute systemic features. Differentiation from an infective granulomatous disorder may be challenging. A few drugs can produce an alcoholic hepatitis–like picture, including typical histologic features (e.g., amiodarone). Other unusual patterns of drug injury have also been described.

7.4 Chronic Liver Disease
Though the large majority of drug-induced hepatic injury is acute or subacute, in a few reactions there is an insidious development of chronic disease. These vary in type.

7.4.1 CHRONIC HEPATITIS
A few agents that induce acute hepatitis are also capable of producing chronic inflammation if drug ingestion continues. Methyldopa and isoniazid are the prime examples. Clinically, biochemically and histologically the reaction may be indistinguishable from idiopathic or immune chronic hepatitis. The disorder typically resolves when the drug intake ceases.

7.4.2 CHRONIC CHOLESTASIS
In rare instances chlorpromazine cholestatic injury becomes prolonged and self-perpetuating even though the drug is discontinued. This can simulate primary biliary cirrhosis, though immunologic features of the latter are lacking.

7.4.3 FIBROSIS/CIRRHOSIS
Insidiously progressive hepatic fibrosis and eventual cirrhosis can occur from methotrexate, some chemotherapeutic agents, and chronic ingestion of arsenicals or vitamin A in megadoses. Scarring typically develops subclinically and with little or no biochemical evidence of hepatic dysfunction. Liver biopsy is therefore the only way to establish the diagnosis. Patients receiving long-term methotrexate therapy for psoriasis or rheumatoid arthritis should generally undergo biopsy after cumulative drug dosage reaches about 1.5 g, and at occasional intervals thereafter.

7.4.4 TUMORS
Prolonged intake of oral contraceptives is associated with an increased risk of developing benign hepatic adenomas. These are usually asymptomatic but occasionally produce an acute abdomen due to intraperitoneal rupture and hemorrhage. In rare instances, oral contraceptive–induced adenomas become malignant.

Other unusual drug-related tumors are known to occur as well – e.g., angiosarcoma from chronic exposure to vinyl chloride.

8. INHERITED LIVER DISEASE / P. Adams

8.1 Hemochromatosis

Hemochromatosis is an iron-storage disorder in which there is an inappropriate increase in the absorption of iron from the gut. This leads to iron deposition in various organs with eventual impairment, especially of the liver, pancreas, heart and pituitary gland. The term *hemochromatosis* is preferred for genetic hemochromatosis, with other diseases associated with iron overload such as thalassemia or a sideroblastic anemia referred to as *secondary iron overload*. The term *hemosiderosis* merely describes the appearance histologically of increased stainable tissue iron.

Genetic hemochromatosis is an inherited disease known to be associated with an abnormal gene tightly linked to the A locus of the HLA complex on chromosome 6. A candidate gene has been described (HLA-H) that encodes for a protein with similarities to MHC class-I proteins. It is one of the most common genetic diseases, inherited as an autosomal recessive trait affecting 1 in 300 of the Caucasian population. The heterozygous individual has normal or minor derangements in iron metabolism that have no clinical significance. The homozygote has continued iron accumulation leading to target organ damage. Normally the body iron content of 3–4 g is maintained such that the absorption of iron is equal to iron loss. In hemochromatosis, the absorption of iron is inappropriate to the needs of the body, resulting in the absorption of 4 mg/day or more. In advanced disease, the total body iron accumulation may be 40–60 g.

Most patients are asymptomatic until the fifth or sixth decade, at which time they may present with nonspecific symptoms of arthritis, diabetes, fatigue or hepatomegaly. Other symptoms include pigmentation of the skin, impotence and dyspnea secondary to congestive heart failure. The classic triad of skin pigmentation, diabetes and liver disease ("bronze diabetes") occurs in a minority of patients and is a late stage of the disease. It more commonly affects males than females because of the regular menstrual blood loss in women. The dark skin color in hemochromatosis is attributed to melanin deposition but evolves in tandem with iron deposition in the skin.

A patient with suspected hemochromatosis or unexplained liver disease should be screened for the disease with a serum ferritin and transferrin saturation (serum iron/TIBC). These test abnormalities increase with age and are more abnormal in males than females because of the regular menstrual blood loss in women. The diagnosis is confirmed by a liver biopsy that demonstrates marked parenchymal iron deposition with iron staining of the tissue. The hepatic iron concentration and the hepatic iron index (hepatic iron concentration/age) are the most helpful in distinguishing genetic hemochromatosis from the increased iron overload that is seen in other chronic liver diseases such as alcoholic liver disease and chronic hepatitis C. CT and MRI scanning can detect moderate to marked iron overload in the liver but lack the sensitivity to detect early disease and do not replace the need for liver biopsy.

The treatment of hemochromatosis involves the removal of excess body iron and supportive treatment of the damaged organs. Iron is best removed from the body by weekly or twice-weekly phlebotomy of 500 mL of blood until the body iron stores are within normal limits. The duration of treatment varies with the age and sex of the patient, but older males may require weekly venesections for more than three years. Serum ferritin is measured every three months to assess progress. When the serum ferritin is in the low normal range the frequency of venesections is decreased to three or four per year. The goal of therapy is to prevent any further tissue damage. Unfortunately, many of the symptoms do not improve following iron depletion. The most common cause of death is liver failure and/or hepatocellular carcinoma.

Siblings of the patient with hemochromatosis must be screened with serum ferritin and transferrin saturation, as the siblings have a 1 in 4 chance of being affected. Screening should begin in the teenage years. Screening of the general population for hemochromatosis has been demonstrated to be cost-effective but has not been widely implemented. The development of a low-cost true genetic test for hemochromatosis could lead to more widespread screening. Chelating agents such as deferoxamine (parenteral) or deferiprone (oral) are reserved for the patient with iron overload secondary to an iron-loading anemia such as thalassemia.

8.2 Alpha$_1$-Antitrypsin Deficiency

Alpha$_1$-antitrypsin, a glycoprotein produced by the liver, constitutes the majority of the α_1 globulin fraction seen on protein electrophoresis. Its deficiency is inherited, resulting in pulmonary emphysema and hepatic disease. Various presentations are possible, including neonatal hepatitis, chronic active hepatitis, cirrhosis and hepatocellular carcinoma.

Alpha$_1$-antitrypsin is a protease inhibitor. Its production is controlled by multiple alleles in the Pi system. Normal individuals are PiMM. The inheritance is autosomal codominant. Patients with liver disease most frequently have PiZZ and possess only 20% of the normal amount of serum α_1-antitrypsin.

Diagnosis of α_1-antitrypsin deficiency is suggested by the absence of the α_1 peak on protein electrophoresis and is confirmed by α_1-antitrypsin levels and phenotyping. The characteristic changes seen on liver biopsy include the presence of PAS-positive, diastase-resistant granules in the cytoplasm of the hepatocytes; these granules are α_1-antitrypsin collections within the endoplasmic reticulum. There is an inability to transfer synthesized α_1-antitrypsin from the cytoplasm of the hepatocyte to the serum. Cirrhosis will develop in 10–15% of patients with PiZZ. The risk to heterozygotes of developing liver disease is uncertain. Experimental medical therapies including infusion of recombinant α_1-antitrypsin and gene therapy may become a possibility in the future. Patients with advanced forms of liver disease may be candidates for liver transplantation.

8.3 Wilson's Disease
Wilson's disease is an inherited disorder characterized by the pathological accumulation of copper in the liver, central nervous system and other organs. The disease has a prevalence of 1:30,000. It is an autosomal recessive disease; the gene responsible has been localized to the long arm of chromosome 13 (ATP7B). The gene product is a copper-transporting ATPase that is highly expressed in the liver. It may present as pediatric liver disease or may have a neuropsychiatric presentation in adults. The hepatic presentation of the disease is variable, and may include fulminant hepatic failure (often with hemolysis), chronic active hepatitis and cirrhosis. Copper deposition in the central nervous system results in extrapyramidal symptoms of rigidity, choreoathetoid movements and ataxia. Biochemical abnormalities include a low serum ceruloplasmin and high urinary copper concentration. Liver biopsy is often not diagnostic, and copper stains are unreliable. It is often necessary to measure the hepatic copper concentration. A Kayser-Fleischer ring – a copper deposition in Descemet's membrane of the cornea – is characteristic of the disease, although it can appear in other chronic cholestatic liver diseases. Visual inspection may identify the Kayser-Fleischer ring, but a detailed slit lamp examination by an ophthalmologist is recommended when the disease is suspected. The chelating agent d-penicillamine is recommended on a lifelong basis. Alternative drug therapies are available for those intolerant of penicillamine. Patients with advanced disease can be successfully cured of the disease by liver transplantation.

9. CHOLESTASIS / J. Heathcote

Cholestasis simply means failure of flow of bile. The cause of this failure can arise anywhere in the biliary system, from the liver cell down to the ampulla of Vater. For clinical purposes it is easiest to think of cholestasis as being either intra- or extrahepatic (Table 11).

9.1 Intrahepatic Cholestasis
Drug toxicity is the commonest cause of cholestasis occurring at the cellular

TABLE 11.   Major causes of cholestasis

Intrahepatic
Common
   Viral hepatitis
   Drugs
   Alcoholic hepatitis ± cirrhosis

Less common
   Primary biliary cirrhosis
   Chronic hepatitis ± cirrhosis
   Metastatic carcinoma
   Cholestasis of pregnancy
   Sepsis, TPN, etc.

Extrahepatic
Common
   Common bile duct stone(s)
   Pancreatic/periampullary cancer

Less common
   Benign biliary stricture
   Sclerosing cholangitis
   Bile duct carcinoma
   Benign pancreatic disease
   Extrinsic duct compression

---

level. The injury may be predictable, as with estrogens (for example), or unpredictable, as with most idiopathic drug reactions. (However, as more intracellular mechanisms become understood – e.g., the polymorphic nature of drug-metabolizing enzymes – fewer reactions will be found to be "unpredictable.") Histologically and clinically, cholestatic drug reactions can be considered as "bland" or "inflammatory."

Systemic sepsis is often associated with cholestasis. Endotoxins have been shown to affect both intracellular and canalicular function. If sepsis occurs on a background of cirrhosis, the cholestasis is much more profound.

Most acute and chronic liver diseases exert a cholestatic effect via interruption of intracellular transport mechanisms or damage to the small interlobular bile ducts. Damage to small bile ducts is not at all unusual in acute and chronic hepatitis, particularly with hepatitis C. Cholestasis is also a common feature of relapsing hepatitis A, but does not carry any particular significance.

Several chronic liver diseases specifically target the intrahepatic and sometimes the extrahepatic bile ducts. The diseases of the liver that are associated with paucity of bile ducts are numerous. Primary biliary cirrhosis (PBC) and primary sclerosing cholangitis (PSC) are the best-known examples; other diseases that destroy bile ducts are chronic drug reactions, chronic rejection, graft-versus-host disease and chronic septic cholangitis, to name but a few.

In children, intrahepatic bile duct paucity may be syndromatic (Alagille's) or nonsyndromatic (e.g., postviral, PSC). PSC is commonly misdiagnosed as autoimmune hepatitis in children, as overt cholestasis may be absent. Cystic fibrosis may give rise to focal biliary cirrhosis as a result of inspissated bile in the ducts.

Many infiltrations may cause a biochemical cholestatic pattern of liver disease, generally anicteric – e.g., sarcoidosis, lymphomas, amyloid and granulomas of any etiology.

There is a very rare condition called "benign recurrent cholestasis" whose mechanism is not understood at all. Several rare congenital conditions, often associated with secretion of abnormal bile acids, result in severe chronic cholestasis in infants. In children, total parenteral nutrition is a well-recognised cause of cholestasis that is thought to be due to the amino acid content interrupting bile acid uptake by the liver.

9.2 Extrahepatic Cholestasis

Diseases of the large bile ducts are generally due to stones, strictures or tumors. The AIDS epidemic has brought its own forms of cholestatic problems: fungal, protozoal and viral cholangitis. Malignant tumors causing biliary obstruction now include Kaposi's sarcoma, lymphoma, and the more common pancreatic and bile duct carcinomas.

9.3 Primary Biliary Cirrhosis (PBC)

9.3.1 *DIAGNOSIS*

The more accurate term for this disease is chronic nonsuppurative granulomatous cholangitis. It predominantly affects women in middle age and is frequently associated with autoimmune phenomena outside the liver (renal tubular acidosis, vitiligo, thyroiditis, sicca syndrome, CREST syndrome, rheumatoid arthritis and, less often, glomerulonephritis and vasculitis). It is therefore presumed that PBC is also an autoimmune disease, although the inciting antigen has not been identified.

PBC is rarely diagnosed at the first visit, because one-third or more of patients are asymptomatic. The biochemical pattern seen in PBC is typically cholestatic: elevated alkaline phosphatase, GGT and 5'NT, with modest elevations of the aminotransferases. An elevated bilirubin is associated with progressive, symptomatic disease, indicating a poor prognosis. The most common symptom of this illness is fatigue, very hard to define yet very distress-

TABLE 12. Diagnostic features of primary biliary cirrhosis

Elevated serum alkaline phosphatase
Elevated serum cholesterol
Antimitochondrial antibody positive
Typical liver histology
Normal ERCP

---

ing to the patient. Other symptoms include pruritus, xanthelasma and, later in the course of the disease, ascites, jaundice and encephalopathy. Portal hypertension occurs early in this disease, as it is presinusoidal in nature; thus, variceal hemorrhage may be a presenting symptom. Many patients with PBC present with nonhepatic associations first. Raynaud's osteoporosis, sicca syndrome and rheumatoid arthritis are the most common. Some patients with PBC have been misdiagnosed as having the chronic fatigue syndrome.

The diagnostic hallmarks for PBC include a cholestatic serum biochemistry as described above, elevated serum cholesterol, elevated serum IgM and a positive mitochondrial antibody test. If all these features are present, a diagnostic liver biopsy is not essential. The biopsy is subject to great sampling error and all four "stages" may be seen in one specimen (Table 12).

9.3.2 MANAGEMENT

The management of PBC includes symptomatic, preventive and specific measures.

There is little one can do for the fatigue, although a sympathetic and understanding ear helps. Pruritus can generally be controlled by using the anion exchange resin, cholestyramine. There are, however, many who suffer gastrointestinal side effects from this drug, so rifampin 150 mg b.i.d. or t.i.d. can be tried instead. Ultraviolet light also helps, so that pruritus is less in the summer. A trip down south always helps in the winter!

For the most part, the complications of long-term cholestasis can be prevented, except for the osteoporosis. Once the serum bilirubin is elevated, steatorrhea may occur with subsequent malabsorption of fat-soluble vitamins. Vitamin A and D supplements are available in water-soluble form, and vitamin K is best given parenterally. The fat intake should not be reduced. Although this may reduce the steatorrhea, it will also result in massive weight loss and will not affect the serum cholesterol. Despite the hypercholesterolemia, there is no increase in incidence of ischemic heart disease in PBC. A low-cholesterol diet will not affect the high serum cholesterol as the elevation is due to failure of biliary excretion. So far nothing has been found to help the osteoporosis, which may cause wedging of the vertebrae, although calci-

TABLE 13.   Comparison of PBC and PSC

	PBC	*PSC*
Symptoms	Often none/pruritus	Often none
Biochemistry	Elevated ALP	Elevated ALP
Serum bilirubin	Slow rise	Fluctuates
Non-organ specific Ab	AMA+ve	AMA–ve
Liver histology	Helpful in diagnosis/staging	Helpful in staging
ERCP	Normal	Abnormal

um supplementation of the diet is always recommended in addition to vitamin D supplements.

Many specific therapies for PBC have been tried, none with resounding success. Some are definitely contraindicated – notably prednisone, because it promotes osteoporosis. Recently, treatment with ursodeoxycholic acid (UDCA) has been studied. It has very few side effects and causes a dramatic fall in all the biochemical markers for this disease, and recently has been shown to improve survival in PBC patients. Untreated, the mean survival of symptomatic PBC is 12 years. Treatment with UDCA in a dose of 13–15 mg/kg/day results in a 31% increase in survival after four years of therapy. The survival of those with asymptomatic disease is much longer. The ultimate treatment is liver transplantation; PBC patients do very well, with a 92% one-year survival rate, though recurrence in the allograft has been reported.

9.4 Secondary Biliary Cirrhosis

Any disease that permanently and progressively damages bile ducts and is not caused by PBC may lead to secondary biliary cirrhosis, sometimes (although not usually) in the absence of overt jaundice. The most obvious cause is biliary atresia; other pediatric conditions include the various hypoplastic duct syndromes, other biliary tree abnormalities – Caroli's disease, choledochal cysts, sclerosing cholangitis – and cystic fibrosis, which causes focal biliary cirrhosis. In adults the commonest cause of secondary biliary cirrhosis is probably primary sclerosing cholangitis (PSC), although iatrogenic bile duct strictures also feature.

Primary sclerosing cholangitis is the most common cause of secondary biliary cirrhosis in adults. It affects about 10% of patients with ulcerative colitis or Crohn's colitis, although 30% of patients with PSC have no background of inflammatory bowel disease at the time of presentation. Patients are commonly asymptomatic. Just as with PBC, PSC causes presinusoidal portal hypertension, so variceal bleeding may present early – i.e., prior to the onset of jaundice (Table 13). A cholestatic enzyme pattern in any patient with liver problems should prompt the suspicion of PSC. The diagnosis is made only by ERCP, never by liver biopsy. Because liver biopsy is not helpful diagnostically it is performed only to see if the patient is cirrhotic. If PSC is suspected prior to ERCP, then antibiotic coverage should be given at the time of the procedure. Sepsis is the major complication of this disease and needs to be avoided if possible, as infection outside the liver precludes liver transplantation – the treatment of choice for decompensated disease. Prior to transplantation the only treatment available is symptomatic and/or preventive, as described for PBC. As yet there have been no therapeutic trials of any reasonable size performed in PSC and hence there is no standard therapeutic intervention, although UDCA therapy certainly leads to a fall in the serum markers of cholestasis and theoretically it should improve the bile flow.

9.5 Approach to the Patient with Cholestasis

9.5.1 *DIAGNOSIS*
The history in any patient is always of utmost importance. A complete drug history should be taken, including prescribed and over-the-counter drugs. A past history of cholecystectomy should never be forgotten; common bile duct stones are not unusual, even in the absence of symptoms and/or dilated bile ducts on ultrasound. Manifestations of other autoimmune disease should be sought. A history of chills and fever would make one suspect extrahepatic (nonmalignant) biliary disease.

Examination should make special note of the patient's temperature. Signs of chronic cholestasis include scratch marks, shiny nails, increased skin pigmentation, xanthelasma, xanthomatous neuropathy, and jaundice, which in its later stages takes on a greenish hue. Hepatosplenomegaly is common in PBC, PSC and biliary atresia, and with infiltrations like lymphoma.

9.5.2 *LABORATORY CONFIRMATION*
The standard biochemical tests are most helpful. Liver function tends to remain normal for long periods in patients with anicteric cholestasis, but the enzyme markers – alkaline phosphatase, GGT, 5′NT – are always elevated. In those with prolonged jaundice, coagulation abnormalities (correctable with vitamin K) are common. If the results of these tests confirm the clinical suspicion, then the next step is an ultrasound to look at the bile ducts. If there is jaundice associated with fever or chills, there should be no delay with the ultrasound examination of the abdomen.

9.5.3 *FURTHER MANAGEMENT*
Further management will depend entirely on whether the patient has dilated

ducts. If the ducts are dilated, the management will be interventional. If the ducts are not dilated but there is still a suspicion that the problem lies in the extrahepatic biliary system (common bile duct stones following cholecystectomy, PSC), then an ERCP may still be indicated. In most circumstances, an ERCP is a more helpful and safer method of investigating extrahepatic biliary obstruction, although if the local expertise is not available, a percutaneous cholangiogram (PTC) may be necessary. The true value of magnetic resonance cholangiography (MRC) is yet to be assessed.

If the history, physical and ultrasound all support a diagnosis of intrahepatic cholestasis, then a liver biopsy may be indicated to make a diagnosis, if this is not already obvious at the bedside (e.g., sepsis, drug reactions). Cholestatic drug reactions may take many months to clear after the drug has been withdrawn. A clinical diagnosis of PBC needs to be confirmed by a positive antimitochondrial antibody test +/- a liver biopsy.

There will always be patients in whom no diagnosis can be made immediately. In the absence of jaundice, the physician has time to observe. Granulomas of the liver are the most likely cause of a "missed" diagnosis on biopsy. Electromicroscopy may be helpful when a drug reaction is suspected.

10. CIRRHOSIS OF THE LIVER / J. Heathcote

Cirrhosis is a chronic diffuse liver disease that is characterized by fibrosis and nodule formation. Fibrosis is not synonymous with cirrhosis. Nodule formation with disturbed architecture is essential for the diagnosis of cirrhosis. The condition results from liver cell necrosis and the collapse of hepatic lobules due to many factors such as inflammation or ischemia. Recovery occurs with formation of diffuse fibrous septa and nodular regrowth of hepatocytes. Thus, the ultimate histologic pattern is the same regardless of etiology. Liver cell necrosis is often absent when the liver is ultimately examined either by biopsy or at post mortem.

10.1 Etiology
Known causes of cirrhosis account for about 90–95% of the cases. Most common etiologies include alcoholism, autoimmune chronic hepatitis and chronic viral hepatitis (Table 14). Less common causes include hemochromatosis, primary biliary cirrhosis, sclerosing cholangitis, drug-induced liver disease and chronic biliary obstruction. Other causes include α_1-antitrypsin deficiency, severe steatohepatitis in the morbidly obese and Wilson's disease. The remaining 5–10% of patients with cirrhosis of the liver have no known cause, a condition termed *cryptogenic cirrhosis*. Over the last 10 years, the rate of

TABLE 14.   Causes of cirrhosis

Alcohol

Viral hepatitis
   Hepatitis B
   Hepatitis C
   Hepatitis D

Metabolic
   Hemochromatosis
   Wilson's disease
   α_1-antitrypsin deficiency
   Galactosemia
   Type IV glycogenosis

Cholestatic
   Sclerosing cholangitis

Autoimmune
   Primary biliary cirrhosis
   Chronic active hepatitis

Drug-induced

Congestive

Cystic fibrosis

---

cryptogenic cirrhosis has fallen from 30% to current levels. The most likely cause for this fall has been the availability of testing for hepatitis C.

The etiology of the cirrhosis usually cannot be determined by the pathologic appearance of the liver (with some notable exceptions, including hemochromatosis and α_1-antitrypsin deficiency). Terms previously used such as *portal cirrhosis* or *postnecrotic cirrhosis* have been replaced by classifications that include three anatomic categories.

10.2 Pathology

Micronodular cirrhosis is characterized by thick, regular septa, by regenerating small nodules of uniform size and by involvement of every lobule. Often associated with the persistence of the injurious agent, this may represent the liver's relative impairment for regeneration, as may be seen in alcoholism, old age, ischemia and malnutrition.

Macronodular cirrhosis is characterized by nodules of variable size, some containing large areas of intact or regenerating parenchyma within each large nodule.

FIGURE 12.   Shown is a mixed macronodular and micronodular cirrhosis. The hepatic lobular architecture has been destroyed and replaced by nodular masses of regenerated cells (N). Fibrous tissue surrounds the nodules. (Retic. stain, original magnification × 37)

Mixed macronodular and micronodular cirrhosis may result from vigorous regrowth in a previous micronodular cirrhosis (Figure 12).

10.3 Clinical Features

The clinical features of cirrhosis relate to those features that are peculiar to the cause of the cirrhosis but more importantly to the magnitude of the hepatocellular failure and the presence of portal hypertension, along with the ability of the surviving hepatocytes to compensate for the loss. Thus, patients often are categorized as having latent, compensated disease or active, decompensated disease, each having its own clinical pathologic correlations. In the fully compensated state, there may be no symptoms whatever, the disease being suspected by a finding of an enlarged liver or spleen. With progression of the disease, features of hepatocellular failure and portal hypertension emerge.

With hepatocellular failure, patients may complain of weakness, fatigue, weight loss and a general deterioration of health. Physical examination may reveal the stigmata of chronic liver disease, although these are often missing in those with chronic viral hepatitis (see Section 2).

The ease of diagnosis of cirrhosis is dependent on the degree of liver decompensation. A high index of suspicion is necessary; the condition may be revealed only by a positive history of excess alcohol ingestion along with the finding of hepatomegaly. Thorough inquiry into all the risk factors for acquisition of viral hepatitis needs to be made, including blood transfusion, injection drug use (ever), tattoos, body piercing and multiple sexual partners. In decompensated disease, the diagnosis is much easier; the clinical features of ascites, asterixis, variceal hemorrhage, jaundice and other signs of hepatocellular failure may be present.

Biochemical tests attempt to identify the specific etiology of the liver disease and to assess the degree of hepatocellular dysfunction. With deteriorating hepatic function, albumin falls, serum bilirubin rises and the INR/prothrombin time becomes increased and not correctable by parenteral vitamin K. Liver enzymes, while helpful in assessing ongoing activity, are not of much help in assessment of the functional severity, as serum aminotransferases may be only mildly elevated despite severe liver disease. Alkaline phosphatase is usually raised, but the level does not reflect the degree of hepatic dysfunction. Commonly a normochromic, normocytic anemia is found, with target cells noted in the blood smear. Occasionally a macrocytic anemia presents, but if gastrointestinal bleeding has been occurring, the anemia may be microcytic as a result of iron loss. Depressed leukocyte and platelet counts may be present secondary to hypersplenism. The urine often contains urobilinogen and bilirubin if the patient is jaundiced. Patients with ascites exhibit a marked reduction in urinary sodium excretion. The radioisotope scan will show patchy uptake by the liver with redistribution to the spleen and bone marrow. Increased radioisotope uptake in the bone marrow (on scan) is reflected by uptake in the spine. Ultrasound of the abdomen is the most helpful imaging test and will reveal an inhomogeneous nodular liver with splenomegaly. A CT scan is rarely needed. These tests do not establish the diagnosis of cirrhosis, which can be made only by a liver biopsy with histologic examination. Liver biopsy may also be helpful in establishing an etiology and degree of activity of the underlying process. When a persistent coagulopathy or ascites is present, biopsy via the transjugular route is necessary.

Prognosis depends on the degree of hepatocellular function and the etiology, as well as on whether any causative agents can be removed. Clearly the prognosis is improved if the alcoholic patient can abstain, if the patient with hemochromatosis has iron removed by venesection or if excessive copper is removed in those with Wilson's disease. In addition, vigorous medical care may prolong life and delay or prevent eventual complications such as ascites

TABLE 15.   Criteria for Child-Pugh classification

Group designation	A	B	C
Serum bilirubin (μmol/L)	Below 34.2	34.2–51.3	Over 51.3
Serum albumin (g/L)	Over 35	30–35	Under 30
Ascites	None	Easily controlled	Poorly controlled
Neurological disorder	None	Minimal	Advanced "coma"
Nutrition	Excellent	Good	Poor, "wasting"

and variceal bleeding. All cirrhotics should be advised to avoid aspirin or NSAIDs (which promote GI bleeding and ascites), aminoglycoside antibiotics (which promote renal failure), ACE inhibitors (which promote ascites) and narcotics (which promote encephalopathy). All episodes of infection should be treated promptly, as septicemia leads to rapid deterioration in a cirrhotic. Beta blockers should be considered for prophylaxis against variceal hemorrhage in all cirrhotics with grade II or larger varices. Once decompensated liver disease is present (jaundice, ascites, neurologic impairment, bleeding, coagulopathy, hyponatremia) the prognosis is poor and liver transplant should be considered, if appropriate.

10.4 Treatment

Clearly, where there is a specific treatment for the underlying etiology of the liver disease this should be offered. All patients should consume a healthy, adequate diet and avoid alcohol. Otherwise the management is that of regular surveillance and early detection of hepatocellular failure. Hepatocellular failure or decompensated cirrhosis may be manifested by any of the following: coagulopathy, jaundice (in noncholestatic liver disease), hepatic encephalopathy, variceal bleeding or ascites. The Child-Pugh classification of cirrhosis, which is a very useful guide to calculate the risk of an invasive procedure, takes into account these variables, plus nutritional status (Table 15). Once decompensation occurs, management includes the control of ascites, avoidance of drugs that are poorly metabolized by the liver and the prompt treatment of infection and variceal hemorrhage. Liver transplantation is now becoming the treatment of choice for many with end-stage decompensated liver disease (see Section 15).

11. PORTAL HYPERTENSION / S.S. Lee

Portal hypertension is defined as increased pressure in the portal vein. With the right atrial pressure as a zero reference, normal portal venous pressure is

TABLE 16.   Causes of portal hypertension

Prehepatic	⎫
Splenic AV fistula	
Splenic or portal vein thrombosis	
Massive splenomegaly	
Intrahepatic	
Sarcoidosis	
Schistosomiasis	Presinusoidal
Nodular regenerative hyperplasia	
Congenital hepatic fibrosis	
Idiopathic portal fibrosis	
Early primary biliary cirrhosis	
Chronic active hepatitis	
Myeloproliferative disorders	
Graft-vs-host disease	⎭
Established cirrhosis	⎤ Sinusoidal
Alcoholic hepatitis	⎦
Alcoholic terminal hyaline sclerosis	⎫
Veno-occlusive disease	
Posthepatic	Postsinusoidal
Budd-Chiari syndrome	
Membranous IVC web	
Right heart failure	
Constrictive pericarditis	⎭

approximately 4–8 mm Hg. The portal vein is formed by the confluence of the splenic and superior mesenteric veins. Its flow rate normally averages about 1–1.2 L/min. The simple phenomenon of increased pressure in this venous circulation unleashes a wide array of hemodynamic and metabolic consequences, including some of the most lethal and distressing complications of chronic liver disease.

11.1 Etiology

The causes of portal hypertension are diverse (Table 16). Since portal pressure is the product of portal blood flow and intrahepatic resistance, any condition causing an increase in flow or resistance will increase portal pressure. An example of a "pure" flow increase is postsurgical or traumatic splenic arteriovenous fistula. The marked increase in splenic and thus portal venous flow leads to the development of portal hypertension. Almost all other causes of portal hypertension are mediated predominantly by increasing resistance, although evidence indicates that most high-resistance syndromes are also accompanied by increases in portal venous flow. In many conditions, the cause of the increased resistance is evident: inflammation and fibrosis lead to vascular distortion, architectural disturbance and impingement of the intravascular spaces. Other less evident factors are predominant in other conditions. For example, in acute alcoholic hepatitis, hepatocyte cell swelling and collagen deposition in the space of Disse lead to narrowing and distortion of sinusoidal spaces. The reasons for the increased mesenteric (and thus portal venous) blood flow in high-resistance states remain unclear. One theory postulates that a circulating vasodilatory humoral factor that would normally be inactivated by the liver escapes into the systemic circulation through shunts or hepatocellular insufficiency.

There are two separate and sometimes overlapping classification systems for the causes of portal hypertension, using either the liver or the hepatic sinusoid as the reference point. The former classifies conditions into prehepatic, intrahepatic and posthepatic causes, while the latter divides conditions into presinusoidal, sinusoidal and postsinusoidal causes (Table 16). However, the exact site of increased resistance in many intrahepatic causes of portal hypertension has recently been questioned, and it is likely that the predominant resistance sites could change according to the stage of some disease processes. For example, early primary biliary cirrhosis is thought to produce mainly presinusoidal hypertension, but as dense cirrhosis supervenes, sinusoidal hypertension becomes more important. Similarly, an early lesion of alcoholic liver disease, the central or terminal hyaline sclerosis, characterized by zone 3 fibrosis, would cause postsinuoidal hypertension, with sinusoidal hypertension predominating as cirrhosis becomes established. In practical terms, there are reasons for trying to correctly classify resistance sites. One is for predicting responses to surgical shunting procedures: presinusoidal conditions generally have well-preserved hepatocellular function and thus respond well to diversion of portal blood, whereas sinusoidal and postsinusoidal conditions tend to be associated with varying degrees of hepatic insufficiency. Another is that ascites generally occurs only with sinusoidal and postsinusoidal hypertension.

11.2 Pathophysiology

Portal pressure can be measured by several methods. A catheter inserted into a hepatic vein and then wedged provides a good estimate of the upstream portal venous pressure, unless the site of resistance is proximal to the intrahepatic portal vein (as in portal vein thrombosis wherein the wedged hepatic vein pressure will be normal in the presence of significant portal hypertension). The spleen, liver or portal vein can be directly percutaneously punctured by small-gauge (19–22 gauge) needles to obtain reliable estimates of portal pres-

TABLE 17.   Common sites of portal-systemic collateral formation

Location	Portal circulation	Systemic circulation	Clinical consequence
Proximal stomach and distal esophagus	Coronary vein of stomach	Azygos vein	Submucosal gastroesophageal varices
Anterior abdominal wall	Umbilical vein in falciform ligament	Epigastric abdominal wall veins	Caput medusae
Retroperitoneal	Splenic vein branch Sappey's veins (around liver and diaphragm)	Left renal vein Retzius's vein	Usually none Usually none
Anorectal	Middle and superior hemorrhoidal veins	Inferior hemorrhoidal vein	May be mistaken for hemorrhoids

sure. Measurement of portal pressure is mostly used for research purposes, as its invasiveness precludes wide clinical use.

Portal hypertension leads to many clinical complications. Ascites is directly related to the development of sinusoidal or postsinusoidal hypertension. Portal-systemic collateral vessels form in an attempt to decompress the portal hypertension (Table 17). The most troublesome site of collateral formation is around the proximal stomach and distal esophagus (gastroesophageal varices). Bleeding from such varices (or the gastric mucosa) and hepatocellular failure are the two commonest causes of death in cirrhosis. Indeed the mortality rates for variceal bleeding range from 15–50% depending on the degree of hepatic function: Child-Pugh class A, B and C patients have, respectively, 15%, 20–30% and 40–50% mortality rates when their varices bleed.

The risk of bleeding from gastroesophageal varices is related to several factors. First, a threshold minimum level of portal pressure of approximately 12 mm Hg appears necessary for varices to form. However, above this level it is unclear whether absolute height of portal pressure affects the bleeding risk. Factors such as intrathoracic pressure gradients induced by coughing, straining or sneezing, and damage to the variceal wall by acid reflux into the esophagus appear not to play a role. The two factors most important in determining bleeding risk are variceal size and local variceal wall characteristics. Several studies have shown that small varices almost never bleed, while the bleeding risk of medium-sized varices is approximately 10–15% over two years, and that of large varices, approximately 20–30% over the same period. During the

TABLE 18.   Comparison of portal hypertensive gastropathy and inflammatory gastritis

	Portal hypertensive gastropathy	Inflammatory gastritis
Endoscopic appearance	Mosaic pattern, speckled red spots	Discrete red erosive lesions
Site	Predominantly fundus	Predominantly antrum
Histology	Scant inflammatory cell infiltrate, prominent vascular dilatation, mucosal and submucosal lesions	Heavy inflammatory cell infiltrate, mucosal lesions
Treatment	Surgery, ? beta blockers, ?cytoprotective agents	Acid suppression, cytoprotective agents

past decade, it has become clear that certain varix wall characteristics that are visible through an endoscope are also predictive of high bleeding risk. These are the red and blue color signs. Small localized wall defects such as thin-walled blebs or sacs in the wall look like red spots or streaks and have variously been termed "red wale markings," "cherry-red spots" or "red streaks," while a diffuse pronounced blue color indicates a large varix (vein) with a stretched mucosa covering it.

Approximately 30–50% of upper GI bleeding episodes in patients with portal hypertension originate from nonvariceal sources. Cirrhotic patients have an increased incidence of acid-peptic disease, mostly erosive gastritis. This is probably due to the alcohol abuse that is common in this population. However, it has recently become clear that the majority of nonvariceal upper GI bleeding in cirrhosis is due to a peculiar form of gastropathy seen in the stomach in portal hypertension. Several features distinguish this portal hypertensive gastropathy from the erosive or inflammatory gastritis seen in nonhypertensive patients (Table 18). The major symptom of portal hypertensive gastropathy is bleeding. Pain or dyspepsia is uncommon as a presenting feature of this type of gastropathy. The appropriate treatment for this condition is still unclear, but it probably responds to measures to decrease portal pressure, although a possible role for cytoprotective agents has also been suggested.

11.3 Diagnosis

Diagnosing portal hypertension is usually easy. The patient often has concomitant ascites and splenomegaly, along with the stigmata of chronic liver disease. However, it should be remembered that all the prehepatic and many of the presinusoidal conditions have well-preserved liver function and no ascites.

Abdominal wall collaterals radiate outward from the umbilicus; when they are very prominent, it is easy to see why this condition is termed "caput medusae," after the fearsome creature in Greek mythology with the serpentine hairdo. Dilated abdominal wall veins, especially in the upper abdomen, are common, but caput medusae is rare. Another diagnostic clue may be the presence of anorectal varices masquerading as hemorrhoids. Gastroesophageal variceal bleeding produces large-volume, brisk bleeding with hematemesis and, later, melena or hematochezia. Portal hypertensive gastropathy may also produce brisk bleeding, but can occasionally cause low-volume oozing manifested only by melena.

11.4 Management

Managing the acute bleeding episode consists of the general resuscitative measures such as volume and blood replacement, and specific measures to stop the bleeding. Various pharmacological, mechanical and surgical modes of arresting hemorrhage are used, usually in that order. Vasoconstrictive drugs to stop bleeding include vasopressin and somatostatin or their longer-acting analogues such as glypressin and octreotide, respectively. Vasopressin infusions induce generalized arteriolar and venous constriction, with resultant decreased portal venous flow and thus pressure, and at least temporary cessation of bleeding in 50–80% of cases. However, the generalized vasoconstriction also may result in peripheral vascular ischemia, myocardial ischemia or infarction and renal tubular damage. Concurrent nitrate administration has been suggested to attenuate some of these side effects, but whether it actually docs so is still unproven. A safer alternative may be somatostatin or octreotide. Their mechanism of action is still unclear but probably relates to a suppressive effect on the release of vasodilatory hormones such as glucagon, leading to a net vasoconstrictive effect. Side effects are minimal. Whatever drug is used, it is generally inadvisable to continue drug therapy for more than one to two days.

Mechanical modes of therapy include inflatable balloons for direct tamponade. The Sengstaken-Blakemore tube has both an esophageal and a small gastric balloon; the Linton-Nachlas tube, with only a large gastric balloon, is attached to a small weight to stanch the cephalad flow of blood in the varices. Both tubes carry significant complication rates (15%), especially in inexperienced hands. The most common complications of esophageal balloon therapy for varices include aspiration, esophageal perforation and ischemic (pressure) necrosis of the mucosa.

The most common and probably the most effective nonsurgical therapies are endoscopic variceal sclerotherapy and ligation. Highly irritant solutions such as ethanolamine, polidocanol or even absolute ethanol are injected through endoscopic direct vision into and around the bleeding varix. The subsequent inflammation leads to eventual thrombosis and fibrosis of the varix lumen. Possible complications include chest pain, dysphagia, and esophageal ulceration and stricturing. The injection of irritant solutions that eventually lodge in the pulmonary circulation can result in lung function abnormalities, although these tend to be subclinical. A newer and probably safer method of endoscopic therapy is ligation or banding, similar to the rubber band ligations used to fibrose anorectal hemorrhoids. Initial studies suggest that its efficacy is similar to sclerotherapy, with fewer esophageal complications. The combination of endoscopic therapy and either balloon tamponade or drug therapy to control actively bleeding varices is successful in 80–95% of cases.

When all the above measures fail, emergency surgery may be tried. Emergency portacaval shunt surgery has been abandoned because of a 30–50% operative mortality rate. The simplest and probably best choice in the emergency situation is esophageal transection, in which a mechanical device transects and removes a ring of esophageal tissue, and then staples the ends together. Another type of "surgery" is the transjugular intrahepatic portal-systemic shunt (TIPS). In this procedure, an intrahepatic shunt between branches of the hepatic and portal veins is made by balloon dilation of liver tissue, and then an expandable metal stent of approximately 1 cm diameter is lodged into the fistula. The procedure can be done by a radiologist using fluoroscopy- guided catheterization, and requires only light sedation and local anesthesia.

Once the acute bleeding episode has been treated, how do we reduce the risk of future rebleeding? Before considering any other therapy, some obvious common-sense measures should be taken. For example, patients with cirrhosis caused by alcohol (the cause of approximately 50–60% of cirrhosis in Canada) absolutely must stop drinking; the rebleeding and mortality rates in patients who continue their alcohol use are much higher than in those who remain abstinent.

Prophylactic therapy to prevent bleeding may be divided into primary (to prevent the first bleed in a patient with varices who has never bled) and secondary prophylaxis (to prevent rebleeds). There is still much conflicting literature on these two topics, but for now, the following preliminary recommendations can be made. First, patients with large varices that have never bled should be started on beta blocker therapy at doses sufficient to reduce the resting heart rate by 20–25%. Beta-adrenergic antagonists are thought to produce arteriolar and venous constriction and significantly reduce blood flow through portal-systemic collaterals while modestly reducing portal pressure. Endoscopic sclerotherapy/banding, TIPS and surgery are ineffective and too risky for primary prophylaxis.

The appropriate secondary prophylaxis regimes remain controversial. There is probably a minority subgroup who respond favorably to beta blocker therapy, but they cannot be easily identified. One approach is to perform enough endoscopic sclerotherapy/banding sessions (usually 3–6) to obliterate varices or reduce them to small size. Treatment failures on this regime (e.g., those with recurrent bleeding) could be considered either for TIPS or surgery. TIPS should not be done in patients with a history of, or active, encephalopathy.

Prehepatic causes of portal hypertension such as portal vein thrombosis generally respond well to some type of portal-mesenteric diversion procedure such as mesocaval or portacaval shunting. In these cases, normal liver function protects against the development of encephalopathy or hepatic insufficiency when portal blood is diverted away from the liver.

Of course the definitive treatment for most of the complications of end-stage liver disease, including recurrent GI bleeding due to severe portal hypertension, is orthotopic liver transplantation. Since the presence of a surgical portacaval or mesocaval shunt greatly complicates the transplantation procedure, we have generally abandoned these types of shunting operations in patients with cirrhosis.

12. ASCITES / F. Wong and L. Blendis

Ascites is a detectable collection of free fluid in the peritoneal cavity. Ascitic fluid is derived from the vascular compartment subserving the hepatosplanchnic viscera. Two factors are important in the formation of ascites: an increased total body sodium and water, and increased sinusoidal portal pressure. In cirrhosis, hepatic dysfunction and sinusoidal portal pressure probably both send a message to the kidney to retain excess sodium and fluid, while the portal hypertension serves to localize excess fluid to the peritoneal cavity rather than the periphery. Portal hypertension alone without hepatic dysfunction rarely results in ascites.

The pathogenesis of ascites formation remains controversial. The "underfill" theory proposes that ascites occurs as a primary event. Sequestration of fluid into the peritoneal cavity as a result of changes in Starling's forces within the splanchnic circulation results in a reduction of the circulatory volume. This in turn leads to stimulation of the sympathetic nervous and renin-angiotensin-aldosterone systems, which promote renal sodium and water retention. The "overflow theory," on the other hand, proposes that renal sodium retention occurs as a primary event. This may be due to the increased production of a sodium-retaining factor or the reduced synthesis of a natriuretic factor by the diseased liver. The circulatory volume is expanded. In the presence of abnormal Starling's forces in the splanchnic circulation, the retained fluid is preferentially localized to the peritoneal cavity as ascites. More recently, "the peripheral arterial vasodilation hypothesis," which encompasses features of both the underfill and overflow theories, was put forward. It proposes that in cirrhosis, arterial vasodilation leads to a decrease in splanchnic and systemic vascular resistance with pooling of blood in the splanchnic circulation, leading to a reduction in the effective arterial blood volume. This in turn activates neurohumoral pressor systems, promoting renal sodium and water retention in an attempt to restore the effective arterial blood volume and maintain blood pressure. When increased renal sodium reabsorption cannot compensate for the arterial vasodilation, arterial underfilling occurs. Then the cascade of further activation of various neurohumoral pressor systems leading to increased sodium retention begins, and ultimately ascites is formed (Figure 13).

Arterial vasodilation is also responsible for the hyperdynamic circulation that is often evident in cirrhosis. This clinically manifests as an increased cardiac output, bounding pulse, wide pulse pressure and systemic hypotension. Locally produced vasodilators may be responsible. More recently, it has been proposed that chronic endotoxemia associated with cirrhosis may stimulate the synthesis and release of a potent endothelin-derived relaxing factor, nitric oxide, resulting in splanchnic and systemic vasodilation.

Clinically, the first evidence of ascites is an increase in abdominal girth accompanied by weight gain. Peritoneal fluid of less than 2 L is difficult to detect clinically, and ultrasound is useful in defining small amounts of ascites. The patient is sallow and intravascularly depleted. Muscle wasting is profound. The abdomen is distended, often with fullness in the flanks and an everted umbilicus. Scrotal edema is frequent. Distended abdominal wall veins that radiate from the umbilicus represent the presence of portal-systemic collaterals. The earliest sign of ascites is dullness to percussion in the flanks. Shifting dullness and a fluid thrill mean that more fluid is present.

A pleural effusion is found in a small percentage of patients with ascites, usually on the right side. This is due to the presence of a diaphragmatic defect that allows ascitic fluid to pass into the pleural cavity.

Examination of ascitic fluid by diagnostic paracentesis should be performed at first presentation, or when there is alteration of the patient's clinical state, such as a sudden increase in the amount of ascitic fluid, worsening of encephalopathy or presence of fever. The purpose of the examination is to rule out other complications such as spontaneous bacterial peritonitis, tuberculosis and hepatocellular carcinoma. Ascitic fluid analysis should include a total polymorph count, protein and albumin concentrations and direct inoculation of at least 10 mL of ascitic fluid each into blood culture bottles at the bedside, as this increases the positive culture yield. A serum–ascitic fluid

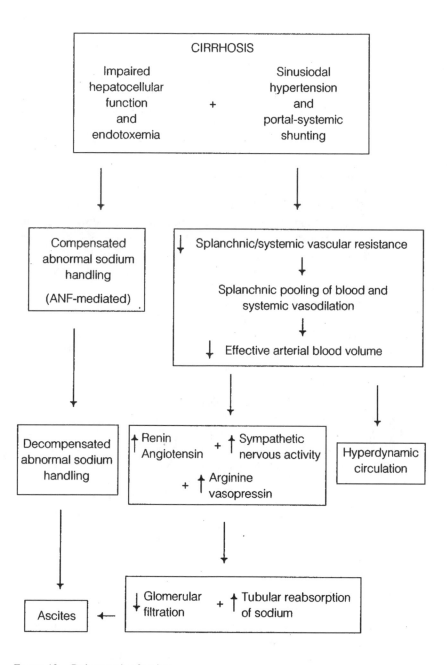

FIGURE 13.   Pathogenesis of ascites.

albumin gradient of greater than 11 g/L represents cirrhotic rather than malignant ascites. A high protein content may be associated with the Budd-Chiari syndrome or seen in pancreatic ascites. A total polymorph count of greater than 250/μL is diagnostic of spontaneous bacterial peritonitis.

Although bed rest will result in a redistribution of body fluid, fluid and salt restriction is required to mobilize the ascites. The patient is usually prescribed a no-added-salt diet containing 2 g (100 mmol) sodium/day, and monitored carefully with daily weights. Measurement of abdominal girth is unreliable, as gaseous distention is common. Too rapid mobilization of fluid will result in worsening of renal function; one should aim at a weight loss of 0.5 kg/day. Patients with peripheral edema can have their fluid mobilized more rapidly, as the edema fluid can easily be absorbed to replenish the intravascular volume.

Diuretic therapy is usually required in addition to salt and fluid restriction. The potassium-sparing diuretic spironolactone can be given in a single daily dose, starting at a dose of 100 mg/day, and may be increased by 100 mg per week up to 400 mg/day if the response is inadequate. Spironolactone has a slow onset of action, and therefore frequent dose adjustments are unnecessary. Its half-life in cirrhotic patients can be as long as 10 days; therefore, it also has a slow offset of action and patients should still be monitored after spironolactone is discontinued. One of its unacceptable side effects is painful gynecomastia. Other potassium-sparing diuretics, such as amiloride and triamterene, are less potent but acceptable alternatives. If there is no diuretic response and the patient is compliant with the sodium intake, a loop diuretic such as furosemide is added. Electrolyte abnormalities are common with diuretic therapy and should be monitored regularly. Hypokalemia and hypochloremic alkalosis can precipitate encephalopathy. Too rapid diuresis can lead to azotemia and the hepatorenal syndrome.

Refractory ascites is defined as ascites unresponsive to 400 mg of spironolactone or 30 mg of amiloride plus up to 120 mg of furosemide daily for two weeks. Noncompliance with sodium restriction is a major and often overlooked cause of resistant ascites, and careful questioning of the patient and the patient's relatives is often required to confirm this. Other causes of resistant ascites include the development of spontaneous bacterial peritonitis, hepatocellular carcinoma and intrinsic renal pathology. Refractory ascites without any underlying cause usually indicates advanced cirrhosis associated with a grave prognosis, with only a 50% survival at two years. Large-volume paracentesis is now recognized as a safe and effective therapy for the treatment of refractory ascites. Removal of ascitic fluid volume of up to 5 L without the simultaneous infusion of plasma expanders such as concentrated albumin is safe in non-edematous patients. Larger volumes can be removed in edematous patients. However, repeated paracenteses may not be practical for all patients with refractory ascites, and a peritoneovenous (LeVeen) shunt should be considered in selected patients with good liver reserve. It may be dramatically effective in resolving the ascites, but in patients with decompensated liver disease it is followed by higher morbidity and mortality. Previous abdominal surgery, spontaneous bacterial peritonitis and large varices are relative contraindications to the procedure. Early complications include pulmonary edema and disseminated intravascular coagulopathy. Late complications include thrombosis of the superior vena cava, infection and blockage or dislodgement of the shunt, all of which require its immediate removal. In suitable patients, the LeVeen shunt, in addition to improved management of ascites, can significantly enhance well-being and nutritional status. More recently, a transjugular intrahepatic portal-systemic shunt (TIPS) has been shown to be an effective means of managing refractory ascites. This method involves creating a communication between a branch of the hepatic vein and a branch of the portal vein held open by a metal stent. Liver transplantation should always be considered as a treatment option in these patients.

12.1 Spontaneous Bacterial Peritonitis

Spontaneous bacterial peritonitis (SBP) is a common and often fatal complication of cirrhosis. In this clinical syndrome, ascites becomes infected in the absence of a recognizable cause of peritonitis. Its increased incidence over the past decade may be due to greater recognition. It is particularly frequent if the patient has severely decompensated cirrhosis with jaundice. In most cases, the infection occurs after admission into hospital. About one-third of cases of SBP are asymptomatic; therefore, the clinician should not hesitate in performing a diagnostic paracentesis. Typically, it presents with fever and/or abdominal pain. It may also present atypically, solely as a worsening of the encephalopathy or renal dysfunction. Diagnosis of SBP is made by paracentesis. Positive culture results may take 48 hours and Gram's stains of ascitic fluid are positive in only 10–50% of infected patients. The "gold standard" for diagnosis of SBP is a polymorphonuclear (PMN) count of >250 cells/µL. A variant of SBP known as *culture-negative neutrocytic ascites* occurs as culture-negative cases of suspected SBP with an ascitic fluid PMN count of >250 cells/µL. The patients with culture-negative neutrocytic ascites have the same clinical presentation and carry the same unfavorable prognosis as those with SBP. Therefore, treatment for suspected SBP should start immediately after the diagnostic PMN count rather than waiting for positive culture results. Gram-negative bacilli account for 70% of cases of SBP. E. coli is the most common pathogen isolated. Other gram-negative organisms include Klebsiella species, Citrobacter freundii, Proteus and Enterobacter. Gram-positive organisms are responsible for 25% of cases;

TABLE 19.   Differentiation between secondary and spontaneous bacterial peritonitis

	Secondary bacterial peritonitis	*Spontaneous bacterial peritonitis*
Organisms	Multiple	Single
Ascitic protein count	>1 g/dL	<1 g/dL
Response to treatment		
PMN count	Continues to rise despite treatment	Falls exponentially
Ascitic culture	Remains positive	Rapidly becomes sterile

these include Streptococcus pneumoniae, Streptococcus viridans, group D streptococci and Staphylococcus aureus. Anaerobic organisms are uncommon causes of SBP, as the oxygen tension in the ascitic fluid is too high for their survival. Among these, Bacteroides species appear to be more common than other anaerobes. Cefotaxime, a broad-spectrum, third-generation cephalosporin, is now recognized as the treatment of choice for SBP. Its spectrum includes most organisms responsible for SBP and it is not nephrotoxic in the therapeutic range. A 5-day course of cefotaxime 2 g IV every 8 hours has been shown to be as effective as a 10-day course. The ascitic fluid PMN count should decrease rapidly, normalizing within 48 hours in response to treatment together with a parallel clinical improvement. Aminoglycosides should not be used since cirrhotic patients are particularly sensitive to their nephrotoxic effects, and monitoring serum levels of aminoglycosides is no guarantee against aminoglycoside-induced nephrotoxicity.

Secondary bacterial peritonitis should be considered as a differential diagnosis if the following features are present: (1) multiple organisms are grown from the ascitic fluid; (2) ascitic fluid protein concentration >1 g/dL; or (3) PMN count remains high despite antibiotic therapy (Table 19). Radiographic examinations are required to exclude perforation of the gastrointestinal tract, with emergency surgery only where perforation is confirmed. Despite successful treatment of SBP, the prognosis of these patients remains poor. SBP recurs frequently in cirrhotic patients. Selective intestinal decontamination to eliminate aerobic gram-negative bacilli with oral nonabsorbable antibiotics has proved effective in reducing the recurrence of SBP. Norfloxacin 400 mg daily has the advantages of rarely causing bacterial resistance and having a low incidence of side effects when administered chronically. The less expensive drug trimethoprim-sulfamethoxazole may be as effective for prophylaxis as norfloxacin. Despite decreased SBP recurrence rates with prophylactic

TABLE 20. Grading of hepatic encephalopathy

Grade	Level of consciousness	Intellectual function	Neurological findings	EEG
1	Lack of awareness Personality change Day/night reversal	Short attention	Incoordination Mild asterixis	Slowing (5–6 cps) Triphasic
2	Lethargic Inappropriate behavior	Disoriented	Asterixis Abnormal reflexes	Slowing Triphasic
3	Asleep Rousable	Loss of meaningful communication	Asterixis Abnormal reflex	Slowing Triphasic
4	Unrousable	Absent	Decerebrate	Very slow (2–3 cps), delta

antibiotics, no change in mortality has been demonstrated as yet. All patients who have experienced one episode of SBP should be considered for liver transplantation.

13. HEPATIC ENCEPHALOPATHY / L.J. Worobetz

Hepatic encephalopathy (HE) is a complex, potentially reversible neuropsychiatric condition that occurs as a consequence of acute or chronic liver disease. It is characterized by changes of personality, consciousness, behavior and neuromuscular function (Table 20). Early features include reversal of sleep pattern, apathy, hypersomnia, irritability and personal neglect. In later stages, delirium and coma may occur. Neurologic signs may include hyperreflexia, rigidity, myoclonus and asterixis. Asterixis is not specific to hepatic encephalopathy and may be present in other causes of metabolic encephalopathy. Seizures and lateralizing signs are uncommon and are more commonly seen in acute than chronic liver failure. Clinically, a number of encephalopathic patterns can be observed: acute, acute recurrent, chronic recurrent and chronic permanent encephalopathy (the last often forms part of the spectrum of acquired hepatocerebral degeneration).

There is no specific biochemical test for hepatic encephalopathy. Blood tests should help to rule out other causes of encephalopathy and detect precipitating factors such as hypoglycemia or electrolyte imbalance. An elevated serum ammonia level is characteristic but not essential, and correlates poorly with the level of encephalopathy. The cerebrospinal fluid is usually normal or may show increased protein with increased GABA levels. Lumbar puncture and CT scan may be necessary to rule out other concomitant CNS pathology. The EEG shows slow, triphasic wave activity found mainly over frontal areas, but this pattern is not specific.

Factors of importance in the pathogenesis of encephalopathy are the shunting of blood around the hepatocytes into the systemic circulation and the presence of hepatocellular dysfunction. Encephalopathy probably results from one or more toxic products of gut origin that are usually metabolized by the liver entering this systemic circulation and reaching the brain. Abnormalities of ammonia metabolism are most frequently implicated in the pathophysiology. The normal gut flora produce a urease that enzymatically cleaves NH_3 from protein in the lumen. Nonionized ammonia is then absorbed into the portal circulation. It reaches the systemic circulation because of shunts and the inability of the liver to metabolize the ammonia. Other hypotheses relate to the findings of increased levels of short-chain fatty acids and increased levels of aromatic amino acids associated with the decreased levels of branched-chain amino acids. As well, the principal neuro-inhibitory neurotransmitter γ-aminobutyric acid (GABA) is increased in encephalopathy. Other concepts include other false neurotransmitters, including an endogenous modulator of GABA receptors, suggesting involvement of the GABA-diazepam receptor complex in the pathogenesis of HE. It is likely that hepatic encephalopathy results from the complicated interplay of many factors, not just one.

Hepatic encephalopathy may arise spontaneously but more commonly will develop as a result of some precipitating factor in the course of acute or chronic liver disease (Table 21). The most important aspect of management is prompt recognition and treatment of these precipitating factors. Exogenous factors include increased dietary protein, administration of certain drugs (such as sedatives), gastrointestinal bleeding, azotemia, electrolyte imbalance from diuretic therapy, hypoxia and infection. Also important is the necessity to provide meticulous care of the confused and often comatose patient. Otherwise, the goal of therapy is to lower the level of toxic substances by reducing or excluding protein from the diet and by cleaning nitrogenous materials from the gut. To this end, constipation is avoided by the use of laxatives and, in more urgent cases, cleansing of the gut with enemas or colonic lavage. A commonly used laxative is lactulose, a synthetic disaccharide that is degraded by intestinal bacteria to produce acidification and an osmotic diarrhea. The acidification of colonic contents reduces ammonia absorption in part by trapping nitrogenous compounds in the lumen. The dosage of lactulose should be titrated to the patient to achieve two to four loose stools per day. The average daily dosages are 45–90 g. Too much diarrhea can result in fluid and electrolyte depletion and can worsen HE and cause renal failure. Its chronic use can

TABLE 21.   Common precipitants of hepatic encephalopathy

Increased nitrogen load
   Gastrointestinal bleeding
   Excess dietary protein
   Azotemia
   Constipation

Electrolyte imbalance
   Hyponatremia
   Hypokalemia
   Metabolic alkalosis/acidosis
   Hypoxia
   Hypovolemia

Drugs
   Narcotics, tranquilizers, sedatives

Miscellaneous
   Infection
   Surgery
   Superimposed acute liver disease
   Progressive liver disease
   Transjugular intrahepatic portal-systemic shunt (TIPS)

---

reduce the frequency of episodes of encephalopathy. Alternatively, antibiotics such as metronidazole may be used; these inhibit urea splitting and deaminating bacteria, reducing the production of ammonia and other potential toxins. The previously commonly used antibiotic neomycin is no longer recommended as it has the potential for ototoxic and nephrotoxic side effects.

Other experimental therapeutic approaches exist, particularly when the encephalopathy becomes refractory. On the basis of increased aromatic amino acids and decreased branched-chain amino acids found in encephalopathy (and the resulting effect on neurotransmitter synthesis), branched-chain amino acids given orally or intravenously have a potentially therapeutic role in improving encephalopathy. Some of the new benzodiazepine-receptor antagonists may be of value. These drugs, which block the benzodiazepine/ GABA-receptor complex, may lead to a decrease in inhibitory GABA-mediated transmission in the brain and lessen the encephalopathy. Based on the possible relationship of a defect in dopaminergic neurotransmission and encephalopathy, both L-dopa and bromocriptine have been tried, with controversial results. Orthotopic liver transplantation should entirely reverse the hepatic encephalopathy. Thus, this should be considered in all patients with

TABLE 22. Diagnosis of hepatorenal syndrome

Chronic liver disease with ascites

Azotemia/oliguria

Tubular function maintained
Urine:plasma osmolarity ratio >1.0
Urine:plasma creatinine ratio >30
Urine [Na⁺] <10 mEq/dL

No sustained benefit by intravascular volume expansion

---

hepatic encephalopathy whose liver disease makes them suitable for liver transplantation.

14. HEPATORENAL SYNDROME / L.J. Worobetz

The hepatorenal syndrome is a syndrome of advancing renal failure in a patient with severe hepatocellular failure, usually advanced cirrhosis. In most instances, the uremia and oliguria that characterize this syndrome arise either spontaneously or in response to changes in blood volume or fluid shifts within body compartments. Patients are seldom admitted with this diagnosis; its development is usually precipitated by events in the hospital, which may include overly vigorous diuretic therapy, diarrhea or GI bleeding. The histology of the kidneys is virtually normal, with the renal failure being a functional failure. Such kidneys have been successfully transplanted and have functioned normally. Conversely, if hepatic function is restored by liver transplantation, kidney function may return to normal. In this syndrome there are abnormalities in renal blood flow, including active renal vasoconstriction, thus decreasing effective renal circulation, especially to the renal cortex. The cause of this is unknown, but is best thought of as an imbalance between systemic vasodilators and renal vasoconstricting mechanisms.

In the early stages, renal dysfunction is characterized by failure to excrete a water load, a reduction in the urinary sodium to <10 mEq/L and a progressive hyponatremia (Table 22). Ascites is usually present. As the syndrome progresses there is increasing azotemia, usually with hepatic failure and increasing difficulty controlling the ascites. Sodium is avidly reabsorbed with increasing urinary osmolality. The patient becomes drowsy, nauseated and thirsty. Terminally, the patient's blood pressure drops, coma deepens and urine volume falls further. The terminal stages may last a few days to weeks.

Clinically, it is important to distinguish hepatorenal syndrome from other causes of renal failure. Iatrogenic renal failure must be ruled out, including drug-induced disease from aminoglycosides and nonsteroidal anti-inflammatory medication. Hepatorenal syndrome must also be distinguished from prerenal azotemia and acute tubular necrosis. Acute tubular necrosis has a high urinary sodium. Although prerenal azotemia may show similar tubular function, this is ruled out by the clinical setting in which hepatorenal syndrome occurs and the lack of sustained benefit by expansion of intravascular volume with colloid replacement. In addition, cirrhosis, especially alcoholic cirrhosis, may leave glomerular mesangial deposits of IgA, which is diagnosed by the presence of proteinuria with microhematuria and casts. Hepatitis B can cause glomerulonephritis, which should be detectable because of red cell casts and proteinuria. Acetaminophen toxicity can also cause concomitant liver and renal failure with high urinary sodium excretion.

Treatment of established hepatorenal syndrome is difficult. Thus, emphasis is toward prevention by avoiding diuretic overdose, treating ascites slowly and recognizing complications early, including electrolyte imbalance, hemorrhage and infection. Conservative management includes the restriction of fluids, sodium and potassium. All potentially nephrotoxic drugs should be withdrawn and a septic workup should be carried out. Volume expansion with albumin results in only transient improvement. Isotonic saline is usually avidly retained, worsening the ascites and possibly precipitating pulmonary edema. Mannitol is not used, as this may lead to intracellular acidosis. Dialysis does not improve survival. The final combination of azotemia, hyponatremia and hypotension is terminal. Liver transplantation should be considered, but presumably would have been offered to the patient earlier in the course of the hepatic illness.

15. **LIVER TRANSPLANTATION** / L.B. Lilly, A.W. Hemming and G.A. Levy

Starzl performed the first human liver transplant in 1963 in a 3-year-old boy with biliary atresia. The first successful liver transplant was not performed until 1967 when a 1½-year-old girl with hepatocellular carcinoma was transplanted; she died of recurrent tumor after 17 months. One-year survival in the early years was 25–35% using methylprednisolone and azathioprine as immunosuppressives; however, with the introduction of cyclosporine in the early 1980s, liver transplantation became a clinical reality and now offers one- and five-year survivals in excess of 80% and 60% respectively.

With the dramatic improvement in results, liver transplantation became the recognized management for end-stage liver disease. The number of liver transplant centers in North America was more than 130 in 1993, and now more than 3,000 liver transplants are performed yearly in the United States alone. In Canada, there are active centers in Halifax, NS; Montreal, PQ; Toronto and London, ON; Edmonton, AB; and Vancouver, BC. Over 300 liver transplants are performed yearly in Canada. One-year survival rates of 80–90% are now expected. The rate-limiting step in the application of transplantation to liver disease has become donor availability.

15.1 Assessment for Transplantation

A patient should be considered for liver transplantation when the diagnosis of irreversible end-stage liver disease is made. The most common indications for liver transplantation in adults and children are listed in Table 23. The selection of appropriate candidates out of a large number of patients with liver disease combined with the relative scarcity of available organs requires a strict individual assessment, which must to a certain extent be tailored to the cause of liver failure. The indications for referral for transplantation in patients with chronic liver disease are outlined in Table 24. Transplantation for hepatitis B remains controversial, and physicians should be aware of their transplant center's policy when considering patients for referral. Exclusion of patients with contraindications to liver transplantation (Table 25) allows the best use of scarce donor resources while maximizing patient benefit.

15.2 Preoperative Workup

The principles behind the liver transplant workup are to definitively establish the etiology of the liver disease and to identify contraindications to surgery. Assessment of patients by a multidisciplinary team that includes medical, surgical, anesthetic, social and psychiatric specialists is done to ensure the success of the transplantation process.

Once the patient is declared a candidate for liver transplantation, he or she goes onto a liver transplant list awaiting a suitable donor. For patients on the waiting list, time to transplantation varies from center to center, but organ allocation for any given patient depends on the length of time that the patient has been on the list as well as the severity of the patient's liver disease. While awaiting organ replacement, transplant candidates may present with complications that require urgent attention, such as gastrointestinal bleeding, spontaneous bacterial peritonitis, hepatic encephalopathy or other complications related or unrelated to the underlying liver disease. In addition, patients may deteriorate in the course of their disease and become too sick to tolerate transplantation. Many programs expect 15–20% of listed patients to die or be delisted before an organ becomes available.

15.3 Timing of Transplantation

With improving results of liver transplantation, patients who once were

TABLE 23.   Liver transplantation: indications

---

1. Chronic liver disease

Cholestatic disorders
Primary biliary cirrhosis
Primary sclerosing cholangitis
Drug-induced cholestasis and biliary cirrhosis

Hepatocellular disease
Chronic viral hepatitis (B ± D, HCV, non-A non-B)
Chronic drug-induced liver disease
Alcoholic liver disease
Autoimmune liver disease
Wilson's disease, hemochromatosis, α_1-antitrypsin deficiency

Vascular disease
Budd-Chiari syndrome
Veno-occlusive disease

2. Fulminant hepatic failure

Viruses
HAV, HBV, (HCV), HDV, HEV, non A–E
HSV, EBV, CMV, HZV, etc.

Drugs and toxins
Acetaminophen, NSAIDs, isoniazid, etc.
Industrial substances, mushrooms

Other etiologies
Metabolic disorders
Hypoperfusion
Microvesicular steatosis
Autoimmune hepatitis
"Surgical" causes

3. Hepatic malignancies (unresectable, confined to liver)

4. Inherited genetic and metabolic disorders

---

transplanted only for treatment of life-threatening complications are now being transplanted earlier in the course of their disease. Today many patients undergo liver transplantation because of quality of life issues such as extreme fatigue, pruritus and inability to hold employment or participate in the activities of daily living. It is clear that transplantation should be considered prior to catastrophic complications and the need for life support,

TABLE 24.   Criteria for referral of patients for transplantation*

Chronic liver disease in general
Portal hypertension with bleeding from esophageal varices or portal gastropathy
Intractable ascites
(Recurrent) spontaneous bacterial peritonitis
Portal-systemic encephalopathy
Malnutrition
Intractable fatigue
Hypoalbuminemia
Rising INR

*Primary biliary cirrhosis and primary sclerosing cholangitis***
Progressive jaundice
Intractable pruritus
Progressive hepatic osteodystrophy
Ascending cholangitis (in PSC)

---

*Assuming no contraindications exist. **In addition to those criteria listed above.

TABLE 25.   Liver transplantation: contraindications

---

1. *Absolute*
Sepsis outside the biliary tree
Extrahepatic malignancy
Advanced cardiopulmonary disease
HIV positivity
Active alcohol and/or substance abuse
Inability to accept the procedure, understand its nature, and cooperate in the medical care
    required following liver transplantation

2. *Relative*
Chronic renal insufficiency
Age
Vascular problems, including prior shunt surgery
Other significant extrahepatic disease(s)

---

although waiting times can be expected to increase as patients are referred
and listed earlier.

15.4 Operative Procedure

Technical details of the procedure are beyond the scope of this discussion;
however, there are several salient points to be reviewed. During the procedure
the liver is mobilized and both inflow to the liver and inferior vena caval

return to the heart are interrupted. This may cause hemodynamic instability, which if not correctable requires the use of venovenous bypass in which IVC and portal blood are diverted through a bypass circuit to the axillary vein. The liver is subsequently removed and the new graft sewn in place. Although the liver is flushed of the high potassium preservation solution prior to reperfusion, there can be significant cardiac abnormalities upon reperfusing the liver. These intraoperative events demand a thorough preoperative assessment of cardiac status.

15.5 Postoperative Management

Issues that must be addressed in the postoperative period include management of fluid and electrolytes, respiratory function, monitoring of neurologic status, immunosuppression and graft function.

In most cases patients are quickly extubated within 24 hours of surgery. However, ventilatory support may be needed for an extended period, particularly when there is delayed graft function, presence of severe pleural effusions, pulmonary infiltrate and diaphragmatic dysfunction or paralysis.

Abnormalities of coagulation are sensitive markers of hepatic dysfunction and correction of coagulation by the administration of exogenous factors is avoided unless active bleeding is ongoing. Coagulation is routinely assessed by measurement of INR/prothrombin time, partial thromboplastin time and/or assay of coagulation factors V or VII. Following successful liver transplantation, coagulation parameters should return to normal levels within 48 hours in most patients. The failure of coagulation parameters to normalize is an ominous sign of graft failure and suggests the need for retransplantation.

Renal insufficiency, occasionally requiring dialysis, is not uncommon postoperatively in liver transplant patients. Renal failure may be due to a combination of factors including pre-existing renal disease, hepatorenal syndrome, intraoperative blood loss and hypotension leading to tubular necrosis, drug-induced nephrotoxicity (especially cyclosporine or FK-506), poor liver function and sepsis.

Most patients wake up within several hours of liver transplantation, whereas patients with fulminant hepatic failure may require one to three days to return to normal neurologic status after liver transplantation. Narcotics and sedatives are kept to a minimum in the immediate postoperative period. Confusion and seizures can occur and are usually related to metabolic disturbances (low serum magnesium levels), but are a known complication of cyclosporine and FK-506. At the University of Toronto all patients are placed on a continuous infusion of magnesium sulfate for the first 72 to 96 hours postoperatively, followed by oral supplementation.

15.6 Immunosuppression

15.6.1 IMMUNOSUPPRESSIVE AGENTS CURRENTLY IN USE

15.6.1.1 Cyclosporine

The introduction of cyclosporine is considered one of the most important factors that has improved the results of liver transplantation. Since its early introduction in late 1978, the one-year graft survival has increased from 30 to >70%. Cyclosporine binds to a specific cell protein, cyclophillin, and through a series of intracellular events prevents activation of T cells and the production of interleukin-2 (IL-2). The drug is given preferentially by the oral route or by slow intravenous infusion. The dosage of cyclosporine is adjusted to maintain a trough cyclosporine level of 300–400 ng/mL (monoclonal radioimmunoassay) in the early postoperative period. Cyclosporine A is lipid-soluble and absorption is dependent upon the availability of bile. Therefore, until adequate bile flow is restored, adequate cyclosporine levels are difficult to obtain. The introduction of a micoemulsion formulation of cyclosporine, Neoral®, which is less bile acid–dependent in its absorption, has all but eliminated the need for the intravenous formulation. Daily monitoring of cyclosporine levels in the immediate postoperative period is mandatory, as the compound has a narrow therapeutic index (efficacy vs toxicity). Cyclosporine interacts with many drugs, such as antibiotics and calcium channel blockers, and caution must therefore be exercised in giving any drug to patients who are taking cyclosporine.

Common side effects of cyclosporine include renal dysfunction, hypertension, increased susceptibility to infections, malignancy (especially post-transplant lymphoproliferative disease), hypertrichosis, tremor, headaches and gum hyperplasia. Other less common side effects include confusion, seizures, agitation, hearing loss, anorexia, diarrhea, nausea and vomiting, abdominal discomfort and gynecomastia.

15.6.1.2 FK-506 (Tacrolimus®; Prograf®)

FK-506 binds to FK-binding protein and subsequently inhibits T-cell activation by blocking IL-2 production in a similar fashion to cyclosporine. Tacrolimus® and Prograf® have been approved by the FDA for liver transplantation in the United States. Tacrolimus® is undergoing evaluation in Canada. Toxicity and efficacy are similar to those of cyclosporine, although recent multicenter trials suggest there may be a slightly decreased incidence of rejection, which to date has not translated to improved graft survival.

15.6.1.3 Corticosteroids

All patients receive methylprednisolone preoperatively. There are probably as many steroid protocols as transplant programs; at the University of Toronto a preoperative dose of 500 mg Solu-Medrol® is given. Subsequently this is reduced rapidly to a dose of 0.3 mg/kg/day. Short-term side effects include an increased incidence of infections (bacterial and fungal), hyperglycemia and impaired wound healing.

15.6.1.4 Antilymphocyte products
Antilymphocyte products can be monoclonal (OKT3) or polyclonal (ALG, RATS, ATG). In either case the aim of therapy is to prevent rejection by depleting lymphocytes. The use of these products has been associated with higher rates of viral infections, in particular cytomegalovirus (CMV) as well as an increased risk of lymphoproliferative disorders. OKT3 has been associated with side effects secondary to the release of tumor necrosis factor and IL-1 that can range from mild flu-like symptoms to life-threatening pulmonary edema and circulatory collapse. In liver transplantation these drugs have shifted from being used for induction of immunosuppression to the treatment of refractory rejection.

15.6.2 NEW IMMUNOSUPPRESSIVE AGENTS

15.6.2.1 Mycophenolate (Mofetil®; Cellcept®)
T and B cells are primarily dependent on the de novo pathway of purine synthesis and have less ability to use the salvage pathway. Mycophenolate inhibits the de novo pathway of purine synthesis and hence should specifically inhibit T and B cell proliferation with little effect on other major organs. Mycophenolate has recently been shown to reduce acute rejection in renal transplantation by 50% and is presently undergoing trials in liver transplantation.

15.6.2.2 Rapamycin
Rapamycin is a new agent that has structural similarities to FK-506. Its mechanism of action, however, is dramatically different in that it appears to block the release of IL-2 at a step after gene transcription and therefore may be synergistic with cyclosporine. Phase I trials in liver transplantation with rapamycin are just beginning.

15.7 Postoperative Complications
Complications common to any surgical procedure can occur with liver transplantation. However, there are several adverse events peculiar to liver transplantation. The most concerning of postoperative complications is *primary nonfunction* (PNF) of the new graft. The incidence of PNF ranges from 2 to

10% and becomes evident by coagulation parameters that worsen and cannot be corrected, increasing acidosis and deterioration in the patient's mental status. The etiology of PNF is unclear, and the treatment is urgent retransplantation. Primary graft dysfunction of a less significant degree has been managed with some success with prostaglandin E_1 and/or N-acetylcysteine.

Vascular thromboses that occur in the early postoperative period are generally technical in nature. Although thrombectomy of both portal vein and hepatic artery has been reported with some success, retransplantation is usually required should these vessels thrombose.

The *bile duct* has been termed the Achilles heel of liver transplantation. Problems occur in 10–30% of cases. Early leaks are secondary to ischemia, sepsis or severe rejection.

Acute allograft rejection occurs in 40–60% of transplant patients, usually in the first three months after transplantation. Rejection is suspected in patients with rising liver enzymes. Patterns of enzyme elevation can be either hepatocellular (high AST) or cholestatic (high bilirubin and alkaline phosphatase). Fever, malaise and right upper quadrant discomfort are late signs and should not be required for diagnosis of rejection. Diagnosis is confirmed by liver biopsy. Histologic findings include periportal inflammation with mononuclear cells and eosinophils, bile duct injury and endophlebitis. Episodes of cellular rejection usually respond to high-dose steroid therapy. Those patients whose rejection fails to respond to steroids are usually treated with a 7–14 day course of antithymocyte globulin (monoclonal or polyclonal). Recently, FK-506 has shown some success in treating rejection refractory to either steroids or OKT3. Failure to respond to immunosuppressive therapy may result in ductopenic rejection (chronic rejection) leading to biliary cirrhosis, which may result in the need for retransplantation in 5–10% of all transplanted patients.

The major cause of death following liver transplantation is related to *infections*. Immunosuppressed patients are at risk for bacterial, viral and fungal infections. Bacterial infections with non-opportunistic organisms are usually seen in the early postoperative period. Opportunistic bacterial infections are seen one to four months or more after transplantation. Wound infections and intra-abdominal sepsis account for the majority of bacterial infections seen in transplanted patients. Viral infections are seen frequently in immunosuppressed patients and usually occur at six weeks or later. Cytomegalovirus (CMV) is present in over half of the population and in non-immunosuppressed patients is virtually nonpathogenic. However, CMV infection in transplanted patients may account for 30% of the infections seen and is a source of morbidity and a small mortality. CMV infection is characterized by high fever, usually associated with anorexia, malaise and arthralgias; the diagnosis is confirmed by viral antigen assay and liver biopsy. The therapy for CMV infection includes the reduction of immunosuppression and the use of anti-viral agents such as ganciclovir or CMV immune globulin. Other viral infections seen in transplanted patients include herpes simplex, Epstein-Barr virus, varicella zoster and adenovirus. Fungal infections have been noted in up to 20% of patients and carry with them a 20–100% mortality rate. Infections in general are usually proportional to the degree of immunosuppression.

15.8 Results of Liver Transplantation

A one-year survival of ≥80% after liver transplantation is now not uncommon. Most mortality occurs within the first 90 days. After one year, few patients or grafts are lost. Furthermore, 60% of patients return to gainful employment, demonstrating that this procedure is not only of benefit to the patient, but to society as a whole. Though there are few reports of cost effectiveness, investigators in Pittsburgh have demonstrated that liver transplantation is less expensive than costs of caring for similar patients treated for complications of cirrhosis. Patients with diseases such as cholestatic liver disease that tend not to recur after liver transplantation have an excellent long-term prognosis (greater than 80% five-year survival). In contrast, patients transplanted for viral hepatitis, and in particular hepatitis B, have a poorer long-term outlook as a result of the problem of recurrent disease. For this reason, hepatitis B patients are generally not candidates for liver transplantation except under experimental protocol. Highly selected patients with asymptomatic small hepatocellular carcinomas can have an excellent long-term survival if they do not have co-existent viral hepatitis B infection.

15.9 Recent Advances and Future Directions

Liver transplantation in the pediatric age group is limited by the shortage of pediatric donors. As a result, reduced-size liver transplantation, where an adult liver is cut down to pediatric size, has been developed. Split liver transplantation, whereby a donor liver is given to two recipients, has been performed with success and is being applied with increasing frequency now that many of the technical hurdles have been overcome. Living-related liver transplantation is performed routinely in some centers with greater than 80% one-year survival.

Isolated hepatocyte transplantation may offer treatment of metabolic liver diseases and has been successful in the laboratory setting. Artificial support systems have shown initial promise in fulminant hepatic failure and may reduce the need for transplantation.

The elusive goal of tolerance has been produced in animal models and if induced in humans would obviate the need for immunosuppression and its associated complications. Xenotransplantation sits on the horizon; the use of transgenic animals may eventually offer a solution to the shortage of donor organs and permit a wider application of liver transplantation to liver disease.

16. NEOPLASMS OF THE LIVER / L.J. Worobetz

Neoplasms of the liver can be divided into benign and malignant, with malignant tumors being either primary or secondary from a cancer that has metastasized from elsewhere. The sites from which metastases occur frequently include lung, colon, pancreas, breast, stomach and ovary. In North America, primary hepatic neoplasms are uncommon and metastatic tumors commonly seen, whereas worldwide, especially in areas such as the Far East, hepatocellular carcinoma (HCC) is much more prevalent than metastatic disease.

16.1 Benign Tumors of the Liver

Benign tumors of in the liver are detected more frequently than in the past, in part as a result of the increased use of diagnostic imaging tests, including ultrasound and CT scanning, for reasons unrelated to the tumors. Benign tumors are divided into three categories: hepatocellular, cholangiocellular and non-epithelial.

Hepatocellular adenomas are benign tumors seen primarily in females in their third and fourth decades. Their increased prevalence paralleled the introduction of the oral contraceptive, suggesting a hormonal influence in their pathogenesis. The tumors may be multiple, usually involving the right lobe, and may be > 10 cm in diameter. Clinical features include an asymptomatic presentation, pain, palpable mass or features of hemorrhage into the tumor. Diagnosis is usually established with imaging techniques including ultrasound, CT scanning, angiography and radionuclear scanning. The tumor is often hypervascular but with hypovascular areas. The risk of malignancy is 10% with an increased risk in the larger, multiple tumors. Management includes stopping oral contraceptives and resection of larger, symptomatic tumors.

Focal nodular hyperplasia differs from the adenoma in that this solid tumor has a fibrous core and includes other cell types such as atypical hepatocytes, Kupffer's cells and inflammatory cells. The lesion is vascular and because of the presence of Kupffer's cells will appear as an area of increased uptake on radionuclear scanning. Although also more common in women, it does not appear related to the oral contraceptive. No treatment is needed if the patient is asymptomatic.

Hemangiomas of the liver are seen in about 0.5–7% of the general population. These are usually detected by imaging techniques done for other reasons. These vascular lesions are usually asymptomatic and are more common in women. The lesion does not require any treatment as there is no malignant potential and hemorrhage is rare. The vascular nature can be confirmed by red blood cell–labeled nuclear scanning.

16.2 Primary Hepatocellular Carcinoma (HCC)

Although HCC is one of the most common tumors worldwide, it represents only 1–2% of malignant tumors in North America. The tumor is more commonly seen in males and usually arises from areas of long-standing liver injury with liver necrosis and repair, as in the cirrhotic liver. The risk of developing HCC is greatest in patients with chronic hepatitis B and C infections, hemochromatosis and cirrhosis from α_1-antitrypsin deficiency. Hepatitis B can predispose to hepatoma in either a cirrhotic or noncirrhotic liver by the integration of the hepatitis B–DNA into portions of the human genome within the hepatocytes where growth-modifying genes are present. Recent studies suggest that in cases of HCC, HCV is substantially more common than HBV. HCC is not often seen in patients with alcoholic cirrhosis who continue to drink, unless the alcoholic has coexisting viral hepatitis. Hepatic co-carcinogens that appear to play a role in HCC include aflatoxin and vinyl chloride.

The clinical recognition of HCC may be difficult, as the tumors often occur in patients with underlying cirrhosis, and the signs and symptoms may suggest progression of underlying liver disease. The more common presentations include deterioration of the known cirrhotic with rapid weight loss, an enlarging liver with a mass, abdominal pain or bloody ascites. A friction rub or bruit may be present over the liver. Patients may present with one of the many paraneoplastic syndromes, including erythrocytosis, hypercalcemia, dysproteinemia or hypoglycemia. Serum α-fetoprotein levels are greater than 500 μg/L in 70–80% of cases. Ultrasound and CT scan imaging are often used to identify the mass, but occasionally radionuclear scanning (using gallium) or x-ray angiography may help further define the nature of the mass lesion and provide important operative details. A biopsy of the mass or examination of the ascitic fluid for cytology may yield a conclusive diagnosis.

Treatment is disappointing. Surgical resection represents the only opportunity for cure, but resection is often complicated by the presence of underlying cirrhosis, the occasional multicentric nature of the tumor and the presence of micrometastases. Up to 70% of patients already have metastatic disease at the time of diagnosis. The mean survival from the time of diagnosis is approximately 6 to 12 months. Liver transplantation may be considered, but recurrence of tumor and presence of metastases after transplantation have limited its usefulness. Other experimental approaches include hepatic artery embolization with chemotherapy, immunotherapy with monoclonal antibodies tagged with chemotherapy and gene therapy with cytotoxic agents.

Screening strategies include ultrasound and/or α-fetoprotein determinations every 6 months in high-risk patients. This approach clearly identifies tumors at an earlier stage but has not yet been shown to improve morbidity or mortality rates.

17. LIVER DISEASE IN PREGNANCY / R.J. Hilsden and E.A. Shaffer

17.1 Normal Pregnancy

The pregnant state normally is mildly cholestatic from the increase in endogenous estrogens. This changes several biochemical tests, but primary liver disease is an uncommon complication. When features of liver disease do occur during pregnancy, prompt evaluation is essential as some conditions, such as acute fatty liver of pregnancy, rapidly progress to become fatal to both mother and fetus.

The anatomic and physiologic changes that accompany pregnancy alter physical findings and liver biochemistries. Yet normal pregnancy does not significantly affect liver metabolism or function.

Pregnancy does not change liver size. In the third trimester, the enlarging uterus displaces the liver superiorly and posteriorly. Therefore, a palpable liver suggests significant hepatomegaly and underlying liver disease. A small amount of peripheral edema is also common during pregnancy, as are some findings that usually connote chronic liver disease, such as spider angiomas and palmar erythema. These findings are signs of high circulating estrogen levels.

Pregnancy does not alter the expected values for serum bilirubin, aminotransferases, γ-glutamyl transpeptidase or 5'-nucleotidase, or the INR/prothrombin time. Dilution from the expanded plasma volume causes a 10 g/L fall in serum albumin and in total protein. Alkaline phosphatase, primarily of placental and skeletal origin, increases 1.5 times normal after the fifth week. Alkaline phosphatase may remain elevated for up to six weeks after delivery. There is an increase in serum globulin, total cholesterol and triglyceride.

Liver diseases occurring during pregnancy can be divided into three categories: (1) acute liver disease coincident with pregnancy; (2) pregnancy occurring in a patient with established chronic liver disease; and (3) liver diseases unique to pregnancy.

17.2 Acute Liver Disease Coincident with Pregnancy

Any liver disease that can afflict young women may arise during pregnancy. Of these, viral hepatitis is the most common cause of jaundice in pregnancy. Pregnancy does not affect the course of viral hepatitis, except for hepatitis E, which occurs as epidemics in underdeveloped countries. In such settings, the combination of pregnancy and hepatitis plus the indigenous malnutrition results in a significant mortality rate (10–40%). In developed areas, hepatitis B poses a high risk of neonatal infection. Neonates born to mothers who are hepatitis B surface antigen (HB$_s$Ag) positive must receive immunoprophylaxis with hyperimmune globulin and hepatitis B vaccine to prevent the long-term sequelae of chronic hepatitis B: cirrhosis and hepatocellular carcinoma.

Gallstones and their complications, and the rupture of a hepatic adenoma, have an increased incidence during pregnancy.

17.3 Pregnancy Occurring in Chronic Liver Disease

Pregnancy is unusual in patients with chronic liver disease. Fertility becomes nearly normal when cirrhosis is well compensated or the active liver disease improves with appropriate therapy (e.g., autoimmune hepatitis on steroids). The degree of hepatic impairment determines the risk for the mother during the pregnancy. Hemorrhage from esophageal varices is the most significant complication of cirrhosis in pregnancy. The increased blood volume and flow through the azygous system that are a part of any normal pregnancy raise the pressure in the esophageal veins; in established cirrhosis this increases variceal size and the likelihood of bleeding.

17.4 Liver Diseases Unique to Pregnancy

17.4.1 ACUTE FATTY LIVER OF PREGNANCY

Acute fatty liver of pregnancy is characterized by fatty infiltration of the liver. It may rapidly progress to hepatic failure and death. Acute fatty liver may be uncommon (1 in 13,328 deliveries), but is important, having a maternal mortality of 18% and fetal mortality of 23%. The etiology is unknown, but the microvesicular fat that accumulates in hepatocytes probably represents disordered intermediary fat metabolism, perhaps related to mitochondrial injury.

Acute fatty liver of pregnancy almost invariably presents in the third trimester, with a peak frequency around 36–37 weeks gestation. Occasionally, it will become apparent only after delivery. There is an association with nulliparity, twin gestations, male fetus and pre-eclampsia or eclampsia. Presentation can vary from nonspecific symptoms to fulminant hepatic failure. Nausea and vomiting with or without abdominal pain are common. Examination may reveal a tender liver. Pruritus is uncommon and would suggest the possibility of a different liver problem such as intrahepatic cholestasis of pregnancy. Progressive hepatic failure then rapidly supervenes, with the development of jaundice, generalized bleeding from coagulopathy, hypoglycemia, hepatic encephalopathy and renal failure. Such severe cases have an inexorable downhill course unless the fetus is delivered; even then, deterioration may continue for a further 48 to 72 hours.

Laboratory features include a moderately elevated aminotransferase, which is usually around 300 IU/L but may range from normal to 1,000 IU/L. Alkaline phosphatase and serum bilirubin are elevated. Liver biopsy reveals tiny droplets of fat (microvesicular fat) inside hepatocytes.

Diagnosis requires a high degree of suspicion, as the presentation is often nonspecific. Acute fatty liver of pregnancy should be considered whenever marked nausea and vomiting develop in the third trimester of pregnancy. Suspicion increases with a twin pregnancy, nulliparity or signs of toxemia. Ultrasound or CT scans may detect the increased fat in the liver and help exclude complications such as a subcapsular hematoma or another entity such as choledocholithiasis. Liver biopsy is diagnostic. Biopsy even via the transvenous route (necessary when a coagulopathy makes percutaneous liver biopsy hazardous) should be done if the results will alter management. For example, differentiation of acute viral hepatitis from acute fatty liver is important to determine whether rapid delivery is indicated. Delivery can be life-saving in acute fatty liver.

Management involves aggressive supportive care. The only definitive treatment for the condition is prompt delivery. The risk of acute fatty liver of pregnancy is not increased in subsequent pregnancies.

17.4.2 INTRAHEPATIC CHOLESTASIS OF PREGNANCY

Intrahepatic cholestasis of pregnancy accounts for 20–25% of cases of jaundice during pregnancy. The etiology is unknown. There is a clear genetic predisposition, likely autosomal dominant, with an increased frequency in women of Scandinavian or Chilean descent. The cholestasis (failure of bile formation) represents an exaggerated response of the liver to the normal increase in endogenous estrogens during pregnancy.

Presentation typically is in the third trimester with the insidious onset of pruritus. In half of these patients, jaundice follows. Other cholestatic features include dark urine and, occasionally, pale stool. Otherwise women generally feel well, without nausea, vomiting or abdominal pain. Serum alkaline phosphatase and cholesterol rise, but aminotransferases are only modestly elevated. Ultrasound and cholangiography are normal. The evaluation of the pregnant woman with cholestasis involves excluding other causes of jaundice and pruritus including viral hepatitis, primary biliary cirrhosis and biliary tract disease by the appropriate laboratory and ultrasound investigations. Liver biopsy, which shows only cholestasis without inflammation, may be necessary in some atypical cases.

Although a benign condition for the mother (other than the inexorable pruritus), intrahepatic cholestasis may decrease fetal survival and increase the risk of prematurity. Treatment is supportive with bile salt–binding agents such as cholestyramine. Ursodeoxycholic acid therapy improves bile formation, perhaps washing out "toxic" bile acids and pruritogenic agents. *S*-adenosyl-methionine, which alters membrane fluidity, and rifampin, which increases the excretion of pruritogenic agents, also work. Treatment for cholestasis and pruritus, however, generally is unsatisfactory. Delivery should occur as soon as fetal lung maturity is documented, to prevent the increased risk of stillbirth. Parenteral vitamin K may be needed to correct a prothrombin deficiency.

Symptoms usually abate within two weeks of delivery. There is a significant risk of recurrence with subsequent pregnancies and with the use of oral contraceptives or other estrogens.

17.4.3 *PREGNANCY TOXEMIAS AND THE HELLP SYNDROME*
In severe pre-eclampsia or eclampsia, liver involvement is evident by abdominal tenderness and abnormal liver biochemistry. Hepatocellular necrosis can occur from endothelial damage and platelet and fibrin deposition in the sinusoids. Subcapsular hematoma and hepatic rupture rarely develop.

The HELLP syndrome (hemolysis, elevated liver enzymes, low platelets) is usually associated with pre-eclampsia; occasionally, it may arise in the absence of either hypertension or proteinuria. Liver complications are similar to those in pre-eclampsia. Differentiation of acute fatty liver of pregnancy from the HELLP syndrome may be clinically difficult, but the treatment – prompt delivery and supportive care – is identical for both.

18. **VASCULAR DISORDERS OF THE LIVER** / L.J. Worobetz

The most frequent abnormality of circulation to affect the liver is congestive heart failure, which leads to reduced outflow of blood from the liver. Other causes of hepatic congestion include constrictive pericarditis, obstruction of the inferior vena cava and hepatic veins (Budd-Chiari syndrome) and occlusion of the small hepatic veins (veno-occlusive disease). Increased resistance to hepatic venous outflow results in congestive hepatomegaly, dilation of hepatic venules and sinusoids, and hypoxia. The hypoxia in turn leads to hepatocyte damage with possible fibrosis and cirrhosis, the latter termed cardiac cirrhosis.

18.1 **Congestive Heart Failure**
The clinical features of congestive heart failure include tender hepatomegaly and abdominal discomfort. In tricuspid insufficiency, the liver may be pulsatile. Ascites, which may be present, often involves exudate with a high protein

content. Characteristic biochemical abnormalities are mild hyperbilirubine-mia with a moderate elevation of aminotransferases (<300) and a mild eleva-tion of alkaline phosphatase, especially in acute congestion. In ischemic liver damage, aminotransferase can be quite high (from the necrosis), simulating hepatitis – hence the term *ischemic hepatitis*. The prognosis is directly relat-ed to the severity and the response to therapy of the underlying heart failure.

18.2 Hepatic Vein Thrombosis (Budd-Chiari Syndrome)

Hepatic vein thrombosis is a rare disorder that may occur alone or in associa-tion with inferior vena cava thrombosis. It may be associated with poly-cythemia vera, paroxysmal nocturnal hemoglobinuria, hypercoagulability, use of oral contraceptives or neoplasia, or it may be secondary to obstruction by a membranous web. The presentation may be acute, with rapidly developing hepatomegaly, ascites, and abdominal pain leading to liver failure and coma. The chronic presentation is usually that of progressive ascites. The degree of aminotransferase elevation is variable, depending on the rapidity of the onset. The liver biopsy shows large hemorrhagic areas with congestion, atrophy and necrosis around the center of the lobule. Diagnosis may be assisted by liver-spleen colloid scan showing decreased uptake in areas that are otherwise nor-mally drained by the hepatic vein. The caudate lobe demonstrates a normal uptake in that it has a different drainage, that being directly into the vena cava. Hepatic vein Doppler studies clarify the impaired venous blood flow. The con-clusive study is IVC hepatic venography revealing blocked hepatic veins. Assuming absence of a correctable lesion such as a membranous web, treat-ment by anticoagulants and streptokinase is rarely successful. With acute thrombosis, most patients die of liver failure and hepatic coma. Occasionally helpful is a portacaval or mesocaval shunt to allow decompression.

18.3 Veno-occlusive Disease

Veno-occlusive disease refers to the obstruction of small and medium-sized intrahepatic veins. Causal factors include pyrroline alkaloids, hepatic irradia-tion, azathioprine and graft-versus-host disease related to bone marrow trans-plantation. The presentation mimics the Budd-Chiari syndrome. In the acute form, presentation may include hepatomegaly, ascites and liver failure. The chronic form leads to cirrhosis and portal hypertension with esophageal varices. The liver biopsy characteristically shows intense congestion around the hepatic venule with thickened obstructive hepatic veins. There is no effec-tive therapy available. Control of the ascites may be required. Some patients have a spontaneous recovery, while others develop cirrhosis with sequelae of portal hypertension, varices and ascites. Liver transplantation may be the only hope for many.

18.4 Portal Vein Thrombosis

Thrombosis of the portal venous system may result from trauma, pancreatitis, neoplasia (e.g., hepatoma), neonatal umbilical sepsis, pylephlebitis or a complication of cirrhosis, or may be idiopathic. Patients usually present with massive hematemesis that is recurrent. Splenomegaly is present. Biochemical tests of the liver are normal or only mildly elevated. Because liver function is usually normal, ascites and encephalopathy are uncommon and bleeding episodes are better tolerated. Diagnosis may be confirmed by special Doppler ultrasound studies of the portal vein, splenoportogram and/or a venous phase of hepatic angiography. If treatment is required for recurrent hematemesis from esophageal varices, sclerotherapy may be necessary. Because of normal liver parenchyma, surgical approaches such as mesocaval shunt may be considered and are generally better tolerated than by patients with chronic liver disease.

SUGGESTED READING LIST

General
Schiff L, Schiff ER (eds.). Diseases of the liver. 7th ed. Philadelphia: JB Lippincott, 1993.
Sherlock S, Dooley J (eds.). Diseases of the liver and biliary system. 9th ed. Oxford: Blackwell Scientific Publications, 1993.

Section 2 Approach to the Patient with Liver Disease
Frank BB. Clinical evaluation of jaundice. JAMA 1989; 262:3031–3034.
Gollan JL (ed.). Pathobiology of bilirubin and jaundice. Semin Liver Dis 1988; 8:105–199.
Reichling JJ, Kaplan MM. Clinical use of serum enzymes in liver disease. Dig Dis Sci 1988; 33:1601–1614.

Section 3 Congenital Hyperbilirubinemia
Sorrentino D, Anthony JE, Berk PD. Familial hyperbilirubinemia syndromes: kinetic approaches. Baillieres Clin Gastroenterol 1989; 3:313–336.
Watson KJ and Gollan JL. Gilbert's syndrome. Baillieres Clin Gastroenterol 1989; 3:337–355.

Section 4 Acute Viral Hepatitis
Alter HJ, Purcell RH, Shih JW, et al. Detection of antibody to hepatitis C virus in prospectively followed recipients with acute and chronic non-A, non-B transfusion hepatitis. N Engl J Med 1989; 321:1494–1500.
Hollinger FB, Lin HJ. Community-acquired hepatitis C virus infection. Gastroenterology 1992; 102:1426–1429.
Hoofnagle JH, Di Bisceglie AM. Serologic diagnosis of acute and chronic viral hepatitis. Semin Liver Dis 1991; 11:73–84.
Krugman S, Overby LR, Mushahwar IK, et al. Viral hepatitis, type B: studies on natural history and prevention re-examined. N Engl J Med 1979; 300:101–106.

Section 5 Chronic Hepatitis
Autoimmune Chronic Hepatitis
Johnson PJ, McFarlane IG, Eddleston AL. The natural course and heterogeneity of autoimmune-type chronic active hepatitis. Semin Liver Dis 1991; 11:187–196.
Ludwig J. The nomenclature of chronic active hepatitis: an obituary. Gastroenterology 1993; 105:274–278.

Viral Hepatitis
Aagh RD, Stevens CE, Hollinger FB, et al. Hepatitis C virus infection in post-transfusion hepatitis: an analysis with first- and second-generation assays. N Engl J Med 1991; 325:1325–1329.
Alter MJ, Margolis HS, Krawczynski K, et al. The natural history of community-acquired hepatitis C in the United States. N Engl J Med 1992; 327:1899–1905.
Hoofnagle JH, Di Bisceglie AM, Shindo M. Antiviral therapy of hepatitis C – present and future. J Hepatol 1993; 17:130–136.
Katkov WN, Dienstag JL. Prevention and therapy of viral hepatitis. Semin Liver Dis 1991; 11:165–174.
Perrillo RP. Antiviral therapy of chronic hepatitis B: past, present, and future. J Hepatol 1993; 17:56–63.
Rizzetto M, Verme G. Delta hepatitis – present status. J Hepatol 1985; 1:187–193.
Seeff LB, Koff RS. Evolving concepts of the clinical and serologic consequences of hepatitis B virus infection. Semin Liver Dis 1986; 6:11–22.

Fatty Liver
Powell EE, Cooksley WG, Hanson R, Searle J, Halliday JW, Powell LW. The natural history of nonalcoholic steatohepatitis: a follow-up study of forty-two patients for up to 21 years. Hepatology 1990; 11:74–80.

Section 6 Alcoholic Liver Disease
Fleming KA, McGee JO. Alcohol induced liver disease. J Clin Pathol 1984; 37:721–733.
Lieber CS. Alcoholic liver disease: a public health issue in need of a public health approach. Semin Liver Dis 1993; 13:105–107.
Mendenhall CL: Alcoholic hepatitis. In: Schiff L, Schiff ER (eds.), Diseases of the liver. 7th ed. Philadelphia: JB Lippincott, 1993:856–874.

Section 7 Drug-Induced Liver Disease
Kaplowitz N (ed.). Recent advances in drug metabolism and hepatotoxicity. Semin Liver Dis 1990; 10 (special issue): 234–338.
Ludwig J, Axelsen R. Drug effects on the liver: an updated tabular compilation of drugs and drug-related hepatic diseases. Dig Dis Sci 1983; 28:651–666.
Zimmerman HJ. Update of hepatotoxicity due to classes of drugs in common clinical use: non-steroidal drugs, anti-inflammatory drugs, antibiotics, antihypertensives, and cardiac and psychotropic agents. Semin Liver Dis 1990; 10:322–338.

Section 8 Inherited Liver Disease
Hemochromatosis
Adams PC, Kertesz AE, Valberg LS. Clinical presentation of hemochromatosis: a changing scene. Am J Med 1991; 90:445–449.

Adams PC, Speechley M, Kertesz AE. Long-term survival analysis in hereditary hemochromatosis. Gastroenterology 1991; 101:368–372.

Crosby WH. Hemochromatosis: current concepts and management. Hosp Pract 1987; 22:173–177, 181–192.

Edwards CQ, Kushner JP. Screening for hemochromatosis. N Engl J Med 1993; 328:1616–1620.

Alpha₁-Antitrypsin Deficiency

Fisher RL, Taylor L, Sherlock S. Alpha-1-antitrypsin deficiency in liver disease: the extent of the problem. Gastroenterology 1976; 71:646–651.

Wilson's Disease

Brewer GJ, Yuzbasiyan-Gurkan V. Wilson's disease: an update, with emphasis on new approaches to treatment. Dig Dis 1989; 7:178–193.

Nazer H, Ede RJ, Mowat AP, et al. Wilson's disease: clinical presentation and use of prognostic index. Gut 1986; 27:1377.

Scheinberg IH, Sternlieb I. Wilson's disease. Major problems in internal medicine, vol. 23. Philadelphia: WB Saunders, 1984.

Tanzi RE, Petrukhin, K, Chernov I, et al. The Wilson disease gene is a copper transporting ATPase with homology to the Menkes disease gene. Nature Genetics 1993; 5:344–350.

Section 9 Cholestasis

Favrant M, Williams R. Natural history and prognosis in primary sclerosing cholangitis. Eur J Gastroenterol Hepatol 1992; 4:272–275.

Kaplan MM. Primary biliary cirrhosis. N Engl J Med 1987; 316:521–528.

Lester R (ed.). The pathogenesis of cholestasis: past and future trends. Semin Liver Dis 1993; 13 (special issue): 219–316.

Vierling JM. Immune disorder of the liver and bile duct. Gastroenterol Clin North Am 1992; 21:427–449.

Section 10 Cirrhosis of the Liver

D'Amico G, Morabito A, Pogliaro L, et al. Survival and prognostic indicators in compensated and decompensated cirrhosis. Dig Dis Sci 1986; 31:468.

MacSween RNM, Anthony PP, Scheuer PJ. Pathology of the liver. 2d ed. Edinburgh: Churchill Livingstone, 1987.

Section 11 Portal Hypertension

De Franchis R, Primignani M. Why do varices bleed? Gastroenterol Clin North Am 1992; 21:85–96.

Hilsden RJ, Lee SS. Suspecting variceal bleeding in portal hypertensive patients. Can J Diag 1993; 10:91–103.

Polio J, Groszmann RJ. Hemodynamic factors involved in the development and rupture of esophageal varices: a pathophysiologic approach to treatment. Semin Liver Dis 1986; 6:318–331.

Stiegmann GV, Goff JS, Michaletz-Onody PA, et al. Endoscopic sclerotherapy as compared with endoscopic ligation for bleeding esophageal varices. N Engl J Med 1992; 326:1527–1532.

Triger DR, Hosking SW. The gastric mucosa in portal hypertension. J Hepatol 1989; 8:267–272.

Sections 12 and 14 Ascites/Hepatorenal Syndrome
Epstein M (ed.). The kidney in liver disease. 3d ed. Baltimore: Williams and Wilkins, 1988:3.
Epstein M. The sodium retention of cirrhosis: a reappraisal. Hepatology 1986; 6:312.
Henriksen JH, Ring-Larsen H. Ascites formation in liver cirrhosis: the how and the why. Dig Dis 1990; 8:152.

Section 13 Hepatic Encephalopathy
Butterworth RF. Pathogenesis and treatment of portal-systemic encephalopathy: an update. Dig Dis Sci 1992; 37:321–327.
Ferenc P, Puspok A, Steindl P. Current concepts in the pathophysiology of hepatic encephalopathy. Eur J Clin Invest 1992; 22:573–581.

Section 15 Liver Transplantation
Kirby RM, McMaster P, Clents D, et al. Orthotopic liver transplantation: postoperative complications and their management. Br J Surg 1987; 74:3–11.
Krom RAF, Wiesner RH, Rettke SR, et al. The first 100 liver transplantations at the Mayo Clinic. Symposium on liver transplantation part 1. Mayo Clinic Proc 1989; 64:84–94.
Maddrey WC, Van Thiel DH. Liver transplantation: an overview. Hepatology 1988; 8:948–959.
Sheiner PA, Greig PD, Levy GA. Perioperative management of the liver transplant patient. In: Vincent JL (ed.), Update in intensive care and emergency medicine, update 1990. Berlin: Springer-Verlag, 1990:706–717.

Section 16 Neoplasms of the Liver
Okuda K. Diagnosis and nonsurgical treatment of hepatocellular carcinoma. Hepato-Gastroenterology 1990; 37:159–164.
Rustgi VK. Epidemiology of hepatocellular carcinoma [Review]. Gastroenterol Clin North Am 1987; 16:545–551.

Section 17 Liver Disease in Pregnancy
Riely CA, Abell TL (eds.). Gastrointestinal and liver problems in pregnancy. Gastroenterol Clin North Am 1992; 21:873–921, 937–958.

Section 18 Vascular Disorders of the Liver
Gibson PR, Dudley FJ. Ischemic hepatitis: clinical features, diagnosis and prognosis. Aust NZ J Med 1984; 14:822.
Klein AS, Sitzmann JV, Coleman J, et al. Current management of the Budd-Chiari syndrome. Ann Surg 1990; 212:144.

ACKNOWLEDGMENT

The authors would like to acknowledge the assistance of Dr. Emma Lew, Department of Pathology, University of Saskatchewan, in the preparation of the pathology pictures.

OBJECTIVES

Jaundice/Ascites/Hepatic Encephalopathy/Liver Failure

1. Describe normal bilirubin metabolism.
2. Describe pathophysiologic mechanisms of jaundice.
3. Outline the diagnostic tests used in approaching patients with jaundice and discuss liver function tests.
4. Define jaundice.
5. Describe mechanisms of ascites formation.
6. List five conditions that associate with ascites.
7. Describe the techniques and diagnostic tests used to detect ascites.
8. Discuss the indication of abdominal paracentesis and interpret the findings.
9. Recognize the complications of ascites.
10. Outline the management of ascites.
11. Give indications for LeVeen's shunt.
12. Interpret serum and urinary electrolytes in patients with ascites.
13. Discuss the mechanisms of action and side effects of drugs used in the treatment of ascites.
14. Demonstrate clinical skills in approaching patients with hepatic encephalopathy and hepatic failure.
15. List the stigmata of chronic liver disease.
16. List neurotransmitters that possibly have pathogenetic roles in hepatic encephalopathy.
17. List precipitating factors of hepatic encephalopathy.
18. Discuss the use of ammonia blood level in hepatic encephalopathy.
19. Outline the management of hepatic encephalopathy.
20. Discuss the mechanisms of action of lactulose and metronidazole in the treatment of hepatic encephalopathy.
21. Discuss the role of liver transplantation.
22. Differentiate between hepatorenal failure and prerenal azotemia.
23. Discuss the management of hepatorenal failure.

Cirrhosis

1. List underlying causes of cirrhosis.
2. List complications of cirrhosis.
3. List major mechanisms contributing to portal hypertension.
4. Discuss diagnostic methods used in patients with cirrhosis.
5. Describe complications of liver biopsy.
6. Classify portal hypertension.
7. List the consequences of portal hypertension.

8. Describe the management of patients with bleeding esophageal varices.
9. Discuss the use of the Sengstaken-Blakemore tube in patients with bleeding esophageal varices.
10. Discuss the efficacy, mechanisms of action and side effects of vasopressin and somatostatin used in treating bleeding esophageal varices.
11. Discuss the role of sclerotherapy and banding in patients with bleeding esophageal varices.
12. List major complications of sclerotherapy and banding.
13. Discuss the surgical management of portal hypertension.

Hepatitis
1. List causative agents for acute hepatitis.
2. Discuss serologic tests used in hepatitis.
3. Discuss the significance of delta agent.
4. Give indications for hepatitis A and B vaccination.
5. Discuss the clinical manifestations of hepatitis A and hepatitis B infections.
6. Discuss the clinical manifestations of hepatitis C.
7. List causes of chronic liver disease.
8. Describe histologic features of mild, moderate and severe chronic hepatitis.
9. Discuss the role of corticosteroids and/or azathioprine in the treatment of chronic liver disease.
10. List possible complications of corticosteroids.
11. Describe major drug-metabolizing pathways of the liver.
12. List five drugs that cause chronic liver disease.
13. Describe alcohol metabolism.
14. Give the spectrum of alcohol-related liver diseases.
15. Discuss clinical manifestations of alcoholic hepatitis.
16. Discuss the management of alcoholic hepatitis.

Cholestasis/PBC/Hemochromatosis/Wilson's Disease
1. Define cholestasis.
2. List conditions associated with cholestasis.
3. Discuss the approach to neonatal jaundice.
4. Discuss diagnostic tests used in patients with cholestasis.
5. Define primary biliary cirrhosis.
6. Discuss the clinical manifestations of primary biliary cirrhosis and diagnostic tests.
7. Give histologic staging of primary biliary cirrhosis.

8. Discuss the treatment of PBC.
9. List the complications of PBC.
10. Discuss normal iron metabolism.
11. Describe salient clinical features of hemochromatosis.
12. Discuss diagnostic tests used in hemochromatosis.
13. Differentiate homozygotes for hemochromatosis from heterozygotes for hemochromatosis.
14. Discuss the management of hemochromatosis.
15. Define Wilson's disease.
16. Describe clinical manifestations of Wilson's disease.
17. Discuss the diagnostic tests for Wilson's disease.
18. Discuss the use and side effects of penicillamine in treating Wilson's disease.
19. List the diagnostic methods that differentiate liver abscesses, neoplasms and cysts.

Jaundice and Liver Disease in Children
1. Understand bilirubin metabolism in the neonate. Understand the significance of bilirubin metabolism in the fetus, and the changes that occur during the first 72 hours after birth.
2. Understand "physiologic jaundice of the newborn."
   a. Why does it occur?
   b. What brings it to an end?
   c. Under what circumstances will it be "unphysiologic"?
   d. What treatment modalities are available to modify and treat this disorder?
3. Understand the importance of careful choice of drugs in the newborn and in the nursing mother.
4. Understand the significance of unconjugated versus conjugated bilirubin in the plasma.
5. Be aware of kernicterus and its various manifestations.
6. Be aware of "hydrops fetalis," "RhoGAM®," Rh and ABO immunization.
7. Be aware of "neonatal hepatitis syndrome," and understand that it is a spectrum of specific and nonspecific disorders of the liver.
8. Know the normal age presentation.
9. Be aware of "giant cell hepatitis," including its histologic abnormality.
10. Be aware of "biliary atresia," including its pathology.
11. Be aware that a number of metabolic disorders may present as "neonatal hepatitis syndrome," including galactosemia; α_1-antitrypsin deficiency; tyrosinemia; cystic fibrosis.

12. Be aware that a number of perinatal infections may present as "neonatal hepatitis syndrome," including first-degree cytomegalovirus infection and rubella.
13. Understand the significance in investigation of:
    a. HIDA scan
    b. Liver biopsy
    c. Mini lap and operative cholangiogram
    d. Alpha-fetoprotein
14. Know the prognosis of giant cell hepatitis and biliary atresia.
15. Be aware of the Kasai procedure and liver transplantation.

15

Manifestations of Gastrointestinal Disease in the Child

R.B. Scott, G. Withers, D.J. Morrison, S.A. Zamora,
H.G. Parsons, J.D. Butzner, R.A. Schreiber,
H. Machida and S.R. Martin

1. RECURRENT ABDOMINAL PAIN / R.B. Scott

1.1 Definition

Recurrent abdominal pain (RAP) is defined as at least three episodes of pain occurring over a period of at least three months in children 3 years of age or older, and which are of sufficient severity that the discomfort interferes with their activities. The overall incidence of recurrent abdominal pain is 10.8%, with 12.3% of girls and 9.5% of boys being affected. The prevalence of RAP at any given age is quite constant in school-age boys, but in girls prevalence reaches a peak between the ages of 8 and 10.

1.2 History

The discomfort of RAP is typically localized in the periumbilical region and is nonradiating. In almost all other respects it is variable in character from patient to patient – often vague and ill-defined, a dull ache or a crampy feeling, but occasionally a sharp and colicky pain. It is generally mild to moderate in intensity; the child will stop playing, sit or lie down, but in a minority of affected children the pain will be sufficiently severe to cause crying. The temporal occurrence, frequency and duration of pain are also highly variable. Pain may occur at any time of the day, be reported upon awaking, or be present until the child falls asleep. However, the discomfort will only rarely awaken the child from sleep at night. The occurrence of pain generally bears no consistent relation to the ingestion of specific foods or to meals, physical activity, defecation, urination or (in girls) menstruation. Episodes may occur infrequently or several times a day, and last from a few minutes to several hours at a time. Although aggravating factors are frequently absent, a relationship between recurrent attacks of abdominal pain and stressful situations is reported in approximately one-third of affected children. A brief rest is often cited as a relieving factor. Characteristically, treatment with antacids, anticholinergics, H_2 antagonists, barbiturates and analgesics provides no consistent relief. Episodes of RAP are commonly associated with nonspecific symptoms: pallor, nausea, headaches, limb or "growing" pains and drowsiness after attacks. Sporadic vomiting may occur, but repetitive or bilious emesis should suggest the possibility of an organic disorder. Diarrhea and documented elevation of temperature are occasionally reported but are atypical, and should also suggest an alternative etiology. Characteristically, the children are otherwise well and active between episodes.

There is nothing specific or diagnostic with respect to the past or family history of the child who presents with RAP. However, as a group, the parents and siblings of children with RAP are much more likely than those of unaffected children or those with organic disease to experience somatization of stress and to provide a history of recurrent abdominal pain/irritable bowel syndrome, peptic ulcer, severe headaches and disorders that were in the past very loosely labeled as "nervous breakdown."

1.3 Physical Signs
Except for subjective abdominal tenderness, the physical examination of children with RAP is striking in its normality. Plots of the previous and currently measured heights and weights demonstrate a normal growth velocity, and objective physical signs of disease are absent.

1.4 Psychosocial Factors
The intellectual abilities of children with RAP are identical to those of unaffected children, but certain personality traits are more commonly recognized in children with RAP than in those without. These children have been described as overachievers, overconscientious, high-strung, fussy or particular, anxious, and timid or apprehensive – generalizations that do not always apply in the individual case, however.

There is a close association between emotional status and function of the gastrointestinal tract, and the literature contains numerous anecdotal reports of children presenting with recurrent abdominal pain in whom there is (1) no organic cause, (2) a temporal relationship between discomfort and a specific stress, and (3) resolution of the pain in response to measures that relieve the stress. However, objective evidence of psychological difficulties – and not just the absence of an organic etiology – is necessary before a "psychogenic" label is applied. Using these criteria, psychological or emotional disturbance will be a primary diagnosis in only a very small number of children presenting with RAP.

1.5 Differential Diagnosis and Approach to Investigation

Although the differential diagnosis of abdominal pain is extensive, a complete history and physical examination with limited laboratory investigations should enable the physician to make a positive diagnosis of recurrent abdominal pain. In 90–95% of affected children, RAP is functional; organic disease is identified in only 5–10%. The approach to diagnosis should not be one of extensive investigation to exclude organic disease. In the majority of cases of recurrent abdominal pain, the extent of appropriate investigation should be limited to a complete blood count, urinalysis, and perhaps a stool occult blood test. Comprehensive lists of organic causes of chronic abdominal pain are available but need be referred to only when features of the history and physical examination, or the CBC and urinalysis, strongly suggest an organic problem that is not readily apparent. Specific aspects of the history that should signal concern on the part of the physician include significant recurrent pain in a child under the age of 3; consistent localization of pain away from the umbilicus; frequently being woken from sleep by pain; repetitive or bilious emesis; and any constellation of symptoms and signs that are typical of a specific organic etiology.

Urogenital and alimentary disorders are the most common organic causes of RAP. Genitourinary diseases such as recurrent infection and hydronephrosis or obstructive uropathy can present with abdominal pain. In patients with these disorders who present without urinary tract symptoms, an abnormal urinalysis and pyuria will frequently bring attention to the underlying problem.

Constipation is a common disorder and patients may experience crampy abdominal discomfort in association with the urge to defecate. A suggestive history and the demonstration on physical examination of bulky stool retained in the rectum should initiate a trial of appropriate treatment.

A history of abdominal pain, bloating, flatus and watery diarrhea that occurs with heavy ingestion of "sugarless" gums or confections suggests the possibility of malabsorption of nonabsorbable carbohydrates. The same history occurring with milk intake in individuals whose ethnic background might predispose to lactase deficiency (oriental, black or peri-Mediterranean) suggests lactose malabsorption.

Pernicious vomiting or bilious emesis in the presence of abdominal pain should always alert the clinician to the possibility of an intestinal obstruction. Malrotation or incomplete rotation of the mid-gut is a disorder that may present as a bowel obstruction and also predisposes to intestinal volvulus. Whenever malrotation is suspected an upper gastrointestinal series should be performed to determine the position of the duodenojejunal flexure, and a barium enema may be required to ensure proper location of the cecum in the lower right quadrant.

Primary peptic ulcer disease is much less common in children than in adults and frequently lacks the typical meal-related characteristics that are common with the adult presentation. A family history of peptic ulcer disease, vomiting, nighttime awakening with pain, hematemesis or melena, or unexplained anemia should suggest the diagnosis.

1.6 Pathophysiology and Treatment

A thorough history, careful physical examination and a minimum of laboratory examinations are essential to provide the data that allow a physician to reach a positive diagnosis of RAP. This care and thoroughness are crucial to the success of subsequent management because they demonstrate that the complaint has been seriously evaluated by the physician and lend credibility to the diagnosis that is subsequently rendered. Having made a positive diagnosis, it is then important to cease investigation and to educate and reassure the patient and parents. If this is not done the parents' perception that there is a significant probability of an underlying organic problem may be reinforced. On the other hand, reassurance in the absence of explanation (i.e., simply saying "Don't worry") is of little value.

It must be made clear that the discomfort of RAP is genuine, not imagined or manufactured for gain or manipulation. It is important to point out that this is a common complaint. Identify for the parent those criteria upon which you based the diagnosis of RAP: the periumbilical location of the discomfort, the absence of any constellation of historical or objective physical findings that suggest underlying organic disease, continued normal growth and development (show the parents the growth chart), continued general well-being between episodes, and a family history of similar functional complaints, if that exists. In those cases where they can be identified note the positive association of RAP with stressful situations or events and any characteristics of the child's personality that might serve to exaggerate the stress. Try to elicit and allay any specific concerns on the part of the child or parents (e.g., "Does my child have appendicitis?").

Encourage the parents to discuss potential stressful contributing events with the child, and recommend a positive approach to coping that includes a return to all normal activities. Insist on attendance at school. Discuss the prognosis of this condition with the parents and provide reassurance by offering to reassess the child should there be any change in the symptoms.

Patient education is generally very effective in relieving the parents' anxiety. Drugs, and specifically analgesics or sedatives, are not considered effective or appropriate. However, a recent prospective, double-blind, randomized control trial demonstrated a significant decrease in RAP in children given additional dietary fiber as compared to placebo.

1.7 Prognosis

Many children and their parents experience considerable immediate relief at having organic disease excluded. In the long term one-third of patients managed in this fashion are completely free of pain as adults, one-third experience continuing abdominal pain, and one-third develop alternative symptomatology such as headaches. Almost all lead unrestricted lives. The goal of management should be to develop, through education, the increased understanding and constructive coping mechanisms that will prevent symptoms from generating dysfunctional behavior.

2. VOMITING AND REGURGITATION / G. Withers and R.B. Scott

2.1 Definitions
Gastroesophageal reflux is the apparently effortless passage of gastric contents into the esophagus due to impairment of the antireflux mechanism at the gastroesophageal junction. Reflux is facilitated by the presence of a gradient in pressure between the positive pressure within the abdominal cavity and the negative pressure within the intrathoracic cavity. Vomiting, however, is a complex coordinated reflex mechanism that may occur in response to a variety of stimuli and results in forceful expulsion of gastric contents through the mouth. The vomiting reflex is controlled by the nervous system, specifically via the vomiting center in the brainstem.

2.2 The Vomiting Child

2.2.1 *INTRODUCTION*
The approach to the vomiting child is one of the most difficult problems in pediatrics, as the differential diagnosis is not limited to the gastrointestinal tract and includes conditions that are pediatric emergencies. In addition, persistent vomiting can lead to complications such as dehydration, electrolyte abnormalities, Mallory-Weiss tears and aspiration of gastric contents. The following comments on history, examination, diagnosis and management provide guidance as to the approach to the vomiting child, but cannot substitute for a broad knowledge of pediatrics and clinical experience that allows differentiation of the sick child from the child that is less unwell.

2.2.2 *HISTORY*
A number of features of the history are particuarly helpful in reaching a diagnosis:

2.2.2.1 *Age*
Vomiting in the neonatal and early infant period may frequently be due to structural abnormalities of the bowel, inborn errors of metabolism and withdrawal secondary to maternal drug addictions (Table 1). A complete history of the pregnancy (including drug history, past pregnancies and abortions), deliv-

TABLE 1. Causes of vomiting according to age of presentation

Neonate/infancy	
Gastrointestinal disorders	*Nongastrointestinal disorders*
Common	Common
Gastroenteritis	Upper respiratory tract infection
Gastroesophageal reflux	Septicemia/meningitis
Pyloric stenosis	Pneumonia
Intussusception	Urinary tract infection
Anatomic obstruction	
Atresia – esophagus, small intestine	
Malrotation and volvulus	
Hirschsprung's disease	
Rare	Rare
Meconium ileus	Inborn error of metabolism
	Raised intracranial pressure –
	tumor/hydrocephalus
	Endocrine deficiency – adrenal, thyroid
	Renal tubular acidosis
	Genetic syndromes (trisomy 21, 13, 18)

Child/adolescent	
Gastrointestinal disorders	*Nongastrointestinal disorders*
Common	Common
Gastroenteritis	Infection – URTI, OM, UTI
Appendicitis	Toxin/drug ingestion
Intussusception	Bulemia
Pancreatitis	Pregnancy
Celiac disease	
Inflammatory bowel disease	
Rare	Rare
Hepatitis	Cyclic vomiting syndrome/migraine
Intestinal obstruction	Brain tumor
Peptic ulcer	Testicular torsion
Achalasia	Ovarian cyst/salpingitis
Reye's syndrome	

ery and postpartum period is vital. Some conditions will occur in specific age ranges: pyloric stenosis at 2 to 8 weeks of age; intussusception at 3 to 18 months. Appendicitis is rare before the age of 12 months. In older children, other conditions, especially gastroenteritis, otitis media and respiratory tract infections are more common.

2.2.2.2 Diet
Food allergy, the most common cause being cow's milk protein intolerance,

occurs primarily in formula-fed infants. Infant celiac disease presents only after prolonged exposure to gluten in the diet. Enzyme-deficiency diseases such as galactosemia and fructosemia manifest only after the introduction of the offending sugar into the diet.

2.2.2.3 *Nature of the vomitus*
Bile-stained vomitus suggests intestinal obstruction distal to the second part of the duodenum, while hematemesis suggests esophageal, gastric or duodenal mucosal disease.

2.2.2.4 *Onset and duration of vomiting*
Acute onset and short duration suggest a transient illness, while a longer history of vomiting suggests chronic disease, especially if associated with growth failure.

2.2.2.5 *Associated symptoms*
Diarrhea is a common feature accompanying gastrointestinal infection, but some looseness of stools can be found in association with other conditions such as urinary tract infections. A bloody stool resembling red currant jelly is seen classically in intussusception. If abdominal pain is present, the nature, severity and location are important. Obstruction of the GI tract often presents with central, colicky, intermittent pain, as do the cramps of gastroenteritis. Colicky pain may be accompanied by pallor, especially in intussusception. Other conditions are associated with a more constant pain, or pain in specific locations – eg., in the right iliac fossa with appendicitis, epigastric/central pain radiating to the back with pancreatitis. Fever suggests an infectious origin, and foci outside the GI tract as in meningitis should be considered. Neurological symptoms such as headache, confusion and loss of developmental skills may indicate a primary CNS pathology.

2.2.3 *EXAMINATION*
A complete physical assessment is required, for it is important to determine whether the child is well or sick. An initial assessment is often possible by careful observation from the end of the bed. The height, weight and head circumference should be plotted (with past recordings if possible) on a growth chart to determine whether there has been a fall-off in recent months. A rapidly expanding head circumference suggests intracranial pathology. An assessment of dehydration (including tissue turgor, mucous membranes, capillary return, pulse and blood pressure) as well as a thorough examination of each system is essential. When examining the abdomen, it is particularly important to detect any distention, masses, tenderness and especially rigidity or guarding that suggests the need for urgent surgical review.

2.2.4 *INVESTIGATION*

Investigation of the vomiting child is dependent on the history and the results of physical examination. An acutely ill febrile neonate requires different investigation than an older child. Investigation may include:

2.2.4.1 *Blood tests*

A complete blood count may show an elevated white cell count with infection or inflammation, but is relatively nonspecific. Anemia may be present and be secondary to an acute bleed, or be of a long-term nature in the presence of chronic disease (normochromic) or ongoing blood loss (hypochromic, microcytic). Electrolytes, urea, creatinine and anion gap provide information regarding fluid balance and metabolic status. Generally, frequent vomiting results in hypochloremic, hypokalemic alkalosis; however, acidosis may occur if dehydration is severe or secondary to an underlying metabolic disorder. Abnormalities of urea are found in dehydration (high) and in urea cycle disorders (low). Hypo- or hypernatremia may occur if inappropriate fluid replacement is given.

2.2.4.2 *Radiology*

Any child with symptoms that suggest a surgical problem such as intestinal obstruction requires an urgent radiograph of the abdomen with both supine and erect films. Intestinal obstruction is suggested by dilated loops of bowel with air-fluid levels, although a similar appearance can occur with an ileus accompanying gastroenteritis. The history and examination usually allow differentiation. Other conditions have more specific appearances, such as the right upper quadrant mass in intussusception, the double-bubble appearance of duodenal atresia and a distended loop of bowel with volvulus. An abdominal ultrasound may be of help in the diagnosis of pyloric stenosis (hypertrophic mass at outlet of stomach), liver disease (gallstones and thickened gallbladder wall in cholecystitis, liver enlargement in hepatitis), pancreatitis (swollen, edematous pancreas), renal disease (hydronephrosis or small kidneys). A child who presents with persistent bile-stained emesis requires an upper GI contrast study to exclude anatomical causes of obstruction including intestinal malrotation, webs, rings and strictures. The contrast study may include a follow-through of the small intestine to identify more distal problems such as terminal Crohn's disease.

2.2.4.3 *Microbiology*

Urinalysis is important to exclude urinary pathology such as infection. Stool examinations for bacterial culture, ova and parasites, and viruses are indicated if diarrhea is present, and for Clostridium difficile toxin if there is a recent history of antibiotic use. In the severely ill and/or febrile child with emesis and suspected sepsis or meningitis, cultures of the blood and cerebrospinal fluid are required.

2.2.4.4 *Endoscopy*
Upper gastrointestinal endoscopy may be employed to exclude mucosal disease in the esophagus (esophagitis), stomach (H. pylori gastritis, ulceration) or duodenum (ulceration, Crohn's disease, celiac disease).

2.2.5 *MANAGEMENT*
Management of the vomiting child centers on establishing an accurate diagnosis and stabilizing the patient's condition with regard to fluid and electrolyte abnormalities. Specific conditions require specific treatment, such as surgery for appendicitis and antibiotics for meningitis. Acute management of dehydration requires an accurate assessment as mild (<5%), moderate (5–10%) or severe (>10%). Fluid requirements are then calculated to replace the deficit (usually over 8, 12 or 24 hours), provide maintenance fluids (age-dependent), and replace continuing GI losses. Mild to moderate dehydration can usually be managed via the oral route unless contraindicated (e.g., preoperative conditions such as appendicitis or intestinal obstruction), while severe dehydration usually requires intravenous replacement, often with colloid as well as crystalloid solutions.

2.3 Gastroesophageal Reflux Disease (GERD)

2.3.1 *INTRODUCTION*
Effortless reflux of stomach contents is noted in approximately 50% of healthy newborn infants. In the majority of affected children it resolves over the first year of life, especially in the second six months when the dietary intake of solids increases and sitting and standing are achieved. In all children, occasional reflux after a meal is a normal event. Pathological reflux is defined as being secondary to an underlying disorder or when the reflux is complicated by failure to thrive, esophagitis or respiratory conditions such as asthma or aspiration pneumonia.

2.3.2 *PATHOGENESIS*
Reflux of gastric contents into the esophagus is prevented by the antireflux mechanism at the gastroesophageal junction, which consists primarily of the diaphragmatic crura and the lower esophageal sphincter (LES). The LES is a physiologically defined region of the lower esophagus that is maintained in a partial contractile condition to create a high-pressure zone, but relaxes as part of the swallowing reflex to allow food passage into the stomach. The primary cause of reflux is transient relaxation of the LES unrelated to swallowing,

rather than a consistently low pressure of the sphincter. Although gastric volume and composition of gastric contents are important influences, the mechanism of this transient relaxation is not understood. Other factors important in the prevention of complications of reflux include esophageal peristalsis, which clears refluxed contents from the esophagus; salivary secretions, which assist in neutralizing refluxed gastric acid; esophageal mucosal resistance; and the protective pulmonary reflexes that prevent reflux into the respiratory tree.

2.3.3 CLINICAL FEATURES

A thorough history and physical examination are required to establish if possible whether the child is refluxing or vomiting. Gastroesophageal reflux is often effortless and vomiting forceful, but some overlap occurs. The onset of gastroesophageal reflux in infants is usually soon after birth. A sudden onset of reflux in a child with no past history or bilious emesis requires a search for a secondary cause. Feeding history is important. Feeds of inappropriately large volume are more likely to be refluxed. The physician should always determine whether the child is otherwise well and if not, identify symptoms or signs that suggest an underlying disorder or predispose to reflux or vomiting (Table 1). The frequency and volume of the reflux episodes should be established and any symptoms or signs of complications of gastroesophageal reflux sought.

2.3.4 COMPLICATIONS OF GASTROESOPHAGEAL REFLUX (Table 2)

2.3.4.1 Failure to thrive

Failure to thrive occurs in association with gastroesophageal reflux when caloric intake is insufficient as a result of the loss of milk through reflux, or when children with esophagitis limit intake due to pain or dysphagia associated with feeding.

2.3.4.2 Esophagitis

Esophagitis may be indicated by dysphagia, hematemesis, anemia, hypoalbuminemia and thrombocytosis. While dysphagia may occur secondary to esophageal ulceration or strictures, it may also be secondary to the impaired motility that is associated with esophagitis and often presents as food sticking.

2.3.4.3 Respiratory complications

Aspiration of gastric contents causing pneumonia is relatively common in the neurologically impaired child, but aspiration of food during its ingestion may also occur as a result of incoordinate swallowing. Some children with asthma, especially nocturnal asthma, may have symptoms secondary to reflux. Gas-

TABLE 2. Complications of GER

Systemic
Failure to thrive

Esophageal
Pain
Esophagitis
Hematemesis
Anemia
Hypoproteinemia
Dysphagia secondary to stricture or dysmotility
Sandifer's syndrome – an unusual posturing of head and
   upper body in infants with reflux esophagitis

Respiratory
Apnea
Bronchospasm
Laryngospasm
Aspiration pneumonia

---

troesophageal reflux is a less common cause of apnea in premature infants, most apnea in this age group being of central origin. Gastroesophageal reflux is not responsible for SIDS.

2.3.5 *INVESTIGATION*
The vast majority of infants with gastroesophageal reflux do not require additional investigation. Infants whose reflux is persistent, severe or associated with symptoms or signs of an underlying disorder require further investigation. Initial investigations should include a complete blood count, electrolytes, urea, anion gap, urinalysis and, in older infants, liver function tests and a lipase or amylase. An upper gastrointestinal contrast study (upper GI) should be performed to exclude predisposing anatomic abnormalities such as malrotation or strictures. Reflux seen during this test is a poor indicator of pathologic reflux. If the infant or child is suspected of having a complication of gastroesophageal reflux, then more extensive investigation may be required. These tests are usually available only at a tertiary center and include 24-hour pH probe monitoring of the distal esophagus to quantify the frequency, duration and pattern (postprandial, nocturnal) of reflux episodes and their association with other events. A pH probe is best performed in conjunction with respiratory monitoring to determine whether respiratory symptoms such as apnea or wheezing coincide with reflux.

Esophageal manometry may be performed to exclude motor disorders of the esophagus such as achalasia, and nuclear medicine gastric emptying studies can document those children in whom delayed gastric emptying contributes to reflux. To determine if esophagitis is present, esophageal mucosal tissue may be obtained either by endoscopic or suction biopsy. Features of esophagitis on biopsy include esophageal inflammatory infiltrate (especially an increased number of eosinophils), increased thickness of the basal layer, increased papillary height and ulceration with a neutrophil infiltrate. Bronchoscopy and bronchial-alveolar lavage to look for lipid-laden macrophages may be of help in the diagnosis of reflux-related respiratory infection.

2.3.6 MANAGEMENT

Management of most children with gastroesophageal reflux often requires no more than an explanation to parents that reflux is a normal phenomenon in infants. Conservative measures may be helpful. These include positioning the infant and smaller, more frequent thickened feedings; rarely, continuous drip feedings may be necessary. Positioning the child in a head-elevated prone position after feeds can be useful, but the use of infant seats has been shown to make reflux worse. Thickening of feeds (usually with rice formula) decreases the number of emeses and time crying, but has not been shown to decrease the time spent refluxing, as shown by esophageal pH monitoring.

For those children with complicated or severe reflux unresponsive to conservative management, drug therapy may be necessary. This usually entails the use of a prokinetic agent and/or an acid suppressant. Cisapride is the prokinetic agent of choice as it lacks the neurological and respiratory side effects of other prokinetic agents such as metoclopramide and bethanechol. Cisapride acts peripherally to increase the release of acetylcholine from the intestinal myenteric plexus and has been shown to be effective in the treatment of gastroesophageal reflux in children. It is given orally approximately 30 minutes prior to feedings at a dose of 0.2mg/kg/dose q.i.d. up to a maximal dose of 0.3 mg/kg/dose. It is well tolerated and side effects are generally limited to an increased stool frequency. However, recent reports have shown that cisapride can induce life-threatening ventricular arrhythmias in individuals with conduction abnormalities such as a prolonged Q–T interval; it should be used with extreme caution in such patients. Acid suppression is helpful in those patients with evidence of esophagitis or reflux-associated pain. An H_2 antagonist such as ranitidine or cimetidine is often sufficient for pain relief, but patients with esophagitis may require more powerful acid suppression with a proton pump inhibitor such as omeprazole to achieve healing.

Surgery may be necessary in patients with gastroesophageal reflux who fail medical therapy or who have life-threatening reflux-associated apnea. Nissen fundoplication, where the fundus of the stomach is wrapped 360° around the lower esophagus to produce an esophageal high-pressure zone, is the operation of choice. Fundoplication is effective, and a successful clinical outcome is seen in almost 90% of patients at five years, but major complications such as postoperative adhesions, wound infection and pneumonia occur in approximately 10–20% of patients. Fundoplication is less successful in controlling reflux in neurologically impaired children, where clinical success rates are of the order of 50–60% and complication rates are higher. Recently, newer surgical techniques such as partial wraps (<360°) and laparoscopic fundoplication have become available, but it is not yet known whether the long-term success rates or complications of these procedures differ from the open Nissen technique.

3. COLIC / D.J. Morrison

The term *colic* is used to describe intense or excessive crying or fussiness in an otherwise healthy infant. This typically starts in the second or third week of life and resolves by three to four months (although it can persist longer). A variety of definitions of excessive crying have been used. Perhaps the most useful is Wessel's "rule of threes": more than three hours per day for more than three days per week for more than three weeks. The most common time of day seems to be early evening. In extreme cases the crying may occur throughout the day and night. Prospective studies have shown that colic is common. Dr. T.B. Brazleton, using crying diaries kept by parents, found that 35% of 6-week-old infants cried for more than three hours per day. Typically these infants cry longer, though not more frequently, than other infants and are more difficult to console.

The etiology of colic is unknown. The fact that it occurs in healthy babies, follows the crying pattern of normal infants and resolves without later sequelae has prompted its description as a disorder of development.

Colic occurs with equal frequency in breastfed and formula-fed infants. The question of milk intolerance as a possible cause of colic is frequently raised, and formula changes are a commonly tried intervention. Cow's milk protein sensitivity probably does cause colic in a small subgroup of infants. These infants may also experience weight loss, vomiting and diarrhea. With such a history, a trial of casein-hydrolyzed formula would be appropriate. The incidence of lactose or carbohydrate malabsorption does not appear to be different in patients with colic compared to those without.

Intestinal immaturity with delayed development of normal patterns of intestinal motor activity and resulting poor propulsion has been proposed as an etiology. Many infants with colic appear uncomfortable, draw their legs up and pass wind. This may be secondary to air swallowing with crying. Antispasmodics and antiflatulents have generally not been shown to help. There is evidence that one antispasmodic, dicylomine hydrochloride, may be effective; however, concern regarding respiratory distress and apnea preclude its use.

Intestinal hormones may play a role in colic; this role is incompletely under-stood at this time, however.

At one time, colic was blamed on "overanxious mothers," but there is no scientific confirmation of this etiology. Certainly, prolonged crying in an infant can itself give rise to anxiety in parents.

In the evaluation of a patient with colic it is first essential to take a thorough history to rule out pathological causes of crying, inquire about feeding prac-tices (including formula preparation and burping procedure) and soothing techniques. For an accurate description of duration of crying it is useful to have the mother keep a diary over a few days. A thorough physical examina-tion must be performed to assess growth and development as well as rule out illness (particularly infection) or intestinal obstruction.

If no apparent cause is found for the crying it is first essential to relieve parental guilt and reassure parents that they do not cause the colic. Explaining the natural history of colic (frequency and duration) can be very helpful. Tri-als of soothing techniques (carrying the baby in a body carrier, car rides or automatic rockers) may be useful. Advising parents on obtaining relief – babysitting or even a weekend away – is often the best intervention. Finally, a trial of casein-hydrolyzed formula for the infant or a milk-free diet for the breastfeeding mother may be useful, particularly if additional symptoms sug-gesting food allergy are present.

4. CHRONIC CONSTIPATION, ENCOPRESIS AND SOILING / R.B. Scott

4.1 Definition
Constipation is a symptom indicative of an abnormality in stool or its elimina-tion: the stool is too large or too hard; passage is too infrequent, painful or incomplete. There is an extremely wide range in what constitutes normal bowel habit, and this changes markedly between birth and adolescence. As a generalization, stool frequency is less in the formula-fed than in the breastfed infant. The formula-fed infant tends to pass 3 to 5 bowel motions per day; breastfed infants, however, can be very well and pass soft stool without diffi-culty with a frequency that may range from 10 stools per day to 1 stool every 10 days. At 2 to 3 years of age the modal frequency of defecation is 2 bowel motions per day. From age 3 to adulthood bowel motions are passed between 3 times per day and 3 times per week in 96% of individuals. One-quarter of all cases of chronic constipation begin during the first year of life, but the majority of children affected develop problems in the preschool years. Chron-ic constipation is a very common cause of referral to pediatric gastroenterol-ogy practices and tends to affect males slightly more often than females (by a ratio of 1.5:1).

Encopresis is a term that has become synonymous with a voluntary or involuntary passage of stool in an inappropriate place (usually the underclothing). *Soiling* refers to the constant involuntary seepage of stool associated with fecal impaction. Chronic constipation complicated by encopresis or soiling is reported to make up 3% of referrals to large teaching hospital clinics. It occurs in 1–2% of 7-year-old primary school children, and is more prevalent in males than females (by a ratio of 5:1).

4.2 **Pathophysiology**
The colon absorbs water and electrolytes, and collects and packages indigestible residue as a formed stool for later evacuation. Colonic motor function is specialized to perform these functions. Repeated ring contractions or haustral contractions cause to-and-fro shuttling of luminal contents, delaying their transit and enhancing absorption. One to three times a day mass movements transport colonic contents distally. Normal defecation is a combination of autonomic and voluntary functions. Distention of the rectum is the stimulus that initiates reflex defecation. When the fecal bolus distends the rectum, sensory receptors in the rectal wall are stimulated, leading to conscious perception of rectal distention and involuntary relaxation of the internal anal sphincter. In the absence of voluntary contraction of the puborectalis muscle and the external anal sphincter, the fecal bolus is expelled.

Intestinal transit time is closely related to defecation frequency. The reduction of frequency of defecation with age is associated with an increase in intestinal transit time. In the first month of life transit time is 8 hours, at age 2 it is 16 hours, between 3 and 13 years it is 26 hours and in an adult it is 48 hours or more. Transit time is largely influenced by the amount of fiber in the diet. Fiber-rich diets favor the retention of water and result in increased stool weight and volume, shorter transit time and more frequent defecation. Normal stools have a water content of 60–85% of mass. An increase or decrease in volume of stool water of as little as 100 mL in the adult can represent diarrhea or constipation, respectively. In constipation the increased desiccation of colonic contents is due to increased duration of mucosal contact rather than an alteration of mucosal absorptive function.

4.3 **Differential Diagnosis**
In the child who presents as having a difficulty with elimination, the physician must determine whether the problem is functional, organic or a parental misinterpretation of symptoms. Examples of the latter include the healthy, breastfed infant who passes a soft stool without difficulty once every 10 days and the normal infant who passes soft stools on a regular basis but frequently becomes fussy, cries or turns red and grunts while defecating. Similarly, 1- to 2-year-old children will interrupt their other activities, become flushed, stand

in a rigid posture, and appear to be concentrating on the passage of a bowel motion that is difficult to pass. Often there is no difficulty and these children are in fact attempting to utilize a newly acquired skill and withhold passage of a bowel movement.

Organic constipation may be the result of mechanical obstruction, perianal difficulties causing painful defecation, metabolic or medical disorders, neuromuscular disorders or medications that favor the development of constipation. Mechanical obstruction may occur as a result of congenital, post-surgical or inflammatory stenosis at the level of the anal canal; obstruction by an intrinsic mass such as adenocarcinoma in the adult; or obstruction by an extrinsic mass such as neoplasia or pregnancy. Painful defecation may result from trauma or surgery to the anorectal region, anal fissures, thrombosed hemorrhoids or a perianal abscess/infection. Metabolic and medical disorders that have been associated with organic constipation include hypercalcemia, hypokalemia, hypothyroidism, porphyria and conditions leading to polyurea and dehydration, including diabetes insipidus, diabetes mellitus and chronic renal failure. Organic constipation can result from dysfunction at all levels of the neuromuscular axis: central nervous disorders such as cerebral palsy or stroke; abnormalities of the peripheral nervous system, including myelomeningocele, trauma, polio or diabetic nephropathy; conditions affecting the enteric nervous system such as Hirschsprung's disease; and skeletal or smooth-muscle myopathies. Medications known to predispose to constipation include the opiates, anticholinergics, tricyclic antidepressants and phenothiazines, aluminum-containing antacids, diuretics, iron and vincristine.

Precipitants of functional constipation include decreased fluid intake or increased fluid losses; decreased physical activity; a diet that is low in fiber, contains excessive milk or is nutritionally insufficient; and anything that leads to chronic involuntary inhibition of defecation. Imposed schedules and some children's reluctance to use different facilities are examples of the latter; children may also be simply too busy to attend to the urge to defecate.

In the child who presents with encopresis, the physician must consider whether the incontinence of stool is due to a congenital or acquired neuromuscular disorder, or a behavioral disturbance. However, most of these children have soiling secondary to chronic fecal impaction and overflow. In such cases children may have secondary behavioral disturbance but their primary problem is one of gross rectal distention with loss of the rectal–anorectal angle and the continence function of the puborectalis sling. Whenever there is a mass movement the only residual continence mechanism in these children is the external voluntary anal sphincter, which rapidly fatigues, leading to involuntary soiling. It is not unusual for younger children to deny any knowledge that this is occurring, because if they admit to awareness their parents often expect

TABLE 3. Differentiating features of functional constipation and aganglionic megacolon
(Hirschsprung's disease)

	Functional constipation	Hirschsprung's disease
Age of onset	Acquired sometime after birth	Present from birth
Growth	Normal	Poor
History	Coercive bowel training Colicky abdominal pain Rarely abdominal distention Periodic voluminous stools Soiling	Lack of coercive bowel training Rarely abdominal pain Abdomen distended Pellet-like or ribbon-like stools No soiling
Past history	No episodes of intestinal obstruction	Frequent episodes of intestinal obstruction
Physical exam	Well child Feces-packed, capacious rectum	Nutritional status poor Empty rectum
Barium enema	Absence of transition zone and a distended distal colon	Presence of transition zone
Manometry	Rectoanal inhibitory reflex intact	Absent rectoanal inhibitory reflex
Biopsy	Normal	Absence of ganglia in myenteric plexus and hypertrophy of nerve trunks
Course	Negligible mortality Variable morbidity	High mortality, depending on promptness of diagnosis, and variable morbidity, depending on type and outcome of surgical management

them to be able to prevent soiling. Such children will regain continence only
if their gross rectal distention is relieved.

4.3.1 DIFFERENTIATION OF CHRONIC FECAL RETENTION FROM HIRSCHSPRUNG'S DISEASE

The most frequently considered organic problem in the differential diagnosis
of patients presenting with functional constipation is Hirschsprung's disease.
These two conditions can frequently be distinguished by significant differences in the history and physical examination. These are detailed in Table 3.

4.4 Treatment

If an organic cause of constipation is suspected, it should be investigated and treated; however, most patients with constipation have no underlying organic abnormality. In patients with mild constipation, dietary modification with an increase in fluid or fiber intake, establishment of a regular bowel habit with a prompt response to the urge to defecate, and appropriate physical activity may be a sufficient remedy. Many individuals will require a laxative in addition. Patients whose constipation is complicated by fecal impaction and soiling require very aggressive management, including education, clearing of the impaction, establishment of a regular bowel habit, laxative therapy titrated to achieve the passage of a soft bowel motion daily, appropriate diet and exercise, and (in younger children) positive reinforcement for appropriate behavior. Therapy must be aggressive and persist for three to six months until the distended and dysfunctional colon has an opportunity to return to normal caliber, tone and sensitivity.

The fecal impaction can generally be cleared by administration of Fleet® enemas at intervals of 12 hours (generally 2–4 are sufficient). There is a variety of laxatives on the market whose mechanism of action includes hydrophilic (dietary fiber), lubricant (mineral oil), osmotic (glycerin suppositories, lactulose, magnesium citrate/sulfate and sodium phosphate/biphosphate), secretory (ricinoleic acid, free hydroxy fatty acids, dihydroxy bile acids, and dioctyl sodium sulfosuccinate) and motor stimulants (anthraquinones and diphenylmethene derivatives). Natural bran, methylcellulose, polycarbophil and psyllium are all forms of fiber that by virtue of their ability to bind water within their structure lead to an increase in stool bulk and weight, and are associated with more rapid transit and more frequent bowel motions. These are safe and effective in children if sufficient amounts are taken, but children's compliance is often poor. Mineral oil is the lubricant laxative of choice in the pediatric age group because of better compliance. It is an indigestible, tasteless oil that adds bulk, softens and lubricates the stool and exerts an additional osmotic effect. Its aspiration can lead to lipoid pneumonia; therefore this form of treatment should be avoided in patients known to aspirate or with a history of reflux. Taken with meals mineral oil will result in a degree of fat-soluble vitamin malabsorption. This problem can be addressed by giving it as a single dose several hours after the evening meal. Properly used, mineral oil is an inexpensive, well-tolerated, effective and safe children's laxative. In those children who refuse mineral oil the osmotic agent lactulose is a more expensive but effective alternative.

Constipation in the very young infant can often be managed by adding prune juice to the diet or brown sugar to the formula, or by feeding the infant purées with a natural laxative action (containing prunes, for example). Mineral oil is frequently not a good choice in this age group because of the frequency of gastroesophageal reflux.

5. **GROWTH FAILURE AND MALNUTRITION /** S.A. Zamora and
   H.G. Parsons

5.1 **Definitions:**

Failure to thrive (FTT), a widely used term in industrialized countries, is not distinct from protein-energy malnutrition encountered in children in developing countries (1). Both terms describe a spectrum of pathologic states resulting from childhood undernutrition. FTT accounts for 1–5% of tertiary hospital admissions for infants and is reported in about 10% of low-income preschool children seen in community-based settings.

FTT is used to describe infants and young children whose growth is substantially less than that of their peers. Although no consensus exists on anthropometric indicators of FTT (2), most commonly used systems for selection of samples of FTT in hospital or clinic studies include children with a weight less than the 5th percentile on reference growth charts (1). The key to the identification of FTT is ascertainment of longitudinal progression of growth with serial measurements over time. A weight decrement of more than two major channels of growth (centiles) from a previously established growth channel or the loss of 10% of an infant's weight is evidence of FTT (1,3). A reduction in growth velocity is a particularly helpful indicator of abnormality in the 5% of otherwise normal children who plot out below the 5th percentile, but follow a growth channel parallel to the normal growth curves.

Acute malnutrition typically results in "wasting," where weight is depressed out of proportion to height. Chronic malnutrition will also affect height and may lead to "stunting," in which weight and height are proportionally decreased. Head circumference is the last parameter to be affected by malnutrition.

Extreme conditions of protein-energy malnutrition are rarely encountered in industrialized countries. Marasmus occurs after severe deprivation, primarily of calories, and is characterized by growth retardation and wasting of muscle and subcutaneous fat. Kwashiorkor results from a protein deficiency exceeding the calorie deficiency and is manifested by edema (secondary to hypoalbuminemia) and muscle wasting.

5.2 **Diagnostic Categories**

FTT can be categorized as organic, nonorganic, or of mixed etiology. Organic FTT involves children who have a specific diagnosable disorder implicated in the failure to grow and accounts for a minority of cases: about 20–30% of children hospitalized for FTT (5, 6) and a lower proportion of children seen in outpatient clinics. Organic causes of FTT can be attributed to prenatal influences (congenital anomalies, in utero insults such as infections or toxins, prematurity) or to ongoing or recurring illnesses after the neonatal period. Non-organic FTT suggests that the cause is primarily external to the infant; it accounts for the majority of cases. It may result from the individual temperament of the child (sickly, difficult child), difficult interactions between the child and the caregiver, nonfeeding, family poverty, stress or loss.

For both organic and nonorganic FTT, the main pathophysiologic denominator resulting in growth delay is an imbalance between nutrient availability and requirements. This imbalance results from a suboptimal intake (psychosocial factors, organic disease interfering with feeding); increased losses (gastroesophageal reflux, vomiting, diarrhea) or malabsorption of nutrients; and more rarely, increased needs (hyperkinetic states, hyperthyroidism). Inborn errors of metabolism may result in FTT despite an adequate balance between nutrient availability and requirements.

A useful diagnostic approach recognizes three types of FTT according to the deviance of head circumference, height and weight on growth charts (8) (Table 4).

5.2.1 TYPE I
Head circumference is normal and weight is reduced out of proportion to height (Figure 1). This pattern results from an imbalance between calorie availability and requirements. The majority of patients with FTT fall into this category; adverse psychosocial factors are the most frequent contributors.

5.2.2 TYPE II
Head circumference is normal or enlarged and weight is reduced in proportion to (or slightly more than) the reduction in height (Figure 2). This pattern is mainly represented by children with constitutional growth delay, familial short stature or endocrinopathies. Chronic malnutrition resulting in stunting may also fall into this group (celiac disease). Comparison of the children's height age and bone age with chronologic age (see Section 5.4.2) further identifies three subgroups:

Type IIa – Most frequently bone age and height age are proportionally delayed beyond chronologic age (e.g., constitutional growth delay).

Type IIb – Bone age is in accordance with chronologic age but height age is retarded (e.g., familial short stature).

Type IIc – Bone age is significantly more delayed than chronologic age (e.g., malnutrition).

5.2.3 TYPE III
Head circumference is subnormal and weight and height are proportionally reduced (Figure 3). These children are frequently described as dysmorphic and may present with associated developmental delay or seizures. Patients in

TABLE 4. Differential diagnosis of failure to thrive based on anthropometric criteria

Type I – HC normal	*W reduction >>> H reduction*
Inadequate caloric intake	
Nonorganic FTT (psychosocial factors)*	Genitourinary diseases (e.g., UTI)
Neurologic and neuromuscular diseases	Malignancy
Chronic infection	Cardiovascular disorders
Increased losses	
Gastroesophageal reflux or vomiting	
Diarrhea	
Malabsorption	
Cystic fibrosis	Parasitic infestation
Milk protein enteropathy	Immunodeficiency
Celiac disease	Inflammatory bowel disease
Shwachman syndrome	Hepatobiliary disorders
Short gut	Intermittent midgut volvulus
Impaired caloric utilization	
Glycogen storage disease	Chronic infection
Galactosemia	Renal disease
Fructose intolerance	Malignancy
Phenylketonuria	Anemia
Increased metabolic requirements	
Hyperthyroidism	Hyperkinesia (attention deficit disor-
Diencephalic syndrome	ders, athetoid cerebral palsy)
Type II – HC normal or enlarged	*W reduction = or > H reduction*
a. Bone age delay = height age delay	
Constitutional growth delay	Metabolic disease
Celiac disease	Chronic diseases
b. Bone age not delayed; height age delayed	
Familial short stature	
c. Bone age delay >>> height age delay	
Endocrine disorder (growth hormone deficiency,	Maternal deprivation syndrome
hypothyroidism, hypopituitarism)	(deprivation dwarfism)
Type III – HC subnormal	*W reduction = H reduction*
Dysmorphic	
Chromosomal abnormalities	Birth asphyxia
Congenital infections	CNS abnormalities
Toxic intrauterine exposure (alcohol, drugs,	Familial
anticonvulsants)	

FTT = failure to thrive; HC = head circumference; W = weight; H = height or length
*Environmental causes are the most common source of problems.
SOURCE: Adapted from Roy CC, Silverman A, Alagille D (eds.). Pediatric clinical gastroenterology. 4th ed. St. Louis: Mosby-Year Book, 1995:5–10.

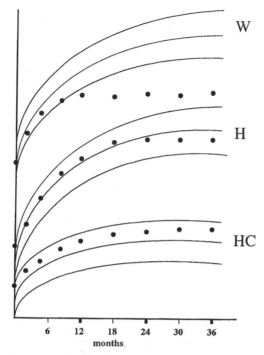

FIGURE 1.   Type I failure to thrive. *W* refers to weight, *H* to height or length, *HC* to head circumference.

this category may have chromosomal abnormalities, intrauterine or perinatal insults (congenital infections, alcohol, drug or anticonvulsant exposure during pregnancy, severe prematurity, birth asphyxia), CNS abnormalities and more rarely a familial phenotype.

5.3 Pitfalls in Diagnosis

The size of an infant at birth is more related to maternal size and intrauterine influences than to genetic factors. Consequently, growth across percentiles (increased or decreased growth velocity) between birth and 2 years of age is to be expected in some children owing to genetic adjustment. Patterns of normal growth in the first two years of life can then present as factitious FTT (2): familial short stature and constitutional growth delay. Term infants born small for gestational age and premature infants can also present diagnostic problems.

5.3.1 *FAMILIAL (GENETIC) SHORT STATURE*

Familial short stature is genetically determined, and these children are short

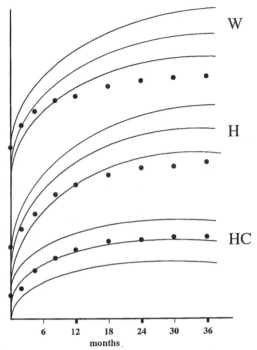

FIGURE 2.   Type II failure to thrive. *W* refers to weight, *H* to height or length, *HC* to head circumference.

throughout life. The final height is determined by mid-parental height, and a readjustment with drop in percentiles may take place in the first two years of age. After this deceleration phase, these children grow normally at constant rates and enter puberty at an appropriate age. Weight in these children is usually proportional to length, and they have no bone age delay. The diagnosis of familial short stature is confirmed on the basis of a normal history and physical examination and if, during follow-up, the child maintains the new growth channel appropriate to his or her genetic potential.

5.3.2 CONSTITUTIONAL GROWTH DELAY
Children with constitutional growth delays are "slow growers" and "late bloomers." They present with marked deceleration of growth in the first three years of life and then follow a lower growth channel into adolescence, when a late pubertal growth spurt occurs and they catch up to their original growth channel (4). The deceleration begins usually between 3 and 6 months, will be greatest in the first two years of life and frequently results in these children

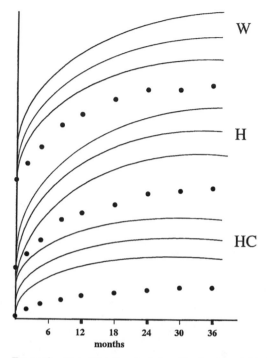

FIGURE 3.   Type III failure to thrive. *W* refers to weight, *H* to height or length, *HC* to head circumference.

falling well below the 5th percentile both for weight and height. These children have a two- to four-year delay in skeletal maturation and will enter puberty late. There is frequently a family history of this type of delayed growth and pubertal development.

5.3.3 *SMALL FOR GESTATIONAL AGE AND PREMATURE INFANTS*
Small for gestational age infants are a heterogeneous group who fail to grow in utero (intrauterine growth retardation, or IUGR) as a result of environmental, maternal, placental or fetal factors. Asymmetric IUGR (birth weight disproportionally more depressed than length or head circumference) frequently results from placental insufficiency. These newborns have a good prognosis for catch-up growth if they are provided with enhanced postnatal nutrition. Symmetric IUGR may result from intrauterine infections, chromosomal abnormalities or prenatal exposure to toxins such as alcohol, drugs or anticonvulsants. Infants who are symmetrically growth retarded at birth have a poor prognosis for later growth. Because of the initial small size, the weight gain and growth progression of these patients may give the false impression

of FTT; however, if the patient doubles the birth weight by 4 months of age and triples it by 1 year of age, FTT must be excluded.

In premature infants corrected age should be used in growth monitoring or they will be inappropriately labeled as FTT. The age at measurement should be corrected for the number of weeks the child was premature (the difference between 40 weeks and gestational age). Corrected age should be used to 18 months for head circumference, 24 months for weight and 40 months for height (5). Premature infants without serious medical problems may show catch-up growth in the first year of life, whereas more severely affected premature infants may not show catch-up growth but should at least parallel reference curves (1).

5.4 Assessment of FTT

Assessment of infants with FTT always demands a very careful history and physical examination in order to minimize the need for investigations. Particularly important are a thorough dietary assessment, documentation of adverse psychosocial factors and an anthropometric evaluation.

5.4.1 DIETARY HISTORY AND PSYCHOSOCIAL FACTORS

The dietary history should document the child's feeding history (breastfeeding and/or method of formula preparation, concentration and volume of formula consumed, age at introduction and acceptance of solids, ability to feed independently), food allergies and difficulties in chewing or swallowing. A three- to seven-day dietary record should ideally be evaluated by a nutritionist or dietitian for adequacy of calories, protein intake and micronutrients. Parents' misconceptions about nutrition may be detrimental. Families concerned with cardiovascular diseases or obesity may restrict and limit the nutritional intake of the infants (through use of skim milk or restriction of sweet food). "Therapeutic fasting" for treatment of diarrhea and elimination diets employed in suspected cases of "food allergy" may also result in caloric insufficiency. Excessive fruit juice intake may result in an unbalanced diet with decreased consumption of milk and snacks.

Considering that the majority of cases of FTT have no organic basis, contributing psychosocial factors should be evaluated in detail: poverty, familial dysfunction, disordered parent–child interaction, chronic illness, depression or intellectual impairment of the caregiver. A feeding disorder is best appreciated by direct observation of a meal. Is the child correctly positioned? Are there inappropriate distractions? Is the interaction between child and caregiver appropriate?

5.4.2 ANTHROPOMETRIC EVALUATION

Repeated, rather than cross-sectional, accurate anthropometric measurements are essential in establishing FTT. Head circumference should always be recorded in children of less than 36 months. Length should be measured recumbent before 2 years of age. Extrapolation of weight and length horizontally to the 50th percentile on growth charts will define the child's weight age and height age, which can be compared to chronologic age and bone age (skeletal maturation). Parental heights and weights will give an idea of the child's genetic growth potential. Mid-parental height is obtained by averaging the parents' height and then adding 6.5 cm for boys or subtracting 6.5 cm for girls.

The most accurate technique for classifying growth deficiency uses Z scores, where the deviance from the median reference value is expressed in units of standard deviations for that population:

$$Z \text{ score} = \frac{\text{actual measured value} - \text{median reference value}}{\text{standard deviation for age of reference population}}$$

A Z score of 0.00 is equivalent to the 50th percentile. A Z score of -2.00 SD corresponds to a percentile of 2.3 and is currently recommended by the WHO as a cut-off value for growth deficiencies (1). Z scores are very sensitive to growth deviances but their calculation necessitates the use of computer software (6).

Other systems commonly used to categorize malnutrition express the child's weight as a percent of the median weight-for-age (Table 5) or as a percent of the median weight-for-height (Table 6). Percent of the median weight- (or height-) for-age is obtained by dividing the actual measurement by the median value for that age. Median weight-for-height (ideal weight for height) is obtained by extrapolating height horizontally to the 50th percentile and taking the median weight for that age. Comparing the child's height to the median height-for-age gives an idea of the severity of stunting or chronic malnutrition. It must be noticed that these methods applied to the same population may classify children in different grades of malnutrition (7). Therefore, appreciation of the severity of malnutrition should not rely exclusively on these ratios.

On physical examination a clinical appreciation of nutritional status is readily available by inspecting the child's buttocks (flat in malnutrition) and subscapular and limb muscles. Evaluation of the triceps skin fold (index of fat tissue) and mid-arm muscle circumference requires the use of published nomograms and reference tables (8,9). Among other physical signs that may be associated with malnutrition are a distended abdomen (malabsorptive states), edema (hypoalbuminemia) and clubbing (chronic disease). More severe cases may show pallor (anemia), glossitis-stomatitis, pellagroid dermatitis, ecchymosis (vitamin K deficiency) and bone deformities (vitamin D deficiency).

TABLE 5.   Classification of severity of underweight

Grade of malnutrition	Percent of median weight-for-age
Normal	90–110
I. Mild	75–89
II. Moderate	60–74
III. Severe	<60

SOURCE: Data from Gomez F et al. Malnutrition in infancy and childhood, with special reference to kwashiorkor. Advance Pediat 1955; 7:131–169.

TABLE 6.   Classification of severity of wasting and stunting

Grade of malnutrition	Percent of median weight-for-height (wasting)	Percent of median height-for-age (stunting)
Normal	90–110	95
I. Mild	80–89	90–94
II. Moderate	70–79	85–89
III. Severe	<70	<85

SOURCE: Data from Waterlow JC. Classification and definition of protein-calorie malnutrition. BMJ 1972; 3:566–569.

5.5 Investigations

Because poor nutrition and psychosocial factors are the major contributors to FTT, investigations are of very limited diagnostic help. Large series of hospitalized children have documented that only about 1% of laboratory studies performed helped identify an organic etiology to FTT. Furthermore, no test was useful in the absence of a specific indication from the history and physical exam. If the clinical evaluation is normal, children with decreased growth should be followed at regular intervals without extensive investigations; frequently, one of the physiologic variations of growth (Table 4) will be identified. Basic tests may be indicated: urine analysis, CBC and differential, albumin, calcium, phosphorus and alkaline phosphatase. Particularly useful is a stool smear for fat. In cases of moderate and severe malnutrition, nutrient deficiencies should be documented (especially iron, zinc, vitamin D).

5.6 Management

Management of FTT generally necessitates a multidisciplinary approach to address both psychosocial and medical factors (nutritionist and/or dietitian, physician and/or nurse, social worker and/or psychologist). Parental education regarding the infant's nutritional needs is essential. Financial difficulties and family dysfunction should be addressed in order to obtain compliance with treatment. The goal of nutritional treatment is to promote compensatory catch-up growth, which is achieved only if the child receives nutrients in excess of the normal requirements for age. Daily caloric needs may be estimated in calories per kilogram as follows:

$$\text{kcal/kg} = \frac{120 \text{ kcal/kg} \times \text{median weight for current height}}{\text{current weight (kg)}}$$

Protein intake should be 1.5–2 times the RDNI[1] for age. As it is not generally possible for a child to eat twice the normal volume, the usual diet must be fortified to increase nutrient density. This is achieved in infants by increasing the caloric density of the formula (normal dilution = 20 kcal/oz or 0.67 kcal/mL) to 24 kcal/oz (by increasing the formula concentration) or 28–30 kcal/oz (by adding polycose or oil). In toddlers, food preferred by the child should be enriched by adding cheese, peanut butter, butter, vegetable oil or carbohydrate additives. Small frequent feedings should be offered. In cases of moderate and severe malnutrition a multivitamin supplement containing iron and zinc should be prescribed routinely during nutritional rehabilitation.

Management of severe malnutrition should be done in hospital with close monitoring of electrolytes and fluid imbalances, which can be lethal if not managed prospectively. Potassium and phosphorus depletion are particularly worrisome. Levels should be monitored daily. Phosphorus supplementation should be routinely instituted with refeeding. Initial caloric intakes should be low, 25 kcal/kg in infants and 50 kcal/kg in children, and advanced daily in 25 kcal/kg increments if tolerated (1).

5.7 Prognosis

Provided that intervention is early and effective, and depending on the primary underlying psychosocial or organic factors, there is a potential for catch-up growth in children with FTT. Long-term follow-up studies on children hospitalized for FTT demonstrate impairment of both physical and mental development in a substantial number. Malnutrition produces functional alterations of behavior at any age, but the brain is particularly vulnerable during the critical period of brain growth that extends from mid-gestation to 3 years of life. In the absence of any organic disease, the duration of malnutrition in the first year of life and the disturbed environment in which the child remains seem to determine the adverse long-term sequelae.

---

[1] Recommended daily nutritional intake (RDNI) identifies the adequate intake of essential nutrients judged to meet the needs of all healthy people in Canada. Except for energy, the RDNI is established at two standard deviations above the estimated mean requirements.

6. ACUTE DIARRHEA IN CHILDREN / J.D. Butzner

6.1 Introduction

A North American child will develop between 6 and 12 episodes of acute diarrhea before the age of 5. This contributes to approximately 12% of childhood hospitalizations and approximately 300 deaths per year. Worldwide, acute diarrheal disease is the leading cause of childhood morbidity and mortality, accounting for three million deaths each year. Most deaths are caused by failure to treat acute dehydration properly and to correct electrolyte imbalances. Studies from both the developing and developed world demonstrate that hospitalization can be avoided and morbidity and mortality can be drastically reduced by the prompt introduction of two simple treatments: oral rehydration therapy and early refeeding. In spite of recommendations to use oral rehydration therapy and to continue or resume feeding early in mild to moderate diarrheal illnesses, the use of unsuitable treatments persists. These include unnecessary intravenous therapy, inappropriate oral fluids (unbalanced sugar-electrolyte solutions), prolonged starvation with a slow introduction of limited feeds, and the inappropriate use of antibiotics as well as antimotility and antidiarrheal agents.

6.2 Pathophysiology of Acute Diarrheal Disease

An understanding of the physiology of intestinal fluid, electrolyte and nutrient transport provides a basis for understanding the mechanisms of acute diarrheal disease and successful oral rehydration therapy. Water absorption occurs primarily in the small intestine, driven by osmotic gradients that depend on the transport of the electrolytes sodium and chloride, as well as nutrients such as glucose and amino acids. Sodium, glucose and several amino acids are transported through the apical membranes of intestinal epithelial cells by sodium-dependent nutrient cotransporters. Sodium is then transported from the cell across the basolateral membrane to the extracellular space by the enzyme Na^+/K^+-ATPase. This enzyme utilizes energy to reduce the intracellular sodium concentration, which produces a negative extracellular electrical charge. The resultant electrochemical gradient facilitates sodium absorption by the epithelial cell, which drives the sodium-dependent nutrient cotransporters. The anion chloride is absorbed to maintain electrical neutrality across the epithelium, and water is passively absorbed in response to the transport of these electrolytes and nutrients. Successful oral rehydration therapy with balanced sugar-salt solutions depends upon these simple physiologic principles.

Diarrhea associated with small intestinal injury in infants and children is caused by four major mechanisms. These include (1) increased osmotic fluid losses, (2) inappropriate secretion, (3) inflammation associated with exudative fluid and protein losses and finally, (4) altered intestinal motility. The most frequent cause of osmotic diarrhea and acute infectious diarrhea worldwide is viral enteritis due to the rotavirus. This virus stimulates the shedding of mature absorptive epithelial cells from the small intestinal villi. These cells are replaced by immature cells with inadequately developed transporters, including the sodium-dependent glucose cotransporter and Na^+/K^+-ATPase. When unbalanced sugar-electrolyte solutions such as fruit juice, soda pop and broth are provided as treatments, the intestine's immature transport capacity is overwhelmed. The osmotic forces created by nonabsorbed nutrients that remain in the lumen stimulate watery diarrheal fluid losses. Children with intestinal injury caused by an acute enteritis may also develop secondary disaccharidase deficiencies, which contribute to osmotic diarrhea by the malabsorption of the disaccharides lactose and sucrose. Interestingly, the frequency of this complication has been markedly decreased in children with mild to moderate dehydration by the prompt implementation of treatment protocols that stress oral rehydration and early refeeding. Osmotic diarrhea is also caused by infections due to Giardia lamblia, Cryptosporidium, Salmonella and enteroadherent E. coli. Medications that contain nonabsorbable sugars such as sorbitol, lactulose and mannitol and poorly absorbable ions such as magnesium, sulfate, phosphate and citrate may also provoke osmotic diarrhea. Healthy children who ingest excessive quantities of fruit juice, soda pop or sugar-free products such as sorbitol-containing gum or mints may develop osmotic diarrhea due to the malabsorption of the fructose and sorbitol found in these products. This is a major cause of chronic nonspecific diarrhea of childhood.

The second major mechanism of diarrheal disease results from the active secretion of the anions chloride and bicarbonate, followed by passive water secretion. Luminal secretagogues include bacterial enterotoxins produced by V. cholerae, heat-labile and heat-stable E. coli, staphylococcal enterotoxins, Clostridium perfringens and Bacillus cereus, as well as hydroxy fatty acids from malabsorbed dietary lipids and nonabsorbed bile acids. Recently, investigators described rotavirus-induced intestinal secretion. Endogenous secretagogues include hormones secreted by intestinal tumors and inflammatory mediators released in response to food allergy, inflammatory bowel disease and systemic infections. These mediators include histamine, eicosanoids, platelet-activating factor, serotonin and IL-1. They are released after direct activation of inflammatory cells or through stimulation of these cells by the enteric nervous system. Cholera toxin was the first described and remains the classic cause of secretory diarrhea. The B subunit of this toxin binds to the luminal surface of the microvillus membrane of the enterocyte. The A subunit is then internalized and irreversibly activates adenylate cyclase, which stimulates the formation of cyclic adenosine monophosphate (cAMP). This activates protein phosphorylation, which triggers chloride secretion and impairs Na^+Cl^- absorption. In secretory diarrhea no morphologic epithelial injury is present and the sodium-dependent glucose transporter and the enzyme Na^+/K^+-ATPase function normally. This permits successful oral rehydration therapy in the face of ongoing intestinal secretion.

The third mechanism causing diarrhea results from exudation of fluid and protein secondary to inflammation and ulceration of intestinal or colonic mucosa. This results in bloody diarrhea or dysentery caused by the bacteria Shigella, Campylobacter jejuni, Salmonella, Yersinia enterocolitica, enteroinvasive and enterohemorrhagic E. coli, as well as the protozoa Entamoeba histolytica. This type of diarrhea is also seen in inflammatory bowel disease, particularly ulcerative colitis. The diarrheal stools contain mucus, exudate and blood. As mentioned above, the release of inflammatory mediators also stimulates fluid secretion.

Finally, both hyper- and hypomotility result in diarrheal fluid losses. Hypermotility occurs in intestinal infections, hyperthyroidism, functioning tumors and irritative-type laxative abuse. Hypomotility is observed in the intestinal pseudo-obstructive syndromes and with partial anatomic obstruction that results in the intestinal blind loop syndrome. With decreased motility, bacterial contamination develops with resultant malabsorption of nutrients and stimulation of secretory diarrheal fluid losses.

6.3 Clinical Assessment

The infant or child with an acute watery diarrheal illness has most likely contacted a viral enteritis. However, these symptoms can be presenting features of other gastrointestinal and nongastrointestinal illnesses, including otitis media, urinary tract infection, bacterial sepsis, meningitis, pneumonia, allergy and toxic ingestion. Children who develop loose, watery stools in conjunction with infections such as those involving the middle ear or urinary tract usually do not become dehydrated. This is known as "parental diarrhea" and is likely due to the release of inflammatory mediators. A careful history and physical examination play a crucial role in differentiating an acute gastroenteritis from the other causes of acute diarrhea. In addition, accurate assessment of the degree of dehydration, ongoing fluid losses and the ability to drink are required to ensure adequate fluid replacement and maintenance of intake.

6.3.1 *HISTORY*

Specific questions about the frequency, volume and duration of vomiting and diarrhea are required to determine the severity of fluid deficit and electrolyte imbalance. Significant dehydration can also be manifested by a decreased activity level, reduced urine volume and weight loss. A summary of the assessment of dehydration appears in Table 7. Information about the consistency of stool as well as the presence and quantity of blood aids in establishing a diagnosis and in determining appropriate investigation. In infants sus-

TABLE 7. Dehydration assessment and management

Degree of dehydration; % deficit	General	Thirst	Eyes; tears	Mouth	Skin	Urine	Rehydration therapy within 4 hrs.	Replacement of fluid losses
None; <2%	Well, alert	Drinks normally	Normal; tears present	Moist	Normal	Normal	Not required; proceed with maintenance and replacement of ongoing losses	10 mL/hr or $^1/_2$–1 cup of ORS for each diarrheal stool; 2–5 mL/kg for each emesis
Mild; 3–5%	Well	Drinks eagerly	Normal; decreased tears	Decreased moisture	Normal	Decreased	ORS 50 mL/kg	As above
Moderate; 6–9%	Restless, irritable	Drinks eagerly	Sunken; absent	Dry	Pallor; delayed capillary refill; tenting < 2 sec.	Absent	ORS 100 mL/kg	As above
Severe; ≥ 10%	Lethargy, floppy, decreased consciousness, rapid weak pulse, rapid breathing	Drinks poorly or not able to drink	Very sunken and dry; absent	Very dry	Pallor; delayed capillary refill; tenting > 2 sec.	Absent	IV fluids (normal saline, Ringer's lactate) 20 mL/kg/hr until pulse and mental status return to normal; then ORS 50–100 mL/kg	As above

SOURCE: Modified from Butzner JD. Acute vomiting and diarrhea. In: Walker-Smith JA, Walker WA, Hamilton JR (eds.), Practical pediatric gastroenterology. 2d ed. Toronto: BC Decker, 1996:51–69.

pected of having a gastrointestinal infection, a history of illness among contacts, including playmates, siblings and day-care attendees, as well as exposure to visiting travelers may provide clues to the source of infection. Mild upper respiratory infections in parents or older children may result in acute vomiting and diarrhea in the infant or toddler. In addition to person-to-person contact, exposure to animals and contaminated drinking water and food may lead to enteric infections. Foods cause acute vomiting and diarrhea by multiple mechanisms. These include immunologic reactions resulting in food allergies as well as metabolic, pharmacologic and toxin-induced reactions to food and its contaminants. Lactose intolerance due to adult-onset lactase deficiency; "Chinese restaurant syndrome" due to monosodium glutamate ingestion; and staphylococcal food poisoning occurring one to six hours after the ingestion of preformed toxins are examples of the nonimmunologic causes of food poisoning. Infants who suffer an acute diarrheal illness in the first few weeks of life are more likely to have a congenital anatomic abnormality of the GI tract or an inherited metabolic disease such as abetalipoproteinemia, cystic fibrosis or one of the rare intestinal transporter deficiencies.

6.3.2 PHYSICAL EXAMINATION
The inaccurate assessment of fluid deficits and ongoing fluid losses is the most important cause of the morbidity and mortality associated with acute vomiting and diarrhea in children. Infants are particularly susceptible to the development of dehydration for they sustain greater fluid losses because of an increased intestinal surface area per kilogram of body weight compared to adults. An immature renal concentrating ability, increased metabolic rate and dependence on others to provide fluids also contribute to the rapid development of severe fluid deficits in the pediatric patient. An immediate pre-illness weight provides the most sensitive mechanism of determining severity of dehydration. Unfortunately, this is rarely available. A weight should be obtained at the time of initiation of treatment in order to judge ongoing losses and gauge successful therapy. As outlined in Table 7, the severity of dehydration used to gauge the level of rehydration therapy can be assessed rapidly with history and physical examination. Watery diarrhea sometimes is mistaken for urine in the diaper. This may result in an underestimation of fluid losses. Evidence of particulant matter or a positive dipstick for sugar or protein suggests watery stool. Rapid, deep breathing may suggest an uncomplicated metabolic acidosis. In the child with a distended abdomen, auscultation of bowel sounds should be performed to rule out a paralytic ileus, and a rectal exam should be performed to determine if fluid is being third-spaced in the gut lumen. Examination of the stool for blood, white blood cells, reducing substances, pH, fat and fatty acid crystals may provide valuable clues about the etiology of a diarrheal illness.

6.3.3 INVESTIGATIONS

The majority of episodes of acute watery diarrhea in previously healthy children are self-limited and associated with only mild dehydration. In this situation, the performance of biochemical or microbiologic examination is rarely required. When an advanced stage of dehydration is suspected, assessment of serum electrolytes, urea nitrogen, and acid/base chemistry will aid in tailoring ongoing rehydration therapy. Virologic and microbiologic examination should be performed only when results will be utilized to alter patient management or treat patient contacts, or for the protection of other hospitalized patients. Examples that require further investigation include an outbreak of diarrheal disease in a day-care center or hospital, diarrhea in a patient with a recent history of travel to an area of endemic diarrheal disease, and evaluation of the immunocompromised patient or of the patient where initial therapeutic measures are unsuccessful. In the infant or child with bloody diarrhea, stool cultures and antibiotic sensitivities should be performed to guide appropriate antibiotic therapy, if treatment is indicated. In areas where enterohemorrhagic E. coli causes bloody diarrhea, additional laboratory investigations including a CBC with a platelet count, blood smear for evidence of intravascular hemolysis, serum electrolytes, serum creatinine and serial urinalyses are warranted to aid in the diagnosis and management of hemolytic-uremic syndrome, the leading cause of acute renal failure in children under the age of 6.

6.4 Management – Oral Rehydration Therapy

6.4.1 ORAL REHYDRATION

In children with acute diarrhea associated with mild to moderate dehydration, the administration of a balanced oral rehydration solution (ORS) should be immediately instituted as described in Table 7. Parents should be instructed in the proper administration of oral rehydration therapy as part of preventive health care. An oral rehydration solution with a carbohydrate-to-sodium ratio of less than 2:1 and an osmolality that is similar to or slightly less than plasma is recommended. In North America, most oral rehydration solutions have a sodium content of 45–75 mmol/L because stool sodium losses (approximately 35–45 mmol/L) in viral enteritis are much less than those in secretory diarrheas such as cholera (90–140 mmol/L). For children with continued high purging rates (>10 mL/kg/hr), solutions with a higher sodium content may be required. When solutions with a sodium content of >60 mmol/L are used for maintenance, low-sodium fluids such as breast milk, infant formula, diluted juice or water must be provided simultaneously to prevent the development of hypernatremia. In North America, intravenous electrolyte solutions are used to manage children with severe dehydration because of their wide availability and high degree of success. In the developing world, children suffering from severe dehydration can usually be successfully rehydrated with oral solutions. More than 90% of vomiting infants can be successfully rehydrated and maintained with oral hydration providing 5–10 mL every 2 to 3 minutes and gradually increasing the amount administered.

About 5–10% of children fail initial oral rehydration therapy as a result of either persistent vomiting or a persistently high stooling rate of > 10 mL/kg/hr. Parents should be instructed to seek further care if the child develops (1) irritability or lethargy that inhibits drinking, (2) intractable vomiting, (3) worsening fluid deficits associated with persistent diarrhea, (4) bloody diarrhea, or (5) decreased urinary output. These children require re-evaluation and intravenous rehydration similar to that provided for the severely dehydrated child. Their hydration status should be monitored, and when rehydration is complete, maintenance therapy to replace ongoing losses can be commenced. If dehydration persists, the fluid deficit should be recalculated and rehydration therapy continued for an additional 2 to 4 hours with ongoing assessment of fluid losses.

There are only a few contraindications to the use of oral rehydration therapy for the initial management of acute diarrheal disease. These include (1) severe (>10%) dehydration associated with hemodynamic instability, (2) refusal to drink due to extreme irritability, lethargy, stupor or coma, and (3) intestinal ileus. These children should be managed initially with intravenous fluids and switched to oral rehydration therapy when they can safely drink. Homemade oral rehydration solutions are not recommended because electrolyte abnormalities caused by inappropriate mixing are a well-recognized complication.

6.4.2 EARLY REFEEDING

Recommendations for the dietary management of acute diarrheal disease stress the importance of continued breastfeeding throughout the illness and early refeeding of the formula-fed infant and older child. Continued feeding throughout a diarrheal illness improves nutritional status, stimulates intestinal repair, and diminishes the severity as well as the duration of illness. Breastfed infants should be allowed to nurse as often and as long as they want throughout a diarrheal illness. The refeeding of the non-breastfed infant remains somewhat controversial. Recent evidence suggests that the infant with mild to moderate dehydration should receive the full-strength infant formula that was fed prior to illness. There is no need to routinely switch to a lactose-free milk or to refeed with dilute formula. Treatment failure rates of 10–15% when refeeding is carried out in this manner are no higher than with more cautious approaches. Infants with severe dehydration, pre-existing intestinal injury and severe malnutrition, and those who have failed initial refeeding, should receive a lactose-free formula; they occasionally require a more predigested formula during refeeding.

The older child, who is established on a wider variety of foods, should receive a well-balanced, energy-rich, and easily digestible diet. Complex carbohydrates including rice, noodles, potatoes, toast, crackers and bananas should be offered initially, with the rapid addition of vegetables and cooked meats. Foods to avoid include those high in simple sugars such as soft drinks, undiluted fruit juice, caffeinated beverages, presweetened gelatins and sugar-coated cereals. Foods high in fat may be poorly tolerated because of delayed gastric emptying that results in increased vomiting. In some children watery stools will persist for longer than 10 days, but not to the extent where they cause recurrent dehydration. In these cases infection should be excluded and stools examined for reducing substances to rule ongoing carbohydrate malabsorption.

6.4.3 *USE OF MEDICATIONS*
The prescription of antiemetic, antimotility and antidiarrheal agents for the treatment of acute diarrhea seldom benefits the child and may be associated with serious complications. In children with acute diarrheal disease, these agents do not reduce stool volume or duration of illness. They often have anorexic or sedating effects, which prevent successful oral rehydration therapy. Their use results in a third spacing of fluid, which leads to an underestimation of ongoing losses. This results in inadequate fluid replacement therapy.

Antibiotics should be used in the treatment of diarrheal disease only when specifically indicated. Antibiotics are not effective for the treatment of viral enteritis. Giardiasis should be treated when the diarrheal illness persists and when cysts or trophozoites are identified in the stool. There is no benefit to treating asymptomatic carriers of Giardia lamblia. Antibiotic therapy for the bacterial diarrheas remains controversial because most infections are self-limiting and antibiotic therapy does not shorten the duration of illness. Antibiotic therapy is indicated (1) when a treatable pathogen has been identified, (2) in the immunocompromised host, (3) as an adjunctive therapy in the treatment of cholera and (4) in infants less than 3 months of age with positive stool cultures. Infants at this age are at increased risk to develop septicemia. Infants and children with diarrhea who display signs of septicemia should be treated with parenteral antibiotics.

7. MALABSORPTION / R.A. Schreiber

7.1 Introduction
Growth and development are fundamental to the general health and well-being of any infant, child or adolescent. In order to achieve a normal growth velocity, the pediatric patient requires a sufficient intake of appropriate dietary

FIGURE 4. Digestion and absorption of triglycerides, proteins and carbohydrates.
SOURCE: Adapted from Silverman A, Roy CC. Pediatric clinical gastroenterology. 3d ed. St. Louis: CV Mosby, 1983:250.

nutrients as well as an intact and functional digestive system. In North America, failure to thrive occurs most often because of an inadequate intake of calories. Malabsorption, however, is another important cause of failure to thrive in the pediatric population.

Malabsorption may be defined as a clinical syndrome characterized by defective digestion and absorption of any dietary constituent. A large number of diseases can cause malabsorption. Moreover, the clinical manifestations of this syndrome may be quite diverse, depending upon the dietary constituents that are malabsorbed. The following section reviews the mechanisms for normal digestion and absorption and presents a practical approach to the evaluation of the pediatric patient with malabsorption.

7.2 Physiology and Pathophysiology of Digestion and Absorption

The normal process of intestinal digestion can be divided into three phases (Figure 4). During the intraluminal phase, ingested carbohydrates, proteins and lipids are hydrolyzed within the intestinal lumen by enzymes released by the salivary glands, the stomach and the pancreas. In the intestinal phase, further digestion of peptides and disaccharides continues at the level of the intestinal brush border and the resulting amino acids, small peptides, monosaccharides, monoglycerides and fatty acids are subsequently absorbed into the enterocyte. The movement of nutrients from the intestinal epithelial cell into the vascular or lymphatic circulation defines the delivery phase. The overall absorptive capacity of the intestinal tract depends upon its length and available surface epithelium. In addition, some dietary substances have specific intestinal sites of uptake. Bile acids, for example, are absorbed in the ileum. Vitamin B_{12} first binds to intrinsic factor secreted by the gastric parietal cell and is then absorbed by a specific receptor-mediated process on ileal enterocytes.

An understanding of the determinants of the digestion and absorption of dietary products can provide a basic framework for the clinical approach to the pediatric patient with malabsorption.

7.2.1 CARBOHYDRATES

Dietary carbohydrates are comprised of polysaccharides (starch), disaccharides (sucrose and lactose) and traces of monosaccharides. Polysaccharides first undergo intraluminal digestion by salivary and pancreatic amylases. The hydrolysis of disaccharides occurs at the intestinal brush border by the disaccharidases sucrase-isomaltase, maltase and lactase. The monosaccharides glucose, galactose and fructose are then absorbed into the enterocyte by simple or facilitated diffusion or by a sodium carrier–mediated active transport. From the enterocyte, monosaccharides diffuse into the vascular circulation.

Symptoms of carbohydrate malabsorption are characterized by gaseous distention, borborygmi, cramps and watery nonbloody diarrhea having an acidic pH (4.0–5.5) and containing unabsorbed reducing sugars. The most common cause of carbohydrate malabsorption in infancy is lactase deficiency secondary to viral gastroenteritis. However, lactase deficiency may also complicate any disease that disrupts the small intestinal brush border, including celiac disease, Crohn's disease and HIV enteropathy. Congenital lactase deficiency, sucrase-isomaltase deficiency and other inherited deficiencies of brush-border enzymes are extremely rare. In each case simply excluding the malabsorbed carbohydrate from the diet will promptly resolve the symptoms.

7.2.2 PROTEIN

Protein digestion begins in the stomach, where gastric acid causes protein denaturation and activates pepsin. In the small intestine brush border, enterokinase converts pancreatic trypsinogen into trypsin which, in turn, activates the pancreatic enzymes chymotrypsin and elastase. Digested protein in the form of free amino acids, di- and tripeptides is rapidly absorbed into the enterocyte and then into the circulation. In contrast to carbohydrate malabsorption, diseases that significantly disrupt the intestinal mucosa do not result in protein malabsorption. Rather, in cases of severe gastroenteropathy, intestinal protein loss develops because of a "back-leak" of protein from the sys-

Dietary   Delivery
Components   Intraluminal Phase   Intestinal Phase   Phase

FIGURE 5. Phases in the digestion of lipids.
SOURCE: Adapted from Silverman A, Roy CC. Pediatric clinical gastroenterology. 3d ed. St. Louis: CV Mosby, 1983:250.

temic circulation across the damaged bowel wall into the intestinal lumen – aptly termed a protein-losing enteropathy.

7.2.3 FAT

The digestion of fat begins in the stomach, where fundal lipase hydrolyzes medium- and long-chain fats. This phase of fat digestion is particularly important in neonates whose pancreatic lipase activity is relatively low compared with the mature adult. In the duodenum, hydrophobic long-chain triglycerides are first emulsified by bile salts and then hydrolyzed by pancreatic lipase. Free fatty acids and monoglycerides solubilize into micelles and approach the luminal surface, where they then diffuse across the enterocyte cell membrane. In the enterocyte the free fatty acids and monoglycerides are re-esterified and packaged along with apoprotein B-48 into chylomicrons. Chylomicrons are excreted via the intercellular spaces into the lymphatic circulation, and then through the thoracic duct into the systemic circulation. In contrast to long-chain fats, medium-chain triglycerides are water-soluble and are absorbed by the enterocyte directly into the bloodstream. Medium-chain triglycerides therefore do not require bile salts for digestion or an intact lymphatic system for circulation.

With fat malabsorption the stools are greasy, soft but not liquid, foul smelling and bulky. Growth failure is a dominant feature, because the intestinal loss of high-energy fat nutrients (9 kcal/g of fat) leads to a profound deficiency in the total calories absorbed daily. In addition to the steatorrhea and failure to thrive, the clinical manifestations of fat-soluble vitamin deficiency (vitamins A, D, E, K) may also be present.

Fat digestion is a complex process involving many organ systems (Figure 5). It is not surprising that a variety of disease states can present with signs and symptoms of fat malabsorption. Impaired bile salt excretion associated with any cholestatic liver disease or disorders of bile salt metabolism including bacterial overgrowth, ileal Crohn's disease or the short gut syndrome can lead to fat malabsorption. Pancreatic insufficiency associated with cystic fibrosis or with the Shwachman syndrome, intestinal mucosal abnormalities such as celiac disease and cow's milk protein intolerance, and rare conditions like abetalipoproteinemia and lymphangiectasia are other important causes of fat malabsorption.

7.3 Diagnosis

A complete history and thorough physical examination are the necessary first steps for establishing a diagnosis of malabsorption and sorting out the potential etiologies. Diarrhea is often a principal clinical symptom, and it is important to determine by the history whether steatorrhea is present. The duration, fluidity, frequency, size, consistency and color of the stools should be documented. Another cardinal presenting symptom for malabsorption is weight loss. However, since failure to thrive in infancy is most often secondary to poor dietary intake, it is critical to obtain a complete dietary history. The physician should ask about the quantity and type of formula the infant is receiving or whether the child is breastfed. The age at which new foods were introduced should be established and the physician should try to ascertain whether there is any correlation between the onset of symptoms and the dietary modifications. The average daily caloric intake should be estimated. Consultation with a pediatric dietitian can be very helpful with this assessment. The physician should inquire about the child's growth and review the record of the child's weight and height. These should be plotted on standard infant growth curves.

A complete birth history should also be obtained. All neonatal complications or prior abdominal surgery should be documented. For a patient who presents with a family history of similar gastrointestinal complaints or with gastrointestinal complaints and a background of consanguinity, an underlying genetic disorder should be considered. Information about travel or recent contacts may help to exclude infectious etiologies. A history of frequent infections may point to an underlying immunodeficiency disorder. Recurrent pulmonary disease might suggest a diagnosis of cystic fibrosis.

On physical examination, accurate measurements of the child's current weight, height and head circumference should be obtained and plotted on a standard pediatric growth curve graph along with all previous measurements. The physician should examine the head, eyes, mouth and tongue, looking for features of fat-soluble or water-soluble vitamin or trace mineral deficiencies. For example, pallor and cheilosis might implicate an iron deficiency anemia.

Alopecia may be a feature of zinc deficiency. The cardiovascular and pulmonary examination should be thorough. Abdominal distention may be a manifestation of organomegaly or intestinal gas. Buttock wasting and excess skin folds, particularly in the groin, are features of subcutaneous fat loss. Edema of the lower extremities may develop with hypoalbuminemia. Clubbing may occur in celiac disease or inflammatory bowel disease.

7.4 Laboratory Tests

7.4.1 BASELINE STUDIES
The stools should be analyzed for leukocytes and blood which, if present, suggest a colitis. Determination of the stool pH and a search for reducing substances will support or exclude a diagnosis of carbohydrate malabsorption. A stool smear staining positively for fat globules or fat crystals suggests the presence of fat malabsorption. It is useful to obtain a complete blood count. Iron deficiency anemia may be associated with celiac disease, inflammatory bowel disease or cow's milk protein intolerance. Megaloblastic anemia is a feature of folate or B_{12} deficiency. Acanthocytes are the hallmark of abetalipoproteinemia. The presence of eosinophilia may support a diagnosis of milk protein intolerance. Low serum protein and albumin are features of a protein-losing enteropathy. A urinalysis and urine culture should be obtained to exclude an occult urinary tract infection. Infants and children who present with failure to thrive despite a sufficient caloric intake should have a sweat test to screen for cystic fibrosis.

7.4.2 72-HOUR STOOL FAT COLLECTION
If fat malabsorption is suspected, the gold standard test is a 72-hour stool collection for fat. In this instance a complete and accurate 72-hour dietary history must be obtained concomitantly with the three-day stool collection so that the coefficient of fat absorption can be calculated. Infants less than 6 months of age should absorb >85% of fat intake. By one year of age the fat absorption should be at an adult level of >95%.

7.4.3 D-XYLOSE
D-xylose is a sugar that is absorbed by the intestinal enterocyte independent of brush-border enzymes or pancreatic function. The D-xylose test is used to assess the integrity of the intestinal mucosa. A standard dose of D-xylose is given by mouth, and a serum level is drawn one hour later. A level greater than 25 mg/dL is normal. A low one-hour serum level suggests mucosal damage. The usefulness of this test in the evaluation of malabsorption is controversial.

7.4.4 BREATH HYDROGEN TEST

The breath hydrogen test is most often used to diagnose lactose malabsorption. In this instance a standard dose of lactose is given by mouth and serial breath samples are obtained. If lactose is malabsorbed, colonic bacteria ferment the sugar, producing hydrogen ion, which is subsequently absorbed by the colon into the blood, circulated to the lungs and then exhaled. A significant rise in breath hydrogen 60–90 minutes after lactose ingestion is consistent with incomplete lactose absorption. Hydrogen breath tests may also be used for the diagnosis of sucrase deficiency or small intestinal bacterial overgrowth.

7.4.5 IMAGING STUDIES

Contrast radiographic studies are useful to exclude congenital anatomical abnormalities of the gastrointestinal tract as a cause for the malabsorption. Ulceration and strictures are features of Crohn's disease. Intestinal dilation and hypomotility support a diagnosis of bacterial overgrowth.

7.4.6 ENDOSCOPY

Upper endoscopy with multiple biopsies permits both gross and microscopic assessment of the intestinal mucosa. The histologic features of a small intestinal biopsy may be highly indicative or even diagnostic for the etiology of the malabsorption. The diagnosis of celiac disease is established only by an intestinal biopsy. The presence of fat-laden vacuoles in intestinal villus cells suggests a disorder in the delivery phase of fat digestion, such as abetalipoproteinemia or hypobetalipoproteinemia. The histological presence of dilated lacteals is a feature of lymphangiectasia.

7.5 Management

There are a few basic principles to the management of the pediatric patient who presents with a malabsorption syndrome. First, it is important to determine the cause of the disorder and direct treatment accordingly. For example, patients with celiac disease recover on a gluten-free diet. Infants with cow's milk protein allergy respond to a modification of the protein in the diet. The manifestations of secondary lactase deficiency will resolve with a lactose-free formula or with the use of enzyme supplements (Lactaid®). The fat malabsorption in cystic fibrosis is corrected with pancreatic enzyme replacement. Second, it is usually necessary to provide ample supplemental calories in order to achieve catch-up growth. A good supply of extra calories is especially important for the young infant with marked failure to thrive. High-calorie formulas are frequently introduced early, often before a specific diagnosis has been established. Third, any vitamin, mineral and trace element deficiencies should be corrected. Anemias are treated with the appropriate supplements.

Fat-soluble vitamins are required for infants with ongoing steatorrhea, especially those with cholestatic liver disease. Vitamin B_{12} supplementation may be necessary for patients with ileal resection.

7.6 Summary
The malabsorption syndrome is characterized by a constellation of signs and symptoms associated with a wide variety of disorders, each having a distinct etiopathogenesis. Two common manifestations of this syndrome in the pediatric population are diarrhea and failure to thrive. A careful evaluation of the infant with malabsorption based on a thorough knowledge of the normal physiology of digestion will help the physician to secure a diagnosis and institute an appropriate management plan. The judicious treatment of an infant with malabsorption should lead to a rapid resolution of the symptoms. The reestablishment of a normal growth velocity is ultimately required in order to ensure the healthy development of any infant, child or adolescent.

8. CYSTIC FIBROSIS / H. Machida

Cystic fibrosis (CF) is an autosomal recessive disease that causes chronic morbidity and decreases the life-span of most affected individuals. Because of a defect at a single gene locus that encodes a protein, the cystic fibrosis transmembrane regulator (CFTR), individuals with cystic fibrosis have defective cyclic adenosine monophosphate–regulated chloride transport in epithelial cells of exocrine organs. Although the exact pathophysiology remains to be clarified for each involved organ, there is an accumulation of viscous secretions associated with progressive obstruction and subsequent destruction of excretory ducts.

Chronic pulmonary disease is the major cause of morbidity in the majority of patients. These individuals have progressive bronchiectasis and associated bacterial endobronchial infections, most often secondary to Pseudomonas species.

Although the pulmonary disease is most prominent, the GI manifestations of cystic fibrosis are extensive and contribute to significant morbidity and even mortality. This section will review the clinical problems related to the gastrointestinal tract, particularly the pancreatic insufficiency and hepatic disease in cystic fibrosis.

8.1 Pancreatic Insufficiency
Approximately 80% of patients with cystic fibrosis are born with pancreatic insufficiency, and another 5–10% develop pancreatic insufficiency in subsequent years. These patients have marked impairment of pancreatic exocrine function, including decreased secretion of water, bicarbonate, lipase, amylase

and proteinases from the pancreas into the duodenum. In the very young, the endocrine function of the pancreas is usually normal, but many gradually develop evidence of glucose intolerance; a small number develop clinical diabetes requiring insulin therapy. Patients with pancreatic insufficiency may present with any of the following clinical entities with or without pulmonary disease.

8.1.1 *MECONIUM ILEUS*

Meconium ileus is partial or complete obstruction of the intestine, commonly the ileum, with thick inspissated meconium. This occurs in approximately 15% of infants with cystic fibrosis. Any infant with meconium ileus must have cystic fibrosis excluded. These infants may present with delayed passage of meconium, abdominal distention, vomiting or other signs of obstruction. Meconium ileus may be complicated by antenatal or postnatal volvulus, atresia, perforation of the bowel and meconium peritonitis. In cases with complications, infants may require surgery shortly after birth. Extensive bowel resection may leave them with the short bowel syndrome.

These infants are investigated initially with a plain abdominal x-ray for evidence of obstruction or perforation. If the bowel perforates in utero the perforation often seals, and the x-ray may show calcifications from the meconium in the peritoneum. If meconium ileus is a possibility, surgery should be considered immediately. As long as the x-ray shows no evidence of free air (implying a perforation), most infants are given a gentle water-soluble contrast enema to attempt to relieve the obstruction or at least outline the obstruction for the surgeon. These enemas can cause significant fluid shifts in small neonates, so an IV must be running during the procedure. If the procedure is unsuccessful, surgery is required. The majority of infants with meconium ileus also have pancreatic insufficiency, but this condition can occur in pancreatic-sufficient patients as well.

8.1.2 *CHRONIC DIARRHEA*

After the neonatal period, chronic diarrhea with or without failure to thrive is common. These infants have loose stools essentially from birth, and one may obtain a history of delay in the passage of meconium. The parents may describe the diarrheal stools as being pale, foul smelling, fatty and/or soupy. The diarrhea is primarily secondary to fat malabsorption because of the pancreatic insufficiency. However, infants who have had small bowel resection, such as for bowel atresia secondary to meconium ileus, may have mucosal disease secondary to bacterial overgrowth. This will contribute significantly to the diarrhea and may cause it to become more watery. Initially, if they do not have respiratory problems, infants with cystic fibrosis tend to have a relatively good appetite and can in some cases compensate for the extreme loss of nutrients by increasing their intake. As they develop pulmonary symptoms or become gradually malnourished, however, their appetite will decrease.

8.1.3 *FAILURE TO THRIVE*

In cystic fibrosis, failure to thrive is usually a result of a combination of decreased intake, loss of fat in the stools and increased metabolic requirements. The requirements of the average cystic fibrosis patient have been reported to be 120% of normal. Nevertheless, some patients have essentially normal caloric requirements, and others may have requirements in excess of 150% of normal. Many in the early childhood years are able to maintain their nutritional status well with pancreatic enzyme supplementation and good nutrition. Unfortunately, the increased caloric requirements of puberty coupled with deteriorating lung function often make it impossible for the most severely affected patients to maintain their nutrition and normal growth. In addition, CF patients may have anorexia of chronic disease and difficulty eating due to chronic cough. They present with a gradual decrease in growth percentiles, first of the weight and subsequently of the height. Puberty may be delayed or arrested in the early stages. At this time, nutritional supplementation becomes extremely important. Pancreatic enzyme supplementation must be maximized, and nutritional supplementation given either orally or by enteral tube feeding. Total parenteral nutrition is rarely required. If enteral feeds are needed, we use nasogastric tubes in all our patients except those who have nasal polyps. These patients are taught to put their nasogastric tubes down five to six nights a week to obtain 10 hours of nocturnal supplementary feedings. We have had patients as young as 4 years of age who are able to put their own tubes down. The optimal supplement to use is still being debated. We have been most successful with regular high-calorie formula such as Ensure® with fiber, particularly in patients who have evidence of glucose intolerance. Some centers do not give pancreatic enzyme supplements with the tube feeding; others give enteric-coated enzymes at the initiation of tube feeds; still others add pancreatic enzyme powder to the feeds. We have had the most success with the last approach. With infants, we use the enteral tube feeds in those who present with significant failure to thrive and are unable to take enough calories for catch-up growth, and also in those who have had small bowel resections. Generally, these infants will require the tube feeding only for several weeks to months. We have had only two children between the ages of 2 and 9 who have needed enteral tube feeding. In the adolescent group who require enteral feeding supplementation, we find that about 50% require the supplementation for only a transient period of six months to two years while they are experiencing the significant growth of puberty. A small number of our patients have had to remain on the enteral tube feeding program for years in order to maintain their weight and nutritional status.

8.1.4 *FAT-SOLUBLE VITAMIN DEFICIENCY*

As a result of significant malabsorption prior to treatment, patients may present with overt evidence of bruising or bleeding due to vitamin K deficiency. We have seen one infant female who presented with this condition as well as evidence of xerophthalmia, apparently due to vitamin A deficiency. The clinical effects of vitamin E deficiencies in cystic fibrosis are not well documented, but this vitamin must be given to patients in a supplement and in adequate doses. We also supplement with vitamin D, although vitamin D deficiency, particularly evidence of rickets, is very uncommon in patients with cystic fibrosis.

8.1.5 *HYPOALBUMINEMIA AND EDEMA*

In spite of their pancreatic insufficiency, most patients with cystic fibrosis do not have difficulty with hypoalbuminemia secondary to protein malabsorption. Protein malabsorption, however, is a problem in infants who are fed a soy protein formula, and sometimes in those who are breastfed. These infants will present with significant hypoalbuminemia, edema and usually a history of diarrhea. We have had at least one infant who presented with heart failure secondary to severe hypoalbuminemia. Feeding with soy formula must be discontinued, but often those who are receiving breast milk may have their albumin corrected with pancreatic enzyme supplementation. Older patients with severe malnutrition or cor pulmonale may also develop hypoalbuminemia.

8.1.6 *RECTAL PROLAPSE*

An infant with untreated pancreatic insufficiency becomes increasingly malnourished and continues to pass numerous stools, and thus may begin to have regular rectal prolapse. This is not infrequently the complaint that brings the infant to medical attention. In these cases, a diagnosis of cystic fibrosis must be made quickly and the child renourished. The prolapse will resolve with appropriate nutrition and pancreatic enzyme supplementation to decrease the stooling. In most of these infants the rectal prolapse reduces spontaneously. If it does not, it must be gently reduced manually.

8.1.7 *DISTAL INTESTINAL OBSTRUCTION SYNDROME*

The distal intestinal obstruction syndrome (DIOS), also known as meconium ileus equivalent, is partial or complete obstruction of the bowel resulting from fecal masses, usually in the cecum. This can occur in any age of child with cystic fibrosis, but we find it most often in the older child. Younger children with DIOS present with decreased appetite, decreased stooling, distention and often vomiting. Older patients complain of grumbling or crampy abdominal pain and a gradual decrease in stooling. In most patients, the fecal masses are easily palpated and an x-ray is not always required. If the diagnosis is made early, most can be treated with N-acetylcysteine given orally. We give a loading dose in a cola drink and 3 subsequent doses (1 dose every 6 hours over 24 hours). Fluids must be encouraged during this time. If there is evidence of marked obstruction, we admit the patients to hospital and give them polyethylene glycol–salt solution (GoLYTELY™) orally or by nasogastric tube. This completely clears the obstructive fecal masses. It is essential to ensure that patients with DIOS get adequate enzymes, as the syndrome seems to occur most often in patients who are not getting enough enzymes or in whom the duodenal pH is too low for optimal efficacy of the enzymes.

8.1.8 PANCREATITIS

Five to 10% of patients with cystic fibrosis will remain pancreatic-sufficient throughout their life. Unfortunately, some pancreatic-sufficient patients develop pancreatitis, which may present with vomiting and acute pain that radiates to the back or with recurrent low-grade abdominal pain and perhaps a change in appetite. Those who present with acute pancreatitis should be treated as any other patient with pancreatitis. The bowel is rested until the enzymes return essentially to normal and the patient is asymptomatic. In patients who are found to have mild abdominal pain and only slight increase in enzymes, management is less definitive. We have treated these patients with pancreatic enzymes to try to decrease the amount of stimulation of the pancreas. Unfortunately, the pancreatitis tends to be a recurrent problem in some individuals.

8.2 Hepatobiliary Disease

Hepatobiliary disease in cystic fibrosis is well documented. Fortunately, although a significant number of patients have subtle manifestation of hepatobiliary abnormalities, only a small number have severe liver disease. Given the increasing life expectancy of patients with cystic fibrosis there may be an increasing need to manage patients with severe liver problems. The following briefly outlines the clinical features of some of the hepatobiliary problems associated with cystic fibrosis.

8.2.1 NEONATAL JAUNDICE

Prolonged conjugated hyperbilirubinemia is reported to occur in neonates with cystic fibrosis. In some cases, the hyperbilirubinemia may be secondary to a problem unrelated to the cystic fibrosis; nevertheless, any infant with conjugated hyperbilirubinemia of unknown origin should be investigated for cystic fibrosis.

8.2.2 ELEVATED LIVER ENZYMES

A significant portion of patients with cystic fibrosis have mildly elevated liver enzymes, including alkaline phosphatase, γ-glutamyl transferase (GGT), aspartate aminotransferase (AST) and alanine aminotransferase (ALT). This is not uncommon in patients who had a meconium ileus as a neonate and are pancreatic-insufficient. In most of these patients, the enzymes either normalize or remain slightly elevated throughout their life. A small proportion develop serious liver disease.

8.2.3 HEPATOSPLENOMEGALY

Many patients with cystic fibrosis have a slightly large liver secondary to fatty infiltration, probably because of poor nutrition. In these patients, the liver is smooth and soft. In those who develop progressive liver disease, the liver is initially large; it gradually begins to feel hard and often nodular. Splenomegaly is usually not detected until the patient is aged 6 or older. On histologic examination, these patients have multinodular or biliary cirrhosis. The liver disease tends to progress slowly and the prominent clinical problems are secondary to hypersplenism. It can be years before there are changes in the albumin, INR/PT or PTT, or an elevation of the bilirubin. With the significant portal hypertension, the patients are at risk for bleeding from esophageal or small bowel varices. As the life-span of patients with cystic fibrosis increases, one would expect to see increasing morbidity and mortality from liver failure.

In very recent years, ursodeoxycholic acid has been used to try to improve the liver disease in cystic fibrosis. Short-term studies report that patients treated with ursodeoxycholic acid show improvement in their liver enzymes and, in some cases, in liver function studies. It has yet to be determined whether long-term treatment will actually prevent progression of the liver disease and perhaps protect some children from developing cirrhosis.

8.3 Management of Pancreatic Insufficiency

As there are numerous gastrointestinal problems in cystic fibrosis and their interrelationship can be quite complex, it is beyond the scope of this section to discuss the management in detail. In the majority of cases, the problem must be identified, assessed and managed as in patients without cystic fibrosis. Nevertheless, because the pancreatic insufficiency causes most of the gastrointestinal problems, an approach to its management will be outlined.

There are several indirect methods that assess pancreatic insufficiency, but the only direct measurement of pancreatic function is a pancreatic stimulation test. Unfortunately, this test requires intubation of the duodenum, it is invasive and uncomfortable for the patient, and generally it will not contribute significantly to the patient's management. Therefore, this test is usually reserved for complicated cases. We usually assess the pancreatic insufficiency by a 72-hour fecal fat collection, which measures the percentage of fat lost in the stools daily. If possible, this test is done before the patient is placed on pancreatic enzyme supplementation and post-enzyme supplementation.

Once the pancreatic insufficiency is diagnosed, it is treated with supplementary pancreatic enzymes. The aim of treatment is to control the fat malabsorption so that the patient has normal growth and good nutrition. (In the majority of cases it is impossible to reduce fecal fat loss to less than 12%, even on optimal enzyme supplementation.) Commonly, the enzymes given are in capsule form and contain enteric-coated spheres of lipase, amylase and proteinases. These enteric-coated spheres are released in the alkaline environment of the duodenum. The strength of these preparations varies; usually the dosage is expressed in lipase units. We find that the appropriate dosage of lipase is best determined empirically.

We begin giving infants under 6 months of age at diagnosis 1 enteric-coated capsule with 4,000 units of lipase per feed. By 1 year of age, the majority will be on 8,000 to 10,000 lipase units per feed and 4,000 per small snack. Subsequently, the enzymes are evaluated and increased as the patient grows and whenever there is evidence of increasing malabsorption. By age 8 the majority of patients with pancreatic insufficiency will require 80,000 to 100,000 lipase units per meal. In most cases an increase in lipase above this level does not improve their fat absorption. In older children, we generally use capsules containing 20,000 lipase units each, so that the child can take fewer capsules per meal. The disadvantage with this is that the child may be taking more enzymes than required for small meals or snacks.

With the lack of bicarbonate secretion from the pancreas, the duodenal pH may be too low for optimal activity of the pancreatic enzyme supplements. In patients in whom the number of enzymes seems maximal for age and weight, ranitidine is started at 2 mg/kg b.i.d. to enhance the efficacy of the enzymes.

8.4 Summary
The gastrointestinal effects of cystic fibrosis are extensive. Most of the prominent problems are secondary to the pancreatic disease. Once this is treated adequately with enzymes, vitamin replacement and adequate nutrition, many problems will resolve. Severe liver disease is less common; it can be devastating in the patients in whom it occurs and may be of more concern as the lifespan of the patients increases. Research into the pathophysiology of the liver disease and into pharmacologic agents such as ursodeoxycholic acid is ongoing. Because failure to thrive and liver disease can present insidiously, it is essential to monitor these patients on a regular basis, including documentation of height and weight, a complete physical examination and a regular biochemical evaluation.

9. APPROACH TO THE JAUNDICED NEONATE / S.R. Martin

Jaundice is caused by the deposition of bile pigment in the skin and other tissues as a result of an elevated serum bilirubin concentration. Bilirubin is formed from the degradation of hemoglobin as well as other heme-containing

TABLE 8.   Factors contributing to physiological jaundice in the neonate

Absence of placental bilirubin metabolism
Reduced hepatic blood flow via ductus venosus shunting
Decreased red blood cell survival
Increased red blood cell mass
Reduced enteric bacterial flora
Presence of intestinal β-glucuronidase
Immature liver function
Delayed oral feeding

proteins, mainly within cells of the reticuloendothelial system. Bilirubin is carried in the circulation bound to albumin and taken up in the liver by the hepatocytes, where it is conjugated with glucuronic acid before being secreted into bile. Conjugated bilirubin is then converted to urobilirubins by intestinal bacteria, preventing its reabsorption and permitting its excretion in the feces. Jaundice in the neonatal period (<1 month) is present in up to 60% of full-term and 80% of premature infants; usually it is a physiological phenomenon related to the developmental nature of bilirubin metabolism. Infants of certain racial background (oriental, Greek, North American native) may be particularly susceptible.

9.1 Physiological Jaundice
Physiological jaundice generally appears around the third to fifth day, rises by no more than 85 μmol/L/day and resolves by the end of the second week of life. Hyperbilirubinemia is always of the unconjugated fraction. Peak levels rarely exceed 150 μmol/L in full-term infants, although in premature infants levels of 200 μmol/L are not uncommon and the resolution may be slower. Several mechanisms that contribute to the development of physiological jaundice, including increased bilirubin load and decreased capacity to process bilirubin, are shown in Table 8.

After birth the placenta is no longer available for bilirubin metabolism and the immature liver has a limited capacity for uptake of bilirubin from plasma and for its binding, conjugation and secretion into bile. Blood flow may not immediately favor hepatic perfusion (shunting via the ductus venosus). An increased bilirubin load derives from the neonate's elevated hematocrit combined with a reduced red blood cell life-span. Delayed feedings result in retention of meconium containing significant amounts of bilirubin within the intestine, which initially has reduced bacterial flora. This limits the conversion of conjugated bilirubin into urobilinogens. Also present is β-glucuronidase, which converts conjugated bilirubin into a reabsorbable form.

9.2 **Pathological Jaundice**

Jaundice is quantified by measuring the serum bilirubin composed, in general, of unconjugated and conjugated fractions. Because it is impossible to differentiate visually between jaundice caused by unconjugated hyperbilirubinemia and that caused by conjugated hyperbilirubinemia, each of which has different etiologies, therapies and prognosis, the first step in evaluating a jaundiced baby is to determine the total and conjugated bilirubin concentrations. Potentially life-threatening illnesses may present with neonatal jaundice, so it is important that the initial evaluation distinguish between physiological and pathological causes of jaundice in order to start any therapy without delay. Pathological jaundice is suggested and requires investigation when any of the following conditions arises:

1. jaundice appearing within the first 24 hours;
2. a rate of rise of more than 85 μmol/L/24 hours;
3. total bilirubin >250 μmol/L in breastfed infants, or >200 μmol/L in formula-fed infants;
4. persistence of jaundice beyond 2 weeks of age; or
5. a conjugated fraction >34 μmol/L, or >15% of the total bilirubin concentration.

9.2.1 *UNCONJUGATED HYPERBILIRUBINEMIA*

In practice, jaundice is caused either by increased production or decreased clearance of bilirubin by the liver. The pathological causes of unconjugated hyperbilirubinemia are shown in Table 9.

9.2.1.1 *Increased bilirubin production*

Any process that presents a greater bilirubin load to the liver than can be processed will result in hyperbilirubinemia. Thus, red blood cell hemolysis from a variety of causes, including maternal–infant blood group incompatibility (Rh, ABO, minor groups), membrane defects, red cell enzyme deficiencies and toxic effects of drugs, increases the load of unconjugated bilirubin presented to the liver. Hemoglobinopathies rarely present in the neonatal period because of the presence of a large proportion of the relatively stable fetal hemoglobin (Hgb F). Massive hemolysis may occasionally also raise *conjugated* bilirubin levels to 25–30% of the total, possibly resulting from the toxic effects of bilirubin secretion into bile. Conditions resulting in increased red cell breakdown, especially hematomas, elevate the serum bilirubin; these are relatively more important in smaller premature infants. Finally, some conditions accentuate the normally high neonatal hemoglobin, resulting in polycythemia. Examples are maternal–infant transfusion, delayed umbilical

TABLE 9. Causes of unconjugated hyperbilirubinemia in the neonate

---

Increased bilirubin production
Hemolytic disease
  Blood group incompatibility (Rh, ABO, minor groups)
  Membrane defects (spherocytosis, elliptocytosis, infantile pyknocytosis)
  Enzyme deficits (G6-PD, hexokinase, pyruvate kinase)
  Drugs (oxytocin, vitamin K)

Increased breakdown
  Infection
  Hematoma, swallowed maternal blood

Increased RBC mass
  Polycythemia (maternal diabetes, delayed cord clamp, small for gestational age, altitude)

Decreased bilirubin metabolism
Reduced uptake
  Portacaval shunt, hypoxia, sepsis, acidosis, congenital heart disease

Decreased conjugation
  Crigler-Najjar type I, II
  Gilbert's syndrome
  Lucey-Driscoll syndrome
  hypothyroidism
  panhypopituitarism

Altered enterohepatic circulation
Breastfeeding
  Free fatty acids, steroids, breast milk β-glucuronidase
Intestinal hypomotility
  Retained meconium
Reduced intestinal flora
  Newborn, antibiotic use

---

cord clamping at birth, and conditions that result in relative intrauterine hypoxia (maternal diabetes mellitus, high altitude, newborn small for gestational age).

9.2.1.2 *Altered bilirubin metabolism*

At any stage in the processing of bilirubin – uptake, transport, conjugation, excretion – abnormalities may affect the unconjugated bilirubin concentration. The Crigler-Najjar syndrome is an inherited disorder characterized by absent or low hepatic glucuronyl transferase activity. Type I is associated with very high levels of bilirubin and with kernicterus, whereas type II has lower bilirubin levels and is responsive to enzyme induction with phenobarbital to lower the serum bilirubin. Gilbert's syndrome, an autosomal dominant condition, is a mild form of elevated bilirubin with reduced glucuronyl transferase activity, in which jaundice (which is rarely observed in the newborn) is often provoked by stress or fasting. It requires no treatment. The Lucey-Driscoll syndrome is a transient form of acquired reduction in glucuronyl transferase activity in the newborn, caused by a factor in maternal serum. Endocrine disorders such as panhypopituitarism and hypothyroidism affect bile conjugation by unclear mechanisms.

9.2.1.3 *Altered enterohepatic circulation*
Jaundice induced by breast milk occurs in approximately 1 in 200 infants. Jaundice may present in the first week in the early form or after the first week in the late form, which is associated with higher bilirubin levels. The degree of hyperbilirubinemia is quite variable (171–462 μmol/L) and may last from 3 to 10 weeks. Despite the occasional presence of very elevated unconjugated bilirubin levels, kernicterus has not been reported in normal term newborns with breast milk–induced jaundice. Several breast milk components have been implicated, including free fatty acids, an isomer of naturally occurring steroids and β-glucuronidase. Hyperbilirubinemia may also be caused by antibiotic-induced reductions in intestinal flora that increase the level of intestinal conjugated bilirubin, the preferred substrate for β-glucuronidase, whose action produces unconjugated bilirubin that is readily absorbed.

9.2.1.4 *Kernicterus*
The importance of determining an etiology for unconjugated hyperbilirubinemia lies in directing appropriate treatment to prevent kernicterus. Severe unconjugated hyperbilirubinemia is associated with brain toxicity possibly secondary to cellular hypoxia induced by bilirubin. Early symptoms are nonspecific – e.g., lethargy, vomiting, poor feeding and loss of the Moro reflex. Progressive injury leads to respiratory difficulties, bulging fontanelles, a high-pitched cry, loss of deep tendon reflexes and opisthotonos, finally resulting in gaze paresis, convulsions and death. In survivors long-term sequelae include choreoathetosis, spasticity, seizures and sensorineural hearing loss.

Although the lowest level of bilirubin predictive of kernicterus is not known, it is almost universal at levels >500 μmol/L, present in one-third of full-term infants >342 μmol/L, and rare below this latter level. However, numerous factors play a role in increasing bilirubin toxicity at lower levels. Some concern exists that more subtle long-term effects may occur in any infant with raised unconjugated bilirubin concentration; motor development may be affected by levels greater than 255 μmol/L. Bilirubin toxicity may be increased by factors that reduce binding to albumin, such as hypoproteinemia, acidosis, hypothermia, hypoglycemia-induced elevations of plasma free fatty acids and drugs (sulfa, salicylates, heparin, hematin, ceftriaxone, sodium benzoate), or by factors affecting the permeability of the blood–brain barrier, such as prematurity, asphyxia, hyperosmolarity, infection, respiratory distress syndrome, acidosis and intraventricular hemorrhage. Such factors are frequent in very low birth weight infants, in whom kernicterus may occur at unconjugated bilirubin levels as low as 255 µmol/L.

9.2.1.5 *Management*
In contrast to cholestatic infants, those with unconjugated hyperbilirubinemia have normal colored stools, the urine is not dark and the liver is only rarely enlarged and is not firm or nodular. When unconjugated hyperbilirubinemia is confirmed, initial management should identify maternal and infant risk factors according to the causes shown in Table 9. Correction of underlying illnesses (sepsis, hypothermia, acidosis, hypoxia) should be initiated. Specific investigations should include maternal and infant blood group, Coombs' test, hemoglobin or hematocrit, red cell indices and morphology to identify polycythemia, hemolysis or red blood cell disorders. Early feedings should be instituted where possible. For high-risk infants with early jaundice (appearing within the first 24 hours), rapidly rising levels of bilirubin (>85 µmol/L/24 hours) or elevated levels of bilirubin (>250 µmol/L in breastfed or >200 µmol/L in formula-fed infants), specific therapy usually includes phototherapy, exchange transfusion or occasionally oral administration of bilirubin binding agents such as charcoal or agar. Phenobarbital may be given to stimulate the enzymes responsible for bilirubin conjugation. Inhibition of bilirubin formation from its heme precursors may in the future be achieved with agents like tin-protoporphyrin, an inhibitor of heme oxygenase. Breast milk jaundice usually does not require treatment other than maintaining good hydration of the infant with more frequent feedings and occasionally supplemental water or formula, as well as periodic serum bilirubin determinations. Cessation of breast milk feedings for 36 to 48 hours will significantly reduce bilirubin levels that are of concern.

9.2.2 *CONJUGATED HYPERBILIRUBINEMIA IN THE NEONATE*
Conjugated hyperbilirubinemia in the newborn is a sign of cholestasis and always requires further investigation. Because cholestasis implies impairment of bile flow at any point from its formation in the hepatocyte to its excretion from the common bile duct, the causes of neonatal cholestasis are many. However, therapeutic interventions that will significantly affect the outcome are relatively few. For certain conditions, notably infections, some metabolic and endocrine disorders and biliary atresia, early intervention is associated with better outcome. The goal, therefore, is to identify treatable causes as early as possible.

The more common causes of cholestatic jaundice in the neonate are out-

TABLE 10. Causes of conjugated hyperbilirubinemia in the neonate

Infection
Bacterial urinary tract infection/sepsis
Cytomegalovirus
Rubella
Herpes viruses: simplex; type 6
Toxoplasmosis
Syphilis
Other viruses: adenovirus, Coxsackie virus, echovirus, parvovirus B19

Metabolic
Galactosemia
Fructosemia
Tyrosinemia
Peroxisomal disorders
Bile acid synthesis disorders
α_1-antitrypsin deficiency
Cystic fibrosis
Niemann-Pick disease
Endocrine disorders: hypopituitarism, hypothyroidism
Neonatal hemochromatosis

Bile duct disorders
Extrahepatic
    Biliary atresia
    Bile duct perforation, stenosis
    Neonatal sclerosing cholangitis
    Choledochal cyst
    Cholelithiasis
    Intra/extrahepatic masses
    Inspissated bile/bile plug

Intrahepatic
    Alagille's syndrome
    Byler's disease (familial progressive cholestasis)
    Nonsyndromic bile duct paucity

Miscellaneous
Parenteral nutrition
Intestinal obstruction
Shock
Trisomy 21

lined in Table 10. Although several groups of illnesses are recognized (infectious, metabolic/endocrine, disorders of the bile ducts, cholestatic syndromes), in practice the diagnostic approach consists initially of differentiating biliary obstruction (which requires surgical intervention) from intrahepatic causes of cholestasis. Idiopathic neonatal cholestasis is commonly, but less precisely (because true hepatitis is not often present), referred to as neonatal hepatitis. Neonatal hepatitis is used as a general name for a wide variety of different disorders that present similarly and together with biliary atresia account for 70–80% of all neonatal cholestasis. As specific diseases are elucidated the proportion accounted for by true idiopathic neonatal hepatitis appears to be diminishing. A possible diagnostic approach is shown in Figure 6.

A maternal history of unexplained illness, rash, exposure to cats or uncooked meat may provide clues to infectious causes. A history of blood transfusion or intravenous drug abuse should be sought, although cholestasis is unusual in the neonate with vertically transmitted hepatitis B or C, or human immunodeficiency virus. The family history is especially important for metabolic disorders such as galactosemia, fructosemia, tyrosinemia, Niemann-Pick, α_1-antitrypsin deficiency, peroxisomal disorders or cystic fibrosis as well as familial disorders such as Alagille's syndrome or familial progressive intrahepatic cholestasis (Byler's disease). A history of previous infant deaths in the family due to unexplained liver disease may be important now that previously lethal familial diseases (such as bile acid synthesis defects) can be successfully treated.

The infant's presentation may also suggest a particular etiology. Lethargy, poor feeding or vomiting may signify sepsis or hypoglycemia associated with pituitary dysfunction. Forceful vomiting may indicate intestinal obstruction, but may also occur with galactosemia and fructosemia. While the normal neonate usually does not have fructose in the diet, several medications have a sucrose-based vehicle that is metabolized to fructose. Jaundice with acholic stools in the first 24 hours of life may suggest a bile duct lesion (stone, stricture, perforation). A well appearing infant of full-term gestation and normal birth weight with gradual onset of persistently acholic stools is likely to have extrahepatic biliary atresia.

The physical examination frequently may guide subsequent investigations. The particular facies and high-pitched cry associated with the murmur of peripheral pulmonic stenosis may suggest Alagille's syndrome. A small for gestational age infant with petechiae, rash, retinal lesions, hepatosplenomegaly and adenopathy portrays the clinical appearance of congenital viral infection. An enlarged, firm and/or nodular liver suggests fibrosis, most commonly due to biliary atresia. Biliary atresia also may be associated with situs inversus and a murmur of congenital heart disease. A palpable right upper quadrant mass may signify a choledochal cyst. A micropenis in the male, optic disk atrophy or midline facial defects such as cleft lip may be a clue to hypopituitarism. Severe hypotonia is associated with peroxisomal disorders. Finally the rectal examination may provide stool to determine the presence or absence of bile.

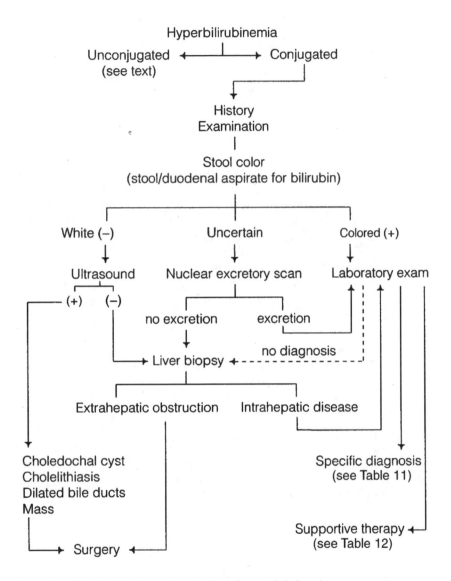

FIGURE 6.   Algorithm for diagnostic evaluation of neonatal cholestasis.

9.2.2.1 *Management*

If the stool is persistently white, investigations should be directed toward possible extrahepatic biliary obstruction. Although acholic stools may occasionally occur with severe intrahepatic disease, Alagille's syndrome and cystic fibrosis, additional clinical features and laboratory investigations usually are diagnostic. An abdominal ultrasound will detect a choledochal cyst, cholelithiasis, dilated bile ducts from obstruction or stenosis, and intrahepatic or extrahepatic masses. Elements of the polysplenia syndrome (preduodenal portal vein, situs inversus, abnormal inferior vena cava), associated with biliary atresia, may also be detected. At this stage it would be appropriate to refer to a pediatric surgeon for surgery and intraoperative cholangiogram. Sometimes the color of the stool is uncertain and tests for bilirubin in the stool (Ictotest®) are equivocal. (Confusion may arise because yellow secretions or urine will color otherwise acholic stools. This often can be avoided by obtaining stool by rectal examination or by breaking open the stool to reveal its true color.) In such cases hepatobiliary scintigraphy using a ^{99m}Tc-labeled iminodiacetic acid derivative, following five days of treatment with phenobarbital to enhance excretion, may demonstrate patency of the biliary tree. If excretion into the intestine is demonstrated, further diagnostic laboratory investigations are indicated. The absence of excretion is less specific and may arise with intrahepatic cholestasis, as previously mentioned.

A percutaneous liver biopsy will usually differentiate extrahepatic biliary obstruction, particularly biliary atresia, from intrahepatic causes of cholestasis. Typically, biliary atresia is associated with fibrous expansion of the portal tracts, bile ductular proliferation and portal bile plugs. Idiopathic neonatal cholestasis is characterized by disorganization of the structure of the lobule, mononuclear cell infiltration, focal hepatocyte necrosis and more diffuse presence of giant cells than found with other disorders. Bile duct paucity is suggested by absence of intralobular bile ducts, but an adequate number of portal spaces must be present to confirm the diagnosis. Early biopsies may suggest idiopathic cholestasis, requiring clinical suspicion and repeat biopsy to arrive at the correct diagnosis. The less common nonsyndromic forms of bile duct paucity may ultimately be shown to be secondary forms because the list of diseases associated with this histological picture appears to be increasing with time.

Laboratory investigations useful in the evaluation of the cholestatic neonate are outlined in Table 11. Serum bilirubin measures the degree of cholestasis. Alkaline phosphatase and γ-glutamyl transpeptidase (GGT) are greatly elevated with biliary obstruction. However, with prolonged cholestasis alkaline phosphatase may be elevated on the basis of the effects of vitamin D malabsorption on bone; γ-glutamyl transpeptidase is normally elevated in the neonatal period. A measure of hepatic synthetic function is provided by INR/prothrombin time, serum albumin and, where available, factor V levels. The most urgent investigations search for possible bacterial infection and certain metabolic/endocrine disorders for which prompt therapy will reverse the cholestasis as well as treat the underlying disease state. Thus, bacterial cultures of the

TABLE 11.   Laboratory evaluation of conjugated hyperbilirubinemia

---

Total and direct serum bilirubin
Alkaline phosphatase, aminotransferases, γ-glutamyl transpeptidase
Prothrombin time or INR, serum albumin (factor V levels, if available)
Complete blood cell count, differential
Urine culture (blood/cerebrospinal fluid, if indicated)
Serology for cytomegalovirus, rubella, herpes simplex, herpes type 6, toxoplasmosis, syphilis
    (adenovirus, Coxsackie virus, reovirus III, parvovirus B19, if available)
Urine for reducing substances, serum galactose-1-phosphate uridyltransferase, serum/urine
    amino acids and organic acids
Sweat chloride
α_1-antitrypsin level and Pi phenotype
Urine for bile acid metabolites
Ophthalmologic examination
Radiograph of vertebral column, long bones, skull
Serum ferritin

---

urine and/or blood; urine for reducing substances (while the infant is ingesting lactose in the form of breast milk or lactose-based formula) or serum galactose-1-phosphate uridyltransferase to diagnose galactosemia; and tests of pituitary function (thyroxin, thyroid stimulating hormone, cortisol and growth hormone levels), in the appropriate clinical setting, are indicated. Serum for very long chain fatty acids may aid in the diagnosis of peroxisomal disorders. Recently, bile acid synthesis defects have been described that respond to specific bile acid replacement therapy if begun early in the course. The presentation and liver biopsy resemble idiopathic neonatal cholestasis (neonatal hepatitis), although the GGT is normal. The diagnosis requires bile acid metabolite analysis of the urine, a technique available in only a few tertiary pediatric centers. The only other cause of neonatal cholestasis with normal or low GGT is progressive familial intrahepatic cholestasis (Byler's disease). The diagnosis of many infections is made serologically, particularly with specific IgM antibody titers. Maternal titers may be required to interpret elevated IgG titers in the face of possible placental transfer. The sweat chloride test is specific for cystic fibrosis but requires a sufficient collection of sweat to be interpretable. Ophthalmologic evaluation may detect the chorioretinitis common in congenital infections, cataracts that develop with galactosemia or the posterior embryotoxon of Alagille's syndrome. Vertebral radiographs may demonstrate the butterfly vertebrae of Alagille's syndrome and long bone radiographs may be abnormal in some congenital infections. Intracranial calcifications that accompany congenital infections may be detected with skull films, ultrasound or CT scan.

TABLE 12.   Management of chronic cholestasis

Malnutrition
Increase caloric intake, if necessary by enteral feedings
Supplement with medium-chain triglycerides
Supplement with water-soluble vitamins and minerals

Fat-soluble vitamin deficiency
Vitamin A 5,000–25,000 IU po qd as Aquasol® A, or 50,000 IU IM/month where available
Vitamin E 50–100 IU po qd (polyethylene glycol–based form)
Vitamin K_1 2.5–5.0 mg po qd, or 10 mg IM twice monthly
Vitamin D_2 5,000–8,000 IU po qd, or preferably 5 mg IM/3 months where available, or 3,000
   IU IV/1–4 weeks with crystalline cholecalciferol IV

Pruritus
Hydroxyzine
Ursodeoxycholic acid
Rifampin
Cholestyramine
Ultraviolet B light therapy
Biliary diversion

9.2.3 *TREATMENT*

Treatment for many of these disorders is supportive. Ensuring optimal caloric intake for growth may at times require nasogastric tube feeding to supplement a poor intake. Fat malabsorption is common as a result of lack of intestinal luminal bile acids; it may be treated with supplemental medium-chain triglycerides, which can be absorbed in the absence of luminal bile acids. Supplemental fat-soluble vitamins are required to prevent rickets (vitamin D), coagulopathy (vitamin K), peripheral neuropathy (vitamin E) or xerophthalmia (vitamin A). Only vitamin E is available in a well-absorbed oral form (d-alpha-tocopheryl polyethylene glycol succinate); intramuscular administration of other fat-soluble vitamins is frequently necessary. Pruritus is treated with variable success with the agents and procedures listed in Table 12. Progression of cholestasis requires monitoring the child for the development of cirrhosis and treating its complications of ascites, portal hypertension and liver failure.

REFERENCES

Section 5 Growth Failure and Malnutrition
1.   Peterson KE. Failure to thrive. In: Queen PM, Lang CE (eds.), Handbook of pediatric nutrition. Gaithersburg, MD: Aspen, 1993:366–383.

2. Wilcox WD, Nieburg P, Miller DS. Failure to thrive: a continuing problem of definition. Clin Pediatr 1989; 28:391–394.
3. Maggioni A, Lifshitz F. Nutritional management of failure to thrive. Ped Clin North Am 1995; 42:791–810.
4. Horner JM, Thorsson AV, Hintz RL. Growth deceleration patterns in children with constitutional short stature: an aid to diagnosis. Pediatrics 1978; 62:529–534.
5. Altagiani M, Murphy JF, Newcombe RG, Gray OP. Catch-up growth in preterm infants. Acta Paediatr Scand 1989; 357(Suppl):3–19.
6. Dean AG, Dean JA, Burton AH, Dicker RC. Epi Info, V.5: a word processing, database, and statistics program for epidemiology on microcomputers. Stone Mountain, GA: USD, 1990.
7. Wright JA, Ashenburg CA, Whitaker RC. Comparison of methods to categorize undernutrition in children. J Pediatr 1994; 124:944–946.
8. Gurney JM, Jelliffe DB. Arm anthropometry in nutritional assessment: nomogram for rapid calculation of muscle circumference and cross-sectional muscle and fat areas. Am J Clin Nutr 1973; 26:912–915.
9. Frisancho AR. New norms of upper limb fat and muscle areas for assessment of nutritional status. Am J Clin Nutr 1981; 34:2540–2545.

SUGGESTED READING LIST

Section 1 Recurrent Abdominal Pain
Boyle JT. Chronic abdominal pain. In: Walker WA, Durie PR, Hamilton JR, Walker-Smith JA, Watkins JB (eds.), Pediatric gastrointestinal disease: pathophysiology, diagnosis and management. Toronto: BC Decker, 1991:45–54.

Section 2 Vomiting and Regurgitation
Sondheimer JM. Vomiting. In: Walker WA, Durie PR, Hamilton JR, Walker-Smith JA, Watkins JB (eds.), Pediatric gastrointestinal disease: pathophysiology, diagnosis and management. 2d ed. St. Louis: Mosby-Year Book, 1996:195–205.
Orenstein SR. Gastroesophageal reflux. In: Hyman PE (ed.), Pediatric motility disorders. New York: Academy Professional Services, 1994.

Section 3 Colic
Barr RG. Colic. In: Walker WA, Durie PR, Hamilton JR, Walker-Smith JA, Watkins JB (eds.), Pediatric gastrointestinal disease: pathophysiology, diagnosis and management, vol. 1. 2d ed. St. Louis: Mosby-Year Book, 1996:241–250.
Symptoms. In: Roy CC, Silverman A, Alagille D (eds.), Pediatric clinical gastroenterology. 4th ed. St. Louis: Mosby-Year Book, 1995:39–43.

Section 4 Chronic Constipation, Encopresis and Soiling
Read NW, Timms JM. Defecation and the pathophysiology of constipation. Clin Gastroenterol 1986; 15:937–965.
Leoning-Baucke V. Chronic constipation in children. Gastroenterology 1993; 105:1557–1564.

Section 6 Acute Diarrhea in Children
Jin S, Kilgore PE, Holman RC, Clarke MJ, Gangarosa EJ, Glass RI. Trends in hospitalizations for diarrhea in United States children from 1979 through 1992: estimates of the morbidity associated with rotavirus. Pediatr Infect Dis J 1996; 15:397–404.
Centers for Disease Control. The management of acute diarrhea in children: oral rehydration, maintenance, and nutritional therapy. MMWR 1992; 41(RR-16):1–20.
Canadian Pediatric Society. Oral rehydration therapy and early refeeding in the management of childhood enteritis. Can J Pediatr 1994; 1:160–164.
Nazarian LF, Berman JH, Brown G, et al. Practice parameter: the management of acute gastroenteritis in young children. Pediatrics 1996; 97:424–435.
Butzner JD. Acute vomiting and diarrhea. In: Walker-Smith JA, Walker WA, Hamilton JR (eds.), Practical pediatric gastroenterology. 2d ed. Toronto: BC Decker, 1996:51–69.
Field M, Semrad CE. Toxigenic diarrheas, congenital diarrheas, and cystic fibrosis: disorders of intestinal ion transport. Ann Rev Physiol 1993; 55:631–655.
Cohen M. Etiology and mechanisms of acute infectious diarrhea in infants in the United States. J Pediatr 1991; 118:S34–S39.
Mackenzie A, Barnes G, Shann F. Clinical signs of dehydration in children. Lancet 1989; 2:605–607.
Brown KH, Peerson JM, Fontaine O. Use of nonhuman milks in the dietary management of young children with acute diarrhea: a meta-analysis of clinical trials. Pediatrics 1994; 93:17–27.
Wolf DC, Giannella RA. Antibiotic therapy for bacterial enterocolitis: a comprehensive review. Am J Gastroenterol 1993; 88:1667–1683.

Section 7 Malabsorption
Malabsorption. In: Roy CC, Silverman A, Alagille D (eds.), Pediatric clinical gastroenterology. 4th ed. Toronto: CV Mosby, 1995:299–362.

Section 9 Approach to the Jaundiced Neonate
Keating JP. Jaundice. In: Walker WA, Durie PR, Hamilton JR, Walker-Smith JA, Watkins JB (eds.), Pediatric gastrointestinal disease: pathophysiology, diagnosis and management. 2d ed. Toronto: CV Mosby, 1996:395–401.
Dellert SF, Balistreri WF. Neonatal cholestasis. In: Walker WA, Durie PR, Hamilton JR, Walker-Smith JA, Watkins JB (eds.), Pediatric gastrointestinal disease: pathophysiology, diagnosis and management. 2d ed. Toronto: CV Mosby, 1996:999–1015.

OBJECTIVES

Recurrent Abdominal Pain

1. Recognize the characteristic clinical presentations (history, physical exam, psychosocial factors) of benign recurrent functional abdominal pain in the child.
2. Be aware of the common organic causes of abdominal pain in children.
3. Be able to identify features of the history or physical exam that are not consistent with functional pain and suggest an organic basis.

4. Understand the approach to the investigation and management of recurrent abdominal pain in children.

Vomiting and Regurgitation

1. Understand the definitions of, and distinction between, vomiting and regurgitation.
2. Be aware of the range of gastrointestinal and nongastrointestinal causes of vomiting characteristic of neonates, infants, children and adolescents.
3. Be aware of an age- and presentation-appropriate approach to the investigation and management of vomiting in neonates, infants, children and adolescents.
4. Be aware of the pathophysiology and natural history of gastroesophageal reflux in infancy, the potential complications of gastroesophageal reflux, the features of history and physical exam that suggest GER-induced disease, available investigations and appropriate treatment of GERD.

Colic

1. Understand that colic describes a pattern of crying or fussiness the etiology of which is not yet clear.
2. Know the possible etiologies for colic that have been proposed.
3. Develop an approach to history taking, physical exam and management of the infant presenting with colic.

Chronic Constipation, Encopresis and Soiling

1. Understand the definitions of constipation, encopresis and soiling.
2. Understand the role of age, colonic motility, dietary fiber and transit time in determining defecation frequency, fecal water and electrolyte content.
3. Recognize normal variations in patterns of elimination in infants (e.g., breastfed vs formula-fed babies).
4. Be aware of the functional and organic causes of constipation.
5. Be able to differentiate chronic fecal retention from Hirschsprung's disease.
6. Understand the mechanism(s) and management of functional constipation and soiling.

Growth Failure and Malnutrition

1. Define the terms *failure to thrive* and *malnutrition*.
2. Learn to categorize failure to thrive in order to facilitate diagnoses.
3. Review appropriate methods for the assessment and management of failure to thrive.

Acute Diarrhea in Children

1. Understand the pathophysiology of acute diarrheal disease in the pediatric patient.
2. Be able to assess severity of dehydration in infants and children.
3. Understand the use of oral rehydration therapy for the management of acute diarrheal disease.

Malabsorption

1. Understand the physiology of digestion and absorption in order to develop an approach to the clinical evaluation of a pediatric patient with the malabsorption syndrome.
2. Be aware of the role of history and physical examination in the assessment of children with the malabsorption syndrome, and in particular, the importance of the dietary record, growth parameters and the need to plot growth curves.
3. Be aware of the various laboratory tests used for the evaluation of children with malabsorption.
4. Understand basic concepts regarding the management of the infant with failure to thrive.

Approach to the Jaundiced Neonate

1. Be aware of the factors contributing to physiological jaundice in the newborn.
2. Be aware of the various causes of unconjugated hyperbilirubinemia in infancy. Know the symptoms and sequelae of unconjugated hyperbilirubinemia. Be aware of options for management.
3. Be aware of the various causes of neonatal conjugated hyperbilirubinemia.
4. Be aware of an approach (algorithm) for the investigation and management of neonatal hyperbilirubinemia.

List of Contributors

ADAMS, P., London Health Sciences Centre, University Campus, 339 Windermere Rd., P.O. Box 5339, London, ON N6A 5A5. Tel: (519) 663-3513, Fax: (519) 663-3232.

ARCHAMBAULT, A., Université de Montréal, Hôpital Maisonneuve-Rosemont, 5415, boul de l'Assomption # 305, Montréal, QC H1T 2M4. Tel: (514) 252-3400 ext. 3367, Fax: (514) 252-3486.

BAIN, V.G., University of Alberta, 2E3.27 W.M.C., 8440 112th St., Edmonton, AB T6G 2R7. Tel: (403) 492-7238, Fax: (403) 492-2504.

BECK, I.T., Director, Gastrointestinal Diseases Research Unit, Queen's University, 166 Brock St., Kingston, ON K7L 5G2. Tel: (613) 544-0225 or 544-3310 ext. 2289, Fax: (613) 544-3114.

BLENDIS, L.M., The Toronto Hospital, General Division, 200 Elizabeth St., Toronto, ON M5G 2C4. Tel: (416) 340-3834, Fax: (416) 340-5019.

BURNSTEIN, M., St. Michael's Hospital, 38 Shuter St., Suite 504, Toronto, ON M5B 1A6. Tel: (416) 864-6050, Fax: (416) 864-5668.

BURSEY, R.F., Memorial University of Newfoundland, Faculty of Medicine, Health Sciences Centre, 300 Prince Philip Dr., St. John's, NF A1B 3V6. Tel: (709) 737-6960, Fax: (709) 737-3605.

BUTZNER, J.D., Dept. of Paediatrics, University of Calgary Health Sciences Centre, 3330 Hospital Dr. NW, Calgary, AB T2N 4N1. Tel: (403) 220-4561, Fax: (403) 283-3028.

CHAMPION, M.C., Division of Gastroenterology, GI Unit A1, Ottawa Civic Hospital, 1053 Carling Ave., Ottawa, ON K1Y 4E9. Tel: (613) 761-4674, Fax: (613) 761-5269.

FARDY, J.M., Memorial University of Newfoundland, Faculty of Medicine,

Health Sciences Centre, 300 Prince Philip Dr., St. John's, NF A1B 3V6. Tel: (709) 737-7064, Fax: (709) 737-3605.

FEAGAN, B.G., University of Western Ontario, Faculty of Medicine, London Health Sciences Centre, University Campus, P.O. Box 5339, London, ON N6A 5A5. Tel: (519) 663-3589, Fax: (519) 663-3232.

FEDORAK, R.N., University of Alberta, 519 Newton Research Building, 11315-87 Ave., Edmonton, AB T6G 2C2. Tel: (403) 492-6941, Fax: (403) 492-3744.

FREEMAN, H.J., Room F-274, 2211 Wesbrook, Vancouver, BC V6T 1W5. Tel: (604) 822-7216, Fax: (604) 822-7236.

GILLIES, R.R., Ottawa Civic Hospital, 1053 Carling Ave., Ottawa, ON K1Y 4E9. Tel: (613) 761-4603 or (613) 729-8926 (home), Fax: (613) 761-5269.

GRÉGOIRE, S., Ottawa General Hospital, 311 McArthur Rd., Suite 203, Vanier, ON K1L 6P1. Tel: (613) 744-8180, Fax: (613) 744-7982.

HABAL, F., The Toronto Hospital, General Division, 200 Elizabeth St., EN9-229, Toronto, ON M5G 2C4. Tel: (416) 340-5023, Fax: (416) 595-5251.

HEATHCOTE, J., The Toronto Hospital, Western Division, 399 Bathurst St., 4th Floor, West Wing, Room 828, Toronto, ON M5T 2S8. Tel: (416) 603-5914, Fax: (416) 603-9195.

HEMMING, A.W., The Toronto Hospital, 621 University Ave., NU10-145, Toronto, ON M5G 2C4. Tel: (416) 340-4912, Fax: (416) 340-3492.

HILSDEN, R.J., Department of Community Health Sciences, University of Calgary, 3330 Hospital Dr. NW, Calgary, AB T2N 4N1. Tel: (403) 220-6536, Fax: (403) 270-7287.

HUNT, R.H., McMaster University Medical Centre, 1200 Main St. W, Room 4W8, Hamilton, ON L8N 3Z5. Tel: (905) 521-2100 ext. 6404, Fax: (905) 521-5072.

LEE, S.S., Dept. of Medicine, University of Calgary Health Sciences Centre, 3330 Hospital Dr. NW, Calgary, AB T2N 4N1. Tel: (403) 220-3245, Fax: (403) 270-0995.

LEMOYNE, M., Hôpital Saint-Luc, 1058, rue Saint-Denis, Montréal, QC H2X 3J4. Tel: (514) 281-2121, Fax: (514) 281-3564.

LEVY, G.A., The Toronto Hospital, 621 University Ave., NU10-151, Toronto, ON M5G 2C4. Tel: (416) 340-5166, Fax: (416) 340-3492.

LILLY, L.B., The Toronto Hospital, 621 University Ave., NU10-162, Toronto, ON M5G 2C4. Tel: (416) 340-4629 Fax: (416) 340-3492.

MA, M., University of Alberta, 2E1.04 W.M.C., 8440 112th St., Edmonton, AB T6G 2R7. Tel: (403) 492-5318, Fax: (403) 492-3340.

MacDONALD, P.H., Hotel Dieu Hospital, 166 Brock St., Kingston, ON K7L 5G2. Tel: (613) 544-3400 ext. 3116, Fax: (613) 546-4854.

MacINTOSH, D.G., Memorial University of Newfoundland, Faculty of Medicine, Health Sciences Centre, 300 Prince Philip Dr., St. John's, NF A1B 3V6. Tel: (709) 737-5070, Fax: (709) 737-3605.

MACHIDA, H., Alberta Children's Hospital, 1820 Richmond Rd. SW, Calgary, AB T2T 5C7. Tel: (403) 229-7211, Fax: (403) 229-7221.

MARTIN, S.R., Hôpital Sainte-Justine, Université de Montréal, 3175, Côte Sainte-Catherine, Montréal, QC H3T 1C5. Tel: (514) 345-4871, Fax: (514) 345-4999.

MAY, G.R., University of Calgary Health Sciences Centre, Room 701, 3330 Hospital Dr. NW, Calgary, AB T2N 4N1. Tel: (403) 220-4557, Fax: (403) 220-8747.

MAYRAND, S., GI Division, Montreal General Hospital, D7120 - 1650, av Cedar, Montréal, QC H3G 1A4. Tel: (514) 934-8307, Fax: (514) 934-8375.

MEBAN, S., Division of General Surgery, Ottawa Civic Hospital, 1053 Carling Ave., Ottawa, ON K1Y 4E9. Tel: (613) 761-4660.

MORRISON, D.J., Alberta Children's Hospital, 1820 Richmond Rd. SW, Calgary, AB T2T 5C7. Tel: (403) 229-7211, Fax: (403) 229-7649.

PARÉ, P., Hôtel-Dieu de Québec, 11, Côte du Palais, 7th Floor, Québec, QC G1R 2J6. Tel: (418) 691-5252, Fax: (418) 691-5348.

PARSONS, H.G., University of Calgary Health Sciences Centre, 3330 Hospital Dr. NW, Calgary, AB T2N 4N1. Tel: (403) 220-7496, Fax: (403) 283-3028.

PATEL, D.G., Division of Gastroenterology, Ottawa Civic Hospital, 1053 Carling Ave., Ottawa, ON K1Y 4E9. Tel: (613) 761-4501, Fax: (613) 761-5269.

PATERSON, W.G., GI Division, Hotel Dieu Hospital, 166 Brock St., Kingston, ON K7L 5G2. Tel: (613) 544-3310 ext. 2332 or 3376, Fax: (613) 544-3114.

SALENA, B.J., McMaster University Medical Centre, 1200 Main St. W, Room 4W8, Hamilton, ON L8N 3Z5. Tel: (905) 521-2100 ext. 6782, Fax: (905) 521-4958.

SCHREIBER, R.A., B.C. Children's Hospital, 4480 Oak St., Vancouver, BC V6H 3V4. Tel: (604) 875-2332, Fax: (604) 875-3244.

SCOTT, R.B., Dept. of Paediatrics, Faculty of Medicine, University of Calgary Health Sciences Centre, 3330 Hospital Dr. NW, Calgary, AB T2N 4N1. Tel: (403) 220-4556, Fax: (403) 283-3028.

SCULLY, L.J., Division of Gastroenterology, GI Unit A1, Ottawa Civic Hospital, 1053 Carling Avenue, Ottawa, ON K1Y 4E9. Tel: (613) 761-4830, Fax: (613) 761-5269.

SEKAR, A.S.C., Division of Gastroenterology, Ottawa Civic Hospital, 1053

Carling Avenue, Ottawa, ON K1Y 4E9. Tel: (613) 729-3179, Fax: (613) 761-5269.

SHAFFER, E.A., Director, Dept. of Medicine, Foothills Hospital, 1403-29 St. NW, Room C210, Calgary, AB T2N 2T9. Tel: (403) 670-1500, Fax: (403) 670-1095.

SIDOROV, J.J., Victoria Medical Building, 307-1669 Victoria St., Prince George, BC V2L 2L5. Tel: (250) 564-2182, Fax: (250) 964-6110.

SIMON, J.B., Hotel Dieu Hospital, 166 Brock St., Kingston, ON K7L 5G2. Tel: (613) 544-3310 ext. 2483, Fax: (613) 544-3114.

STEINBRECHER, U.P., Room 3300, 950 West 10th Ave., Vancouver, BC V5Z 4E3. Tel: (604) 875-5862, Fax: (604) 875-5447.

THOMPSON, W.G., Division of Gastroenterology, Ottawa Civic Hospital, 1053 Carling Ave., Ottawa, ON K1Y 4E9. Tel: (613) 761-4147, Fax: (613) 761-5269.

THOMSON, A.B.R., University of Alberta, 519 Newton Research Building, 11315-87 Ave., Edmonton, AB T6G 2C2. Tel: (403) 492-6490, Fax: (403) 492-7964.

TURNBULL, G.K., Queen Elizabeth II Health Sciences Centre, Victoria General Hospital Site, Room 9018, 1278 Tower Rd., Halifax, NS B3H 2Y1. Tel: (902) 473-3620, Fax: (902) 473-4406.

VANNER, S.J., Hotel Dieu Hospital, 166 Brock St., Kingston, ON K7L 5G2. Tel: (613) 544-3310 ext. 2473, Fax: (613) 544-3114.

WHITTAKER, J.S., St. Paul's Hospital, 1081 Burrard St., Vancouver, BC V6Z 1Y6. Tel: (604) 631-5034, Fax: (604) 631-5338.

WITHERS, G., Dept. of Paediatrics, University of Calgary Health Sciences Centre, 3330 Hospital Drive NW, Calgary, AB T2N 4N1. Tel: (403) 220-4556, Fax: (403) 283-3028.

WONG, F., The Toronto Hospital, General Division, 200 Elizabeth St., Toronto, ON M5G 2C4. Tel: (416) 340-3834, Fax: (416) 340-5019.

WOROBETZ, L.J., Dept. of Gastroenterology, Royal University Hospital, University of Saskatchewan, 103 Hospital Dr., Saskatoon, SK S7N 0W8. Tel: (306) 966-7964, Fax: (306) 966-8021.

ZAMORA, S.A., Dept. of Paediatrics, University of Calgary Health Sciences Centre, 3330 Hospital Drive NW, Calgary, AB T2N 4N1. Tel: (403) 220-4556, Fax: (403) 283-3028.

Index

The bold letter **t** following a page reference indicates a table. The bold letter **f** indicates a figure.

aneurysm, aortic, 26
angiodysplasia, 34t, 35t, 393-94
angioedema, 489
angioma, 259
angiomatosis, 301
angioplasty, balloon, 276
angiosarcoma, 57t, 511
angiotensin converting enzyme (ACE)
    inhibitors, 524
anismus, 371
ankylosing spondylitis, 311t, 313, 327, 339t,
    343
anorectal spaces, 379
anorexia: about, 14-15; in acute abdomen,
    27; in celiac disease, 243; in cholecystitis,
    450; in Crohn's disease, 310t; in gastritis,
    168; in gastroenteritis, 229; in liver dis-
    ease, 31, 33, 466t, 467, 485, 503-4; in
    malassimilation, 64t, 206, 212; in malnu-
    trition, 25, 57, 58t; in ulcerative colitis,
    326, 333; nutritional intervention, 68
anoscopy, 384
antacids: causing diarrhea, 22, 23t, 223t, 233,
    234t, 235, 241t; in liver transplantation,
    545; to treat esophagitis, 111; to treat
    GERD, 7, 107t, 108; to treat pancreatitis,
    424; to treat PUD, 155, 157, 159
anthraquinones, 582
antiarrhythmics, 233
antibiotics: causing diarrhea, 23t, 24, 223t,
    231-33, 241t; causing esophagitis, 113;
    and Clostridium infection, 373; to treat
    bacterial overgrowth, 253; to treat bile duct
    disease, 456, 458; to treat cholangitis, 459;
    to treat cholecystitis, 451; to treat colonic
    infection, 372-75; to treat Crohn's disease,
    318; to treat cystic fibrosis, 433; to treat
    diarrhea, 166, 229, 600; to treat diverticu-
    losis, 357; to treat esophagitis, 112; to treat
    H. pylori infection, 179; to treat hepatic
    encephalopathy, 539; to treat HIV-associ-
    ated infection, 291, 292t-93t; to treat
    ischemia, 272; to treat pancreatitis, 418; to
    treat pseudo-obstruction, 257; to treat
    PUD, 155; to treat Whipple's disease, 256
anticholinergics: affect LES, 108t, 113, 143;
    to treat chest pain, 123; to treat gastrino-
    ma, 163; to treat gastritis, 171; to treat irri-
    table bowel, 364t; to treat PUD, 155, 159;
    to treat pyloric stenosis, 176
anticoagulants, 276
antidepressants, 19t, 364t
antifungal agents, 295
antigastrin agents, 155

antihistamines, 14
anti-inflammatory agents, 319
antilymphocyte products, 547
antimetabolites, 23t, 233, 241t
antimitochondrial antibody tests, 472
antimotility agents, 364t
antinuclear factor test, 472
antiretroviral drugs, 289-90, 301
antismooth muscle antibody test, 472
antithymocyte globulin, 548
alpha$_1$-antitrypsin deficiency, 476, 493, 495t,
    513-14, 521t, 521, 551
antituberculous drugs, 293-94
antral G-cell hyperfunction, 147
antrectomy, 161, 165, 167
antrum, retained, 150, 160-61, 165
anxiety, 4-5
aorto-SMA graft, 259
aortovisceral bypass, 276
apathy, 56, 212
aperistalsis, 117
apnea, 575t, 575
apolipoproteins, 52
apoprotein, 465
appendicitis, 27-28
appetite, 14-15, 208t
arachidonic acid, 144
areflexia, 59t
arginine, 205
arsenicals, 57t, 511
arterial reconstruction, 274
arthralgia, 95, 256
arthritis: and gastric secretions, 150; in
    inflammatory bowel disease, 311t, 313,
    327, 339t, 343; in liver disease, 489, 501,
    512, 516-17; in PUD, 160-61
artificial sweeteners, 21, 23t, 233, 235t
ASA, 35, 144, 146, 524
5-ASA see mesalamine
ascites: about, 33-34, 531-32, 533f; dietary
    therapy, 65-66; examining for, 47-48; in
    congestive heart failure, 555-56; in hepatic
    vein thrombosis, 556; in liver disease,
    466t, 467, 504, 517, 523-24, 527-28, 531-
    37, 551; in veno-occlusive disease, 556;
    pancreatic, 420
ascorbic acid see vitamin C
aspartate aminotransferase, 470-71
aspiration: children, 569; in deglutition disor-
    ders, 115; in esophageal neoplasms, 126;
    in GERD, 97, 109-10; in Zenker's diverticu-
    lum, 130
assimilation see absorption; digestion
asterixis, 537